T0177619

OXFORD MEDICAL PUBLICATIONS

Oxford Handbook of
Humanitarian Medicine

Published and forthcoming Oxford Handbooks

Oxford Handbook for the Foundation Programme 5e
Oxford Handbook of Acute Medicine 3e
Oxford Handbook of Anaesthesia 4e
Oxford Handbook of Cardiology 2e
Oxford Handbook of Clinical and Healthcare Research
Oxford Handbook of Clinical and Laboratory Investigation 4e
Oxford Handbook of Clinical Dentistry 6e
Oxford Handbook of Clinical Diagnosis 3e
Oxford Handbook of Clinical Examination and Practical Skills 2e
Oxford Handbook of Clinical Haematology 4e
Oxford Handbook of Clinical Immunology and Allergy 3e
Oxford Handbook of Clinical Medicine – Mini Edition 9e
Oxford Handbook of Clinical Medicine 10e
Oxford Handbook of Clinical Pathology
Oxford Handbook of Clinical Pharmacy 3e
Oxford Handbook of Clinical Specialties 10e
Oxford Handbook of Clinical Surgery 4e
Oxford Handbook of Complementary Medicine
Oxford Handbook of Critical Care 3e
Oxford Handbook of Dental Patient Care
Oxford Handbook of Dialysis 4e
Oxford Handbook of Emergency Medicine 4e
Oxford Handbook of Endocrinology and Diabetes 3e
Oxford Handbook of ENT and Head and Neck Surgery 2e
Oxford Handbook of Epidemiology for Clinicians
Oxford Handbook of Expedition and Wilderness Medicine 2e
Oxford Handbook of Forensic Medicine
Oxford Handbook of Gastroenterology & Hepatology 2e
Oxford Handbook of General Practice 4e
Oxford Handbook of Genetics
Oxford Handbook of Genitourinary Medicine, HIV, and Sexual Health 2e
Oxford Handbook of Geriatric Medicine 3e

Oxford Handbook of Infectious Diseases and Microbiology 2e
Oxford Handbook of Integrated Dental Biosciences 2e
Oxford Handbook of Humanitarian Medicine
Oxford Handbook of Key Clinical Evidence 2e
Oxford Handbook of Medical Dermatology 2e
Oxford Handbook of Medical Imaging
Oxford Handbook of Medical Sciences 2e
Oxford Handbook for Medical School
Oxford Handbook of Medical Statistics
Oxford Handbook of Neonatology 2e
Oxford Handbook of Nephrology and Hypertension 2e
Oxford Handbook of Neurology 2e
Oxford Handbook of Nutrition and Dietetics 2e
Oxford Handbook of Obstetrics and Gynaecology 3e
Oxford Handbook of Occupational Health 2e
Oxford Handbook of Oncology 3e
Oxford Handbook of Operative Surgery 3e
Oxford Handbook of Ophthalmology 4e
Oxford Handbook of Oral and Maxillofacial Surgery 2e
Oxford Handbook of Orthopaedics and Trauma
Oxford Handbook of Paediatrics 2e
Oxford Handbook of Pain Management
Oxford Handbook of Palliative Care 3e
Oxford Handbook of Practical Drug Therapy 2e
Oxford Handbook of Pre-Hospital Care
Oxford Handbook of Psychiatry 3e
Oxford Handbook of Public Health Practice 3e
Oxford Handbook of Rehabilitation Medicine 3e
Oxford Handbook of Reproductive Medicine & Family Planning 2e
Oxford Handbook of Respiratory Medicine 3e
Oxford Handbook of Rheumatology 4e
Oxford Handbook of Sport and Exercise Medicine 2e
Handbook of Surgical Consent
Oxford Handbook of Tropical Medicine 4e
Oxford Handbook of Urology 4e

Oxford Handbook of
Humanitarian Medicine

Edited by

Amy S. Kravitz

Medical Officer, United States Agency for International
Development (USAID), Washington, DC, USA

Associate Editor

Alexander van Tulleken

Institute of International Humanitarian Affairs, USA

OXFORD
UNIVERSITY PRESS

OXFORD
UNIVERSITY PRESS

Great Clarendon Street, Oxford, OX2 6DP,
United Kingdom

Oxford University Press is a department of the University of Oxford.
It furthers the University's objective of excellence in research, scholarship,
and education by publishing worldwide. Oxford is a registered trade mark of
Oxford University Press in the UK and in certain other countries

First Edition published in 2019

Impression: 1

Published in the United States of America by Oxford University Press
198 Madison Avenue, New York, NY 10016, United States of America

British Library Cataloguing in Publication Data
Data available

Library of Congress Control Number: 2018949667

ISBN 978–0–19–956527–6

Printed and bound in China by
C&C Offset Printing Co., Ltd.

Foreword

Now seen as a branch of clinical practice which deals collectively with human misfortunes that affect health beyond the individual, Humanitarian Medicine embraces the predicaments of groups of people with shared experiences in facing calamities: calamities that are either immediately apparent—or waiting to strike.

Despite intense media exposure and ostensible political support by disinterested parties, in truth many campaigns in Humanitarian Medicine have proved social misfits lacking loyal and authoritative parents; judged retrospectively as they must be, their effects signal bitter political failure.

With the *Oxford Handbook of Humanitarian Medicine*, Dr Amy Kravitz and her contributors have authored a unique and original guide: not simply to the practical relief of critical and fast-emerging 'ground' emergencies with plague, pestilences, starvation, torture and war-related human disasters of every possible kind, but to essential strategic measures. The authors succinctly explore the need to predict, to resource, as well as develop tailor-made advocacy for political and economic solutions to the unique conflation of forces that can drive populations ineluctably to doom.

This handbook goes beyond simple therapy; it seeks to promote, provide, and instruct. Within the ethical framework of conventional medicine, it offers support those who holistically improve well-being and health of populations while conforming to the Charter of the United Nations, the Universal Declaration of Human Rights, the Red Cross and Crescent Conventions, and other accepted canons of practice. Naturally there is a complex political dimension in this field; and the practitioner of Humanitarian Medicine must at all costs operate systematically with discretion to avoid neo-colonial dominance and dependence at all costs. At the same time, there is really no place for the 'parachute mentality' related to theatrical international emergencies apparently promulgated in global media. Usually local conditions of healthcare are fractured and, after military intervention and colonization, wayward and permanently starved of resources. Not only is diplomacy and sharing of resources and responsibility between multiple agencies crucial; but the need for ethical refinement and disinterested investment, is paramount.

After the immediate crisis has resolved, resources for sustaining parachute missions quickly recede and many humanitarian workers withdraw from the penumbra of conflict. In this first-edition of the wide-ranging Oxford Handbook, Dr Kravitz and her glittering team of experienced co-authors and practitioners show not only how to move to the best standards of care but to settle realistically for what can be sustainably offered for the public health of the entire residual population. This extraordinary book has much to offer directly for those who wish to learn and engage with the innumerable complexities of Humanitarian Medicine: its weight lies in its focused but comprehensive treatment and the profound vision needed strategically to resolve every human disaster.

Timothy M. Cox
Professor of Medicine Emeritus
Director of Research
Honorary Consultant Physician
Addenbrooke's Hospital, Cambridge

Preface

Welcome to the first edition of the *Oxford Handbook of Humanitarian Medicine* (*OHHM*).

This book was conceived as a way to share the accumulated experiences and wisdom of the most experienced humanitarian practitioners from across disciplines. It includes clinical guidance aimed at conflict, displacement, and low-resource settings, by authors who have first-hand experience. *OHHM* goes beyond the clinical domain, however, to include detailed information on important socioeconomic and political drivers, as well as the voices of allied disciplines such as logistics, epidemiology, law, and security.

Humanitarian medicine is, by nature, variable and nuanced. There can be no guide to definitively tell a reader exactly what to do in complicated situations of conflict or natural disaster, especially where additional socioeconomic and political intricacies are often present. It is our hope, however, that this book helps to provide the framework and guidance necessary for the humanitarian practitioner to make the best decisions possible in these challenging settings.

Humanitarian medicine is a practice that is needed now more than ever. The United Nations Office for the Coordination of Humanitarian Affairs (OCHA) estimates that at least 128 million people in 33 countries will need humanitarian assistance in 2017—the highest level in history. Protracted conflicts and man-made crises have caused complex humanitarian emergencies and have contributed to unprecedented levels of displacement. The Office of the United Nations High Commissioner for Refugees (UNHCR) reports an estimated 65.5 million people forcibly displaced worldwide in 2016, another all-time record-breaking high. In other words, nearly 1% of the global population is currently internally displaced, a refugee, or an asylum seeker. Indeed, this is a critical time in the humanitarian sphere. The increase in needs has grown faster than available funding and has stretched the capacity of the humanitarian sector to the limit.

Concurrently, there have been increased violations against international humanitarian and human rights law, and lack of respect for the protection of civilians, humanitarian and medical workers, and civilian infrastructure. Médecins Sans Frontières (MSF), for example, reports the bombing of more than 60 of their health structures since 2015, and the indiscriminate and disproportionate targeting of civilians. No longer is conflict fought on a battlefield. Despite the clear violations of international law, perpetrators have not been held accountable and have largely escaped consequences.

Humanitarian response is guided by medical ethics and the principles outlined in international humanitarian law: humanity, neutrality, impartiality, and independence. When nations and warring parties disregard the international obligations and the protections in place for impartial provision of healthcare, humanitarian action itself is threatened. This message, a component of the #NotATarget campaign, launched by MSF in 2015, was also part of the 2017 agenda for the United Nations World Humanitarian Day, and in an affiliated petition 'demanding that global leaders do more to ensure the rules of war are upheld and civilians are protected in armed conflicts'. At present, however, there lacks much substantive commitment by global leaders to support the rhetoric.

At this critical time when the global community is at a crossroads, today's geopolitical context portends uncertainty. The global governance no longer has any appearance of solidarity, and the traditions of humanitarianism that once ran deep in world politics are often reduced to strategic interests. The view has turned decidedly inward, and the moral responsibilities of world leaders are no longer assumed.

Those practising humanitarian medicine, indeed the readers of this book, are holding onto those general principles of humanity. Their work goes beyond the therapeutic acts of relieving suffering and saving lives, as by also bearing witness and demanding accountability, they help to restore dignity for those impacted by crises.

It is truly a privilege to bring this book to print. On behalf of the all the dedicated humanitarians in the world, and those countless million whose voices are often unheard, we hope that this book serves to both inform and inspire. Now more than ever, it is critical.

Amy S. Kravitz
January, 2017

Acknowledgements

First, I thank Alex van Tulleken, my co-editor. We joined forces many years ago with a similar vision, and I am so proud that we are coming out the other end together. Without his clarity of vision and initiative in getting this project off the ground, this book never would have been a reality. I am also deeply grateful, of course, to Michael Hawkes. Through the years, and what must amount to thousands of emails and phone calls, his unwavering support and guidance has been the foundation upon which this book was built.

I am also grateful to those who have supported me and my work over the years. The list is too long to include, but I would be remiss to not extend a personal thanks to Mr Allan McRobie and Professor Timothy Cox. Their mentorship, support, and encouragement have had a profound impact on my life, and I am deeply grateful to have had the good fortune to cross their paths.

Last, but certainly not least, I thank my family for their support with this project. At times, 'the book' evoked a sentiment similar to that of a visiting houseguest who refused to leave, and I am grateful to Alvaro for never considering if it was time to kick them out. Now with two small boys who grew at an exponentially faster pace than I could muster this book to do, I dedicate this book to them, in the hopes that one day they can see the value in perseverance and be proud to have been part of this journey.

Amy S. Kravitz
2018

I owe a huge debt of gratitude to a number of people. Anton Bilton for his tremendously generous support almost a decade ago; John Fraser and all the Fraser MacCallum family; Brendan Cahill and Helen Hamlyn; Andrew Cavey; and my own family, especially my son Julian.

Two people deserve a special mention. First, Michael Hawkes at OUP for his patience, dedication, and for sticking with the project for almost a decade. Finally, and most importantly, I have to thank Amy Kravitz who understood the vision of the book from our first conversation. Ours is not a normal partnership: she has worked tirelessly with the contributors, without help from me, for the last 3 years of this project and she has shaped every aspect of the content. It is hard to exaggerate how difficult this book was to create and it owes existence to her determination and brilliance. I am lucky to have been able to work alongside her.

Alexander van Tulleken
2018

The editors would also like to extend a tremendous thanks to *Dr Raghu Venugopal*. We appreciate all of his input, and are very grateful for his assistance with persuading some of the most experienced and dedicated humanitarians to take time from their work to contribute to this book. Without his assistance, this book would not be what it is today.

We would like to specifically thank *Dr Tammam Aloudat* for his contributions to the book. In addition to co-authoring two chapters, he also develop a third chapter which although ultimately was not able to be included, did help to inform the introduction of *OHHM*. His thoughtful contributions are most appreciated.

We would also like to extend our sincere appreciation to *Dr Sydney Wong, Dr Sandrine Tiller, Dr Ester Casas*, and *Dr Aditya (Adi) Nadimpalli*. Each of them went above and beyond what we could reasonably expect to help provide expert reviews of the manuscript. We thank them for their time and input.

We would like to thank *Dr Benjamin Black* as well for his excellent assistance in reviewing the manuscript.

Last, but certainly not least, we would like to thank *Dr Jennifer Turnbull*. Jennifer is not only an author in *OHHM*, but also helped in numerous other ways, including by serving as co-editor for the following three chapters: Chapter 1, 'Introduction to humanitarian medicine'; Chapter 3, 'Health priorities in displacement'; and Chapter 17, 'Approach to paediatric care'. We thank her not only for her skilful editorial assistance, but also for her perseverance and commitment in helping to bring this book to print (even while balancing a newborn!).

These are the people who personify the ideal image of the humanitarian doctor—dedicated, determined, and brilliant.

Contents

Contributors

Tammam Aloudat
(Chapter 3: Health priorities in displacement; Chapter 46: Chronic non-communicable diseases)
Deputy Medical Director, Medical Department, Médecins Sans Frontières, Geneva, Switzerland

Elizabeth Ashley
(Chapter 29: Malaria)
Director of Clinical Research, Myanmar Oxford Clinical Research Unit, Yangon, Myanmar; Centre for Tropical Medicine and Global Health, University of Oxford, UK

Anne Aspler
(Chapter 25: Oedema)
Emergency Medicine, University of Toronto, Canada

Nathalie Avril
(Chapter 3: Health priorities in displacement)
Nutrition Advisor, Médecins Sans Frontières Operational Centre, Geneva, Switzerland

Marco Baldan
(Chapter 49: Medical management of the surgical abdomen)
General Surgeon, Delegate Regional Surgeon for the Near and Middle East, International Committee of the Red Cross, Beirut, Lebanon

Aaron L. Berkowitz
(Chapter 39: Neurology)
Director, Global Neurology Program, Brigham and Women's Hospital, Boston, MA, USA
Associate Professor of Neurology, Harvard Medical School, Boston, MA, USA
Health and Policy Advisor in Neurology, Partners in Health, Boston, MA, USA

Catherine Berry
(Chapter 34: Global impact of antimicrobial resistance)
Clinical Advisor, Médecins Sans Frontières-UK, Chancery Exchange, London, UK

Massey Beveridge
(Chapter 49: Medical management of the surgical abdomen; Chapter 50: Wound care and minor surgical procedures; Chapter 51: Burns)
Adjunct Assistant Professor of Surgery, University of Toronto, Canada

Axel Bex *(Chapter 40: Urology)*
Urologic Surgeon, Division of Surgical Oncology, Department of Urology, Netherlands Cancer Institute, Amsterdam, Netherlands

Benjamin Oren Black
(Chapter 42: Obstetric care)
Obstetrician and Gynaecologist, London, UK Obstetric Technical Lead, UK-Med and UK Emergency Medical Team, UK Association member, Médecins Sans Frontières-UK, London, UK

Laurent Bonnardot
(Chapter 45: Ear, nose, and throat)
ENT and Emergency Physician, Médecins Sans Frontières, Paris, France

Marie Claude Bottineau
(Chapter 43: Neonatology)
Pediatrician and Neonatology,
MSF International Pediatrics
Working Group Leader, MSF-CH
Women & Children Health Pool
Leader, Médecins sans Frontières
Operational Centre, Geneva,
Switzerland

Françoise Bouchet-Saulnier
*(Chapter 3: Health priorities
in displacement; Chapter 9:
International Law for
Healthcare Workers)*
Doctor of Law and Magistrate,
International Legal Director
of Médecins sans Frontières,
Paris, France

Philippa Boulle
*(Chapter 3: Health priorities
in displacement; Chapter 37:
Respiratory illness; Chapter 46:
Chronic non-communicable diseases)*
Chronic Non-Communicable
Disease Advisor; Chronic
Conditions Team Leader,
Médecins sans Frontières,
Geneva, Switzerland

Vincent Buard *(Chapter 27:
Diarrhoea and vomiting)*
General Practitioner,
Médecins Sans Frontières (MSF),
Angers, France

Jorge Castilla Echenique
(Chapter 4: Health systems design)
Senior Health Advisor,
Emergency Operations, WHO
Health Emergencies Programme,
World Health Organization,
Geneva, Switzerland

Vanessa Cavallera
*(Chapter 6: Mental health in
humanitarian emergencies)*
Independent Consultant

Kevin Chan *(Chapter 19: Fever;
Chapter 28: Malnutrition)*
Chair, Pediatrics, Memorial
University and Clinical
Chief, Children's Health,
Eastern Health, St. John's,
Newfoundland, Canada

Bernard Chomilier
*(Chapter 12: Medical logistics in
humanitarian settings)*
Logistics Expert, retired

Christine Chomilier
*(Chapter 12: Medical logistics in
humanitarian settings)*
Logistics Expert, retired

Iza Ciglenecki
*(Chapter 3: Health priorities in
displacement)*
Operational Research
Coordinator, Médecins Sans
Frontières Operational Centre,
Geneva, Switzerland

Gustavo Fernandez
*(Chapter 3: Health priorities in
displacement)*
Migration Senior Project
Manager, Médecins Sans
Frontières Operational Centre,
Geneva, Switzerland
Deputy Head, Humanitarian
Representation Team,
Humanitarian Representative
in Geneva, Médecins sans
Frontières International

Sheri Fink
*(Chapter 1: Introduction to
humanitarian medicine)*
Fellow, FXB Center for Health
and Human Rights, Harvard T.H.
Chan School of Public Health,
Boston, MA, USA

Christos Giannou
(Chapter 15: Mass casualty triage)
Honorary Lecturer, Queen
Mary & Barts, Blizard Institute,
University of London, UK
Former Head Surgeon,
International Committee of the
Red Cross, retired

Sarah Giles *(Chapter 45: Ear,
nose, and throat)*
Assistant Clinical Professor,
Department of Family Medicine,
Faculty of Medicine, University of
Ottawa, Ottawa, Canada. Member,
Médecins sans Frontières, Canada

P. Gregg Greenough
(Chapter 7: Epidemiology)
Assistant Professor, Global
Health & Population, Harvard
T.H. Chan School of Public
Health; Faculty, Harvard
Humanitarian Initiative,
Cambridge, MA, USA

Andre Griekspoor
(Chapter 4: Health systems design)
Senior Humanitarian Policy
Adviser, Emergency Operations,
WHO Health Emergencies
Programme, World Health
Organization, Geneva, Switzerland

Monique Gueguen
(Chapter 54: Blood transfusion)
Medical Laboratory Advisor,
Médecins sans Frontières,
Paris, France

Jan Hajek
*(Chapter 30: Neglected tropical
diseases)*
Clinical Assistant Professor,
Department of Medicine,
Division of Infectious Diseases,
University of British Columbia,
Vancouver, Canada

Ingo Hartlapp
(Chapter 38: Gastrointestinal Illness)
Senior Physician, Specialist
for Internal Medicine/
Gastroenterology/Infectiology/
Oncology, Würzburg University
Hospital, Germany
Member, Médecins sans
Frontières Telemedicine
Program, Germany

Laura Hawryluck
(Chapter 18: Shock)
Associate Professor Critical
Care Medicine, University of
Toronto, Canada
Physician Lead, Critical
Care Rapid Response Team,
University Health Network,
Toronto, Canada
Member, Médecins Sans
Frontières Telemedicine
Program, Canada

Laurent Hiffler
*(Chapter 17: Approach to
paediatric care)*
Paediatric Advisor, MSF
Operational Center, Barcelona,
Athens, Dakar, Senegal

Chris Houston
(Chapter 10: Security)
Senior Program Officer
(Humanitarian), Grand
Challenges Canada
Board member, Médecins sans
Frontières, Canada
Module Lead, Global Health
Education Initiative, Postgraduate
Medical Education, University of
Toronto, Canada

Tim Jagatic
*(Chapter 32: Clinical suspicion
of Ebola)*
Physician, Médecins Sans
Frontières, Ontario, Canada

Kiran Jobanputra
(Chapter 3: Health priorities in displacement)
Head of Manson Unit, Médecins Sans Frontières, London, UK

Lynne Jones (Chapter 6: Mental health in humanitarian emergencies)
Fellow, FXB Center for Health and Human Rights, Harvard University, Boston, MA, USA
Honorary Consultant Child and Adolescent Psychiatrist, Cornwall Partnership NHS Foundation Trust, Cornwall, UK and South London and Maudsley NHS Foundation Trust, London, UK

Jaap Karsten
(Chapter 17: Approach to paediatric care)
Médecins Sans Frontières, Amsterdam, The Netherlands

Saleem Kassam
(Chapter 36: Cardiac conditions)
Consultant, Director, Cardiac Catheterization Laboratory, Rouge Valley Health System, Toronto, Canada
Vice President, Médecins Sans Frontières, Canada

Jocelyn T.D. Kelly
(Chapter 5: Gender-based violence in humanitarian crises)
Director, Women in War Program, Harvard Humanitarian Initiative, Cambridge, MA, USA

Hyo Jeong Kim
(Chapter 4: Health systems design)
Technical Officer, Emergency Operations, WHO Health Emergencies Programme, Geneva, Switzerland

Cara Kosack
(Chapter 53: Laboratory; Chapter 54: Blood transfusion)
Leader, Diagnostic Network, Médecins sans Frontières, Amsterdam, The Netherlands

Alena Koscalova
(Chapter 3: Health priorities in displacement)
Tropical Medicine Adviser, Médecins sans Frontières, Operational Centre, Geneva, Switzerland

Amy S. Kravitz
(Chapter 1: Introduction to humanitarian medicine)
Medical Officer, United States Agency for International Development (USAID), Washington, DC, USA

W. Ted Kuhn
(Chapter 55: Ultrasound)
Former Director, International Medicine, Co-director, Ultrasound Fellowship, Medical College of Georgia, Augusta University, GA, USA

Kenneth Lavelle
(Chapter 11: Medical care under fire: a perspective from the international medical organization Médecins Sans Frontières)
Deputy Director of Operations, Médecins Sans Frontières, Geneva, Switzerland

Matthew Lyon
(Chapter 55: Ultrasound)
Executive Director, Center for Ultrasound Education, Medical College of Georgia, Augusta University, GA, USA

Anna MacDonald
(Chapter 23: Lymphadenopathy)
Emergency Physician, St
Michael's Hospital, North
York General Hospital,
Toronto, Canada

Peter Maes *(Chapter 56: Water,
sanitation, and hygiene; Chapter 57:
Medical waste management)*
Water, Hygiene and Sanitation
Unit Coordinator, Water,
Hygiene & Sanitation Unit,
Médecins Sans Frontières – O.C.
Brussels, Belgium

Olivier Malard
(Chapter 45: Ear, nose, and throat)
ENT – Head and Neck Surgery
Department, Centre Hospitalier
Universitaire de Nantes, France

William Mapham
(Chapter 44: Ophthalmology)
Ophthalmologist, Stellenbosch
University, South Africa

Daniel Martinez Garcia
*(Chapter 17: Approach to
paediatric care)*
Paediatric Advisor, Medical
Department, Médecins Sans
Frontières, OCG Women &
Child Health Unit, Geneva,
Switzerland

James Maskalyk
*(Chapter 26: Patient with
unintentional weight loss)*
Emergency Physician, Assistant
Professor, University of
Toronto, Canada

Pierre Maury
*(Chapter 3: Health priorities in
displacement)*
Médecins Sans Frontières,
Geneva, Switzerland

Camille Michel
*(Chapter 11: Medical care under
fire: a perspective from the
international medical organization
Médecins Sans Frontières)*
Legal Advisor for International
Humanitarian Law and
Medicolegal Issues, Médecins
Sans Frontières, Geneva,
Switzerland

Rose Leonard Molina
*(Chapter 5: Gender-based violence
in humanitarian crises)*
Assistant Professor of
Obstetrics, Gynecology and
Reproductive Biology, Harvard
Medical School, Boston,
MA, USA
Faculty Physician, Division of
Global and Community Health,
Department of Obstetrics
and Gynecology, Beth Israel
Deaconess Medical Center,
Boston, MA, USA
Associate Scientist, Division of
Women's Health, Brigham and
Women's Hospital, Boston,
MA, USA

Peter Moons
*(Chapter 16: Medical triage;
Chapter 27: Diarrhoea and
vomiting)*
Consultant Paediatrician,
Academic Pediatric Center
Suriname, Paramaribo,
Suriname

Lily Muldoon
(Chapter 20: Anaemia)
Emergency Medicine Resident,
Department of Emergency
Medicine, University of
California San Francisco,
CA, USA

Veronique Mulloni
(Chapter 3: Health priorities in displacement)
Water, Hygiene and Sanitation Technical Referent, Technical Support to the Operations, Médecins Sans Frontières, Geneva, Switzerland

Aditya Nadimpalli
(Chapter 37: Respiratory illness)
Primary Care Ultrasound Fellow, School of Medicine, University of South Carolina, Columbia, SC, USA

Thomas Nierle
(Chapter 11: Medical care under fire: a perspective from the international medical organization Médecins Sans Frontières)
Former President, Médecins Sans Frontières, Geneva, Switzerland

David Nott *(Chapter 48: Major trauma)*
Consultant Surgeon, Imperial College, London, UK

Dirk-Jan Omtzigt
(Chapter 8: Understanding economic effects of humanitarian intervention)
Analyst, UNOCHA Regional Office for Southern and Eastern Africa

Joseph O'Neill
(Chapter 21: Pain; Chapter 24: Cough and breathlessness; Chapter 47: Palliative care)
Palliative Medicine, University of Maryland/Shore Regional Health, Easton, MD, USA

James Orbinski
(Humanitarianism Today)
Professor and Director, Dahdaleh Institute for Global Health Research, York University, Toronto, Canada

Susan Ann O'Toole
(Chapter 42: Obstetric care)
Obstetrician-Gynaecologist, Collingwood, ON, Canada

AnneMarie Pegg
(Chapter 35: Response to epidemic disease)
Clinical Lead, Epidemic Response and Vaccination, Médecins Sans Frontières, Paris, France
Associate Clinical Faculty, University of Calgary, Department of Family Medicine, Calgary, Canada

Max Ritzenberg
(Chapter 20: Anaemia)
Clinical Instructor, Department of Emergency Medicine, Faculty Affiliate, Institute for Global Health Sciences, University of California, San Francisco, CA, USA

Patrick Robitaille
(Chapter 2: Responders and responses)
Independent Consultant

David Rowley
(Chapter 52: Orthopaedics and limb injuries)
Emeritus Professor, University of Dundee, UK

Monica Rull *(Chapter 3: Health priorities in displacement)*
Operations Health Coordinator Médecins Sans Frontières, Geneva, Switzerland

Margaret Salmon
(Chapter 20: Anaemia)
Director and Innovator at
InnovationsCZ, Attending:
Valley Emergency Physicians,
San Francisco, CA

Peter Saranchuk
*(Chapter 31: Tuberculosis and HIV
in humanitarian contexts)*
TB/HIV Adviser, Southern Africa
Medical Unit (SAMU), Médecins
Sans Frontières, Cape Town,
South Africa
Medical Technical Advisor, Seva
Foundation, Berkeley, USA
Practicing Clinician, Bridges
Community Health Centre, Fort
Erie, Canada

Elisabeth Sauvaget
*(Chapter 45: Ear, nose,
and throat)*
Chief of ENT – Head and Neck
surgery department, Hôpital
Saint Joseph, Paris, France

Laura Sauve
(Chapter 19: Fever)
Pediatric Infectious Diseases
Specialist, BC Children's
Hospital; Clinical Assistant
Professor, Division of Infectious
Diseases, Department of
Pediatrics, University of British
Columbia, Vancouver, Canada

Jennifer Scott
*(Chapter 5: Gender-based violence
in humanitarian crises)*
Director, Division of Global and
Community Health, Department
of Obstetrics and Gynecology,
Beth Israel Deaconess Medical
Center, Boston, MA, USA
Associate Scientist, Division of
Women's Health, Brigham and
Women's Hospital, Boston,
MA, USA
Instructor, Harvard Medical
School, Boston, MA, USA

Norman Sheehan
(Chapter 10: Security)
Risk Management Consultant

Jonathan Spector
(Chapter 43: Neonatology)
Executive Director, Global
Health, Novartis Institutes
for BioMedical Research,
Cambridge, MA, USA

Craig Spencer
*(Chapter 32: Clinical suspicion
of Ebola)*
Director of Global Health in
Emergency Medicine,
New York-Presbyterian/
Columbia University
Medical Center,
New York, NY, USA
Assistant Professor of Medicine
and Population and Family
Health, Columbia University
Medical Center, New York,
NY, USA

Miroslav Stavel
(Chapter 18: Shock)
Staff Paediatrician and
Neonatologist, Royal
Columbian Hospital, New
Westminster, Canada

Marianne Stephen
(*Chapter 41: Reproductive health*)
Specialist Registrar Obstetrics
and Gynaecology; Field Doctor,
Médecins Sans Frontières

Ana Maria Tijerino
(Chapter 3: Health priorities in displacement)
Mental Health Advisor, MSFCH – Médecins Sans Frontières, Geneva, Switzerland

Sandrine Tiller
(Chapter 2: Responders and responses)
Strategic Adviser, Médecins Sans Frontières, London, UK

Michelle Tubman
(Chapter 22: Jaundice)
Attending Physician, Emergency Medicine, Alberta Health Services, Edmonton, Canada
Clinical Lecturer, Department of Emergency Medicine, University of Alberta, Edmonton, Canada

Jennifer Turnbull
(Chapter 15: Mass casualty triage; Chapter 28: Malnutrition; co-editor of Chapter 1: Introduction to humanitarian medicine; Chapter 3: Health priorities in displacement
Attending Physician, Division of Pediatric Emergency Medicine, McGill University Health Centre, Montreal Children's Hospital, Canada
Assistant Professor, Department of Pediatrics, McGill University, Montreal, Canada

Rafael Van den Bergh
(Chapter 56: Water, sanitation, and hygiene; Chapter 57: Medical waste management)
Senior Operational Research and Technical Support Officer, LUX-OR, Médecins Sans Frontières Operational Centre, Brussels, Belgium

Joos Van den Noortgate
(Chapter 56: Water, sanitation, and hygiene; Chapter 57: Medical waste management)
Responsible Innovation & Training, Water, Hygiene & Sanitation Unit, Médecins Sans Frontières Operational Centre, Brussels, Belgium

Peter Ventevogel
(Chapter 6: Mental health in humanitarian emergencies)
Senior Mental Health Officer, UNHCR, Geneva, Switzerland

Raghu Venugopal
(Chapter 14: Approach to clinical care in humanitarian contexts); Chapter 27: Diarrhoea and vomiting)
Médecins Sans Frontières Telemedicine Coordinator
Assistant Professor of Medicine, University of Toronto, Canada
Attending Physician, Department of Emergency Medicine, University Health Network, Toronto, Canada

Isabelle Voiret
(Chapter 3: Health priorities in displacement)
Médecins Sans Frontières, Geneva, Switzerland

Rod Volway
(Chapter 13: Working for international organizations)
Humanitarian Development Professional

David A. Warrell
(Chapter 33: Venomous animal bites and stings and marine poisoning
Emeritus Professor of Tropical Medicine and Honorary Fellow of St Cross College, University of Oxford, UK

Inka Weissbecker
(Chapter 6: Mental health in humanitarian emergencies)
Senior Global Mental Health and Psychosocial Support Advisor, International Medical Corps, Washington, DC, USA

Andrew James Willis
(Chapter 7: Epidemiology)
Epidemiologist, Médecins Sans Frontières, Montreal, Canada

Symbols and abbreviations

➔	cross-reference
⌘	website
±	with or without
↑	increased
↓	decreased
~	approximately
ACT	artemisinin-based combination therapy
AEC	antiepileptic drug
AFB	acid-fast bacilli
AIDS	acquired immunodeficiency syndrome
ALT	alanine transaminase
AMI	acute myocardial infarction
AP	Additional Protocol
ART	antiretroviral therapy
AST	aspartate transaminase
ATFC	ambulatory therapeutic feeding centre
ATLS®	Advanced Trauma Life Support®
AVPU	alert, voice, pain, unresponsive
BCG	bacillus Calmette–Guérin
BEmONC	basic emergency obstetric and newborn care
BMI	body mass index
BPD	biparietal diameter
BPH	benign prostatic hyperplasia
bpm	beats per minute
CAD	coronary artery disease
CCm	cryptococcal meningitis
CDC	Centers for Disease Control and Prevention
CEmONC	comprehensive emergency obstetric and newborn care
CFR	case-fatality rate
CHB	chronic hepatitis B
CHC	chronic hepatitis C
CHF	congestive heart failure
CHW	community health worker
CMV	Cytomegalovirus
CNS	central nervous system
COPD	chronic obstructive pulmonary disease

CrAg	cryptococcal antigen
CS	caesarean section
CSF	cerebrospinal fluid
CVP	central venous pressure
DHMT	district health management team
DIC	disseminated intravascular coagulation
DKA	diabetic ketoacidosis
DPT	diphtheria, pertussis, and tetanus
DR-TB	drug-resistant tuberculosis
DST	drug susceptibility testing
DVT	deep vein thrombosis
EBV	Epstein–Barr virus
EC	emergency contraception
ECG	electrocardiography/electrocardiogram
EEG	electroencephalography
EHEC	enterohaemorrhagic Escherichia coli
EP	ectopic pregnancy
EPI	Expanded Programme on Immunization
EPTB	extrapulmonary tuberculosis
ETAT	Emergency Triage, Assessment, and Treatment
EU	European Union
EWARS	early warning alert and response system
FAST	focused assessment with sonography in trauma
FEV1	forced expiratory volume in 1 second
FGC	female genital cutting
FGM	female genital mutilation
FNA	fine-needle aspiration
FVC	forced vital capacity
G6PD	glucose-6-phosphate dehydrogenase
GAM	global acute malnutrition
GBV	gender-based violence
GCS	Glasgow Coma Scale
GFR	glomerular filtration rate
GI	gastrointestinal
GN	glomerulonephritis
GNI	gross national income
HAT	human African trypanosomiasis
Hb	haemoglobin
HbA1c	glycated haemoglobin
HBsAG	hepatitis B virus surface antigen

HBV	hepatitis B virus
Hct	haematocrit
HCV	hepatitis C virus
HEOC	health emergency operations centre
HIC	high-income countries
HIG	Humanitarian Intervention Guide
HIV	human innunodeficiency virus
HL	hearing loss
HPV	human papilloma virus
HQ	headquarters
HTC	HIV testing and counselling
HUS	haemolytic–uraemic syndrome
IAC	international armed conflict
IASC	Inter-Agency Standing Committee
IBD	inflammatory bowel disease
ICP	intracranial pressure
ICRC	International Committee of the Red Cross
ICU	intensive care unit
IDA	iron deficiency anaemia
IDP	internally displaced person
IFRC	International Federation of Red Cross and Red Crescent Societies
Ig	immunoglobulin
IHL	International humanitarian law
IHP+	International Health Partnership
IHR	International Health Regulations
IM	intramuscular
IMCI	Integrated Management of Childhood Illness
iNGO	international non-governmental organization
IPC	infection prevention and control
IPT	isoniazid preventive therapy
IRIS	immune reconstitution inflammatory syndrome
ITFC	inpatient therapeutic feeding centre
IUCD	intrauterine contraceptive device
IV	intravenous
IVC	inferior vena cava
JVP	jugular venous pressure
LIC	low-income countries
LRTI	lower respiratory tract infection
LUQ	left upper quadrant

LV	left ventricular
mcg	microgram
MDA	mass drug administration
MDG	Millennium Development Goal
MDR	multidrug resistant
mhGAP	Mental Health Gap Action Programme
MHPSS	mental health and psychosocial support
MIC	middle-income countries
MISP	Minimum Initial Service Package
MMR	maternal mortality ratio
MNS	mental, neurological, and substance use
MOH	Ministry of Health
MRI	magnetic resonance imaging
MROP	manual removal of placenta
MSF	Médecins Sans Frontières
MTB/RIF	Mycobacterium tuberculosis and resistance to rifampin
MUAC	mid-upper arm circumference
MVA	manual vacuum aspiration
NCD	non-communicable disease
NDMA	National Disaster Management Authority
NG	nasogastric
NGO	non-governmental organization
NIAC	non-international armed conflict
NSAID	non-steroidal anti-inflammatory drug
NTD	neglected tropical disease
OCHA	Office for the Coordination of Humanitarian Affairs
ODA	overseas development assistance
OECD	Organisation for Economic Co-operation and Development
OHHM	Oxford Handbook of Humanitarian Medicine
ONS	optic nerve sheath
ORS	oral rehydration salts
PAT	Paediatric Assessment Triangle
PCR	polymerase chain reaction
PEP	post-exposure prophylaxis
PLHIV	people living with human immunodeficiency virus
PO	orally
PPH	postpartum haemorrhage
PPI	proton pump inhibitor
PPV	positive pressure ventilation

PRN	pro re nata (as required)
PTB	pulmonary tuberculosis
PTSD	post-traumatic stress disorder
PV	per vagina
RBC	red blood cell
RDT	rapid diagnostic test
ReSoMal	rehydation solution for malnutrition
RPR	rapid plasma reagin
RUQ	right upper quadrant
RUTF	ready-to-use therapeutic food
SAM	severe acute malnutrition
SCD	sickle cell disease
SCF	Save the Children
SD	standard deviation
SOB	shortness of breath
SP	sulfadoxine–pyrimethamine
SRM	sexual and reproductive health
SSD	silver sulfadiazine
STD	sexually transmitted disease
STI	sexually transmitted infection
T3	triiodothyronine
T4	thyroxine
TB	tuberculosis
TBSA	total body surface area
TM	tympanic membrane
TOP	termination of pregnancy
TSH	thyroid-stimulating hormone
TTI	transfusion-transmissible infection
UK	United Kingdom
UN	United Nations
UNDAC	United Nations Disaster Assessment and Coordination
UNFPA	United Nations Population Fund
UNHCR	United Nations High Commissioner for Refugees
UNICEF	United Nations International Children's Fund
URI	upper respiratory infection
US	United States
UTI	urinary tract infection
VDRL	Venereal Disease Research Laboratory
VHF	very high frequency
VPD	vaccine-preventable disease

WASH	water, sanitation, and hygiene
WBC	white blood cell
WFP	World Food Programme
WHO	World Health Organization

Humanitarianism Today

This welcome and comprehensive volume offers deep and very rich expertise on the technical realities and practical challenges of medical humanitarian action. It draws on the expertise and wisdom of some of the most experienced and best humanitarian practitioners in the world. Seven years in the making, it is a bold step forward in contributing to greater clarity around the nature and challenges of medical humanitarian action.

Placing this work in a broader context, humanitarianism in its fullest conception is fluid in its forms and difficult to define. While humanitarianism makes or aspires to universalist claims, there is no clear universal definition of humanitarianism, humanitarian action or space, or of the humanitarian system, and nor is there absolute clarity on where boundaries do or may lie. Yet, the formal international system (to date) is mainly the Western-funded humanitarian system which works closely within or in coordination with the international authority of the United Nations (UN) and the Red Cross. This formal system is very good and getting better at rapid responses to major sudden-onset disasters, and it is now very big.

Most recent estimates suggest that there are 4480 humanitarian organizations operating around the world, 80% of which are local or national non-governmental organizations (NGOs) working only inside their own countries. Today, the vast majority of humanitarians are not among the some 450,000 professionals now working in this formal system. They are most importantly, among the millions of community and nationally based people who are largely volunteers, and who are the most significant first responders. They are also the most enduring, who remain long after the acute phase of a crisis has passed and with it, the attention and resources of the formal humanitarian system. The most important political reality too, is the persistent and formal authority of states—an authority that is often tested in crisis, and contested in war. Medical technical skill and knowledge, and evidence and standards of care have practical meaning only when applied with adaptability and flexibility to actual and rapidly changing social and political realities. And the world is and will be changing, and indeed be challenging.

Geopolitics

We are now well into the second decade of the twenty-first century, and we are witnessing a major shift in great power politics. Our world is volatile, uncertain, complex, and ambiguous, so that the future appears discontinuous with the past. There is massive and widening inequity. Globally, we face multiple and converging crises in climate, ecology, energy, food, finance, and economy, and in emerging and re-emerging infectious diseases. Our population is explosive at 7.5 billion—already at four times the carrying capacity of the planet—and likely to reach 8.5 billion in 15 years. Humans are urbanizing at a rate portending revolutions in how we live, work, play, and govern locally. Governance is our greatest challenge, especially for the collective problems of the global commons. Since its founding, the UN has never been more needed as a forum for collective problem-solving, yet it has been weakened by neglect, and effectively sidelined by other governance platforms such as the G7 and the G20, and in many other respects by bilateralism, and unilateralism.

The United States' Trump administration may well abandon Pax Americana,* calling into question the liberal international order with its emphasis on consensus, openness, and rule-based relations enshrined in intergovernmental organizations (IGOs) and institutions such as the UN. Deeply alarming are the potential impacts of the Trump Effect on geopolitical stability; on climate change mitigation and adaptation; on water and biodiversity protections; on financing for vitally important IGOs such as the World Health Organization and the Joint United Nations Programme on HIV and AIDS (UNAIDS), and UN humanitarian agencies such as the United Nations High Commissioner for Refugees (UNHCR), Office for the Coordination of Humanitarian Affairs (OCHA), World Food Programme (WFP), and United Nations Development Programme (UNDP), and on research, trade, pricing, and access to healthcare technologies such as medicines, diagnostics, vaccines, and medical devices. Globally, the very notion of human rights is under increasing attack. Given policy assertions such as a return to the use of torture, and the rhetorical assaults on minorities, refugees, and Muslims during the 2016 US presidential campaign and beyond, the potential practical and normative effects on human rights and dignity, on respect for refugee law, the right to asylum and protection, and for respect for the laws of war, are deeply concerning.

Changing humanitarian need

In the last 25 years, increasing refugee and forced migration flows, violent extremism, a rise in regional wars and conflicts, as well as climate-related disasters have changed the global humanitarian landscape. Humanitarian needs in the world are both changing and increasing. OCHA projects that at least 128 million people in 33 countries will need humanitarian assistance and protection in 2017. The international humanitarian system is larger in absolute financial resources than it has ever been. However, need continues to grow and vastly outstrip the growth in funding and so it remains structurally incapable of meeting the global humanitarian demand. While funding to UN humanitarian agencies has increased and is more coordinated and accountable than ever before, there is a profound mismatch between growing needs and donor funds provided. Between 2012 and 2015, the average amount of aid contributed per recipient dropped by 26%. Despite massive media attention and multiple appeals, of the 20.1 billion USD required for UN interagency humanitarian assistance and protection in 2016, there was a crippling shortfall of 10.7 billion USD—or 53%—in actual donor state funding.

Protection and forced migration

By 2016, there were 65 million people who were either internally displaced or refuges, and half were children. This is more than at any time since the end of World War II. With refugees and asylum seekers attempting access by land or sea to Europe by the hundreds of thousands, forced migration is now recognized as a global crisis. Each dead person drowned in Mediterranean waters is the definition of a refugee. That this must be stated illuminates just how far humanitarianism and human rights have penetrated beyond the 'Never Again' of the Holocaust. *The Economist* declared on its

---

* Pax Americana refers to the historical concept of relative world peace and international order resulting from the preponderance of power of the United States post World War II.

23 April 2015 cover: 'Europe's boat people [are] a moral and political disgrace' for Europe and the world.

Despite a global media emphasis on a European 'refugee and migrant crisis', as of 2015 the Global South hosted 86% of the world's refugees and 89% of the world's internally displaced people (IDPs). Colombia has the largest number of IDPs in the world, with 6.9 million. Lebanon has the highest ratio in the world of refugees to population (one in every five people), while Turkey has the highest overall number of refugees (2.5 million). Both in economic terms and demographic terms, the 'developing' countries are bearing a disproportionately large impact.

The protectionist political responses to this global migration crisis—as manifest by European walls, the nefarious European Union (EU)–Turkey migrant deal, the anti-refugee rhetoric in Britain, the US, and across the EU, and the off shore detention centres administered by the Australian government—demonstrate utter disregard of international refugee law.

A messy mix with other global health challenges
Forced migration is intimately linked to violent conflict, but also to other often related global health issues such as health emergencies, hunger, climate-related migration, or development-induced displacement. These have complex origins, often rooted in inequity, social disruption, poverty, and environmental collapse. To cite but a few examples, the deliberate disruption of essential health services and conflict-related displacement has facilitated epidemics (e.g. cholera in Zimbabwe, measles in the Democratic Republic of Congo, yellow fever in Angola, or polio in Somalia, Afghanistan, Pakistan, and Syria), interfered with vaccination campaigns, and posed immediate threats to, and imposed long-term burdens on, national and regional health security. In Africa, the worst drought in 35 years—due to the combined effects of El-Nino and climate change—left some 36 million people hungry and in need of food assistance over 2016–2017. More generally, declining or poor access to land, food, fuel, and safe water forces people, often women, to travel further for resources or shelter, eroding human and ecological resilience. The residual effects of recent civil wars in Sierra Leone and Liberia, including fragile healthcare systems and deep distrust of governments, substantially hampered the capacity to respond to the Ebola virus disease crisis.

Medical standards and their limits

Medical standards are a codification and an extension of technical competencies and knowledge to the full range of humanitarian actors, but not necessarily to the full range of circumstances and contexts in which they work. As humanitarian actors strive to implement programmes according to rigorous standards, they should not underestimate the fluidity of the political context, and the possibility of being manipulated by opposing political factions or belligerents in war.

Medical humanitarian practice must be both reactive and adaptive to the changing nature, technologies, and impacts of war and conflict. Learning lessons and applying them to future situations can improve the effectiveness and scope of humanitarian medicine. Yet, these practices must continually react and adapt or they risk becoming rarefied and fossilized, and potentially irrelevant to the many who need assistance and protection.

Standards most often derive from and apply to situations that can be standardized, as with grouped populations in relatively stable circumstances where humanitarian space is possible and largely uncontested (e.g. following a natural disaster, or in long-term refugee settlements). But their universality, or applicability to all situations, cannot always be implied. Particularly in areas lacking respect for the provisions and protection of humanitarian space, technical standards may have limited use.

In more complex situations such as active war in Afghanistan or the Democratic Republic of Congo, or in regionalized conflict as in the Middle East today, changing and multiplying political and military actors make it difficult to locate legitimate and accountable authority. In the Middle East region, for example, massive and egregious violations of international humanitarian law have occurred including the use of siege and starvation tactics, the use of biochemical weapons, and bombings of hospitals and medical sites. Compounding this reality is that rather than a consensus of international consternation, there can actually be complicity. For example, in 2016, while 15 nation states were bombing in Syria, four of them were actually veto-holding permanent members of the UN Security Council who are charged with upholding international peace and security, and international humanitarian law. This duplicity renders UN Security Council resolutions on humanitarianism not only hypocritical, but effectively meaningless. In such contexts, with lack of international protections and recognized humanitarian space, the application of rigorous medical humanitarian standards is all but impossible.

Aiming to apply standards of care to humanitarian settings is a goal which implies and promotes accountability. While accountability is rarely negative, in humanitarian settings, it requires a nuanced understanding to prevent it from being a proverbial double-edged sword. This is because humanitarian actors who fail to meet a standard of care may be medically incompetent, or other factors might be at play. The distinction is an important one. If accountability implies responsibility, then this must not be misplaced, or the burden of responsibility for a viable humanitarian space shifts, from belligerents to humanitarian actors, thus allowing the former to avoid accountability for their failure.

Humanitarians must also not be silenced or co-opted in a way that allows states or parties to a conflict to avoid their duty to respect or uphold relevant international law. NGOs, other humanitarian actors, donor states, and peripheral states often share immediate interests and goals in a particular situation, but not always. Donor states typically preferentially support humanitarian programme coordination and extended coverage. This is usually good, but not always. Indeed, the UNHCR recently led a protest against the EU–Turkey refugee repatriation agreement that it and other humanitarian actors were expected to support with coordination and programming. It was a protest quickly joined by Médecins Sans Frontières, the International Rescue Committee, the Norwegian Refugee Council, and Save the Children. All five refused to be involved in what they saw as the blanket expulsion of refugees and the contravention of international humanitarian law—most especially the protection needs of asylum seekers and migrants.

Principles and evidence-based guidelines which support humanitarian medicine are the means, not the ends to which humanitarians aspire.

Principles and guidelines should be used to steer action that is responsive and adaptive to reality 'as it is'. Where needs exist but standards cannot be met, this must not preclude solidarity-based actions. The 'gold standard' is to see the dignity of the other—the victim—and to respond in word and in action, however imperfectly and however difficult the circumstances.

Governance challenges

Ours is a world in 'post-normal times' with ongoing and escalating governance and humanitarian crises. There is no humanitarian organization or coalition of organizations or current system big enough to cope with this kind of need. These are twenty-first-century problems being confronted by a failing mid-twentieth-century global governance architecture. An attempt at addressing the challenges in the global governance of humanitarianism was the World Humanitarian Summit, held in mid 2016, which was unfortunately a great disappointment for its failure to adapt to the contemporary reality in which humanitarian needs are emerging. Yet, one encouraging aspect was that various reports published in preparation for the summit, showed a distinct focus on recognizing that 'people affected by crises should be at the heart of humanitarian action' and local people are 'the primary agents of their own response'. One report (World Humanitarian Summit Secretariat (2016): 'Restoring Humanity: Synthesis of the Consultation Process for the World Humanitarian Summit'), called for 'a fundamental change in the humanitarian enterprise, from one driven by the impulses of charity to one driven by the imperative of solidarity'. It called for a 'conceptual shift' to recognize that 'autonomy and dignity of people affected by crisis' are given priority—in contrast to priorities or plans of donors or international agencies. This is consistent with the 2015 ALNAP *The State of the Humanitarian System* report that questioned the performance of the formal humanitarian system, and argued that its 'one size fits all approach doesn't work', and that the system 'has reached its limits'.

Concluding thoughts

We are in a time when humanitarian principles risk becoming ever more rhetorically noble, while formalized humanitarian action is ever more hobbled in its practical response to the type, scale, and scope of human suffering. In this context, we must remain loyal to the purpose of humanitarianism, and engage in the struggles required to achieve this. The key to meaningful humanitarianism has been independence from political influence; impartial assessment of needs and provision of support; remaining neutral to the causes of conflict or crisis, but ever-vigilant about the conditions of conflict; and for some, a willingness to speak out against violations of human rights, war crimes, crimes against humanity, and genocide. Indeed, humanitarian action must always stand in solidarity with the victim, and be prepared to be reactive to the failures or misuses of power.

For me, humanitarian action is an act of solidarity, of protest, and of initiative. It is not a substitute for the responsibility of states. It is a beginning and can demonstrate what might be, if only we so choose. Sometimes the smallest act has the greatest meaning. And sometimes too, it takes the greatest ambition to do the smallest thing. This may well be that time.

James Orbinski OC, MSC, BSc, MD, MA, MCFP

Dr Orbinski has over 30 years of international experience in humanitarian medicine, having worked in situations of war, genocide, famine, and epidemic disease. He was international president of Médecins Sans Frontières/Doctors Without Borders (MSF) from 1998 to 2001. He is Professor and Director of the Dahdaleh Institute for Global Health Research at York University, Toronto, Canada, and Professor at the Dalla Lana School of Public Health, University of Toronto. He researches humanitarian medicine, emerging and re-emerging infectious diseases, and the global health impacts of climate change.

Part I

Practical and professional issues in humanitarian medicine

Introduction to humanitarian medicine

Amy S. Kravitz and Sheri Fink

Why the *Oxford Handbook of Humanitarian Medicine*?

The *Oxford Handbook of Humanitarian Medicine* (OHHM) was conceptualized and developed to recognize the complexity of the sector, the changing contexts of humanitarian emergencies, and the challenges inherent in promoting best practices. With no overarching licensing body or clinical review board for humanitarian settings, identifying and disseminating best practices in humanitarian response and clinical patient management is difficult. There can be no definitive training or certification programme that prepares for the near limitless variability of contexts and scenarios, particularly when circumstances make clinical gold standards difficult or impossible. Further, recognizing that the vast majority of humanitarian workers are national or local staff, available resources should be within their reach, logistically, geographically, and economically, to have an optimal and equitable impact. The *OHHM* was developed to fill that gap.

This evidence-based guide covers all facets of healthcare provision in humanitarian settings. The hope is to continually improve medical humanitarian practice, and to integrate it with responsible development programmes whenever possible. This handbook consolidates the available evidence base. It also draws on the accumulated experience of humanitarian practitioners from a variety of disciplines and contexts to guide the reader through what are often complicated scenarios. The handbook contains essential information and clinical guidelines on cross-cutting issues such as gender-based violence, international law, logistics, epidemiology, mental health, and humanitarian coordination and security. The *OHHM* is written by leading experts from across the world, with years of practical experience. It is intended for humanitarian practitioners, and we have attempted to provide guidance that is clear, practical, and relevant.

As a first edition, the *OHHM* was conceived over 7 years ago, in recognition of the unique challenges faced by healthcare workers in humanitarian and complex emergencies, such as the conflict in Darfur. Awareness of humanitarian medicine was growing at this time, but it remained a sector that seemed abstract to most until the unfortunate arrival of several prominent crises. These included the Ebola outbreak of 2014 and the escalating Middle East conflicts, Syrian conflicts, and related refugee crises. The sudden surge in public awareness, and in some cases the sheer numbers of actors interested in contributing to the humanitarian response, such as the Haitian earthquake of 2010, underscored the importance of bringing this handbook to print.

What is humanitarian medicine?

Humanitarian assistance is universal in that it seeks to assist those whose livelihoods and health are impacted by conflict, disaster, or displacement. However, the backgrounds and expertise of those who provide it and the places in which they work are diverse. Humanitarian medicine differs from the typical practice of medicine, whether locally or 'globally', in that it deals with complex humanitarian emergencies in environments that are inherently resource limited and insecure. The World Health Organization (WHO) defines complex humanitarian emergencies as 'situations of disrupted livelihoods and threats to life produced by warfare, civil disturbance and large-scale movements of people, in which any emergency response has to be conducted in a difficult political and security environment'.

Humanitarian medicine also requires a diversity of skills. To deliver humanitarian relief effectively, disciplines such as law, logistics, security, and epidemiology come into play. Often working without extensive auxiliary or administrative staff, providers of effective humanitarian relief sometimes need to work beyond the traditional confines of their training, while also respecting the principles of medical ethics.

The provision of healthcare in humanitarian crises is complex and can often be characterized by unstable or chaotic settings with high morbidity and mortality and insufficient time and resources. Treating patients in such environments may first require humanitarian workers to negotiate for humanitarian space, sometimes with armed combatants, and to design a clinical practice layout which reflects the security and contextual realities of the community that they are serving. While treating unfamiliar diseases, often with limited medicines and supplies, humanitarian providers need to gain trust within these communities and strive to understand the prominent culturally driven health behaviours. In many cases, this is all done while working through an interpreter and with a population that may be traumatized.

The healthcare provider may be called on to run clinics or nutritional centres, combat epidemics, support surgery, carry out vaccination campaigns, or strengthen hospital management. Further, humanitarian workers must have a nuanced understanding of the specific contexts in which they work, especially in complex emergencies involving armed conflict, in which additional socioeconomic and political intricacies are often present. Working effectively in Borno, Nigeria, requires an understanding of malnutrition, cholera, and malaria and an emphasis on water and sanitation. Working in Yemen, by contrast, involves supporting surgical, maternal, and inpatient care for a population long exposed to conflict and reduced access to healthcare. Treating Syrian refugees in Jordan means a focus on chronic and non-communicable diseases. The nuanced information provided in the *OHHM* recognizes the complexity of humanitarian medicine and its differences from typical care in most countries.

Origin and humanitarian principles

Humanitarian medicine has developed tremendously over the preceding decades, but in a way that still recognizes its origins in the nineteenth-century Red Cross movement. The Red Cross's founder was Henri Dunant, a Swiss businessman who encountered thousands of soldiers of multiple nationalities lying wounded near Solferino, Italy, during the 1859 War of Italian Unification. Dunant assisted the wounded and wrote a book about the experience, highlighting the need for a cadre of pre-trained volunteers ready to assist in emergencies and calling for the establishment of an international relief society.[1] His idea was that aid workers should be allowed to enter the battlefield unharmed as long as they agreed to remain neutral in a conflict. The Red Cross movement was born out of this idea, and Dunant went on to participate in the drafting of the Geneva Conventions that enshrine the concept of rules in war, and of protection for humanitarian assistance. The Red Cross is now universally recognized as the guardian of international humanitarian law.

Humanity, neutrality, impartiality, and independence are widely accepted humanitarian principles, forming the bedrock of humanitarian assistance. The United Nations (UN) Office for the Coordination of Humanitarian Affairs (OCHA) summarizes these key principles as follows:

Humanity: human suffering must be addressed wherever it is found. The purpose of humanitarian action is to protect life and health and ensure respect for human beings.

Neutrality: humanitarian actors must not take sides in hostilities or engage in controversies of a political, racial, religious, or ideological nature.

Impartiality: humanitarian action must be carried out on the basis of need alone, giving priority to the most urgent cases of distress and making no distinctions on the basis of nationality, race, gender, religious belief, class, or political opinions.

Independence: humanitarian action must be autonomous from the political, economic, military, or other objectives that any actor may hold with regard to areas where humanitarian action is being implemented.

The humanitarian response

While states are the primary agents responsible for responding to crises in their territories, they may be overwhelmed and may call to the international community for help, such as in the case of a major natural disaster. In some cases, civil war or international conflict means that a state is no longer able or willing to assist certain populations, which may also lead to a call for international assistance.

Both national and international movements have developed to address humanitarian crises. Under the 1991 UN resolution 46/182, the international community sought to organize a convention for the provision of international assistance led by the UN agencies. Guiding principles of the resolution (and subsequent UN resolutions such as 60/123 in 2006) uphold humanitarian principles as well as the independence and involvement of affected states. While these resolutions legitimize the humanitarian mandate, there has been a concurrent and substantial expansion of humanitarian actors including national and international non-governmental organizations (NGOs). The increasing number of complex humanitarian emergencies in the world has overwhelmed many affected states, opening the door for the growing humanitarian sector.

The number of people engaging in humanitarian relief is steadily increasing and on average, the humanitarian fieldworker population rose by approximately 4–6% per year from 2007 to 2010, with financial contributions to the international emergency response efforts rising nearly threefold.[2] In 2010, the total number of humanitarian workers was estimated to be 274,000, who collectively responded to 103 natural disasters and 43 complex emergencies.[2] By 2014, this had grown to approximately 450,000 humanitarian aid workers[3] working in more than 4480 operational aid organizations. Although international actors attract a great deal of media attention, local and national agencies and authorities deliver the preponderance of assistance in conflict and disaster situations, particularly in the critical early days. Still, and despite approximately $25 billion in expenditures, the humanitarian response remains unable to meet overall global demand.

Throughout the history of humanitarian action, nearly every major response effort has raised questions about how to make the sector more effective, efficient, professional, and ethical. With the diversity of influences, contexts, and needs in terms of skills and competencies, a uniform approach to improve humanitarian assistance is not easy to achieve. Despite the challenges, over the past two decades, great strides have been made to further the effectiveness of humanitarian action.

Coordination

One of the major challenges in the humanitarian sector has been improving coordination. There is no organization that has sufficient capacity to independently address a humanitarian crisis, and promoting collaboration between agencies, host authorities, and affected communities has been a pressing issue. Strategies have included the establishment of OCHA, and the adoption in 2006 of the UN humanitarian cluster system, designed to advance interagency coordination, predictability, accountability, and efficiency. Despite their mixed results, an understanding of these coordination mechanisms, how they work, and the resources they make available, is essential for humanitarian providers.

Standardization

Concurrent attempts have been made to standardize best practices in humanitarian relief. The failure of humanitarian agencies to avert widespread death and suffering among refugee populations in the 1990s (in particular, among Rwandan refugees in what was then Zaire) led to a call for minimum standards in aid, increased qualifications of aid workers, and better research on morbidity and mortality in affected populations.

A result of these coordinated efforts included the SPHERE project, initiated in 1997 to enhance the quality of assistance and increase accountability by the groups providing it. This project led to a handbook on minimum standards in relief which provided tangible guidance for providers in four technical aspects: (1) water supply, sanitation, and hygiene; (2) food security and nutrition; (3) shelter, settlement, and non-food items; and (4) health action. These 'technical standards' were benchmarks in humanitarian action, facilitating the development of the Core Humanitarian Standards on Quality and Accountability (discussed later in this section).

Also in 1997, Médecins Sans Frontières (MSF) published the book *Refugee Health* that established ten top priorities for managing refugee emergencies. Significant changes in the context of humanitarian emergencies over the past two decades have necessitated a reconsideration of these priorities, as outlined comprehensively within the *OHHM*.

A review of the response to the Haiti earthquake revealed the need, as articulated by the WHO, 'to develop principles, criteria and standards for medical teams that respond to emergencies and disasters'. This led to the 'Classification and Minimum Standards for Emergency Medical Teams' in sudden-onset disasters, developed under the auspices of the Global Health Cluster and the WHO, which provides benchmark criteria for foreign medical teams offering their services to affected countries.

While the continual evolution of the standards in the sector has served to help codify best practices and promote accountability, it also underscores the reality of the rapidly changing environment in which humanitarian relief work operates. With pronounced variations in populations and contexts, exact technical standards which apply to all occasions are often infeasible. Rather, as seen in the Core Humanitarian Standards on Quality and Accountability (CHS), launched in 2014 by the collaborative Joint Standards Initiative, there is movement towards utilizing these standards as tools for effectiveness and accountability. With this aim, the CHS consolidated the proliferation of standards in the sector into nine 'commitments', aiming to improve the quality and effectiveness of humanitarian assistance, while also providing affected communities with a framework of what they can expect from those delivering humanitarian assistance.

Evidence-based medicine

In the past, best practices in humanitarian medicine were based upon experience and consensus; however, as in clinical medicine today, data-driven approaches are increasingly being emphasized. There is a challenge, though, with developing an evidence base for a clinical practice that has near limitless contexts, and for which the scope of operations continues to widen. Displacement today, for example, occurs much more frequently in urban areas, necessitating different approaches than those established by the rural precedent set in the previous decades. There is currently a compelling push to further an evidence base for optimal practices in these evolving contexts, and peer-reviewed journal articles and tailored research projects have become more common within the sector. Some such recent initiatives include the compilation of resources on earthquakes by Cochrane and Evidence Aid, MSF's central role in Ebola vaccine trials, and other relevant clinical studies, such as the FEAST trial[4] that examined the administration of intravenous (IV) fluid boluses to children in resource-limited settings. Results have drawn attention to both best practices as well as possible shortcomings in the current approaches used. The humanitarian providers of today need to understand the importance of data-informed practices, be able to easily access the available recommendations, and know how to use population-based applications to guide programming.

Security

By its very nature, humanitarian assistance is carried out in insecure environments. Recently, however, adherence to humanitarian law has lessened in many contexts, associated with a decrease in the respect for humanitarian actors and their work, and an increase in both indirect and targeted attacks on humanitarian workers. Political factors, such as the blurring of the line between military and humanitarian action, are at play in the narrowing of humanitarian space. International humanitarian law must be prioritized, recognized, and respected if the sector is to continue to provide assistance to vulnerable populations without unacceptable risk.

Conclusion

The context and conditions of modern humanitarian medicine have changed considerably since its early origins almost two centuries ago. Despite these changes, the fundamental humanitarian principles of humanity, neutrality, impartiality, and independence continue to be of utmost importance when serving vulnerable populations whose health and livelihoods have been upended by conflict, epidemics, and disasters. As the field of humanitarian medicine grows and evolves, there has been an important shift to a focus on coordination, standardization, and evidence based medicine. This has occurred in a changing and often precarious security environment.

Those working in humanitarian medicine have great challenges, responsibility, and also potentially great rewards. This field requires an extensive skill set and includes the ability to work calmly and effectively while under pressure. Excellent medical skills and a solid understanding of medical ethics and international law are essential. Rather than viewing things from afar, humanitarian workers typically have a deep and up-close understanding of current events, persistent international health problems, and the human implications of political and military decisions. They are often immersed in the emergency, while maintaining a broader sense of the overall context.

Amidst some of the most traumatic environments, inspiration can be found in the dedication and humanity of those providing humanitarian relief. This lends itself to a sense of solidarity within humanitarian workers, and a common sense of understanding among those who have experienced the tremendous professional, emotional, and psychological highs and lows associated with this work.

The *OHHM* aims to support these workers, and to provide evidence-based guidance and support in these complex situations, so that ultimately those suffering in complex humanitarian emergencies can receive the care and support they need and deserve.

References

1. Dunant H. A Memory of Solferino. Geneva: International Committee of the Red Cross; 1986 (first published in 1862). ℰ https://www.icrc.org/en/publication/0361-memory-solferino
2. ALNAP. The State of the Humanitarian System. ALNAP Study. London: ALNAP/Overseas Development Institute; 2012.
3. ALNAP. The State of the Humanitarian System: 2015 Edition. ALNAP Study. London: ALNAP/ Overseas Development Institute; 2015. ℰ https://www.alnap.org/system/files/content/resource/files/main/alnap-sohs-2015-web.pdf
4. Maitland K, Kiguli S, Opoka RO, Engoru C, Olupot-Olupot P, Akech SO, et al. Mortality after fluid bolus in African children with severe infection. N Engl J Med 2011;364(26):2483–95.

Chapter 2

Responses and responders

Patrick Robitaille and Sandrine Tiller

Context

International humanitarian assistance comes in during major emergencies, where the host government is unable or unwilling to provide for the needs of the population. When emergencies strike, it can be difficult for health providers to understand how the humanitarian response is being organized, to know who is in charge, and how to coordinate and collaborate with others. This chapter reviews the different types of international humanitarian crises and the response to them, the main activity sectors, the description of the architecture of the aid system, and the actors involved in the response. It allows the reader to understand how responses to large emergencies are organized, by whom, and how to get more information.

Typology of crises and responses

The origin of the crisis, the type of emergency, and the phase of the operating context all inform the types and speed of the response and the roles assumed.

Origin of the crises

Natural disasters
- *Geological disasters:* e.g. earthquakes, volcano eruptions, and landslides.
- *Meteorological disasters*—e.g. storms such as:
  - cyclones (South Pacific and Indian Ocean)
  - typhoons (in the Northwest Pacific)
  - hurricanes (in the Atlantic and Northeast Pacific).
- *Hydrological disasters:* e.g. tsunamis, floods, and droughts. Meteorological and hydrological disasters are increasing in terms of occurrence and severity due to climate change.
- *Biological hazards:* e.g. epidemics. Infectious disease risk is high in many humanitarian settings due to patient vulnerabilities and inadequate hygiene (see Table 2.1).

Table 2.1 Common or recent epidemics

Name	Considerations
Measles and meningitis	Vaccination should be a primary consideration for displaced populations
Cholera	Mortality can occur very rapidly, sometimes in <24 hours Very easy to prevent (hand washing) and to cure (rehydration) No existing vaccine until very recently
HIV/AIDS	Since 2000, around 38.1 million people have become infected with HIV and 25.3 million people have died of AIDS-related illnesses
Tuberculosis	Kills 2 million people per year
Ebola	The most deadly epidemic with a mortality rate that can be >90%. Was marginal before the 2014–2015 epidemic in West Africa

Non-natural
- *Food crises:* food crises can originate from droughts but are usually compounded with a variety of sociopolitical causes.
- *Conflict and violence:* e.g. civil war, regional or international conflict, urban violence, ethnic-based violence, and genocide.
- *Population displacement:* e.g. refugees, internally displaced people (IDPs), and mass migration. Although population displacement can be caused by natural disasters such as droughts, most are due to conflicts. See ➲ Chapter 3.

Types of emergencies

The origin of a crisis helps to understand the likely and possible needs of the population at the onset. The type of emergency has a huge impact on the speed of the necessary response and the capacity to prepare. For sudden or rapid-onset emergencies, pre-arranged kits and available stockpiles of lifesaving material such as blankets, tarps, and kitchen sets are essential for a quick and efficient response. (See Fig. 2.1.)

- *Sudden onset*: developing within minutes, hours, or days, e.g. an earthquake, and fast developing storms and flash floods, or the outbreak of a cholera epidemic.
- *Rapid onset*: developing over days or weeks, e.g. seasonal floods which can be more or less predicted by the monitoring of rainfalls, or the surge of IDPs/refugees as a consequence of a war.
- *Slow onset*: developing over months, e.g. droughts and food crises.
- *Chronic emergencies*: lasting for years or decades, e.g. civil conflict, structural violence, and a HIV/AIDS epidemic.

Operating contexts

The context in which the crisis originates will inform the needs of the population, to what extent the government and local authorities are to respond, and the support needed for existing health and social systems.

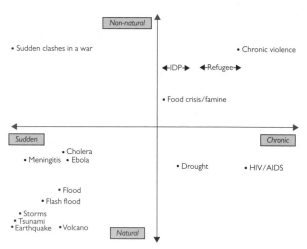

Fig. 2.1 Examples of crises by origin and type of emergencies.

Low- versus middle-income countries

There is a growing trend for humanitarian crises to occur in middle-income countries (MIC), such as violence in the Middle East or storms in South East Asia or in the Caribbean. These contexts can differ from low-income countries (LIC) due to increased capacity of response of the government, better infrastructures and services such as well-functioning hospitals, availability of specialized equipment, and better supply of clean water and electricity.

It can be a challenge in MIC for humanitarians specialized in emergencies to negotiate space as increased capacity in counties with well-established system can be linked to increased regulations and, at times, increased bureaucracy. Further, once access is established, pre-diagnosed morbidities such as chronic diseases may be better recognized, leading to differences in caseloads. This can include patients already being managed with hypertension and diabetes, who need continuity of care in addition to the acute presentations typical in acute emergencies. This variation from what is commonly seen in remote, low-resource settings can lead to differences in clinical concerns, medications, and resource allocation.

Rural versus urban

In preceding decades, aid organizations have been largely responding to needs in LIC, with primarily rural populations. Increasingly, responses in MIC are linked with larger proportions of urban populations. In such settings, there is typically a pre-existing governmental structure which is still functioning, and requires close collaboration with the humanitarian responders. In some situations, however, crises can weaken or even disable those pre-existing social structures, resulting in the humanitarian organizations supporting or even replacing the government infrastructures. This is challenging for humanitarian organizations, and involves an expansion of the typical skill-set associated with crises response.

'In recent decades, there has been a massive increase in the number of people living in cities and who are vulnerable to disasters or conflict. Urban disasters differ in important ways from rural disasters, and force the humanitarian community to rethink fundamental tools, approaches and assumptions when deciding how best to respond.'

(⅋ http://www.alnap.org/what-we-do/urban; also see The Urban Humanitarian Urban portal: ⅋ http://www.urban-response.org/)

Response phases

The acute, active phase of an emergency response is often considered a core activity period of a humanitarian response, but in reality, preparations start well before a possible disaster, and extends well beyond the initial response. Humanitarian action can be seen as a relief-to-development continuum, although lines are often blurred. (See Fig. 2.2.)

Preparedness phase

The objective is to reduce the risks associated with a humanitarian crisis by addressing the source of the vulnerability and likelihood of an event occurring and preparing for the possibility of an unfortunate event to happen.

Short term: relief phase

The first relief is usually done by the population themselves during and immediately after an event. In the days and weeks that follow the onset of the emergency, a coordination mechanism for the aid is put in place by OCHA in agreement with the government.

Intermediate: reconstruction, early recovery

This is the period of time when the focus of the humanitarian actors shifts to starting reconstruction and rehabilitation of the community. During this phase, the government can re-establish the pre-crisis governance mechanism.

Long term: transition to development

This covers the period of gradual exit of the international humanitarian actors and handover of activities to the population and government.

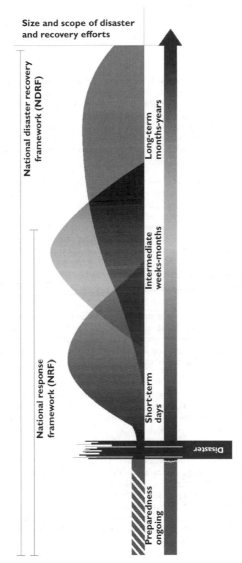

Fig. 2.2 Size and scope of disaster and recovery efforts. Reproduced from FEMA. National Disaster Recovery Framework. P.8. http://www.fema.gov/pdf/recoveryframework/ndrf.pdf with permission from FEMA.

Programme cycle

There are different phases for a humanitarian programme or project. Each phase has to be carefully addressed in order to achieve the intended objectives.

Assessments

At the onset of an emergency, humanitarian actors have to rapidly assess whether or not they should and can intervene. Assessments can be done independently or jointly between government officials, NGOs, and UN organizations, such as the United Nations Disaster Assessment and Coordination (UNDAC), for more efficiency and coherence. Timing can vary, and assessments can be done in the first hours/days of a sudden onset of a disaster, or within weeks and month in the case of a slower onset.

Programme design

The results of the assessment will inform the design of the programme, which refers to the operational structure and focus of the intervention. This must inherently include budget planning, logical framework, logistical and administrative considerations, timeline, local and international human resources, etc. Formulating a programme design can be done very rapidly in case of emergencies, or take place over the course of several months for longer-term responses. In all cases, the development of programme designs should involve the local population to ensure that the activities chosen are coherent with actual needs. A good design is key to avoid problems during the implementation phase.

Implementation

Implementation of the planned activities is the core of any response, and is usually the most visible and most costly aspect of any programme. Despite careful planning, realities on the ground may change, and so it is important that implementation is flexible and adaptable to address any developments or challenges found during the process.

Monitoring

Monitoring is performed throughout the implementation to ensure that the set objectives and indicators agreed upon are tracked and reported internally and also externally to other actors such as the government and coordination bodies.

Evaluation

Evaluations or reviews can be done internally or externally by third parties according to the organization's or donor's policy. They will evaluate the response against agreed benchmarks. The typical criteria established by the Development Assistance Committee (DAC) of the Organisation for Economic Co-operation and Development (OECD) are timeliness, impact, efficiency, coverage, relevance, appropriateness, coherence, connectedness, and effectiveness (℘ http://www.oecd.org/dac/evaluation/daccrit eriaforevaluatingdevelopmentassistance.htm).

Aid architecture and coordination

The humanitarian aid system includes many types of organizations that are working in different ways, with different objectives. In most crises situations, there is usually a UN-led humanitarian coordination mechanism implemented at a local, regional, and national level.

The UN-led humanitarian aid system

The humanitarian aid system is based on an organization framework with the UN serving as the core coordinating body through the in-country Humanitarian Coordination Teams and the cluster system. Established in 1991 through a General Assembly Resolution, this proposed that humanitarian assistance must be provided in accordance with the principles of humanity, neutrality, and impartiality within a coordinated approach among actors. It established the key pillars of the UN-led International humanitarian aid system:

- Creating the position of the Emergency Relief Coordinator who reports to the UN Secretary General and the in-country designation of a Humanitarian Coordinator.
- Establishing the Inter-agency Standing Committee (IASC) as the main policy and decision-making body guiding the international humanitarian response. Its members include key UN agencies, NGOs (Steering Committee for Humanitarian response (SCHR) and International Council of Voluntary Agencies (ICVA), see later in this section), the International Red Cross and Red Crescent Movement, and intergovernmental organizations.
- Setting up the United Nations Office for the Coordination of Humanitarian Affairs (OCHA).
- Proposing a system for international funding appeals.

The cluster system: lead agencies

In 2005, the cluster system was introduced by the UN to improve coordination between agencies for improved efficacy and efficiency (See Fig. 2.3.) It established 11 sectoral clusters, each with one or two cluster lead agencies (from IASC members). The aim of the clusters is to coordinate humanitarian responders in order to avoid duplication, standardize, and to provide information for decision-making.

The Transformative Agenda

Following the large earthquake in Haiti, and the devastating floods in Pakistan in 2010, there was a recognition that there were weaknesses in efficiency and coverage of the humanitarian system. In 2012, the Transformative Agenda was developed, with the aim to improve some key areas of the UN-led humanitarian aid system. It proposes strengthening leadership and coordination by:

- improving accountability for performance
- improving accountability to affected people
- building capacity for preparedness in selected countries
- improving advocacy and communication.

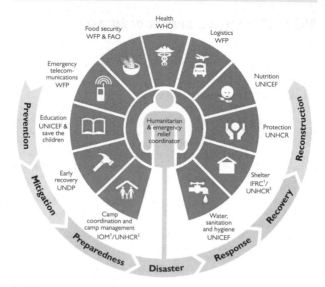

Fig. 2.3 The UN cluster system. Reproduced from OCHA, How are disaster relief efforts organized? – Cluster Approach and Key Actors, Copyright © United Nations 2017.

NGO representation systems

There are many different types of NGOs and they are represented at the IASC in Geneva. This means that NGOs have an input into decisions about the activation and strategy of UN-led responses though two key consortia:

The *ICVA* currently includes 74 NGO members with regional hubs in Bangkok, Amman, and Dakar. It aims to make humanitarian action more principled and effective by working collectively and independently to influence policy and practice.

The *SCHR* has a more limited membership, and comprises nine of the major humanitarian organizations and aims to improve the quality effectiveness and accountability of aid efforts. It has spearheaded initiatives such as the Certification process and the Core Humanitarian Standards (℘ http://chsalliance.org/).

SCHR members include the International Committee of the Red Cross (ICRC), ACT Alliance, CARE International, Caritas Internationalis, International Federation of Red Cross and Red Crescent Societies (IFRC), Lutheran World Federation (LWF), Oxfam GB, Save the Children International, and World Vision International.

Responders

Responding to crises involves a network of national and international actors, which come from private, pubic, and military sectors. The lead in these responses should be from the host government itself, and humanitarian actors should aim to support their response effort and should not undermine their authority. However, at times this is not possible, e.g. for countries where power is contested, or there is an active conflict, the national authorities may not be willing or able to provide assistance directly. This is where there is a clear role for international agencies to step in and provide humanitarian assistance in a neutral and impartial way.

The host governments and national response

National Disaster Management Authorities

National governments have the foremost responsibility to respond to emergencies in their own countries, and many countries prone to natural disasters have established their own National Disaster Management Authorities (NDMAs). These take on the functions of direction, coordination, and implementation of emergency response in their own country and may work closely with the UN in-country management team. NDMAs have the authority to organize the response and may do so according to national legislation.

Domestic facilitation of international disaster relief

Many disaster-prone countries have laws regarding international disaster assistance, stipulating how aid should be organized, and what kind of customs and taxation regimes should be put in place. To assist national authorities in developing these regulations, the IFRC have developed extensive guidance for national authorities, called Guidelines for the domestic facilitation and regulation of international disaster relief and initial recovery assistance' (IDRL Guidelines). These were adopted by the state parties to the Geneva Conventions in 2007.

UN agencies

The UN and other intergovernmental organizations include 32 specialized agencies, all with their own mandates, programmes, and funds. Those with significant humanitarian roles include:

- *OCHA*: OCHA is the part of the UN Secretariat responsible for coordinating responses to emergencies. In-country, OCHA sets up coordination hubs in the capital and in the most affected areas, bringing together key humanitarian actors to plan and organize the humanitarian response. OCHA is also responsible for coordinating the UN's country-based 'strategic response plan' (SRP) which includes response plans by sector. (See Fig 2.4.)
- *World Food Programme (WFP)*: WFP is the central UN agency tasked with providing food aid in emergencies to save lives, protect livelihoods, and to reduce chronic hunger and under-nutrition. WFP is the cluster lead agency for logistics, including establishing communications, infrastructure, and transportations.

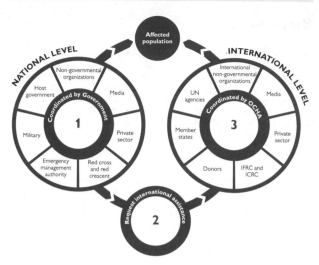

Fig. 2.4 A representation of the actors of the response. Reproduced from OCHA, How are disaster relief efforts organized? – Cluster Approach and Key Actors, Copyright © United Nations 2017.

- *United Nations International Children's Fund (UNICEF)*: UNICEF is the cluster lead agency for nutrition, water, sanitation, and hygiene and the co-lead for education (with Save the Children) and child protection. It coordinates emergency response activities for vaccinations, family reunification, gender-based violence (GBV), and care of child soldiers. UNICEF mainly works through subcontracts with NGOs, and supports national programmes through the host government.
- *World Health Organization (WHO)*: WHO is the UN agency responsible for providing leadership on global health matters, shaping the health research agenda, setting norms and standards, providing technical support, and monitoring health trends. WHO is the lead of the health cluster, and mainly works through national authorities. WHO has special authority to declare a Public Health Emergency of International Concern (PHEIC).
- *United Nations High Commissioner for Refugees (UNHCR)*: UNHCR leads international action to protect refugees and resolve refugee problems worldwide. It provides legal and diplomatic protection for refugees, helps with legal procedures, non-refoulement, and provides assistance to refugees and some IDPs in accessing health, water and sanitation, food, and shelter. UNHCR is also the cluster lead for protection and co-lead for shelter (with IFRC). UNHCR usually implements through national and international NGOs.

The WHO has also organized the implementation of response procedures and flexible national registration mechanisms for Emergency Medical Teams, both governmental (civil and military teams) and non-governmental organizations with either national or international responses. The WHO's new registration system is building a global roster of medical teams, and has set minimum standards for health workers and allows teams to clearly outline their services and skills ensuring a more effective response and better coordination between aid providers and recipients.

Emergency Medical Teams work under the overall guidance of the Classification and Minimum Standards for Emergency Medical Teams in sudden-onset disasters.

- *International Organization for Migration (IOM)*: IOM is an inter-governmental organization that is not formally part of the UN but works to promote humane and orderly migration. It does so by providing services and advice to governments and migrants. It also provides humanitarian assistance to migrants, refugees, and IDPs.
- *Others*: other agencies that have a role in development role and humanitarian aid include the Food and Agriculture Organization (FAO), United Nations Population Fund (UNFPA), United Nations Office for Project Services (UNOPS), and UN Women.

The International Red Cross and Red Crescent Movement

The International Red Cross and Red Crescent Movement has a global network able to respond to natural disasters and conflict emergencies.

It is composed of three parts:

- *International Committee of the Red Cross (ICRC)*: ICRC is a private, Swiss organization, established in 1863 which leads the Movement's response in times of conflict. Its humanitarian mission is based on the Geneva Conventions which stipulates the ability of neutral agencies to provide assistance to the wounded and sick in times of war. It also promotes international humanitarian law in accordance with the Geneva Conventions.
- *International Federation of Red Cross and Red Crescent Societies (IFRC)*: IFRC supports its member societies in times of major natural disasters, including technological disasters, refugee movements, and health emergencies. It provides technical support, emergency response teams, and coordination is done alongside the host National Societies.
- *National societies*: national societies lead coordination in times of peace. There are currently 189 national societies in the world, termed either a National Red Crescent Society or a Red Cross Society depending upon national law. National societies provide a range of services, from first aid, disaster response to social programmes, blood bank management, or youth activities. National societies are auxiliaries to the government so often have a particular role defined in the laws governing the national response to disasters.

International non-governmental organizations

International non-governmental organizations (iNGOs) are non-profit organizations and are the main implementers of international humanitarian responses. The majority of iNGO headquarters are based in the main Western donor countries with funding from three main sources: governments, UN agencies or private donations.

There are a few large organizations who account for the majority of humanitarian responses globally. A small group of iNGOs account for a large percentage of overall humanitarian spending. In 2010, five iNGO federations/organizations (MSF, Catholic Relief Services (CRS), Oxfam, Save the Children, and World Vision) spent approximately $2.8 billion on humanitarian programming. This amounts to 38% of the total humanitarian expenditure by iNGOs.[1]

Some NGOs base their action on the humanitarian principles of impartiality, neutrality, and independence (such as ICRC and MSF) while others work on the basis of the standards set forth by the sector, having more of a technical approach. See ➲ Chapter 13 for more information.

Local NGOs and civil society

There is a wide range of local NGOs and civil society organizations around the world. Local NGOs and civil society organizations are often very well connected, with a deep understanding of local dynamics and can be vital partners for iNGOs. Historically, it has been difficult for local NGOs to access funding independently due to challenging requirements and reporting. There are moves to decentralize the humanitarian aid system and ensure that local NGOs and civil society groups can better access funding and be part of the long-term solutions.

Military

The military have capacities and know-how that are very useful in disaster responses. Militaries can be self-sufficient, deploy at short notice, and take on major logistical tasks such as repairing the infrastructure. It is usually rapid and short-term support. This support can, however, have implications for humanitarian providers particularly in situations when populations lack clarity as to the motivations of military responses, especially in situations when the military is deployed as part of a political action which could include stabilization and reconstruction. As such, militaries can be considered political actors, which can cause problems in the perception of humanitarian action by the local population, which can complicate, and at times endanger, humanitarian responses. Please see the ICRC campaign 'Health Care in Danger' for more information (℗ http://www.healthcareindanger.org).

Donors

Donors are an essential aspect of humanitarian work as they fund the majority of aid responses. Having an understanding of the forms of funding can make the humanitarian aid architecture clearer and help to improve coordination and collaboration. (See Fig. 2.5.)

UN funding

In major emergencies, where more than one UN agency is responding, the UN develops, in coordination with the host government, a SRP (this is part of the UN's Transformative Agenda and replaces the Consolidated Appeals Process (CAP). The SRP outlines the UN's country strategy, as well as more detailed plans by sector. This comes attached with a funding plan towards which donors make pledges.

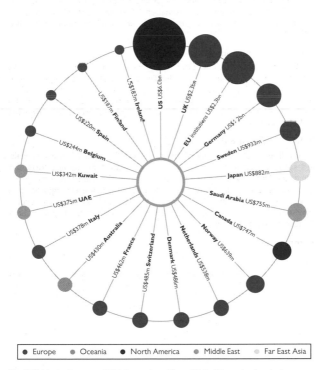

Fig. 2.5 Major donors in 2014. Reproduced from Global Humanitarian Assistance Report 2015 (http://devinit.org/wp-content/uploads/2015/10/GHA2015P_Friendly2.pdf), with permission from DIPR.

The UN has two pooled funds available in times of disaster which are managed by OCHA. They are the:
- Central Emergency Response Fund (CERF): a global fund available only for UN agencies
- Country-based Pooled Funds (CBPF): a fund allocated to NGOs as well as UN agencies.

The UN country team can also issue flash appeals 3–5 days after a sudden-onset disaster and serves as initial planning and funding guidance for donors for the first few months of a disaster.

Development Assistance Committee donors

The DAC of the OECD is composed of 29 members who provide a large proportion of the humanitarian funds. Of the global sum of \$24.5 billion provided for humanitarian assistance in 2014, the US Government (through its USAID programme) provides the greatest funding, followed by the UK (through its Department for International Development (DFID)) and the European Union (through the European Commission's Humanitarian Office (ECHO)).

Private foundations

A number of private foundations are significant contributors with the Bill and Melinda Gates Foundation, a leading grant maker focusing on health and development, providing grants for humanitarian response totalling US\$9.3million in 2014. The other major private foundation is the Sheikh Thani bin Abdullah Foundation for Humanitarian Services which provided US\$41.3 million in 2014.[2]

Public joint appeals

When disaster strikes, many of the major NGOs launch funding appeals, and some do so jointly, in order to consolidate fundraising efforts and minimize duplication. In the UK, for example, the Disasters Emergency Committee (DEC) raises funds from the public for major emergencies as a service to ten major UK NGOs. Funds are disbursed to agencies according to their plans and capacities, and they must spend the funding in a short (9–12 months) time frame.

References

1. ALNAP. The State of the Humanitarian System. ALNAP Study. London: ALNAP/Overseas Development Institute; 2012.
2. Development Initiatives. Global Humanitarian Assistance Report 2015. Bristol: Development Initiatives; 2015, p. 44.

Health priorities in displacement

Gustavo Fernandez, Françoise Bouchet-Saulnier, Alena Koscalova, Kiran Jobanputra, Ana Maria Tijerino, Philippa Boulle, Veronique Mulloni, Iza Ciglenecki, Nathalie Avril, Tammam Aloudat, Monica Rull, Pierre Maury, and Isabelle Voiret

Context

Medical humanitarian action remains a challenge and all the more so in complex emergencies. Displacement occurs in the context of a crisis which affects populations, such as armed conflict or natural disasters. Each displacement situation includes unique sociopolitical and environmental features that require an understanding of the specific context for successful implementation.

Due to the complexities of providing healthcare in displacement, MSF developed the now recognizable refugee handbook in 1997, which outlined the top priorities for such settings. Recognized globally, this handbook has become one of the main sources of guidance for humanitarians in the field. The intent of this chapter is not to reproduce the handbook, but rather to understand the considerations that led to the development of such priorities and how the changing picture of humanitarian crises necessitates adaptation of the priorities outlined two decades ago.

Humanitarian operations today are occurring in increasingly complex environments with increased urban crises, complex hostilities, and the lack of respect and enforcement of humanitarian principles. Given this complexity, the priorities outlined previously can be adapted, based on years of operational experience and acknowledgement of the special circumstances of many of today's humanitarian crises.

The scope

The growing magnitude of displacement is one of the greatest humanitarian crises in the world today. The end of 2015 found an all-time record of 65.3 million people forcibly displaced as a result of conflict, persecution, human rights violations, and violence. This record number comprises 21.3 million refugees, 40.8 million internationally displaced persons, and 3.2 million asylum seekers according to the UN refugee agency (UNHCR). Nevertheless, it does not include those crossing borders for other reasons, such as extreme poverty or simply in search of a better life. In 2015, the International Organization for Migration (IOM) estimated there were 232 million international migrants and 740 internal migrants in the world. Furthermore, unsafe and 'irregular migratory routes' are sometimes the only option available, exposing people to risks such as sexual abuse, forced labour, trafficking, physical and psychological violence, or death.

Key terms in displacement

Refugee

• Refugees share three basic characteristics, as per the UN definition:
  1. They are outside their country of origin or former habitual residence.
  2. They are unable or unwilling to avail themselves of the protection of that country due to fear of persecution.
  3. The persecution feared is based on at least one of five grounds: race, religion, nationality, membership of a particular social group, or political opinion.

- The term 'asylum seeker' refers to a person who has applied for asylum within another country, but whose refugee status has not yet been determined.

Internally displaced person

Persons considered to have been forced to leave their homes due to man-made disaster, including conflict, or natural disaster, but who have not crossed an internationally recognized state border. While IDPs often flee their homes for the same reasons as refugees, they are not eligible for protection under the same international system as refugees because they remain within their own country. There is no single international body entrusted with the protection and assistance and IDPs.

Migrant

With no official or consensus definition, this typically refers to those whose decision to migrate was freely undertaken for reasons of 'personal convenience', including for improvement of their social and economic situation, but without the intervention of a compelling external factor such as those listed in the definition of refugee status.

Poverty is unfortunately not a recognized criterion under the refugee convention, and those fleeing its consequences are often treated as 'illegal' or economic migrants.

The changing picture of displacement

Rural versus urban displacement

Historically, most humanitarian responses for displacement were in rural areas, often involving camp settings, and as such, approaches have evolved specifically for those contexts. Current trends, however, show increased instances of urban displacement that require fundamental differences in responses as compared to rural settings. The capacity for response in urban settings needs to be improved quickly as currently the great majority of tools, approaches, policies, and practices for humanitarian responses are designed for the rural, camp setting.

Challenges in urban response include the following:
- Increased population density, leading to large numbers of people impacted as compared to more sparsely populated rural areas.
- Complexity of dense urban areas requires a deeper knowledge of the spatial and social structure of cities, including shelter and housing rehabilitation, and water and sanitation.
- Disaster situations which impact dense urban areas can have a direct and debilitating impact on the resources, assets, and services normally used for emergency responses, causing delay with reaction times.
- The presence of an increasing number of marginalized communities, including IDPs, refugees, and undocumented migrants, requires additional attention to reach.
- Acute increase in demand for health services by displaced populations can lead to the saturation of pre-existing services and can cause a sense of competition for resources and decreased tolerance between both communities.

Humanitarian assistance in urban settings requires a shift from an individual beneficiary approach towards one with a joint focus on district- or community-based approaches. Further, humanitarian actors working in urban crises need to form stronger partnerships with municipal and national governments, civil society, and communities, which may not have been an emphasis in previous rural responses.

The massive displacement of populations towards Lebanon, as a result of the Syrian civil war, demonstrates the complexity of responding to crises in urban settings. Lacking any clearly established camps, people arriving from Syria settled in urban areas without any clear differentiation with the local population. Not only are the refugees often difficult to locate, but with already established health services in the area, the need for collaboration to prevent redundancy in coverage of services was vital. Further, any activity developed for Syrian refugees was to be carefully balanced with the acute needs of the local population itself in order to avoid a growing sense of disparity in terms of aid provided to those in greatest need.

Causes of displacement

Displacement and the resulting humanitarian crisis happen for many reasons, with the most common causes being natural disasters and armed conflicts.

Natural disasters

Natural disasters can have a profound impact on populations, with acute and medium/long-term consequences, and are one of the primary causes of displacement. According to the Internal Displacement Monitoring Centre (IDMC) there were 19.2 million new displacements associated with disasters in 113 countries in 2015, more than twice as many as for conflict and violence (⌖ http://www.internal-displacement.org/globalreport2016/).

The reported number of natural disasters has steadily increased over the past century (see Fig. 3.1), at least partially attributed to the rising numbers of climate-related disasters, such as floods and storms. In 2014, 518 natural disasters—excluding conflict-related famine, and epidemics—are estimated to have occurred.

The impact of natural disasters from a population perspective
Acute effects
- Injuries from sudden-onset disasters are frequent, and abundant; local capacities and organizations are typically the only possible response to the immediate emergency.
- Population displacement in the aftermath of acute disasters is common, due to fear of living in dwellings rendered hazardous by the disaster. This was observed in the Haiti 2010 earthquake and also occurs following floods after hurricanes and storms.

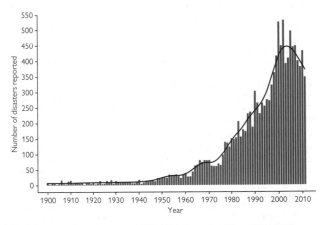

Fig. 3.1 Natural disasters reported 1900–2011. Reproduced from EM-DAT: The OFDA/CRED International Disaster Database, http://www.em-data.net, with permission.

Medium- to long-term effects
- Climatological disasters such as crop failure or prolonged drought leading to famine can also have a protracted effect on the population including starvation, displacement, and violence. The repeated famines in the Horn of Africa and Sahel are clear examples of this phenomenon.
- Long-term effects lead to demographic and socioeconomic changes including the collapse of normal social infrastructure, economic changes, dependency on aid, loss of property, alteration in social and gender roles, and loss of access to education.

Effective aid implementation in natural disasters
Assisting populations displaced by natural disasters requires a clear understanding of the local response mechanism, including the administrative framework and the availability of local and regional resources. The key elements for implementation in natural disasters include the following:
- Preparedness in advance of any emergency, including awareness and harmonization with national emergency response plans.
- Logistic capabilities: this includes issues of access, considering the geographic locations and the quick utilization of air and land resources, as well as in the actual delivery of the aid.
- Close coordination with other responders for quick responses.
- Early service expansion to include basic permanent needs. This includes those not directly arising from the disaster and consequent displacement, such as reproductive care and chronic diseases.

Armed conflicts

Conflict, in the acute phase, generates displacement as the population naturally searches for safety and basic survival services. Typically, the people who compose the most affluent sector of society will leave the conflict zone early. Conversely, the poor are typically the last to leave, and often those trapped in conflict areas are the most vulnerable in a population as they lack the necessary means to leave.

In a conflict, the resources needed by the population may be less available or not safely procured. Population movement towards areas of humanitarian aid activity is common, and in some settings there is reliance on such programmes for basic survival. The ability of humanitarian organizations to respond, however, is often complicated by factors such as donor funding priorities and mechanisms, and the local warring factions' willingness to accept (and respect) aid.

Impact of insecurity in delivering aid to displaced populations
If insecurity prevents the delivery of aid, further displacement by the population is a likely result. In recent years, aid agencies (local and international) have encountered growing difficulty in providing assistance during situations of armed conflict due to increasing security concerns. The result is that many areas are simply out of reach of humanitarian actors.

Keeping humanitarian actors safe and operational is further complicated by the increasing lack of distinction between civil and military operations. Armed forces are frequent actors in relief operations in conflict areas, and this can cause a lack of clarity for the host population. When insecurity prevents the delivery of necessary aid, not only does the population in need not receive the essential assistance for survival, but the result can be further displacement.

Modern conflict has significant differences to that in the historic past. Changes which impact humanitarian security and operations include:
- changing type of conflict, with more urban warfare
- lack of enforcement of international regulations for protection
- lack of distinction between civil and military operations
- general risk aversion in the humanitarian sector.

Implementing effective assistance for a population affected by armed conflict
- Negotiating a 'humanitarian space' is an essential and continuous process. A clear distinction must be maintained between humanitarian actors and military parties.
- Transparency in actions and intent must be clearly displayed and all warring parties should be informed about humanitarian programmes and location of health facilities.
- A dialogue with all armed actors must be maintained to ensure acceptance and understanding of the services provided.

See Chapter 11 for more information.

Key priorities in humanitarian health interventions

The priorities listed below will help you prepare and respond to a complex emergency. These are based on the 1997 MSF book *Refugee Health* whose ten priorities for managing refugee emergencies have become a standard read for those working in this sector. Since the time that *Refugee Health* was written, there have been substantial changes in the picture of displacement and humanitarian responses, as outlined in earlier sections in this chapter.

In light of the changing picture of humanitarian responses today, these top ten priorities have been reconsidered by the MSF team, and outlined here is a revised and reconsidered list, relevant for the state of humanitarian efforts today.

The priorities, as considered today, are:
- I. Assessment, surveillance, monitoring, and evaluation.
- II. Vaccination in humanitarian emergencies.
- III Control of communicable diseases.
- IV. Site planning and shelter.
- V. Water, sanitation, and hygiene (WASH).
- VI. Chronic disease in displacement.
- VII. Food security and nutrition.
- VIII Mental health and psychosocial support (MHPSS).
- IX. Health services: a patient-centred approach.
- X Advocacy and collaboration.

The amount of investment needed for each priority will vary with each situation due to differences in the affected population's health profile, environmental hazards, or availability of pre-existing quality services. While there is no prescribed formula to follow, the points outlined in this chapter will nevertheless provide the humanitarian provider with a foundation to the most important aspects of response to displacement and lead to improved preparedness and response to both traditional and contemporary displacement scenarios.

Each of the points will need to be addressed simultaneously in most scenarios, albeit with varying levels of urgency. It is important to understand the specific context of operations so that these points can be adapted to the particular environment. An essential starting point is a needs assessment, which, based on the outcome, will help determine the allocation of effort and resources. As always, collaboration and coordination are key.

Assessment, surveillance, monitoring, and evaluation

Developing a database related to an intervention is essential to ensure that appropriate aid is delivered to the right areas, in a way that is equitable, efficient, and effective. The mechanisms for this include assessments, surveillance, and monitoring/evaluation.

Assessments

Despite years of experience, one cannot assume in advance what the exact needs will be in a specific displacement situation, as these situations are highly variable and rapidly changing. The aim of an assessment is to understand a situation and identify the problems, their sources, and consequences as a means to determine the best course of response (see Box 3.1).

Box 3.1 Development of an intervention plan

An assessment feeds into the development of an intervention plan which typically includes:
- a summary of the humanitarian situation and context, population needs and vulnerabilities, and existing response activity
- expected impacts (positive and negative) of interventions and assumptions made
- objectives of the intervention
- implementation strategies and resource requirements per objective
- key performance indicators for monitoring progress on each objective and means/frequency for measuring these indicators
- criteria for expanding, changing, or ending the intervention.

A rapid assessment serves to gather the following information:
- The population size in need.
- The current and potential future health needs.
- The vulnerabilities and at-risk groups within the population.
- The available local capacity.

Timing of the assessment
- In rapid-onset crises, an initial rapid assessment should start as soon as possible after identifying the emergency (i.e. within 24–72 hours).
- Timeliness has priority over gathering detailed information that can be done at a later stage.
- In a slow-onset emergency, there may be a more complex assessment process, usually comprising several phases.
- An assessment provides a snapshot picture of the situation, but as emergencies are not static, continuous assessments are needed to spot changes and to help adapt the response accordingly (see Box 3.1).

Surveillance

Surveillance provides an overview of the evolving health status and needs of the population through the ongoing collection, analysis, and utilization of data. Historically, one of the primary purposes of surveillance in displacement was to detect early outbreaks of disease; however, surveillance has a much broader role and surveillance systems need to be tailored to the context, particularly in light of the changing picture of displacement. The initial assessment will help define the essential components to include, which, for example, might be primarily infectious disease reporting in a refugee camp in Burundi, whereas an open IDP setting in Iraq may be more focused on non-communicable diseases (NCDs).

In general, surveillance should aim to:
• collect information on mortality (crude, age, sex, and cause-specific), nutritional status, morbidity, and diseases of epidemic potential
• monitor access to health, food, clean water
• include sufficient information on human rights abuses
• have modelling to allow for recognition of blocked access to healthcare, differential exposure to violence, population movement, obstruction to aid, and/or human rights abuses.

Monitoring and evaluation

The impact of the programme is measured through monitoring and evaluation (M&E). There is no standardized list of what M&E should focus on in displacement, as the specifics monitored will depend on the intervention plan, the objectives, and the indicators defined.

Monitoring is the systematic collection and analysis of information about the response, to enable the response to be adapted and improved.

Evaluation is a more formal, structured process, conducted at the end of or at key points during the intervention; it typically involves determining to what extent the intervention has achieved its initial objectives, based on key performance indicators defined at the start.

Keys to effective monitoring
• Frequency of data collection. Monitoring should be carried out frequently (daily or weekly) in the early stages of the response, but may be less frequent (monthly) as the situation stabilizes.
• Timeliness of reporting. The data should reach the operational teams in a timely manner to enable problems associated with the intervention to be addressed.
• Dissemination of results. Data should be displayed graphically over time, with analysis of trends.
• Detailed analysis. The monitoring should include descriptive analysis of the intervention over time and the challenges faced should supplement the quantitative analysis of the indicators, so that clear lessons can be drawn and recommendations be made for future interventions.

Vaccination in humanitarian emergencies

There is high risk for communicable disease spread in humanitarian emergencies due to mass population movement, overcrowding, decreased access to safe water and sanitation, inadequate shelter, poor nutritional status, and often limited access to healthcare including routine immunization services (Expanded Program of Immunization (EPI)). Minimizing morbidity and mortality from vaccine-preventable diseases (VPDs) is a top priority in all cases of displacement.

Measles

- Preventing measles outbreaks is one of the top priority interventions in humanitarian emergencies and particularly in displacement.
- Camp settings with overcrowding contribute to the fast spread of measles, while associated malnutrition and weak health status contribute to a high case-fatality rate (CFR) (up to 32% has been described in complex emergencies).
- The target group for vaccination may need to be broadened further than Sphere standards (see Box 3.2) as recent outbreaks in refugee settings included >50% of cases who were older than 15 years. Measles epidemiology among the displaced and host populations should be taken into consideration when defining target age groups.

Box 3.2 Sphere standards recommendation for measles

- Mass vaccination campaigns for all children aged 6 months to 14 years of age (children aged 6–9 months need to be revaccinated), if measles vaccine coverage is <90% in children aged 9 months to 5 years or if this coverage is unknown.
- Mass measles vaccination should be accompanied by distribution of vitamin A for children under 5 years of age.

Prevention of epidemics

- Epidemics of other VPDs have been described in complex emergencies including cholera, meningococcal meningitis, poliomyelitis, yellow fever, hepatitis A and E, mumps, and rubella.
- In camp settings especially, such epidemics can spread exponentially and reactive vaccination campaigns might intervene too late to impact the spread of diseases; for this reason, preventive mass vaccination campaigns are preferable.

Mass vaccination campaigns

- To sustain high vaccination coverage, a system should be put into place that ensures immediate vaccination of new arrivals (e.g. in reception centres, if they exist).
- Mass vaccination campaigns allows:
  - a rapid increase in vaccination coverage
  - several vaccines to be combined and accompany other activities to reduce the necessary resources.

- With mass vaccination in place, routine EPI activities should also be implemented within primary health programmes as soon as possible.

Guidance on how to prioritize vaccines in complex emergencies is now available (Box 3.3). The final decision on which vaccines to prioritize should be taken together with the Ministry of Health (MOH), UN agencies (UNICEF, WHO), and other actors who can facilitate rapid deployment.

Box 3.3 WHO's Strategic Advisory Group of Experts (SAGE)

In 2013, the group published a framework for decision-making for prioritization of vaccines for prevention of epidemics as well as routine vaccination in acute humanitarian emergencies, which are based on:
- assessment of the epidemiological risk for each VPD in a given context
- properties of each vaccine
- prioritization in relation to other urgent public health interventions, including ethical principles and contextual factors.

Further information on this can be found at: ℘ http://apps.who.int/iris/bitstream/10665/92462/1/WHO_IVB_13.07_eng.pdf.

Prevention of under-five mortality
- The main causes of mortality among children under 5 years of age in complex emergencies include respiratory tract infections, diarrhoeal diseases, and malaria.
- While routine vaccines are utilized at baseline for the main causes of respiratory tract infections and diarrhoea (i.e. *Haemophilus influenza*, *Pneumococcus*, and *Rotavirus*), coverage is often low in complex emergencies, and in some countries these vaccines have not yet been included in national schedules. By delivering vaccines through mass campaigns, coverage can be rapidly increased in a short time (see Box 3.3 for prioritization of vaccines).

See ➲ Chapter 35 for further information.

Control of communicable diseases

Communicable diseases, including diarrhoeal diseases, acute respiratory tract infections, malaria and measles among children, and HIV and tuberculosis (TB) among adults are some of the major cause of death in complex emergencies. Identifying the risk factors for potential disease outbreaks allows effective ways of preventing and managing outbreaks to be put in place and prevents excess mortality.

General measures for communicable disease control

- Epidemic control means having a good surveillance system in place with an early and appropriate response. Its effectiveness will be enhanced if contingency plans have been drawn up in advance.
- The most effective preventative measures for controlling communicable diseases consist mainly of improving the environment and the living conditions of displaced persons/refugees by:
  - decreasing overcrowding by proper site organization
  - providing shelter
  - ensuring adequate water supply
  - disposing of excreta
  - supplying food
  - controlling vectors, etc.
  - immunization.
- Outreach activities should include home visits for early case finding and active screening with rapid referral of suspected cases.

The most common communicable diseases seen in displaced populations are shown in Table 3.1, along with the factors that impact their transmission and potential prevention measures.

Communicable diseases of importance in emergency situations and their epidemic thresholds are shown in Table 3.2.

Table 3.1 Main diseases with high mortality rates in displacement

Disease	Major contributing factors	Preventive measures
Measles	Overcrowding Low vaccination coverage	Minimum living space standards Immunization of children
Diarrhoeal diseases	Overcrowding Contamination of water and food Lack of hygiene	Adequate living space Safe water supply and sanitation Sufficient quantity of water per person Public health education Good personal and food hygiene Distribution of soap
Acute respiratory infections	Poor housing Lack of blankets and clothing	Minimum living space and proper shelter Distribution of clothes and sufficient blankets
Malaria	Displaced from malaria hypo-endemic area to high transmission zone Stagnant water which becomes a breeding area for mosquitoes	Provision of insecticide-treated long-lasting mosquito nets Destroying mosquito breeding places, larvae, and adult mosquitoes by spraying
Tuberculosis	Poor housing Overcrowding Bad nutrition status Interruption in diagnosis and treatment	Minimum living space and proper shelter Sufficient and balanced food distributions Active case detection, prompt diagnosis and treatment
HIV	Poverty, social instability, violence	Public health education Access to preventive measures (condoms, counselling and testing) Prevention and treatment of sexually transmitted infections (STIs)

Table 3.2 Communicable diseases of potential importance in emergency situations with their epidemic thresholds

Disease	Epidemic threshold → immediate investigation
Measles	1 case (*in closed setting*)
Cholera	1 case (*in closed setting*)
Yellow fever	1 case
Viral haemorrhagic fevers	1 case
Plague	1 case
Typhus	1 case
Relapsing fever	1 case
Meningococcal meningitis (A, C, W135)	*<30,000 inhabitants:* doubling of number of cases over a 3-week period, or 5 cases in one week *>30,000 inhabitants:* 15 cases/100,000 inhabitants/week and in high-risk zone with no epidemic for 5 years, 10 cases/100,000 inhabitants/week
	Alert → immediate investigation
Whooping cough	1 case
Typhoid	1 case of intestinal perforation
Dysentery—shigellosis type A (Sd1)	1 death
Visceral or cutaneous leishmaniasis	1 case
Trypanosomiasis	1 case
Schistosomiasis urinal	1 case
Malaria	Excessive number of cases in relation to prior experience according to place, time of year, and population → comparison of the incidence of the disease with a previous incidence at a similar time of year and in the same population which is usually not possible in regard to refugee/displaced population
Hepatitis A and E	
Tetanus neonatal	
Tetanus in situation of natural catastrophe	
Conjunctivitis	
Scabies	↓ Doubling of number of cases over a 3-week period

Site planning and shelter

In situations of displacement, sites will need to be established for housing and services for the population. Site planning is a top priority as the specifics of the location can have far-reaching consequences for the population, and affect the ability to deliver services.

Site planning

The Sphere handbook provides specific minimum recommended standards for site planning and shelter (see resource link given later in this section). In a general sense, appropriate site planning needs to consider the following:
- Access to water.
- Safety and security.
- Space (both for immediate and prospective needs).
- Infrastructural needs of various programme services (i.e. health, education, water, and sanitation).
- Shelter needs, including consideration of infrastructure, privacy, and provisions of supplies.
- Legal and administrative status of the land or parcel to be used.

The local context is very important in site planning and shelter development. Consider the following:
- A market survey (local material is a plus).
- Importation needs (regulation, custom clearance duration, capacity of transportation).
- Local regulations and/or building codes.
- Skilled and manual worker availability.
- Governance, institutions, and administrative regulations that influence how the site is to be laid out.
- Cultural considerations.

Considering future implications

Needs of the sites change over time, so reassessments should consider the:
- anticipated length of time of displacement, i.e. short term (seasonal) or mid to long term (several years)
- possibility of scaling up the camp for an increased population size.

For further information, the Sphere standards for site planning and shelter can be found at 🔗: http://www.spherehandbook.org/en/1-shelter-and-settlement/.

Water, sanitation, and hygiene

WASH actions are of fundamental importance in situations of displacement because they are among the most effective means of controlling and preventing disease transmission and of reducing disease reservoirs. Countless examples of disease outbreaks, such as cholera and other water-borne diseases, malaria, and hepatitis E, all related to poor living conditions and inadequate water and sanitation, have shown that WASH is an important priority in complex emergencies.

While the range of WASH activities is broad, the focus for displaced populations is generally on ensuring the safe treatment and distribution of potable water, the construction of sanitary facilities, appropriate waste water management, healthcare waste management, vector control, and finally, the promotion of hygiene. Which interventions are prioritized should be considered on a case-by-case basis, and used according to their ability to contribute to the impact on morbidity and mortality.

WASH interventions in displacement

Displaced populations have specific WASH needs, which generally contain both an education and health promotion component ('software component') and technical interventions ('hardware components'). How these elements are implemented can vary based on the population size and distribution:

- *Small population groups* (up to 2000 people) dispersed over a territory (cluster distribution): interventions generally focus on health promotion and education at the community or family level. In the early days of an intervention, an experienced WASH technician should be on the ground to properly train teams that will then train the community. These activities can be complemented with discrete hardware such as household water treatment kits, when appropriate.
- *Medium-size population* (>2000 but <15,000 people): as with smaller populations, early interventions should focus on health promotion using WASH teams educated in a train-the-trainer model. In contrast to small populations, however, the hardware component of WASH implementation is more robust and involves following standardized WASH guidelines and uses pre-existing WASH kits.
- *Large-scale intervention* (>15,000 people): the hardware component may include the need to improve, replace, or complement existing infrastructure, which requires high-level technical skills and a WASH team on site.

See ↪ Chapter 56 for further information.

Chronic disease in displacement

Medical response, particularly for people displaced by conflict or natural disaster, has typically been geared towards acute care and rapid interventions. Pre-existing chronic conditions, whether NCDs such as cardiovascular disease and diabetes, or infectious diseases such as HIV and TB, are actually heavy contributors to mortality and morbidity in low- and middle-income settings and should not be overlooked. This is particularly apparent in situations of displacement such as in the Middle East, where the health profile of the population means that chronic non-communicable conditions constitute a larger proportion of medical consultations. Furthermore, in displacement, treatment interruptions are common, which contributes to exacerbation and deterioration of pre-existing medical conditions.

Addressing chronic diseases

Chronic diseases are not intuitively easy to include in the medical response to displacement, with their requirements for an understanding of continuity of care, longitudinal follow-up, and patient self-management. There is a gap in evidence and knowledge of how to include these diseases in the emergency response and which elements of their care are essential. Despite this, the implications of gaps of continuity of care for these diseases may be even more complicated to manage in situations of displacement. It is therefore crucial to make the conceptual shift required to routinely consider chronic disease when planning for humanitarian response in displacement.

It is important that chronic diseases should not be neglected simply because of the setting—at the very least, it is important to understand any potential harms incurred by the patient due to any changes in continuity of care. Follow-up can be done in a relatively light and flexible manner, with innovative strategies including telephone follow-up and use of community focal points.

See ➜ Chapter 46 for prioritization and specific management guidance on NCDs, and ➜ Chapter 31 for information on those often chronic infectious diseases.

Food security and nutrition

Displaced populations are at risk for both macro- and micronutrient deficiencies via a complex interplay of factors, and may have elevated rates of undernutrition even prior to displacement. Population nutritional status is considered a key indicator of the severity of a humanitarian crisis and is therefore a priority for assessment and intervention.

Assessment

Information on both food security and nutritional status should be part of the general initial assessment of a displaced population. This can occur in two phases: a rapid qualitative assessment, and a more detailed quantitative assessment that will guide intervention types, and will define the severity of the crisis.

The extent of data collection will depend on the role of your organization in nutritional intervention. Information gathered can include the following:

- Food security: this can include food availability, food accessibility, food used, and coping mechanisms (i.e. decreasing the number of meals, selling of livestock).
- Nutrition: global acute malnutrition (GAM) in children aged 6 months to 5 years serves as a marker for overall nutritional status of the population. A survey of a representative sample of the under-five population (see ℘ http://smartmethodology.org/for the standard nutrition survey methodology) can be done rapidly in lieu of a costly and time-consuming evaluation of all children.
- The following factors can affect the nutritional assessment:
  - High mortality rate: may 'hide' the extent of the problem as these deaths are not captured in the nutritional survey.
  - Season: natural variations in food availability and accessibility as well as in health situation (e.g. outbreaks) can raise or lower rates of malnutrition.
  - Quality of available food and of food aid: sufficient calories in available food may yield acceptable levels of GAM, while producing significant micronutrient deficiencies.
  - Rapidly changing population with ongoing population movements: initial surveys can quickly become non-representative.
  - Security and political context: food insecurity and food aid can and have been used as political tools. The security context can directly affect access to food even when food is available.
  - The presence of other factors related to the health and WASH situation (i.e. availability and accessibility to clean water in sufficient quantity, vaccination coverage, availability and accessibility to functional health services, among others) must be considered for the interpretation of the assessment's results as well as for prospect scenario planning. Poor vaccination coverage rates and lack of access to quality water should be interpreted as aggravating factors of the situation.

Intervention

The overall objectives of nutritional intervention are to provide adequate food rations (quantity and quality) to the entire population, to prevent malnutrition in certain vulnerable populations, and to treat moderate and severe malnutrition. Criteria for inclusion in each programme, choice of programme(s), and thresholds to intervene will depend on each organization's specific role in nutritional intervention. Organizations such as the WFP, UNHCR, and host country authorities all play a role, and coordination is essential. Understanding your organization's specific role is key to efficiency and effective intervention.

Surveillance and monitoring

These should be done frequently in the acute phase and focus on food security, nutritional status, health and WASH situation, and evaluation of nutritional programmes.

- All levels of the food ration process should be monitored to ensure quality and quantity of food distributed. Issues of procurement and transport should be planned for in advance. Inequity in food distribution at the population level can sometimes be missed, as the most vulnerable are less visible.
- Other factors influencing food security such as droughts and seasonal changes, market food prices, and the political and security context should be monitored beyond the acute phase.
- Regular nutritional surveys should be performed to monitor nutritional status. The frequency of these surveys depends on the phase of the crisis as well as aggravating factors that may occur such as new population movements and disease outbreaks.
- Health indicator data, i.e. crude mortality rate, under-five mortality, and outbreak and disease surveillance, should be collected in order to interpret nutritional data in the broader context. WASH information (i.e. access to clean water) should also be considered for a comprehensive interpretation of the nutritional data. (For further information, see ⊃ Chapter 56).
- Routine data collection at community and centres levels should be analysed to see trends and changes (such as mid-upper arm circumference (MUAC) screening).
- Specific indicators for nutritional programmes are covered in ⊃ Chapter 28. Areas of concern can be detected early and addressed with interventions such as community education, active case finding, or adjustment of levels of nutritional intervention.

See ⊃ Chapter 28 for more information on diagnosis, management, and programme surveillance.

Mental health and psychosocial support

During and after emergencies, mental health needs increase, while community and professional resources for support are simultaneously greatly reduced. Mental health and psychosocial needs in humanitarian settings include not only those directly related to the emergency, but also pre-existing problems (e.g. chronic mental disorders) and problems that are induced or aggravated by the post-emergency context (displacement, disrupted support systems, dependency from aid). For all these reasons, it is important to prioritize MHPSS issues in humanitarian settings.

People may express psychological distress in various and often indirect ways, e.g. by using culturally salient 'idioms of distress'. Given the considerable stigma and discrimination suffered by people with mental disorders, they may be reluctant to seek help. People with mental health problems may present to health facilities with physical symptoms such as headaches, problems sleeping, and body pains without apparent medical cause.

Access to mental health and psychosocial interventions

In the initial emergency response, the emphasis should be on facilitating healthy coping for adversity and loss, identifying and assisting people who are overwhelmed by acute stress and grief, and protecting and treating people with severe mental disorders.

MHPSS interventions range from (1) providing basic needs in ways that are conducive to well-being (i.e. by ensuring dignity, preventing dependency, and promoting the participation of the emergency affected people), (2) strengthening mutual social and emotional support mechanisms in the affected population ('helping people help themselves'), (3) providing focused psychosocial interventions by trained non-specialists, and (4) providing psychological and psychiatric interventions (see Fig. 3.1). Even when resources are scarce, it is important to pay attention to all layers of this intervention pyramid.

Basic management of mental disorders including psycho-education, psychosocial interventions, and medication prescription can, to a large extent, be done by non-specialists (such as nurses, social workers, and community health workers) provided they are well trained and supervised. Such 'task-sharing approaches' require that mental health specialists dedicate their attention to on-the-job training, clinical supervision, and seeing people with more complicated problems.

How to act

- Ensure delivery of assistance with respect and dignity.
- Facilitate community supportive structures.
- Inform all humanitarian staff (not only the medical staff!) about normal reactions to stressful situations.
- Include mental health in regular health promotion messages.
- Ensure that health facilities are ready to manage people with MHPSS problems: allot extra time for consultations for patients with mental disorders.
- Have staff trained in basic identification and management of priority mental health conditions.

- Ensure availability of psychotropic medications (particularly those on the WHO essential drug list).
- Ensure referral to more specialized mental health services if needed (see Fig. 3.2).

See ➲ Chapter 11 for further information.

Intervention pyramid

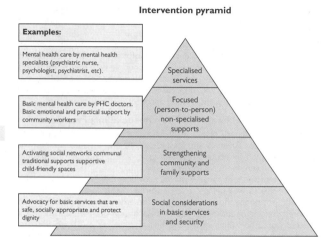

Examples:

Mental health care by mental health specialists (psychiatric nurse, psychologist, psychiatrist, etc.)

Specialised services

Basic mental health care by PHC doctors. Basic emotional and practical support by community workers

Focused (person-to-person) non-specialised supports

Activating social networks communal traditional supports supportive child-friendly spaces

Strengthening community and family supports

Advocacy for basic services that are safe, socially appropriate and protect dignity

Social considerations in basic services and security

Fig. 3.2 Multilayered interventions for mental health and psychosocial support. Reproduced with permission from Inter-Agency Standing Committee (IASC), Mental Health and Psychosocial Support in Humanitarian Emergencies (2010). Geneva. p3.

Health services development

Of the nearly 60 million people who are currently forcibly displaced, many travel to countries that have insufficient pre-existing health infrastructures, making this additional burden difficult to absorb. This is particularly apparent in LIC and MIC, which already deal with 93% of the worldwide disease burden, but have only 11% of global health spending. Addressing the needs of the displaced in such contexts is extremely challenging and there is no single model for setting up health services that is applicable to all contexts.

The health model developed will depend upon the information collected in the assessment phase, including information about:
- pre-existing health structures (quantity, quality, and accessibility)
- population figures (host and displaced)
- population epidemiological profile (host and displaced)
- outbreak history
- human resources available
- national health policies (right to practice, medical protocols, etc.).

When establishing health services, coordination and authorization from the MOH is essential, with a mutually agreed upon understanding of regulations and policies that could impact the service provision (i.e. medical item importation, quality of local drug supply, national medical protocols, etc.). Working closely with health counterparts will optimize coverage, enhance services, and avoid overlaps. Equally, make the link with the population to be served and involve them in the process. Identify the community stakeholders. Consider the impact and perception of the new services on the pre-existing services (i.e. potential competition) and the community. General goals of basic services should include:
- integration of preventative approaches
- capacity to manage most illnesses at the basic level of care
- referral capacity between levels of care
- cultural mediation and translation capacity.

When establishing health services in displacement, it is essential to reinforce local health capacities that will care for both local and displaced populations, as when parallel systems of care are put in place, resentment, competition for resources and a sense of discrimination are common, particularly if displacement is protracted. Medical services set inside a camp may be of a higher standard, with a broader scope of service and be less expensive than what the hosting population has available, which can create resentment. To minimize these tensions, it is important to:
- understand local system of medical care
- not discriminate care based on administrative or other criteria
- coordinate with local health authorities
- coordinate with all health programmes existing in the area of assisted
- communicate clearly to the population what the service is about.

Minimum Initial Service Package

One cross-cutting area which requires special attention in health service development relates to reproductive health. Although there is a justified focus on the major causes of mortality in refugee emergencies (i.e. infectious disease, malnutrition, as outlined in this chapter), aspects of reproductive health should also be addressed in the initial phases of the response to reduce mortality and morbidity, particularly among women.

The Minimum Initial Service Package (MISP) for reproductive health is an internationally recognized minimum standard for priority lifesaving interventions to be put into place at the onset of every emergency. The key objectives of MISP, which should be incorporated into any health system design, as well as some key activities are summarized as follows.

Objectives of the MISP

Objective 1. Identify an organization(s) and individual(s) to lead the implementation of the MISP.

Objective 2. Prevent and manage the consequences of sexual violence:
• Protection systems in place, especially for women and girls.

Objective 3. Reduce transmission of HIV:
• Safe blood transfusion available.
• Standard precautions practised.
• Free condoms available.

Objective 4. Prevent maternal and infant mortality:
• Emergency obstetric and newborn care services available, with 24/7 referral systems.
• Clean delivery kits provided to skilled birth attendants and visibly pregnant women.

Objective 5. Plan for comprehensive reproductive health services integrated into primary healthcare:
• Reproductive health equipment ordered.
• Staff capacity assessed and trainings planned.
• Sites identified for future delivery of comprehensive reproductive health.

Advocacy and collaboration

Health workers in developing countries sometimes hesitate to make noise about injustices faced by their patients, since they risk retribution or find their career opportunities curtailed. This is where human rights organizations and iNGOs can play an important role, with less fear of retribution. In some countries where protest is not possible, international organizations can give a voice to healthcare workers and patients' demands. In this sense, advocacy can be considered an essential aspect of humanitarian work that seeks to highlight and address the root causes of those needs and the obstacles to address them. See ➲ Chapter 9 for more details.

Messages medical aid actors will frequently advocate for:
- Violation of international humanitarian law.
- Right to seek asylum.
- Principle of non-refoulement.
- Call for respect of medical ethics.
- Humanitarian access or access to healthcare.
- Adequacy of the aid system and policy.

> In 1999, MSF initiated a campaign for the access and development of life-saving essential medicines which stirred up the global debate on drug pricing In connection with patient group initiatives. In 2015, this campaign launched 'A Fair Shot', which used social media to highlight the absurdity of pricing pneumonia vaccines according to ability to pay. The vaccine pricing policies of multinational pharmaceutical companies can be challenged when members of the public demand change (🔎 http://www. doctorswithoutborders.org/fair-shot).

Advocacy process
- Different tools and approaches can be used, depending upon the situation, but collaboration, coordination, and partnerships are required for increased effectiveness.
- Advocacy starts with the identification of the problems of the population and the obstacles that lead to these problems.
- It requires planning and strategy—it is not effective if conducted inconsistently.
- The purpose of advocacy is to inform and influence decision-makers with the formal or informal power to make the change happen.
- It is not enough to raise awareness or just educate. The ultimate goal is to achieve desired change at the local, national, or global level.
- Advocacy is stronger when based on evidence. Experience or data to prove the issue is important, and a suggested solution is required.
- Approaches and tools that are most appropriate for the context and environment can vary.

The advocacy cycle

Advocacy is a strategic series of actions designed to influence those who hold governmental, political, economic, or private power to implement public policies and practices that benefit those with less political power and fewer economic resources (the affected group).

Advocacy in medical humanitarian projects (Geneva Centre for Education and Research in Humanitarian Action)

The principles of planning advocacy are similar to those of planning any other programme, with the need for being clear about objectives and targets, and of course monitoring and evaluation. However, because advocacy often involves a political context, with stakeholders having their own agendas and influences, it can be complex.

The advocacy planning cycle (see Fig. 3.3) aims to identify the factors that might influence the outcome of advocacy. It also prepares NGOs to account for factors that have not been identified, as they arise. The cycle can be split into two distinct parts: the first steps are more strategic in nature; the second develop that strategic background into a workable action plan. The advocacy planning cycle will take you, step by step, from identifying the core issues you need to work on through to drawing up a specific action plan to implement your advocacy work. Advocacy planning

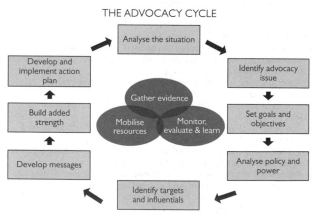

THE ADVOCACY CYCLE

Analyse the situation

Identify advocacy issue

Develop and implement action plan

Set goals and objectives

Gather evidence

Build added strength

Mobilise resources

Monitor, evaluate & learn

Analyse policy and power

Develop messages

Identify targets and influentials

Fig. 3.3 The Advocacy Planning Cycle. Reproduced with permission from http://www.who.int/pmnch/media/events/2013/advocacy.pdf, with permission from The Partnership for Maternal, Newborn & Child Health, www.pmnch.org.

is a cycle because, although there are some sequential steps, some steps run in parallel, or may change sequence according to progress. It is also a repetitive process: ongoing monitoring and review will lead to updating and adjusting the plan, as will different reactions to the advocacy among your targets.

Further reading

Médecins sans Frontières. Refugee Health: An Approach to Emergency Situations. MSF; 1997. ℜ http://refbooks.msf.org/msf_docs/en/refugee_health/rh.pdf

Tearfund. Advocacy Toolkit: ℜ http://tilz.tearfund.org/en/resources/publications/roots/advocacy_toolkit/

Health systems design

Jorge Castilla Echenique, Andre Griekspoor, and Hyo Jeong Kim

Context

Crises can interfere with health service delivery in many ways, including through damage and destruction of health facilities, interruption of health programmes, loss of health staff, and overburdening of clinical and preventive services.

Natural disasters generally cause short-term disruptions of the health systems, but return of services and health system functions back to pre-disaster levels may take several years, as seen in Haiti, in particular if there was significant damage to the health infrastructure. Usually governments plan for such a reconstruction and recovery period from 3 to a maximum of 5 years. The disruption of health systems in conflict-affected countries is generally much more substantial, and even when conflicts come to an end, recovery may take >10 years.[1]

One of the great challenges of humanitarian interventions pertains to how to provide emergency assistance in a way that considers the long-term development goals of the country in which the interventions are taking place. The reality in the field is often chaotic and stressful, where limited resources are stretched to the limit, leading to a focus on interventions that have a short-term life-saving focus, sometimes bypassing the existing health system. In this context, consideration of the longer-term recovery and development goals can get pushed to the back burner—but this is a mistake. Emergency interventions that function as substitutes in the health system may temporarily serve to fill gaps in service coverage for affected populations; however, they may undermine future recovery of the health system by fragmenting existing systems and disempowering the roles of local and national health authorities.

This chapter aims to provide the reader with the necessary background to healthcare systems at baseline and in times of distress. It clarifies what humanitarian healthcare workers can do to ensure effective aid that delivers immediate healthcare relief to patients but at the same time considers connections with the existing healthcare system, and where appropriate strengthens it, during and beyond deployment.

Health systems architecture

Humanitarian interventions can and should support the health system in the country in which they operate. There is considerable variation in health systems, but in general, a health system consists of all organizations, people, and actions whose primary intent is to promote, restore, or maintain health. It includes the totality of preventive and curative health services provided within a country, delivered by both the public and private sectors. In contexts of emergencies or humanitarian settings, effective interventions require a basic understanding of the nature and specific architecture of the healthcare system in which they are operating. Even well-intended programmes can undermine and fragment the existing system, rather than making it more resilient.

The following sections outline the major components of health systems:

WHO health system building blocks

A health system is usually described by its six interdependent building blocks (see Fig. 4.1):

- Good *health services* are those that deliver effective, safe, good quality health interventions to those that need them, when needed, with minimum waste of resources.
- A well-performing *health workforce* works responsibly, fairly, and efficiently to achieve the best health outcomes possible, given available resources and circumstances.
- A well-functioning *health information system* ensures the production, analysis, dissemination, and use of reliable and timely information on health determinants, health systems, and health status.
- A well-functioning health system promotes equitable access to essential *medical products and technologies* of assured quality, safety, efficacy, and cost-effectiveness, and their scientifically sound and cost-effective use.
- A good *health financing system* raises adequate funds for health, in ways that ensure people can use needed services, and are protected from financial catastrophe or impoverishment associated with having to pay for them. It provides incentives for providers and users to be efficient.
- *Leadership and governance* ensures strategic policy frameworks that are combined with effective oversight, coalition building, regulation, attention to system design, and accountability.

These six main elements of health systems can be impacted by crises, with specific considerations to humanitarian providers working in such settings (see guide to WHO building blocks for health systems in Fig. 4.1).

Primary and secondary or higher healthcare

Healthcare systems are generally subdivided into primary (at community or facility levels for basic interventions) and secondary or higher healthcare[2,3] (where more complex cases and life-threatening conditions are referred to). The sources of care may be diverse but most commonly are the state, the private for-profit sector, and the private not-for-profit sector which may include faith-based organizations or NGOs.[4,5]

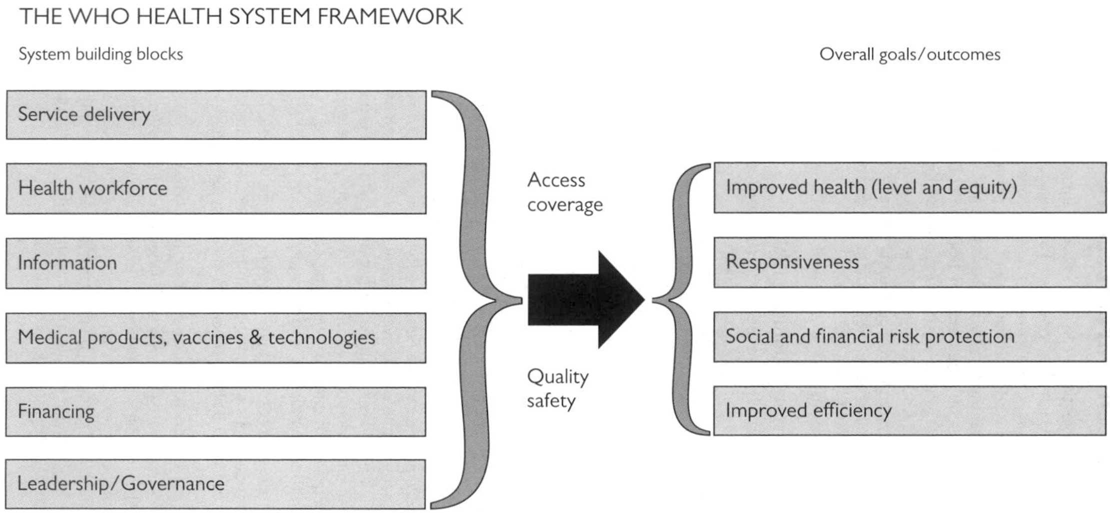

THE WHO HEALTH SYSTEM FRAMEWORK

System building blocks

Fig. 4.1 WHO health systems framework. Reproduced with permission from World Health Organization 2007. Everybody's business. Strengthening health Systems to improve health outcomes. WHO's framework for action. http://www.who.int/healthsystems/strategy/everybodys_business.pdf

Acknowledging the diversity of regional and national healthcare systems globally, WHO defines primary healthcare as 'essential health care made universally accessible to individuals and families in the community by means acceptable to them, through their full participation and at a cost that the community and country can afford. It forms an integral part both of the country's health system of which it is the nucleus and of the overall social and economic development of the community.'

Models of *primary healthcare* vary from country to country. In most cases, they provide a package of health interventions through health centres/posts and related community health workers (CHWs) who connect the healthcare system and the community. Primary healthcare usually consists of:

- community outreach services
- basic healthcare services in fixed or mobile clinics
- health promotion (information, education, and communication).

Secondary[6] and higher-level healthcare is a centralized service providing more advanced healthcare to the population and act as the reference for the primary healthcare level. It deals with clinical management of potentially life-threatening conditions.

Models of secondary care vary from country to country. In all cases it provides a package of services through:

- emergency and outpatient care
- inpatient care (hospitalization)
- surgery and comprehensive emergency obstetric care
- laboratory, X-ray, and blood bank services.

Public and private healthcare provision

In most countries, health services are provided by a mix of public and private providers—the latter can be divided into for-profit and not-for-profit providers and include faith-based organizations, national health NGOs, and traditional healers. In some eligible countries, global health initiatives, such as Gavi, the Vaccine Alliance and the Global Fund to fight Aids, TB and Malaria, can provide significant support to service delivery.

Public health service functions are generally the responsibility of the public sector, such as routine vaccinations, vector control, water quality testing, surveillance and control of epidemics.

Most public sectors aim to provide certain services for free, mostly preventive services such as child vaccination programmes and growth monitoring, or ante- and postnatal care. Depending on the way health services are funded and financed, public providers can charge fees, but usually at a lower subsidized cost compared to the private sector.

Healthcare governance

All countries have MOHs that govern their health sectors. Many MOHs refer to global health policies when setting objectives for their national health development strategic plans, such as the health-related Sustainable Development Goals, Universal Health Coverage 2030, or the International Health Regulations (IHR, 2005).

Depending on different policies that exist around decentralization, different governing functions may be implemented at subnational levels. Most countries have provincial or district health management teams (DHMTs) that manage the health network in their administrative areas. Some countries have explicit policies in place that allow engagement with communities at subnational level, e.g. through their representation in district health or village health committees.

To manage coordination with international health development partners in support of one national health plan through stronger country partnerships, there is the International Health Partnership (IHP+) that supports implementation of the Paris Declaration on Aid Effectiveness in the health sector. For fragile and conflict affected countries, there is the Busan 'New Deal', which is an agreement between the affected states, development partners, and civil society to work together on peace and state building objectives taking into account contextual fragility factors.

Disaster risk management

Most countries are likely to experience a large-scale emergency approximately every 5 years,[7] and some are prone to seasonal hazards (e.g. monsoonal floods, cyclones). Shocks to the health system can undo years of development progress. Having minimal national and community disaster risk management (DRM) capacities in place will help countries to mitigate the effect of unforeseen shocks to the health system and prepare the system to respond and recover more effectively.

DRM programmes address preparedness and disaster risk reduction, and the response to and recovery from an event. (See Fig. 4.2.) Humanitarian response forms part of the DRM programme; as such, it is important for humanitarian providers to understand the concept of

> *Health systems resilience* can be defined as the ability of the health system, community, or society exposed to hazards to resist, absorb, accommodate to, and recover from the effects of a hazard in a timely and efficient manner, including through the preservation and restoration of its essential basic structures and functions. (Reproduced from UNISDR Terminology on disaster risk reduction, 2009.)

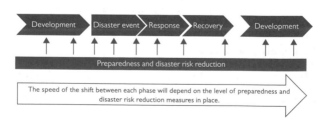

Fig. 4.2 Disaster risk management components.

DRM, make sure their programmes are aligned with existing national plans, and support the strengthening of DRM within the context of their existing programming.

DRM programmes for health use an '*all-hazards approach*' that anticipates the potential health effects of all types of hazards (see Table 4.1 for classification of hazards). A risk analysis identifies which hazards may occur in a certain context, and serves as the foundation for general preparedness and hazard-specific contingency planning. The risks that emergencies pose to communities are directly related to the communities' *exposure to hazards*, their *vulnerabilities to those hazards*, and their *capacities to manage* both. This relationship is well represented by the illustrative formula:

$$\text{Risk } \alpha \ \frac{\text{Hazard} \times \text{Vulnerability}}{\text{Capacity}}$$

Another aspect of DRM programmes for health is the multisectoral nature of the work. Health is not a standalone area but depends heavily on the work of other sectors such as water and sanitation (WASH), nutrition, and logistics. As such, there should be close coordination with other sectors as most disasters require a multisectoral response, including large-scale complex epidemics.

Humanitarian partners and DRM

When entering a country affected by disaster, with a functional DRM programme, international humanitarian partners need to have a basic understanding of what DRM programmes are, and to know better how to offer support complementary to national capacities, while not undermining or bypassing national capacities that have been put in place to manage the risks. When working in a country that is prone to disasters, international humanitarian partners can contribute to building DRM capacity of national and local health authorities and communities. Or, in the context of many humanitarian settings, where the government has limited capacity or may have broken down, they may have to resume responsibility to ensure basic DRM functions and include the required preparedness budgets in their planning.

Table 4.2 shows aspects of a DRM programme linked with health system building blocks from a MOH perspective, considering the contribution by humanitarian partners. Being part of a wider collective response, humanitarian partners need to be aware that when they enter a country, they should register and connect with the coordination structures that are managed under a Health Emergency Operations Centre. When supporting health facilities in a district, humanitarian partners need to know how to assess the damage and functionality of health facilities, so they can feed into sector-wide assessments.

Humanitarian partners often work closely with communities. Strengthening the capacity of the community health workforce to be prepared for, respond to, and recover from emergencies is essential in the overall DRM.

Table 4.1 Hazards classification

Generic groups	1. Natural				2. Human-induced	
Groups	1.1 Geological	1.2 Hydro-meteorological		1.3 Biological	1.4 Extraterrestrial	2.1 Technological	2.2 Societal
Subgroups		1.2.1 Hydrological / 1.2.2 Meteorological	1.2.3 Climatological				
Main types • Subtypes [sub-subtypes]	Earthquake (G1): • Ground shaking • Tsunami Mass movement (G2) Liquefaction (G3)	Flood (H1): • Riverine flood • Flash flood • Coastal flood • Ice jam flood Landslide (H2): • Avalanche [snow, mudflow, debris, rockfall]	Storm (M1): • Extra-tropical storm • Tropical storm • Convective storm [e.g. storm/ surge, tornado, wind, rain, winter storm/blizzard, derecho, lightening/ thunderstorm, hail, sand/dust storm]	Drought (C1) Wild fire (C2): • Land fire [e.g. brush, bush, pasture] • Forest fire Glacial lake outburst (C3)	Emerging diseases (B1) Epidemics and pandemics (B2) Insect infestation (B3): • Grasshopper • Locusts Foodborne outbreaks (B4)	Impact (E1): • Airbust Space weather (E2): • Energetic particles • Geomagnetic storms • Shockwave	Industrial hazards (T1): • Chemical spill, gas leak, collapse, explosion, fire, radiation Structural collapse (T2): • Building collapse, dams/bridge failures Transportation (T3): • Air, road, rail, water Explosions/fire (T4)	Armed conflicts (S1): • International • Non-international Civil unrest (S2) Terrorism (S3) Chemical biological, radiological, nuclear, and explosive weapons (CBRNE) (S4): • Conventional weapons • Unconventional weapons

Volcanic activity (G4):	Wave action (H3):	Extreme temperature (M2):	Air pollution (T5):	Financial crisis (S5):
• Ash fall	• Rogue wave	• Heatwave	• Haze	• Hyperinflation
• Lahar	• Seiche	• Cold wave	Power outage (T6)	• Currency crisis
• Pyroclastic flow		• Severe winter condition [e.g. snow/ice, frost/ freeze]	Hazardous materials in air, soil, water (T7):	
• Lava flow		Fog (M3)	• Biological, chemical, radionuclear	
			Food contamination (T8)	

Reproduced with permission from WHO, Emergency Response Framework, 2nd edition (2017), available from: http://www.who.int/hac/about/erf/en/.

Table 4.2 DRM for health functions and health system resilience

Health system building blocks	Related DRM for health functions
Governance	DRM for health programme in MOH
	IHR capacity-building programme in MOH, including legislation
	Legislation, policy, and strategy on DRM for health
	DRM integrated in national health strategy
	Preparedness plans, and hazard-specific contingency plans[a]
	Create an operational platform, supported by health emergency operations centres (HEOCs) for response and recovery
	Event management system
Health information systems	Risk and vulnerability analysis[a]
	Early warning alert and response system (EWARS) for early detection and surveillance, for epidemics, and other hazards[a]
	Mapping of (functionality of) health facilities[a]
	DRM capacity assessment of the health sector
Service delivery	Preparedness to scale up service delivery capacity especially through primary healthcare services to address overall increased morbidity[a]
	Medical care provision in outbreaks and epidemics[a]
	Mobile clinics, national medical teams, mass casualty management[a]
	Temporary clinics to deal with specific diseases (i.e. Ebola or cholera treatment centres)[a]
	Quality assurance of care delivered in emergencies, including patient safety[a]
	Safe hospitals programme—linked to hospital accreditation, infection prevention and control (IPC) measures, planning, building, and functions
Health workforce	Health workforce capacity building to assess the impact and needs, early detection, surveillance, and respond to and recover from disasters
	Mobilizing health workforce for response, nationally and globally—linked to health workforce planning

Table 4.2 (*Contd.*)

Health system building blocks	Related DRM for health functions
Access to essential medicines	Measures for ensuring/restoring access to essential medicine[a]
	Emergency stockpile of essential medicine as part of contingency plans[a]
	Drug donation guidelines and regulation of donations
	Importation of emergency medicine (linked to international trade and health)
Financing	Emergency financing for response (e.g. when waiving user fees)
	Financing for recovery and transition—linking to health insurance schemes, universal health coverage, etc.
	Financing of preparedness[a]

[a] Functions potentially supported by humanitarian providers.

Health systems and humanitarian interventions

Health emergency interventions should, whenever possible, support the existing national system, filling its gaps and addressing its constraints. Humanitarian providers should only operate in parallel and/or through a vertical approach when existing health services have collapsed, or where populations are not being served by the existing health system. However, during acute emergencies in the field, international aid agencies may need to balance conflicting aims, often perceived as a choice between the humanitarian imperative of saving lives by direct action or strengthening the existing systems to reinforce the local capacity, and support a better local response in the future.

It is possible, however, to develop effective emergency action, and design effective health actions that do not create obstacles for the future betterment of the systems. Within their mandate for saving lives, humanitarian responses need to take into account longer-term consequences and see how interventions can contribute to longer-term recovery and development. This is referred to as early recovery approaches.

Early recovery

Early recovery refers to applying development principles to humanitarian situations to stabilize the local and national capacities from further deterioration to provide a foundation for full recovery.

> '*Early recovery* is an approach that addresses recovery needs that arise *during the humanitarian phase* of an emergency, using humanitarian mechanisms that *align with development principles*. It enables people to use the benefits of humanitarian action to *seize development opportunities*, builds *resilience*, and establishes a sustainable *process of recovery* from crisis.' (Emphasis added; Guidance Note on Inter-Cluster Early Recovery. Global Cluster for Early Recovery, Jan 2016. http://www.earlyrecovery.global/ sites/default/files/Guidance%20Note%20-010816.pdf.)

If there is not a focus on early recovery and building resilience, recurrent emergency action can become common as was seen in Sahel countries after the recurrent droughts. Many low-resource conflict environments with a fragile health system, such as Central African Republic (2014, 2015) require prolonged humanitarian interventions to fill the gaps. After withdrawal, however, often little trace of the efforts is left behind, and with the continued healthcare gaps as a result, emergency actions cannot be stopped without seeing the need of new emergency actions a short time after. Instead, humanitarian partners should establish the foundation for health system recovery during a protracted emergency.

Early recovery principles

Do not impede the life-saving objectives

The work towards an aspirational better future should not come at the expense of attending to the emergency-related needs:

- The transition between emergency and recovery is not clear cut and binary.
- Localized crises with a high mortality risk may remain after the emergency; part of the health development system should include risk management and emergency response preparedness.

Do not undermine the national systems

Emergency project design should reflect upon, not create, obstacles for development:

- It is becoming increasingly recognized that many well-intentioned humanitarian interventions can actually inadvertently serve to weaken the national health system, in part by setting up parallel systems, such as for payments, training, or management.
- Humanitarian intervention should avoid disruption of the national system by using salary grids that can be taken over by the government, or that do not attract health workers out of their public services. Ideally the government should establish standards for salaries or incentives for humanitarian actors to use for local staff which recognize compensation for working in difficult circumstances, but which are not out of touch with the country's economic reality.
- Purchase local medicines *but* only if the local procurement centres have been quality certified and quality is proven by audit.
- Humanitarian actors' training should follow the national guidelines and be linked with training institutions so that the NGOs' and agencies' training is recognized as valid by the government.

Strengthen the national health authorities

Humanitarian providers should work with, and strengthen, national health authorities and partners whenever possible. This could include the following:

- Supporting the development of capacity within the humanitarian mandate (e.g. for contingency planning, EWARSs, DHMTs, and district health committees).
- Participating in joint planning and programming when possible.
- Transferring leadership of projects and coordination functions to national/subnational health authorities.
- Engaging development actors to assume investment in areas that no longer correspond to an emergency, but which require continued support. Humanitarian actors can document the extent and relative severity of the needs, to facilitate prioritization and longer-term programming.

Integrate early recovery approaches from the beginning

From the early stages of any intervention, consider the foundation for longer-term health system recovery and resilience, and support health emergency and DRM capacities:

- Include when possible elements of preparedness planning, and disaster risk reduction into the response programming, ideally complementarily

to a larger national disaster management programme. As an example, if cholera is a risk in an area where actors are responding to an earthquake, contingency plans for cholera should be developed or updated together with those of the health authorities.
- Include elements of local capacity development into projects, e.g. by aligning the package of emergency services with the existing national package of essential health services, and national approaches for district health management and community engagement.

Create a collaborative environment

Consider how development partners can connect from the earliest phases, even during the emergency. This can include the following:
- Make available detailed disaggregated information on the agency's supported facility recurrent costs (staff, medicine, transport, fuel, etc.) so that this can be budgeted for in the development planning.
- Utilize and feed into national formats for epidemiological and service delivery reporting.
- Link blood transfusions to the central blood bank and to the national transfusion system.
- Support, when feasible, programmes run directly by local health authorities such as EPI, TB, HIV, etc., for which international funding is usually available so costs are not a barrier to the national authorities.

See Table 4.3 for examples of early recovery activities that can be introduced during the emergency response and how these may connect with processes applied in recovery and development.

> In many humanitarian interventions, humanitarian service providers are frequently present for only short periods of time, leading to a lack of awareness of overall structure, capacities and gaps of the local health system, the development initiatives, and policies. This can lead to lost opportunities to build on or articulate with the health system.

Supporting Integrated Development Goals

Health partners should support the recovery of the health system from the earliest stages of the humanitarian response. To do so, the initial assessment should include the needs, capacities and gaps between the immediate needs, and the more long-term development goals. The capacities should include development goals related to the health system, classified according to the general system building block which they fall under, outlined as follows.

Infrastructure and service delivery

Infection prevention/control, medical waste management, and community engagement are elements that are frequently not included in the emergency response, but are critical elements. In the 2014–2015 Ebola epidemic, for example, attention to both made it possible to interrupt the transmission of disease at the community level (community engagement), and to protect the health staff from infection (infection control).

Human resources

First responders in any emergency are generally the national staff, and follow-up humanitarian operations are almost always done with the assistance of local providers. It is critical that national staff benefit from capacity-building initiatives and contribute to national disaster risk reduction efforts when the crisis is over.

Financing

High coverage of health services is only possible when communities have geographic and financial access. Free access to health is desirable, but this has costs that the national health authorities may not be able to absorb after the crisis. Health financing mechanisms need to be prioritized, with particular focus on prevention activities and the care of the most vulnerable groups. The current trend is to facilitate universal access in low-resource countries through public funding mechanisms including insurance schemes, social transfers, and external aid.

Essential medical products and technologies

Effective health interventions require quality supplies, and particular attention must be paid to the quality of drugs, and the risks of counterfeit. See ➜ Chapter 12 for more information.

Leadership and governance

Large emergency operations are challenging in terms of coordination, logistics, and staff. Coordination mechanisms should help to avoid duplication, expand coverage, support and monitor quality, and facilitate the improvement of local capacities. Health coordination mechanisms need to be part of the overall support to health interventions.

Health information systems

Early warning systems and surveillance are a priority during an emergency response to detect health hazards, identify needs, and monitor the impact of interventions. Early warning systems can spearhead larger health information systems.

Table 4.3 Examples of early recovery activities

	Early recovery activities in emergency response	Health system recovery, development, and resilience
Leadership and coordination	Humanitarian/emergency coordination: strengthen role of national and subnational health authorities, taking responsibility for the six coordination functions	Health development partner coordination (IHP+, etc.) Recovery coordination for post-conflict recovery and peacebuilding assessments: led by health authorities
	Registration and mapping of all health partners: integrated in mapping of national response capacity, memorandum of understanding with MOH	Coordination for the conflict recovery assessment and planning: led by health authorities
	Subnational emergency coordination: focused capacity building of district health management functions in support of delivery of the essential package of health services (EPHS) and lifesaving functions	Core functions and capacities for DHMTs Decentralization policies, district operational planning
	One or two lead NGOs per district to support DHMT	
	Accountability to affected populations; connect with primary health care (PHC) traditions (district and village health committees)	People-centred and integrated health services Guidance for district, community, and village health committees
	Emergency preparedness and contingency planning Strengthen role of national and subnational health authorities, HEOC, IHR core capacities	Emergency and DRM programme for health (including HEOC and incident management system (IMS)), integrated in national health sector development policy Implementation of IHR core capacities, legislation
Health information system	Simplified morbidity surveillance; aligned with integrated disease surveillance and response system (IDSR)	IDSR
	Mortality and nutrition surveys	Vital statistics

	Rapid health assessments, humanitarian needs overview, multisectoral analysis of needs	Emergency DRM and IHR capacity assessment
	All-hazards risk analysis	All-hazards risk analysis; led by health authorities, connected with National Disaster Management Authority (NDMA)
	EWARS; aligned with national EWARS, IHR core capacities	EWARS
	Health Resources Availability Mapping (HeRAMS); baseline links with service availability and resource assessment (SARA)	SARA
	Selected health information system indicators; harmonized with health management information system (HMIS)	HMIS
Service delivery	Restore lifesaving services; special attention for excluded/marginalized groups	Restore basic services, and address pre-disaster constraints for access and performance
	EPHS; harmonized with basic package of health services (BPHS), and national quality assurance systems (accreditation of national health providers)	BPHS, accreditation, contracting
	Progressive expansion of coverage and quality	Universal health coverage
	Rapid response mechanism; role of health authorities	Preparedness to scale-up service delivery capacity
	Establish temporary treatment centres (e.g. nutrition rehabilitation unit, cholera or Ebola treatment centres); build capacity of MOH in rapid response mechanisms and national medical teams	Safe hospital programme, mass casualty management, national medical teams, mobile clinics
	IPC; aligned with national standards	Risk reduction activities; staff and patient safety, IPC, etc.

(Continued)

Table 4.3 (*Contd.*)

	Early recovery activities in emergency response	Health system recovery, development, and resilience
Pharmaceuticals and equipment	List of core lifesaving pharmaceuticals; aligned with national essential medicine list	Essential medicine lists, by level of health facility
	Drug and equipment donation guidelines; items aligned with national standards	Essential medical equipment lists, by level of health facility
		Standards for diagnostics and laboratory by level
	Stocks of supplies linked with preparedness and contingency plans	Stocks of supplies linked with preparedness and contingency plans; managed by national health authorities
	Quality control of pharmaceuticals procured by international partners	Prequalification of suppliers
		Regulation of private pharmacies
	From kits to procuring bulk items, common logistics through a dedicated procurement partner	Central medical stores for national procurement
Human resources for health	Standardized remuneration/incentives guidelines	A human resources for health unit with responsibility for development and monitoring of policies and plans
	Staffing standards by level of health facility; aligned with national standards	
	Mapping available human resources by type (e.g. through HeRAMS)	

	Scaling up education and employment of integrated teams of PHC workers (including CHWs)	Established national health workforce accounts and health workforce registries to track health workforce stock, distribution, flows, demand, supply, capacity, and remuneration
	Post description aligned to national human resources for health/CHW policy and post descriptions	Bilateral and multilateral agencies that have integrated in their programming health workforce assessments, support, and information exchange
		Training curricula for types of health workers, standard post description, licensing
	Training of health workers; aligned with national curricula, accreditation of training	Training of health workers on emergency risk management and IHR, IMS, etc.
		Training and exercises for emergency response, linked with preparedness plans
		SOPs for repurposing health workers for response
Financing	Services free at point of delivery	Health financing policies, with shifts to pre-payment approaches
	(Temporary) waiving of user fees	Financial protection from catastrophic health expenditures
	Services financed by humanitarian donors/resources	Selective free services (vaccination, antenatal care, etc.)
	Purchasing services in national health facilities (public or private) using pooled health risk funds, or other cash-based programming, to access health services based on prepayment and risk sharing	Emergency fund to reimburse costs for temporary waiving of user fees
		Financing preparedness and risk reduction
	Admin systems connect with national admin for performance-based financing systems	(Performance-based financing), contracting of services

Guide systems in crises

The WHO health system building blocks have a central role in national health system strengthening. Understanding the characteristics of each building block is essential for mitigating the impact of crises. Humanitarian workers should aim to understand the implications of such disruptions, to harmonize their interventions in support of health system strengthening.

I. Service delivery

Characteristics of good service delivery

Effective service delivery includes the following:

- A defined package of services and benefits, with comprehensive clinical and public health interventions that respond to the health problems of their populations.
- Community health and primary healthcare services provided as close to the community as possible, with the back-up of secondary and tertiary specialized hospital services.
- A public health service capable of delivering health risk management services including risk identification, reduction and prevention, and emergency health interventions.
- Standards, norms, and guidance to ensure access and quality, including safety, effectiveness, integration, and continuity.
- Mechanisms to hold providers accountable for access and quality and to ensure consumer voice.

Impacts of crises on service delivery

Most disasters cause direct damage to the health infrastructure and assets, disrupting service delivery. Geographic access to still-functional facilities may be reduced when bridges are destroyed or access roads have flooded. Insecurity and/or discrimination of population groups can further constrain access, at times when demand for health services is often increased.

Implications for humanitarian healthcare workers

In humanitarian crises, service delivery can become fragmented when different facilities provide different packages of services depending on which humanitarian agency provides support. Further, supporting service delivery means providing equitable health interventions that consider the distribution of and access to that service.

Delivery of services requires safe, accessible, and user-friendly health facilities. The process of planning, designing and building, managing, and maintaining this health infrastructure is often expensive and fraught with political considerations that have little to do with health. Humanitarians should aim to consider the functionality of the health system beyond their immediate catchment areas, and strive to ensure the package of services is provided in accordance with the national health plan, and pay particular attention to the distribution of those services to allow equitable access for all.

II. Human resources for health

Characteristics of a high-performing health workforce

An effective workforce is one that is responsive to the needs and expectations of the population and works efficiently given available resources, constraints, and circumstances. To do so requires:

- standards for staffing at the various levels of service delivery
- sufficient numbers of health workers with a mix of competencies
- payment systems that provide the right type of incentives
- regulatory mechanisms to ensure system-wide deployment and distribution in accordance with needs
- in-service training to maintain the quality of service delivery.

Impacts of crises on the health workforce

Even countries not affected by crises face challenges in the development of their health workforce, including in recruitment, education, training, improving productivity, and retention. Disaster situations can further exacerbate these baseline challenges, particularly in prolonged crises. Health workers may themselves suffer from injuries and psychological trauma, and their homes and families may also have been affected. If they are able to report to work, payment of salaries may become disrupted. The health workforce difficulties include the following:

- *Distribution of health workers*: after emergencies, health workers may leave affected areas and concentrate in the capital, affecting the distribution of health personnel and the ability to provide care. Better salaries and working conditions offered by iNGOs may pull health workers from the remaining public system.
- *Shortages in providers*: there can be absolute shortages in providers in emergency and post-emergency settings. For example, in post-conflict Liberia, there were fewer than 20 doctors in the country. Doctors may flee the country entirely, and accredited production of new health workers may come to a halt, as was seen during the decades-long war in South Sudan.
- *Attacks on health workers*: in some conflicts, health workers become targets of violence and/or are imprisoned. Many are fearful to come to work. See ➲ Chapter 11.

Implications for humanitarian healthcare workers

Many of the countries prone to humanitarian crises are those which suffer from human resource limitations at baseline. Humanitarians should be aware of how their recruitment practices may inadvertently drain the public health system, and should provide salary scales in accordance with national guidelines. In the absence of the functioning accreditation programmes in prolonged crises, some international aid agencies have trained (new) cadres of health workers. Be aware that without being able to offer accredited diplomas, countries can be left with significant challenges to absorb these workers when the crisis ends. As such, close collaboration with health authorities is essential throughout the process.

III. Health information systems

Characteristics of good information management

Providing an effective health service depends upon good quality and timely information on health needs, on the context in which the system operates, and on the performance of the health system. To be useful for action, health information must be timely and include:

- health status of the population served
- health risk analysis
- utilization of health services
- access to and availability of care, quality of services provided
- acute hazards to health, such as epidemics and other emergencies, through early warning and alert systems
- progress in meeting defined health objectives and overcoming challenges
- financial expenditures.

Impacts of crises on information management

Most routine data collection systems will be interrupted during the initial phases of a disaster, or when they remain functional, they are not generally adapted to allow decision-making for the emergency response. While some MOHs will have the capacity to introduce simple information systems to track the most important morbidity (i.e. an early warning systems for diseases that are potentially epidemic), and establish mapping of the damage and functionality of health facilities, often the areas without the capacity to produce such information are the worst affected.

In most conflict-affected countries, information systems are disrupted and the quality of information insufficient or absent. In some cases, information from >5 years ago is still used with the risk of making ill-informed decisions.

Implications for humanitarian healthcare workers

Most humanitarian agencies have developed their own assessment methods and simplified information systems that can be quickly introduced in a crisis. Humanitarians should first consider if the MOH has already developed such systems and use these rather than introducing their own. In case new systems do need to be introduced, it is important that all humanitarian health partners apply the same tools, to avoid multiple parallel systems and fragmentation of information, and allow aggregation and joint analysis of data across different areas of operations. This needs to be coordinated under the MOH or by the health cluster if it was activated.

IV. Essential medical products and technologies

Characteristics of reliable therapeutic goods supply systems

Healthcare is dependent on access to affordable essential medicines, vaccines, diagnostics, and health technologies of good quality, which are used in a scientifically sound and cost-effective way.

Medical supplies are the second largest component of most health budgets (after salaries) and the largest component of private health expenditure in LIC and MIC. Key components include:

- a regulatory system of medical products which includes marketing authorization, and safety and quality monitoring

- national lists of essential medicines and other medical products, national diagnostic and treatment protocols, and standardized lists of medicines and equipment per levels of care
- a supply and distribution system to ensure universal access through public and private channels
- guidance for the rational use of drugs.

Impacts of crises on medical supplies

Just as the infrastructure itself can be damaged by a disaster, medical supplies and equipment may be equally impacted. Even without overt physical damage, unseen quality compromise may occur, such as when power outages affect the cold chain. Further, normal supply lines may be affected, preventing the replacement of necessary supplies.

In conflicts, as centrally led procurements systems are interrupted and the regulatory capacity of the government is weakened, access to quality drugs is usually compromised. This leaves an opportunity for the private sectors to fill the gap; however, with a lack of regulatory oversight, this runs the risk of introducing low-quality and/or counterfeit drugs, and the creation of unregulated private drug shops where patients can directly go to buy drugs.

Implications for humanitarian healthcare workers

In the early phases of an emergency, it may be justified to bring in standard international kits for the supply of medicines and equipment to replenish damaged stocks or to meet increased needs. Soon afterwards though, humanitarian workers should then align the further procurement of emergency medical supplies to national standard lists for essential medicines and equipment. Where possible, it is then preferred to procure these supplies from national manufacturers, provided these comply with international quality standards. From the perspective of cost savings and efficiency, procurement should be done by one agency rather than having each humanitarian partner procure their own drugs for their own projects.

> Donations of medicines and equipment, may actually add additional stress to the system when they are not in compliance with the international guidelines for drug donations.[8] After the war ended in the Balkans, for example, excess medical supplies, classified as chemical waste requiring special incineration, had to be destroyed at high costs to the government.

V. Health financing

Characteristics of effective healthcare finance

Health financing is a key policy tool used to improve health and reduce health inequalities. Health financing should:

- raise sufficient public funds for health
- pool financial resources from many sources and inject them appropriately into the health system

- reduce financial barriers to access services and protect from catastrophic health expenditures, based on pre-payment and risk sharing principles
- maintain accountability for funds and prevent corruption (e.g. through regulation, audit, and expenditure review).

Impacts of crises on healthcare finance

Most disasters disproportionally affect poor people, who have limited reserves. When livelihoods are impacted by disaster, the overall ability of households to pay for health services is diminished. In countries whose health financing depends largely on direct out-of-pocket payments, this adds financial barriers for accessing lifesaving services and increased risks for catastrophic health expenditures. When health insurance schemes exist, households may no longer be able to pay the premiums, or reimbursement from the fund to the providers is interrupted. In protracted emergencies where the proportion of government public funding is often low, payment for service providers usually relies mostly on direct out-of-pocket payments.

Implications for healthcare workers

Due to the barriers to life-saving services associated with out-of-pocket payments during crises, and the disproportional impact on the poor, there is now consensus among many in the humanitarian community that services supported by the international aid agencies should be provided for free at the point of delivery.[9] Humanitarians should be aware, however, that this may distort the existing user fee system if applied by public and/or private health providers, as patients no longer go to the clinics where they have to pay, so the health providers have less revenue and in the worst cases have to close their clinic. There is growing experience with the use of cash transfers and/or vouchers that patients can use to cover charges or reduce other indirect financial barriers such as costs for transport. See ➲ Chapter 8 for more information.

VI. Leadership and governance

Characteristics of good healthcare governance

Each country's specific context and history shapes the way governance is exercised, but common aspects of good practice in leadership can be identified, which include:

- national health policies, strategies, and plans that set a clear direction for the entire health sector, established through a transparent and inclusive consultation processes
- adequate emergency health and DRM capacities
- coordination with all health development partners
- subnational health management with community engagement
- effective regulation
- effective policy dialogue with other sectors
- mechanisms to channel donor funding, aligned with country priorities
- Accountability to stakeholders.

Impacts of crises on healthcare governance

During both protracted conflicts and acute disaster settings, the ability of the government to lead the response may be diminished. Disasters may weaken overall governance functions, including the planning and policy processes. In cases of large-scale disasters, where often >200 international health partners arrive to offer support, the capacity of the existing governing bodies may be overwhelmed to manage and task these. In other cases, the governance structure may remain strong but may be compromised by a lack of respect for humanitarian principles or international humanitarian law, such as when governments deliberately exclude populations from services, or put constraints on cross-border or cross-front-line support.

Implications for healthcare workers

When governments are able to coordinate the response with respect to international humanitarian law and humanitarian principles, humanitarians should commit to work with and be coordinated by the national or subnational health authorities. In particular for natural disasters, governments will increasingly insist that international emergency medical teams register with and report to them, and expect that partners are able to adhere to international quality standards.[10] Humanitarians should familiarize themselves with existing national policies, guidelines, and standards, and where appropriate align their work with these.

Performance standards

The third edition of the Sphere handbook published in 2011 defines a set of minimum standards for both health programmes in humanitarian response as well as for the performance of the health system response based on the six building blocks.[11] Adherence to these standards avoids the potential negative impacts humanitarian programming can have on the health system.

Box 4.1 offers an example of the health system standard on service delivery. This includes guidance on facility and room design, planning of human resource needs, and identification of gaps in facilities distribution. Monitoring of provided indicators can lead to programmatic adjustments such as resource allocations, increased collaboration, and resource mobilization.

Box 4.1 Health systems standard 1: health service delivery

Goal: people have equal access to effective, safe and quality health services that are standardized and follow accepted protocols and guidelines.

Key actions
- Provide health services at the appropriate level of the health system: household/community, clinic/health post, health centre, hospital.
- Adopt or establish standardized case management protocols for most common diseases, taking account of national standards and guidelines.
- Establish or strengthen a standardized referral system, and this is utilized by health agencies.
- Establish or strengthen a standardized system of triage at all facilities to ensure those with emergency signs receive immediate treatment.
- Initiate health education and promotion at community and health facility levels.
- Establish and follow safe blood supply and rational use of blood and blood products.
- Ensure that lab services are available and utilized when indicated.
- Avoid the establishment of alternative or parallel health facilities and services, including mobile clinics and field hospitals.
- Design health services in a manner that ensures patients' rights to privacy, confidentiality and informed consent.

Indicators
- There are an adequate number of health facilities to meet the essential health needs of the all the disaster affected population:
  - One basic health unit per 10,000 population.
  - One health centre per 50,000 population.
  - One district/rural hospital per 250,000 population.
  - >10 inpatient and maternity beds per 10,000 people.
- Utilization rates at health facilities are 2–4 new consultations/person/year among disaster-affected population, and 0.5–>1 new consultations/person/year among rural and dispersed populations.

References

1. Pavignani E, Colombo S. Analysing Disrupted Health Sectors: A Modular Manual. Geneva: World Health Organization; 2009. ✍ http://www.int/hac/techguidance/tools/disrupted_sectors/en/
2. ✍ http://ec.europa.eu/echo/files/policies/sectoral/health2014_annex_b_en.pdf
3. ✍ http://ec.europa.eu/echo/files/policies/sectoral/health2014_general_health_guidelines_en.pdf
4. ✍ http://www.who.int/hac/network/global_health_cluster/herams_services_checklist_eng.pdf
5. ✍ https://prezi.com/pv8widffs5i2/
6. ✍ https://prezi.com/nmkultq5hncs/
7. World Health Organization. Global Assessment of National Health Sector Emergency Preparedness and Response. Geneva: World Health Organization; 2008. ✍ http://www.who.int/hac/about/Global_survey_inside.pdf
8. ✍ http://www.who.int/selection_medicines/emergencies/guidelines_medicine_donations/en/
9. ✍ http://www.who.int/hac/global_health_cluster/about/policy_strategy/position_paper_user_fees/en/
10. World Health Organization. Classification and Minimum Standards for Emergency Medical Teams in Sudden Onset Disasters: ✍ http://www.who.int/hac/techguidance/preparedness/foreign_medical_teams/en/
11. The Sphere Project. Humanitarian Charter and Minimum Standards in Humanitarian Response, 3rd ed. The Sphere Project; 2011. ✍ http://www.sphereproject.org/handbook/

References

Gender-based violence in humanitarian crises

Jennifer Scott, Rose Leonard Molina, and Jocelyn T.D. Kelly

Gender-based violence

Gender-based violence (GBV) is one of the most challenging aspects of humanitarian crises and complex emergencies. GBV lies at the intersection of human sexuality, gender norms, cultural customs, reproductive health, and the very social fabric of communities, making it one of the most deeply private, stigmatized, and taboo issues. Due to its hidden nature, GBV is easily overlooked and under-recognized. Women, men, girls, and boys are at risk for GBV, especially in humanitarian crises.

In humanitarian crisis, healthcare providers may:
• be the first to hear the survivors' stories and treat their injuries
• be involved in the direct clinical care at different stages of GBV survivors' recovery
• bear witness to the crimes committed upon survivors
• need to advocate for resources to support the recovery of survivors and to reduce the risk for others.

GBV is an important health and human rights issue and warrants a focused chapter due to its complexity and impact on the health of individuals, families, and communities. This chapter aims to provide the reader with an understanding of this complex topic, guidance for the management of survivors of GBV, and recommendations for a multisectoral approach to GBV programming in humanitarian settings. Provided throughout this text are links to other chapters, including → Chapter 9 ('International law for healthcare workers') and → Chapter 41 ('Reproductive health'), which provide additional information on this subject → Chapter 6 ('the mental health'), → Chapter 31 ('HIV PEP').

Definitions and affected populations

• GBV comprises actual or threatened physical, sexual, and psychological violence perpetrated against a person because of his or her gender, gender identity, or sexual orientation.
• GBV may include sexual harassment and intimidation, physical and/or sexual intimate partner violence, non-partner sexual violence, forced pregnancy, forced sterilization, sexual trafficking, and other forms of exploitation.
• While GBV is most commonly recognized as being directed against women and girls, men and boys also experience GBV. Men may experience abuse in many forms, which are often less commonly referenced than, but as significant as, violence against women.
• Other groups at risk of GBV include children, who are also vulnerable to sexual exploitation and abuse, and harmful traditional practices, such as early marriage. In addition, persons with disabilities are at risk of GBV and may not have access to services.
• In humanitarian crises, women, men, and children are at risk of various forms of GBV. Displaced persons are particularly at risk of GBV. In conflict and post-conflict settings, gang rape and sexual captivity may occur. "In election-related violence, sexual violence may also increase when individuals are targeted for political or ethnic reasons. In many circumstances, the acts of violence may occur in front of family or community members, and those individuals may also suffer as a consequence of witnessing such violence.

Understanding GBV

Global prevalence

- Worldwide, approximately 30% of women aged 15 years or older have experienced intimate partner violence in their lifetimes.[1]
- Globally, 7% of women aged 15 years or older reported non-partner sexual violence.[2]
- It is estimated that one in five female refugees in complex humanitarian emergencies have experienced sexual violence.[3]
- The estimated prevalence of GBV among men is not as well quantified in most areas. Many barriers can prevent accurate reporting of GBV.

Humanitarian context

- GBV, in particular sexual violence, has been a part of humanitarian crises throughout history including recent examples in the former Yugoslavia, Rwanda, Democratic Republic of the Congo (DRC), and South Sudan, among others.
- The context in each case varies but in conflict settings, GBV may be used as a weapon of war.
- However, GBV is not limited to conflict settings, and studies conducted in recent humanitarian crises report a high prevalence of GBV. For example, in post-earthquake Haiti, one study estimated that in Cité Soleil over 50% of women reported sexual violence.[4]
- There are fewer data on intimate partner violence in humanitarian settings, but a growing body of literature suggests that this is the most common form of violence in these settings and often goes unreported and receives less attention than non-partner sexual violence.[5]
- In humanitarian crises where persons are affected by displacement and shortages in natural resources, women and girls, in particular, are at risk of GBV while searching for resources, such as water and firewood.
- Measuring GBV within a community is challenging and it is often under-reported due to shame, stigma, cultural biases, and well-founded concerns about confidentiality.

Studies in recent conflict and post-conflict settings have measured GBV among both women and men. A 2010 study of GBV in eastern DRC, a region of conflict with pervasive violence, found that nearly 40% of women and 24% of men surveyed reported experiencing sexual violence.[6]

Roots in gender inequality

- GBV is rooted in gender inequality which refers to unequal opportunities for socially valued resources and empowerment; thus, women are more likely than men to bear the burden of violence in most contexts. However, it is important to consider that interpersonal violence may result from a myriad of factors beyond gender norms and gender inequality.

- Gender inequitable norms in families, households, and communities allow for GBV to exist. Furthermore, a social tolerance of violence, especially towards women, persists in many communities.
- On a global level, efforts are being made towards achieving gender equality, including the Millennium Development Goal 3 (MDG 3) and the 2015 Sustainable Development Goals (SDGs) which prioritize gender equality and women's rights throughout the 2030 Agenda for Sustainable Development.
- Gender inequality may manifest as violence, but is also reflected in reproductive health disparities. In many contexts around the world, a woman's right to access health services is limited. As an example, in certain contexts, a woman needs to have her husband's consent simply to access care including contraception, or to have more complex procedures such as a tubal ligation.
  - Indicators such as contraception prevalence rate and use of modern contraceptive methods can be indicative of women's status, their access to options, and their decision-making power.
  - Maternal health indicators such as total fertility rate, percentage of births with skilled attendants, and maternal mortality ratio (MMR) provide further understanding about the social expectations of women and the risks that are unique to women, especially in low-income settings.

Important reproductive health indicators

MMR: number of deaths of women resulting from pregnancy-related conditions (including pregnancy, delivery, postpartum, and related complications) per 100,000 live births.

Total fertility rate: estimated number of children a woman has during her reproductive years.

Contraception prevalence rate: usually reported as 'any method' and 'modern method'. Modern methods include barrier methods (condoms), hormonal pills, injectables, implants, intrauterine devices, and male and female sterilization.

GBV and humanitarian crises

GBV exists in all communities of the world; it often takes the form of partner violence, harmful traditional practices, and sexual harassment. In many crises, GBV becomes even more common due to community acceptance of violence, breakdown in law and order, and polarization of gender roles. In conflict, GBV can be used as a means of domination, intimidation, ethnic cleansing, or a strategy of war.

Women and girls, men and boys are at risk of GBV at each stage of the humanitarian crisis. Recognize who is most vulnerable to GBV:

- In Darfur, women were at risk of sexual violence when they ventured from camps for firewood.[7]
- In post-earthquake Haiti, women were at risk for GBV in the camp latrines where lighting and protection were inadequate.[8]
- In conflicts such as in the DRC in which armed groups enter a village and violence is systematic, women are at risk in their own homes.[9]

Specific considerations during the various stages of the humanitarian crises include the following:

Emergency phase

During the initial emergency phase, communities are disrupted, populations are displaced, and usual protection strategies are compromised. Individuals, especially women and children, become vulnerable to GBV due to weakened social norms and loss of family and community supports.

Displacement

Displacement also causes increased propensity for GBV, both at border crossings and in refugee camps. Within the camp setting itself, GBV can be a significant problem due to the concentration of people living in close quarters with diminished security and fewer social protection mechanisms.

During armed conflict

During armed conflict, forms of GBV can include abductions and sexual slavery. In a number of conflict settings in sub-Saharan Africa, women and girls have been abducted into sexual slavery by an armed group. While in captivity, they experience psychological, physical, and sexual abuse.

Post-conflict phase

In the post-crisis phase, GBV can be elevated compared to pre-conflict levels because communities have been destabilized by conflict, and both traditional and formal law enforcement and justice mechanisms break down. As a result, violence that has occurred at baseline in homes and communities can also escalate.

> In humanitarian crises, GBV programming is often integrated into reproductive health programming. While this chapter primarily focuses on GBV, it also underscores aspects of reproductive health related to GBV. For a complete review of reproductive health recommendations in humanitarian settings, please refer to ➔ Chapter 41.

Health systems and programming

Most GBV programming is multifaceted, with a foundation in reproductive health services. The Minimum Initial Service Package (MISP) includes a set of priority reproductive health activities to be implemented from the onset of a humanitarian crisis, specifically to prevent and manage the consequences of sexual violence, prevent excess maternal and newborn morbidity and mortality, reduce HIV transmission, and plan for comprehensive reproductive health services.[8] Providers working in humanitarian contexts should be aware of MISP and inquire about its implementation. In the context of GBV, MISP activities include:

• putting in place measures to protect affected populations, in particular women and girls, from sexual violence
• making clinical care available for survivors of rape
• ensuring community awareness of available clinical services.

The MISP contains a coordination and monitoring checklist that includes emergency contraception (EC), post-exposure prophylaxis (PEP), empiric treatment for sexually transmitted infections (STIs), wound care and tetanus prevention, hepatitis B vaccination, appropriate referrals to support services, and information on post-rape care.[10]

Health system designs

The needs of GBV survivors are often complex and require unique considerations due to the sensitive nature of GBV and the extent of physical and/or psychological trauma endured. As a healthcare provider working in a humanitarian setting, it is important to know the systems, protocols, and programmes in place to care for GBV survivors with attention to:

• triage design, room availability, noise levels, and privacy
• security in the facilities
• human resources considerations such as the gender of medical staff and interpreters
• training on confidentiality for medical staff and interpreters
• specialized services, including availability of testing and forensics
• referral systems
• partnerships with other organizations for legal and psychological support
• support from human rights organizations for documenting war crimes.

These and many other issues need to be considered as part of your institutional policies. Ask about the protocols that your clinical setting or programme has for addressing GBV and for caring for the GBV survivor:

• Evaluate your system and/or programme to consider its gender neutrality.
• Consider gender among the support staff, including interpreters.
• Consider ethnicity among the staff, which is equally important in some contexts.
• Recognize that GBV can affect both women and men. To prevent barriers to accessing care for male survivors, consider the entire process that an individual must undergo to access care, and ensure that it recognizes the needs of both males and females.

Care of sexual violence survivors

How to ask about gender-based violence in the clinical setting

As a provider, if you ask a woman or man whether she or he has experienced GBV, the initial response may be 'no'. However, if the same people are asked whether they have ever been hit by an intimate partner, forced to have sex against their will, or felt physically or emotionally controlled or manipulated, their answers may be very different.

There is no single best way to ask about GBV, but the goal of a provider would be to provide a safe space, which would allow an individual to share his or her experience. Examples of direct questions for confidential screening for intimate partner violence include[11]:

- 'Has your partner ever threatened you or made you feel afraid?'
- 'Has your partner ever hit, choked, or physically hurt you?'
- 'Has your partner ever forced you to do something sexually that you did not want to do, or refused your request to use condoms?'

Keep in mind that in some cases, people who have experienced violence can often present with chief complaints or symptoms that would not necessarily lead to a prompt recognition of GBV. Somatization and some chronic pain syndromes have been associated with a history of violence. To prevent missing such cases, consider asking screening questions about GBV during routine gynaecological care and offer opportunities for survivors to disclose in a safe environment. While GBV screening questions have not been standardized across contexts, there are screening tools and recommendations that could be adapted for various contexts. The approach to screening should be discussed in collaboration with colleagues in each context. Before implementing GBV screening in the clinical setting, it is critical that systems are in place for referral and treatment.

Management approach

The role of the provider is to gather clinical evidence, provide clinical management, and support the physical and psychosocial needs of the survivor. It is not the role of the medical provider to determine whether or not sexual violence has occurred—this is the role of the judicial system.

What should be documented?

- Determine if there is a form for documentation of sexual violence that has been approved by the Ministry of Health or local judicial system.
- Partner with local and international organizations to ensure that consistent standards of documentation are in place for the examination and findings. It is best to obtain this information in advance and not wait until a sexual violence survivor presents for care.
- If a standard form is not available, document the following details, including the medical examination. Sample medical examination forms are available through the UNFPA.[12]

- Obtain a brief history of the event (concise, brief, and in the words of the individual). Document any coercion or threats. Include details of time, date, place, circumstance, use of condoms, and/or information about the perpetrator (e.g. combatant, civilian, and known or unknown to survivor). Document whether the individual reported the incident and/or if GBV care was received.
- Obtain a targeted medical history including obstetric history, last menstrual period, pertinent medical and surgical history, and medication use.
- The WHO and UNFPA have published a checklist of needs for the clinical management of rape survivors, reproduced in Fig. 5.1.[12]

Checklists of needs for clinical management of rape survivors

1 Protocol	Available
▸ Written medical protocol in language of provider*	
2 Personnel	**Available**
▸ Trained (local) health care professionals (on call 24 hours/day)*	
▸ For female survivors, a female health care provider speaking the same language is optimal.	
▸ If this is not possible, a female health worker (or companion) should be in the room during the examination*	
3 Furniture/setting	**Available**
▸ Room (private, quite, accessible, with access to a toilet or latrine)*	
▸ Examination table*	
▸ Light, preferably fixed (a torch may be threatening for children)*	
▸ Magnifying glass (or colposcope)	
▸ Access to an autoclave to sterilise equipment*	
▸ Access to laboratory facilities/microscope/trained technician	
▸ Weighing scales and height chart for children	
4 Supplies	**Available**
▸ "Rape kit" for collection of forensic evidence, could include:	
✓ Speculum* (preferably plastic, disposable, only adult sizes)	
✓ Comb for collecting foreign matter in pubic hair	
✓ Syringes/needles (butterfly for children)/tubes for collecting blood	
✓ Glass slides for preparing wet and/or dry mounts (for sperm)	
✓ Cotton-tipped swabs/applicators/gauze compresses for collecting samples	
✓ Laboratory containers for transporting swabs	
✓ Paper sheet for collecting debris as the survivor undresses	
✓ Tape measure for measuring the size of bruises, lacerations*	
✓ Paper bags for collection of evidence*	
✓ Paper tape for sealing and labelling containers/bags*	

Fig. 5.1 Checklist of needs for clinical management of rape survivors. Reproduced with permission from Clinical Management of Rape Survivors, rev edition © World Health Organization/United Nations High Commissioner for Refugees, 2004: http://apps.who.int/iris/bitstream/10665/43117/1/924159263X.pdf

(Continued)

Checklists of needs for clinical management of rape survivors

▸ Supplies for universal precautions (gloves, box for safe disposal of contaminated and sharp materials, soap)*		
▸ Resuscitation equipment*		
▸ Sterile medical instruments (kit) for repair of tears, and suture material*		
▸ Needles, syringes*		
▸ Gown, cloth or sheet to cover the survivor during the examination		
▸ Spare items of clothing to replace those that are torn or taken for evidence		
▸ Sanitary supplies (pads or local cloths)*		
▸ Pregnancy tests		
▸ Pregnancy calculator disk to determine the gestational age		
5 Drugs		**Available**
▸ For treatment of STIs as per country protocol*		
▸ For post-exposure prophylaxis of HIV transmission (PEP)		
▸ Emergency contraceptive pills and/or copper-bearing intrauterine device (IUD)*		
▸ Tetanus toxoid, tetanus immuno-globulin		
▸ Hepatitis B vaccine		
▸ For pain relief* (e.g. paracetamol)		
▸ Anxiolytic (e.g. diazepam)		
▸ Sedative for children (e.g. diazepam)		
▸ Local anaesthetic for suturing*		
▸ Antibiotics for wound care*		
6 Administrative supplies		**Available**
▸ Medical chart with pictograms*		
▸ Forms for recording post-rape care		
▸ Consent forms*		
▸ Information pamphlets for post-rape care (for survivor)*		
▸ Safe, locked filing space to keep records confidential*		

Items marked with an asterisk are the minimum requirements for examination and treatment of a rape survivor.

Fig. 5.1 (*Contd.*)

Medical examination of the sexual violence survivor

- Any skilled provider trained in the clinical management of sexual violence survivors can provide medical care.
- Maintain privacy and confidentiality, respect the rights of the patient, and obtain consent before the examination.
- If possible, have another colleague who can assist in the medical care and an interpreter present during the examination (ideally of the same sex as the patient).
- If forensic analysis capacity exists, collect physical evidence (clothing, underwear, hair). If the survivor presents for care >120 hours (5 days) after the incident, physical evidence is not necessary.
- Provide a medical certificate documenting that the survivor sought medical care. In most countries, this certificate is a legal requirement.
  - UNFPA has a sample certificate or this may be available through local and regional organizations.[13]
  - The certificate should include the name and signature of the examiner, name of the survivor, date and time of examination, narrative of the incident, clinical examination findings, samples taken, and a conclusion.
  - While the medical certificate is important in most contexts, the obligation is to protect the safety of the survivor. Consider if documentation may cause more harm to the survivor.
- Provide counselling or psychosocial support on site or partner with local and regional organizations that provide this support.

Physical examination

- General appearance (include the state of clothing).
- Systemic examination:
  - Describe the location of injuries, estimated age of injuries, and what may have caused them.
  - Document the physical examination of head, neck, chest, back, abdomen, and extremities.
- Reproductive examination (vaginal or penile examination):
  - For women, describe the external vulva and vagina (document the presence or absence of lacerations or lesions). If possible, visualize the cervix (document the presence or absence of lesions or discharge).
  - For men, describe the skin of the scrotum and penis (document the presence of absence of lacerations or lesions) and document the presence or absence of discharge.
  - Examine the anus in both men and women for lacerations or lesions.

Laboratory tests
- It is not necessary to know the results of tests before providing empiric treatment for STIs, EC, and PEP.
- Commonly obtained laboratory tests include:
  - vaginal swab (yeast, bacterial vaginosis, trichomonas)
  - cervical/vaginal (female) or urethral (male) swab for gonorrhoea, chlamydia
  - urine: urinalysis, urine pregnancy test
  - blood: rapid plasma regain/Venereal Disease Research Laboratory (RPR/VDRL), HIV, haemogram/erythrocyte sedimentation rate, liver and renal function.
- Radiological imaging (if clinically indicated and available).

Treatment of sexual violence survivors

As part of treatment for rape survivors, pregnancy prevention for women and prophylaxis against STIs, including HIV, should be discussed and offered to both women and men.

Contraception

There are oral and intrauterine methods of EC for female rape survivors. The availability of EC methods may vary by districts within a country or region, depending on local laws, healthcare infrastructure, and cultural norms or religious beliefs.

There are currently two recommended options for EC[14]:

- Option 1. Levonorgestrel 0.75 mg: 2 tablets by mouth once (1.5 mg total).
- Option 2. Copper-containing intrauterine device (IUD).

Consider:

- Timing: most effective immediately after unprotected intercourse, but can be effective for up to 120 hours (5 days).
- Mechanism of action: prevention of ovulation, fertilization, and implantation; it is not an abortifacient.
- Contraindications: known pregnancy. Even if taken while pregnant, oral EC should not have a teratogenic effect on pregnancy. It is not necessary to do a pregnancy test prior to giving oral EC. Pregnancy testing prior to insertion of an IUD is recommended.
- Follow-up: if no menses within 2–3 weeks, follow-up with a urine or serum pregnancy test.

Consideration of sexually transmitted infections

- When counselling a patient after GBV, it is important to discuss the possibility of contracting STIs. Most of these infections will not be immediately apparent with clinical symptoms.
- Recommendations in the context of sexual violence include empiric prophylaxis against HIV, chlamydia, gonorrhoea, trichomonas, and bacterial vaginosis.[15]
- Patients should be counselled about possible STI symptoms, and advised to present to medical care if they develop such symptoms. See ➋ Chapter 41 for more information.

Sexually transmitted infection prophylaxis

Prophylaxis against infections after sexual exposure should be discussed and offered to survivors based on existing guidelines.

- Provide an empiric regimen for chlamydia, gonorrhoea, trichomonas, and bacterial vaginosis. (See ➋ Chapter 41.)
- Provide EC as discussed previously in this section under 'Contraception'.
- Provide hepatitis B vaccination if available and not previously immunized to prevent hepatitis B infection. Follow-up vaccinations should be given at 1–2 months and 4–6 months following first dose.
- Consider administration of tetanus toxoid or tetanus immunoglobulin based on vaccination history, age, and status of wounds.

- Start first dose of HIV PEP as early as possible and within 72 hours. Provide a 28-day course if the survivor cannot return to the facility. Provide counselling on PEP. Voluntary counselling and testing is not mandatory to receive PEP. Provide PEP prior to HIV testing to avoid a delay in treatment. HIV testing should be repeated at 6 weeks, 3 months, and 6 months after sexual violence.

Protocols for post-exposure prophylaxis for HIV
See → Chapter 31 for detailed guidance on PEP.

Psychosocial care
- While this chapter is intended to provide guidance for the medical needs arising from GBV, it is important to acknowledge the importance of psychosocial care and sequelae which we are not able to address comprehensively in this chapter.
- It should be noted, however, that holistic recovery for survivors often requires thoughtful programming that integrates medical, psychosocial and economic components. Attitude change at the community level is often also required to help survivors feel empowered to come forward about their experiences. There is much more nuanced management with GBV presentations than with most other medical presentations, primarily because of the psychological impact and social contexts. See → Chapter 6 for more information.

GBV and legal and human rights

GBV is universally under-reported. Survivors of GBV do not report incidents due to self-blame, fear of reprisals, mistrust of authorities, social stigma, and fear of rejection by family and communities. *It is important to ask about it, understand the local judicial capacity, and the international legal and human rights framework.*

- Speaking to women's groups, traditional and religious leaders, and local health providers can help the practitioner understand the 'landscape' of gender roles and vulnerability to GBV in each setting.
- Asking open-ended questions is a good way to begin to understand these complex and sensitive topics.

Relevant international, legal, and human rights frameworks for GBV:
- UDHR—Universal Declaration of Human Rights.
- CRSR—Convention Relating to the Status of Refugees.
- ICESC—International Covenant on Economic, Social and Cultural Rights.
- ICCPR—International Covenant on Civil and Political Rights.
- CEDAW—Convention on the Elimination of All Forms of Discrimination against Women.
- Rome Statute of the International Criminal Court.
- UN Security Council Resolutions 1325 and 1820 on Women, Peace and Security.

For more information on GBV and legal and human rights issues, see Chapter 9, which offers a framework on responding to GBV.

Intersection of GBV and reproductive health

There are community and cultural practices affecting women and girls that are important to consider as part of the discussion of GBV. Gender inequitable practices, such as those referred to as harmful traditional practices, may also be considered as forms of GBV. Health providers may encounter various forms of GBV in their roles in crisis settings, including child and forced marriages, female genital mutilation/cutting, and crimes committed to 'preserve' honour.

Virginity examinations

- In some parts of the world, it is relatively common for medical practitioners to be asked to perform 'virginity exams' for girls to confirm that the hymen is intact prior to marriage.
- Although it is universally known that there is no medical indication or objective value of hymen evaluation, an intact hymen is culturally required for marriage in some cultures.
- There are no standard guidelines for how clinicians should respond to this practice, as healthcare providers work in various cultural contexts. As a general rule, these examinations are not considered evidence-based clinical practice and thus should not be performed as such.

Female genital cutting

In many contexts, and indeed in other chapters of this book, this is referred to as female genital mutilation (FGM). In this chapter, the term female genital cutting (FGC) is preferentially used in an effort to avoid stigmatizing language in what some consider a cultural practice.

- The term refers to the partial or total removal of female external genitalia.
- There are four recognized types of FGC, classified based on the specific tissues removed. (See ➔ 'Female genital mutilation' pp. 732–3 for complete details.)
  - Type 1: cliteroidectomy: partial or total removal of the clitoris.
  - Type 2: excision: partial or total removal of the clitoris and labia minora with or without removal of the labia majora.
  - Type 3: infibulation: narrowing of the vaginal opening.
  - Type 4: other harmful practices not for medical purposes.
- More than 125 million girls and women have undergone FGC worldwide, with high prevalences in Africa and the Middle East.[16]
- This harmful practice is often viewed as a rite of passage within certain communities and is performed between infancy and adolescence.
- No health benefit is derived from FGC.
- Short-term consequences include bleeding, pain, infection, and injury to surrounding organs and tissues.
- Long-term consequences include recurrent bladder and vaginal infections, pain with intercourse, and vaginal surgery to enable childbirth.
- FGC has been widely recognized as a violation of human rights yet the social context behind FGC is complex.

For clinical management guidance of FGC, see ➔ Chapter 41. Also, see ➔ Chapter 9 for legal aspects.

GBV and ethical considerations

Sustained attention to GBV has only occurred in the past several decades as international attention focused on the atrocities committed in the many recent conflicts, demonstrating its global impact. As a result of this increasing recognition, the UN, national governments, and civil society have become increasingly aware of the importance of recognizing and documenting GBV. Clinicians and programmers may be among the first to recognize that GBV is a problem in communities and be engaged in advocacy or research efforts. The information that is gathered through the course of providing services can be invaluable for monitoring and tracking this problem; however, ethical considerations must be paramount.

The WHO has created a set of ethical and safety recommendations for researching, documenting, and monitoring sexual violence in emergencies including the following[17]:

- Efforts to understand the dimensions of GBV in a given crisis should first and foremost respect the dignity and rights of every survivor.
- At each step of the documentation process, privacy and confidentiality are vital considerations.
- A minimum set of services should be available before asking questions about GBV, including clinical and psychosocial resources and a referral network if needed.
- Asking questions about GBV should not endanger the respondent, her or his family, or the community. If working in a clinical capacity, ensure that your organization or facility has a protocol in place for GBV.

References

1. Devries KM, Mak JY, Garcia-Moreno C, Petzold M, Child JC, Falder G, et al. Global health. The global prevalence of intimate partner violence against women. Science 2013;340(6140):1527–8.
2. Abrahams N, Devries K, Watts C, Pallitto C, Petzold M, Shamu S, et al. Worldwide prevalence of non-partner sexual violence: a systematic review. Lancet 2014;383(9929):1648–54.
3. Vu A, Adam A, Wirtz A, Pham K, Rubenstein L, Glass N, et al. The prevalence of sexual violence among female refugees in complex humanitarian emergencies: a systematic review and meta-analysis. PLoS Curr 2014;6:(10)1371.
4. Rahill GJ, Joshi M, Lescano C, Holbert D. Symptoms of PTSD in a sample of female victims of sexual violence in post-earthquake Haiti. J Affect Disord 2015;173:232–8.
5. Humanitarian Practice Network. Preventing and Responding to Gender-Based Violence in Emergencies. London: Overseas Development Institute; 2014.
6. Johnson K, Scott J, Rughita B, Kisielewski M, Asher J, Ong R, et al. Association of sexual violence and human rights violations with physical and mental health in territories of the Eastern Democratic Republic of the Congo. JAMA 2010;304(5):553–62.
7. Tsai AC, Eisa MA, Crosby SS, Sirkin S, Heisler M, Leaning J, et al. Medical evidence of human rights violations against non-Arabic-speaking civilians in Darfur: a cross-sectional study. PLoS Med 2012;9(4):e1001198.
8. Rahill GJ, Joshi M, Lescano C, Holbert D. Symptoms of PTSD in a sample of female victims of sexual violence in post-earthquake Haiti. J Affect Disord 2015;173:232–8.
9. Johnson K, Scott J, Rughita B, Kisielewski M, Asher J, Ong R, et al. Association of sexual violence and human rights violations with physical and mental health in territories of the Eastern Democratic Republic of the Congo. JAMA 2010;304(5):553–62.
10. Women's Refugee Commission. Minimum Initial Service Package for Reproductive Health in Crisis Situations. 2006. (Revised November 2007, revised February 2011 ed.) ℘ http://www.unhcr.org/4e8d6b3b14.html
11. American College of Obstetricians and Gynecologists. The American College of Obstetricians and Gynecologists Committee Opinion: Intimate Partner Violence. 2012. ℘ http://www.acog.org/Resources-And-Publications/Committee-Opinions/Committee-on-Health-Care-for-Underserved-Women/Intimate-Partner-Violence

12. World Health Organization and United Nations High Commissioner for Refugees. Clinical Management of Rape Survivors: Developing Protocols for Use with Refugees and Internally Displaced Persons. 2004. ℘ http://whqlibdoc.who.int/publications/2004/924159263X.pdf

13. World Health Organization and United Nations High Commissioner for Refugees. Clinical Management of Rape Survivors: Developing Protocols for Use with Refugees and Internally Displaced Persons. 2004. ℘ http://whqlibdoc.who.int/publications/2004/924159263X.pdf

14. World Health Organization and United Nations High Commissioner for Refugees. Clinical Management of Rape Survivors: Developing Protocols for Use with Refugees and Internally Displaced Persons. 2004. ℘ http://whqlibdoc.who.int/publications/2004/924159263X.pdf

15. Centers for Disease Control and Prevention. 2010 STD Treatment Guidelines: Sexual Assault and STDs. 2011. ℘ http://www.cdc.gov/std/treatment/2010/sexual-assault.htm

16. Nour NM. Female genital cutting: impact on women's health. Semin Reprod Med 2015;33(1):41–6.

17. World Health Organization. WHO Ethical and Safety Recommendations for Researching, Documenting and Monitoring Sexual Violence in Emergencies. 2007. ℘ http://www.who.int/gender/documents/OMS_Ethics&Safety10Aug07.pdf

Chapter 6

Mental health in humanitarian settings

Vanessa Cavallera, Lynne Jones, Inka Weissbecker, and Peter Ventevogel

Introduction

In humanitarian emergencies many people are distressed. The effects of violence, loss, and forced displacement on the mental health of people can be pervasive and profound. People may have lost their loved ones, their belongings, and their livelihoods. They may have been displaced and have experienced adversity prior to or during flight. Often, protective social environments have broken down. The way people respond to such stressors varies significantly and may affect their mental health and psychosocial well-being.

Support for mental health is often complicated by the breakdown of the health and social services that may have existed before the crisis and humanitarian aid attempts to fill the gaps. Mental health must not be considered less important than other health issues.

In humanitarian settings, the term 'mental health and psychosocial support' (MHPSS) is widely used. MHPSS refers to any type of local or outside support that aims to protect or promote psychosocial well-being and/or prevent or treat mental disorder. Routine humanitarian responses now include programming for MHPSS. This may include support interventions in the health sector, education, community services, and protection. It may include advice to other sectors such as WASH, shelter, and nutrition as to the best ways to provide those services while supporting psychological well-being. While many MHPSS programmes are driven by actors working outside the formal health sector, it is essential that all health providers in humanitarian emergencies understand the fundamental principles of mental health in humanitarian settings.

It is of utmost importance that medical providers realize that the management of MHPSS problems in humanitarian crises cannot be reduced to 'psychiatry'. The majority of distressed people in humanitarian settings will respond to culturally appropriate social and community-based psychosocial interventions. Only a minority will require individual psychological and pharmaceutical interventions.

This chapter provides some basic knowledge that all health workers in humanitarian emergencies should have and includes descriptions of the presenting symptoms and management of common clinical conditions encountered. To carry out effective MHPSS work they should also understand the humanitarian context in which these conditions occur and the absolute necessity of collaboration with non-health actors to address the psychosocial needs of their patients. Key resources that supplement this chapter and make this possible are identified in the following sections.

Context

Mental health in the humanitarian context

Many emotional, cognitive, physical, or behavioural reactions are normal and are more likely to resolve quickly if a supportive family and community environment is available. Unfortunately, in humanitarian settings, many of the protective informal community networks of support may break down. Humanitarian crises are responsible for causing high rates of distress, but only some of those suffering distress will develop mental health problems (see Table 6.1). Those most vulnerable include those who:

• have pre-existing mental health disorders
• experienced difficulties in functioning before the emergency
• experienced cumulative stressors
• have limited social support
• engage in negative coping behaviours (e.g utilizing alcohol or drugs).

Cultural and social factors

• The way people experience and describe mental disorders is highly influenced by factors such as language and culture.
• Worldwide, there are major variations in:
  • perception and labelling of feelings and behaviours
  • beliefs about the causes of mental disorders
  • formal and informal support networks and service provision
  • reception/acceptance of mental problems within communities.

Table 6.1 WHO projections of mental disorders and distress in adult populations affected by emergencies

	Before emergency: 12-month prevalence	After emergency: 12-month prevalence
Severe disorder (e.g. psychosis, severe depression, severely disabling form of anxiety disorder)	2–3%	3–4%
Mild or moderate mental disorder (e.g. mild and moderate forms of depression and anxiety disorders, including mild and moderate PTSD)	10%	15–20%
Normal distress/other psychological reactions (no disorder)	No estimate	Large percentage

Reproduced with permission from World Health Organization (WHO), Assessing Mental Health and Psycho-social Needs and Resources: Toolkit for Humanitarian Settings. Geneva: WHO; 2012. (http://www.who.int/mental_health/resources/toolkit_mh_emergencies/en/)

- In many languages, the terms 'mental disorder' and 'mental illness' have strong negative connotations, and are only used for people with severe mental disorders.
- The way people define 'mental disorder' has major implications for their help-seeking behaviour.
  - In many societies, people are more likely to seek help from traditional healers and religious leaders. This may be because of a belief in spiritual or magical causation, or because Western treatments are seen as ineffective.
  - Mild and moderate forms of mental disorder are not always identified as illness, but rather as social or moral issues, or problems related to weaknesses in a person's character. Those affected often seek help from trusted community members.

Idioms of distress

People often use culturally relevant expressions ('idioms of distress') to communicate feelings and experiences. These may be indicative of psychopathological states that undermine well-being, but do not necessarily imply a mental disorder.

Idioms of distress often focus on a typical symptom or body part or behaviour. Examples include:

- idioms related to thoughts: e.g. 'kufungisisa' ('thinking too much', Shona, Zimbabwe), 'yeyeesi' ('many thoughts', Kakwa, South Sudan, and in many other African countries)
- idioms related to the heart: e.g. 'poil-heart' ('heavy hearted', Krio in Sierra Leone), 'qalb maqboud '(squeezed heart', Arabic)
- idioms related to the head: 'amutwe alluhire' ('my head is tired', Nande in Democratic Republic of Congo).

Health workers should actively try to understand salient idioms in the area where they work and engage with the cultural context. Use can help communication and identification of local coping methods, at times more appropriate than Western interventions.

People with severe mental disorders are at a higher risk for abuse and neglect and discrimination in seeking care. Further, in many humanitarian emergencies, human rights violations are particularly common due to increased vulnerabilities including displacement, breakdown in social structures, violence, and a lack of access to health services.

International guidelines

The following resources provide guidance on providing mental health services and psychosocial support activities in humanitarian contexts. Readers should refer to them for further information, beyond what is provided in this chapter.

mhGAP

The WHO developed the Mental Health Gap Action Programme (mhGAP) to support the global scaling up of services for mental, neurological, and substance use (MNS) disorders, particularly in LIC and MIC. The programme consists of policy tools, instruments for advocacy, and clinical guidance to address priority conditions in non-specialist healthcare settings. The core of mhGAP is the Intervention Guide (2010/2016) that is accompanied by a training curriculum, training materials, workbook, and tips on how to set up a supervision system. In 2015, WHO and UNHCR published a humanitarian version: the mhGAP Humanitarian Intervention Guide (mhGAP-HIG).[1]

Materials are freely available online and have been translated into many languages (℘ http://www.who.int/mental_health/mhgap/en/).

IASC Guidelines on Mental Health and Psychosocial Support in Emergency Settings

The IASC Guidelines on Mental Health and Psychosocial Support in Emergency Settings[2] outline a set of minimum multisectoral responses related to mental health and psychosocial well-being. The guidelines are useful for the planning and coordination of activities and provide organizations from various backgrounds with a common conceptual framework for setting up services. The guidelines include a matrix with key interventions which should be part of the minimum response (during or after an emergency) and comprehensive response (for stabilized phase or during reconstruction) (℘ https://interagencystandingcommittee.org/mental-health-and-psychosocial-support-emergency-settings).

The IASC Reference Group for MHPSS consists of more than 40 members, and fosters a unique collaboration between NGOs and UN and international agencies, promoting best practices in MHPSS.

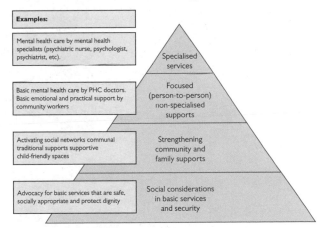

Fig. 6.1 The IASC intervention pyramid for mental health and psychosocial support in emergencies.[2] Reproduced with permission from Inter-Agency Standing Committee (IASC), Mental Health and Psychosocial Support in Humanitarian Emergencies (2010). Geneva. p3.

Sphere Handbook

The Sphere Handbook represents consensus on universal minimum standards in core areas of the humanitarian response. The 2018 version of the Sphere Handbook integrates notions about mental health and psychosocial support throughout the text addressing issues such as self-help, coping, and resilience. The chapter on Protection Principles gives particular attention to mental health ('Assist people to recover from the physical and psychological effects of violence, coercion, or deliberate deprivation') and the chapter on Health contains a separate standard on mental health that has nine key actions.

UNHCR MHPSS guidance for refugee settings

UNHCR has developed operational guidance for MHPSS programming for refugee operations (2013).[3] It is consistent with the IASC guidelines and tailored for refugee contexts. It highlights the need for integrated interventions related to health, community-based protection, child protection, and education.

Approach to clinical conditions

This section aims to provide guidance for non specialized health professionals in humanitarian contexts in the identification and management of
priority mental health conditions. The content is consistent with the clinical
mhGAP-HIG of WHO and UNHCR.

Additional details and more in-depth descriptions of the mental health
interventions outlined in this chapter are available:

- World Health Organization and United Nations High Commissioner
  for Refugees. mhGAP Humanitarian Intervention Guide (mhGAP-
  HIG): Clinical Management Of Mental, Neurological and Substance Use
  Conditions in Humanitarian Emergencies (Version 1.0). Geneva: WHO.
  2015. (℘ http://www.who.int/mental_health/publications/mhgap_
  hig/en/).
- World Health Organization. mhGAP Intervention Guide (mhGAP-IG)
  Version 2.0 for Mental, Neurological and Substance Use Disorders for
  Non-Specialist Health Settings. Geneva: WHO; 2016. (℘ http://www.
  who.int/mental_health/mhgap/mhGAP_intervention_guide_02/en/).

For all conditions listed in this chapter, readers are referred to the mhGAP-
HIG (2015) and mhGAP-IG v2.0 (2016) for further information or specific
details.

Prescribing psychopharmacological treatment

Pharmacological treatment may be prescribed by non-specialists, provided the clinician has been adequately trained and is able to use the
mhGAP-IG or -HIG for guidance on the prescription of psychotropic
medication and is able to do the necessary monitoring and follow-up of
treatment.

General approach

While specific clinical conditions have detailed recommended management
(outlined in the following subsections), it is helpful for providers to approach
each patient with the same general management principles (see Box 6.1).

**Box 6.1 General management principles for all mental
disorders**

- Listen carefully. Do not pressure the person to talk.
- Ask the person about his/her needs and concerns.
- Help the person to address basic needs, access services, and connect
  with social supports.
- Offer additional psychosocial support as needed:
  - Address current psychosocial stressors.
  - Strengthen social support.
  - Teach stress management.
- Protect the person from (further) harm.
- Manage concurrent conditions.
- Provide regular follow-up.
- Refer to appropriate agencies (e.g. protection, tracing, human rights,)
  if needed (with the person's consent).

Communication skills

Good communication skills are essential to ensure effective care of people in distress in emergency contexts.

- Keep consultations brief, flexible, and focused.
- Use empathy as a key aspect of good communication (e.g. 'listening attentively, being respectful and showing understanding of the person's feelings and experiences').
- Involve the person with the MNS condition as much as possible even if the person's functioning is impaired.
- Seek permission to ask relevant assessment questions to the carers, and involve them when the management plan is discussed and agreed.
- If required, use trained interpreters (preferably of the same gender as the person) but be aware that the person with the MNS condition may not fully disclose.
- Do not press the person to discuss or describe potentially traumatic experiences if they do not wish to do so. Simply let them know that you are there to listen.
- Never belittle the person's feelings, preach, or be judgemental.
- If referral to other services is necessary, explain clearly what the next steps will be. Seek the consent of the person to share information with other providers who may be able to help.
- Understand that unusual behaviours may be because of the person's illness. Stay calm and patient.
- Involve their carers or other staff members in creating a calm space. Distressed/agitated patients may need to be seen first.

Conditions specifically related to stress

The most common reactions to stressful events are transient—disappear within a month—and do not impair functioning beyond what is culturally expected. Usually these reactions do not require clinical management and it is sufficient to support the person's needs, address his/her concerns, and conduct follow-up in order to promote natural recovery. However, in the first month after a stressful event, some people develop symptoms that are so severe or disabling they require clinical management: these are called 'significant symptoms of acute stress'.

Acute stress

Clinical features (any of the following can occur)

- Anxiety about threats related to the traumatic events.
- Sleep problems.
- Concentration problems.
- Re-experiencing symptoms: recurring frightening dreams, flashbacks, or intrusive memories of the events.
- Deliberate avoidance of thoughts, memories, activities, or situations that remind the person of the events.
- Hyperarousal symptoms: feeling 'too alert', 'jumpy', or 'on edge'.
- Feeling shocked, dazed, or numb, inability to feel anything.
- Any disturbing thoughts or emotions (e.g. frequent tearfulness, anger).
- Worrisome changes of behaviour such as aggression, social isolation, and withdrawal, risk-taking behaviours in adolescents, or regressive behaviour such as bedwetting and clinginess in children.
- Hyperventilation (e.g. rapid breathing, shortness of breath).
- Unexplained physical complaints (e.g. palpitations, dizziness).
- Dissociative disorders of movement and sensation (e.g. 'pseudoseizures', inability to speak or see).

Assessment

- Has the person recently experienced a potentially traumatic event? (If the potentially traumatic event occurred >1 month ago, then consider other conditions such as depression, or PTSD.)
- If a potentially traumatic event occurred within the last month, does the person have any of the symptoms of acute stress as previously listed under 'Clinical features'?
- Is the person having considerable difficulty with daily functioning because of the symptoms or seeking help for the symptoms?
- Rule out concurrent medical conditions that may explain symptoms.

Management

- Provide general management as outlined in ➲ Box 6.1 p. 107.
- Reassure the person about normal reactions to acute stress and that in most cases, reactions will reduce over time.

Post-traumatic stress disorder

When a characteristic set of symptoms (re-experiencing, avoidance, and heightened sense of current threat) persists for more than a month after a potentially traumatic event and causes considerable difficulty with daily functioning, the person may have developed PTSD. As PTSD-like symptoms may occur in normal acute stress, there has been an overdiagnosis of PTSD in humanitarian settings and much debate about its clinical utility, as well as concern that an overemphasis may divert attention away from other problems and interventions. Therefore, if PTSD is suspected, always make sure to exclude other diagnoses first.

Clinical features

The patient may present with non-specific symptoms including sleep disturbances, irritability, persistent anxious or depressed mood, or multiple, persistent physical symptoms with no clear physical cause (e.g. headaches, pounding heart). However, PTSD cannot be diagnosed unless at least one symptom from each of these three symptom clusters, is present (for definitions see earlier under 'Acute stress'):

1. Re-experiencing symptoms.
2. Avoidance symptoms.
3. Hyper-arousal symptoms.

Plus the patient must be experiencing difficulties in daily functioning.

Management

- General management principles (see ➔ Box 6.1 p. 107).
- Reassure patient that the symptoms are a common reaction, and that many people recover from PTSD over time without treatment, while others need treatment.
- Encourage the person to:
  - continue their normal daily routine as much as possible
  - when ready, talk to trusted people about what happened
  - engage in relaxing activities to reduce anxiety and tension
  - avoid using alcohol or drugs to cope with symptoms
  - if available, consider referring for brief evidence-based interventions.
- When interventions and stress management have no effect or are not available, the prescription of antidepressants (selective serotonin reuptake inhibitors or tricyclic antidepressants) can be considered for adults with PTSD (do not use them in children and adolescents).
- The effectiveness of antidepressants for PTSD is limited, however, and in humanitarian emergencies there is a real risk that antidepressants are prescribed too generously. It is important to monitor the prescribing behaviour of clinicians.

Grief and loss

A common experience in humanitarian emergencies is loss, which can be external (e.g. loss of someone in the family or of a friend, loss of health, loss of home) or internal (e.g. loss of identity, sense of belonging and control). The effect of such losses can be overwhelming and clinicians should differentiate between normal and abnormal grief. However, the extent to which people experience and manifest grief depends on personal, social, and cultural factors, which must be taken into consideration.

Any of the following symptoms can occur in normal grief:

- Sadness, anxiety, anger, despair.
- Yearning and preoccupation with loss.
- Intrusive memories, images and thoughts of the deceased.
- Loss of appetite.
- Loss of energy.
- Sleep problems.
- Concentration problems.
- Social isolation and withdrawal.
- Medically unexplained physical complaints (e.g. palpitations, headaches, generalized aches and pains).
- Culturally specific grief reactions.

Management

- Symptoms of grief may mimic those of moderate severe depression. It is very important to avoid treating grief reactions as depressive illness. Instead, people should be helped to understand and cope with their reactions to loss.
- General management principles (see ➲ Box 6.1 p. 107).
- Educate the person about normal reactions to losses (see ➲ below and Table 6.2).
- Answer questions, provide information.
- Support culturally appropriate burial and mourning rituals.
- Encourage return to previous normal daily routines when possible.

Approaches for a grieving person

- Educate the person about normal reactions to losses:
  - People may react in different ways after major losses. Some people show strong emotions while others do not.
  - Crying does not mean a person is weak.
  - People who do not cry may feel the emotional pain just as deeply as others but have other ways of showing it.
- A person may believe that the sadness and pain felt after this loss will never diminish, but in most cases, these painful feelings do diminish over time.
- Many people find it helpful to talk with someone they trust, others prefer to remain quiet. The person will know what is best for themselves.
- *Do not say*: 'I know how you feel' (you don't!).
- *Do not say*: 'Stop worrying, everything will be all right' (you do not know!).

If the person is a child
- Do not lie to the child.
- Answer the child's questions by providing clear and honest explanations appropriate to the child's level of development.
- Check for and correct 'magical thinking' common in young children (e.g. the child thinks they somehow caused the loss).
- Encourage the child to maintain connection with the lost parent (e.g. through shared good memories, with photographs, or hand-made mementoes).
- Address the need for protection and ensure consistent, supportive caregiving, including socioemotional support (involve protection agencies if necessary).
- Manage concurrent conditions such as sleep problems and regressive behaviour (e.g. bedwetting) (see Box 6.2).

> **Box 6.2 Management approach for bedwetting in distressed children**
> - Confirm that bedwetting started after experiencing a stressful event.
> - Rule out other possible causes (e.g. urinary tract infection).
> - Explain that bedwetting is a common, harmless reaction in children who experience stress.
> - Children should not be punished and the caregiver should avoid embarrassing the child by mentioning bedwetting in public.
> - Train carers on the use of simple behavioural interventions:
>   - Rewarding avoidance of excessive fluid intake before sleep.
>   - Rewarding toileting before sleep.
>   - Rewarding dry nights.

Prolonged grief disorder
Prolonged grief disorder may be suspected if the grief reaction has persisted for >6 months or for a period that is much longer than what is expected in that person's culture, and if in addition there is severe preoccupation with or persistent and pervasive longing for the deceased person accompanied by intense emotional pain. Prolonged grief can cause considerable impairment in daily functioning, and if diagnosed, should be referred to a specialist.

Distinguishing the impact of traumatic events and loss
- In humanitarian emergencies, people may suffer from a combination of potentially traumatic events and losses simultaneously.
- Table 6.2 may help in understanding which reaction predominates and thus guide management.

Table 6.2 Understanding predominating reactions

Reactions to loss	Reactions to traumatic events
Separation anxiety	Anxiety about threat re: traumatic event
Sadness more than anxiety	Anxiety more than sadness
Yearning and preoccupation with loss	Fearful, anxious, and preoccupied with traumatic event
Sense of security intact	Personal sense of safety challenged
Primary relationships disrupted	Primary relationships intact
Intrusive memories are images and thoughts of the deceased	Intrusive memories are of traumatic event plus re-experiencing accompanying emotions
Memories sought after positive and comforting	Uncontrollable intrusions: negative and distressing
Dream of dead person is comforting	Nightmares of event are terrifying
Seek out reminders of loved ones	Hypervigilant, scanning environment for threat
Avoidance of reminders of absence of loved one (denial)	Avoidance of reminders of threat
Anger at loss	Irritable, diffuse, unfocused anger and rage
Guilt at not doing enough	Guilt at surviving
Coping involves reconstructing life without loved one	Coping involves re-establishing sense of safety

Information from: Hendricks J. H., Black, D, Kaplan T. 'When father killed mother: guiding children through trauma and grief.' 2nd edition, Routledge, 2000.

Moderate–severe depressive disorder

The risk for depressive disorders is increased in humanitarian settings. Mild and transient forms of depression do not significantly impair daily functioning, but moderate–severe depression does: it involves persistent symptoms, not secondary to a major loss, within the last 6 months, which impair functioning.

Clinical features

- Core symptoms (at least one symptom for at least 2 weeks):
  - Persistent sadness or depressed mood, anxiety (including irritability for children).
  - Markedly diminished interest in, or pleasure from, normal activities (including reduced sexual desire).
- Additional symptoms (at least three symptoms for at least 2 weeks):
  - Low energy or fatigue.
  - Disturbed sleep (decrease or increase).
  - Significant change in appetite or weight (decrease or increase).
  - Beliefs of worthlessness or excessive guilt.
  - Multiple persistent physical symptoms with no clear cause (e.g. aches and pains).
  - Reduced ability to concentrate and sustain attention on tasks.
  - Indecisiveness.
  - Observable agitation or physical restlessness.
  - Talking or moving more slowly than normal.
  - Hopelessness about the future.
  - Suicidal thoughts or acts.
  - The individual has considerable difficulty with daily functioning in personal, family, social, educational, occupational, or other important domains for at least 2 weeks.

Assessment

- Evaluate for other possible explanations for the symptoms.
- Rule out concurrent physical conditions (e.g. malnutrition, hypothyroidism), normal reactions to major stressors or loss, and prolonged grief disorder.
- Evaluate for any a concurrent MNS condition requiring management.

Management

- In addition to the general management principles (see ➲ Box 6.1 p. 107), educate the person and the carers that depression is common and does not mean weakness or laziness.
- People with depression tend to have unrealistically negative opinions about themselves and so encourage the person to:
  - continue activities that were previously pleasurable
  - maintain regular sleeping and waking times
  - be as physically active as possible
  - eat regularly despite changes in appetite
  - spend time with trusted friends and family
  - participate in community and other social activities.

- If the person experiences thoughts of self-harm or suicide, encourage him/her not to act on them, but to tell a trusted person and come back for help immediately (see ➔ next section on Self-harm of suicide pp. 115–16).
- Pharmacological treatment may be used if the prescribing clinician has been trained in the use of psychotropics and is able to do the necessary monitoring and follow-up of treatment. Before considering the prescription of antidepressants always offer psychoeducation and support as explained previously. There is a serious risk that busy clinicians may erroneously view antidepressants as a quick alternative to psychosocial interventions and brief evidence-based psychotherapy.

Pharmacological treatment of moderate–severe depressive disorder

Fluoxetine

- Adults: 10–20 mg once per day (effective dose 20–40 mg; max. dose 60 mg).
- Adolescents and elderly: 10 mg once per day (effective dose 20 mg; max. dose 40 mg).
- Common side effects: headache, restlessness, nervousness, gastrointestinal disturbances, reversible sexual dysfunction.
- Additional notes: caution—stop immediately if the person develops a manic episode. Occasionally people report an increase in suicidal thoughts. Stop if this occurs.

Amitriptyline

- Adults: 50 mg at bedtime (effective dose 100–150 mg; max. dose 150 mg).
- Elderly: 25 mg at bedtime (effective dose 50–75 mg; max. dose 100 mg).
- Common side effects: orthostatic hypotension (risk of fall), dry mouth, constipation or difficulty urinating, dizziness, blurred vision, sedation.
- Additional notes: caution—stop immediately if the person develops a manic episode (antidepressants may precipitate a maniac episode and/or bipolar disorder).
- *Do not* prescribe for children or adolescents.
- *Do not* prescribe in people with cardiovascular disease.

Self-harm or suicide

Assessment

- Has the person attempted a medically serious act of self-harm?
  - Observe for evidence of self-injury.
  - Ask about recent poisoning or other self-harm.
  - Look for signs/symptoms requiring urgent medical treatment.
- Is there an imminent risk of self-harm/suicide? Ask person and carer about:
  - current thoughts or plans to commit suicide or self-harm
  - history of thoughts or plans of self-harm in the past month or acts of self-harm in the past year
  - access to means of self-harm.

- Look for:
  - severe emotional distress
  - hopelessness
  - extreme agitation
  - violence
  - uncommunicative behaviour
  - social isolation.

Management

- In all cases place the person in a secure and supportive environment at the health facility while being assessed (*do not* leave them alone).
- Care for the person with self-harm.
- Offer and activate psychosocial support.
- Consult a mental health specialist if available.
- Maintain regular contact and follow-up.
- Offer psychoeducation.
- If there is imminent risk of self-harm/suicide:
  - Remove means of self-harm.
  - Create a secure and supportive environment; if possible, offer a separate, quiet room while waiting.
  - Supervise and assign a named staff member or a family member to ensure safety.
  - Attend to mental state and emotional distress.

Substance use disorders

During emergencies, people may self-medicate to cope with stress, resulting in an increased prevalence of substance abuse. Acute emergencies can also disrupt the provision of illegal drugs and alcohol, leading to unexpected life-threatening withdrawal symptoms.

Substance dependence

Clinical features
- Strong desire or compulsion to take the substance.
- Difficulties in controlling onset, termination, or levels of substance use.
- Physiological withdrawal state when substance use has ceased or been reduced, or use of similar substance to relieve symptoms.
- Tolerance (increased doses of substance are required to achieve effects).
- Progressive neglect of alternative pleasures or interests.
- Substance use persisting, despite clear evidence of overtly harmful consequences.

Assessment
- Assess for both harmful alcohol and drug use in the same person as they often occur together.
- Explore level and pattern of consumption, triggers, and any behaviour associated with substance use without sounding judgemental.
- Ask about harm to self or others, medical and social problems.
- Perform a quick general physical examination to look for signs of substance use (gastrointestinal bleeding, liver disease, malnutrition, severe weight loss, evidence of infections).

Management of substance dependence
- General management principles (see ➔ Box 6.1 p. 107).
- Provide medical care for physical consequences of substance use and concurrent mental conditions.
- Motivate the person to either stop or reduce the use of the substance.
- Ask about the perceived benefits and harms of substance use.
- Challenge any exaggerated sense of benefit from substance use.
- Highlight the negative aspects of substance use both in the short term and long term.
- Let the person know you are willing to support them.
- Discuss various ways to reduce or stop harmful use (e.g. do not store substances at home, ask for support from carers and friends, encourage social activities without substances, and connect the person to a self-help group).
- Arrange detoxification if necessary (and treat withdrawal symptoms as necessary).

Alcohol withdrawal

Symptoms of clinical alcohol withdrawal
- Tremor in hands
- Sweating
- Vomiting
- Increased pulse and blood pressure

- Agitation
- Life-threatening features:
  - Convulsions/seizures (within 48 hours)
  - Features of delirium (within 96 hours): acute confusion, disorientation, or hallucinations
  - Alcohol withdrawal can be life-threatening!

Management of alcohol withdrawal
1. Treat with diazepam (initial dose 10–20 mg up to four times/day for 3–7 days to give slight sedation).
2. Maintain hydration (start intravenous (IV) hydration or encourage oral fluid intake of at least 2–3 litres/day).
3. Monitor the withdrawal symptoms every 3–4 hours; gradually decrease diazepam dose and/or frequency as soon as the symptoms improve.
4. If delirium or hallucinations persist despite treatment of other withdrawal symptoms, then consider using antipsychotics such as haloperidol 2.5–5 mg orally up to three times daily.
5. Transfer to the nearest hospital as soon as possible.

Sedative drug overdose

Clinical features
- Unresponsive or minimally responsive.
- Slow respiratory rate (<10 breaths/minute).
- Oxygen saturation <92%.
- Pinpoint pupils (opioid overdose).

Management
- Treat airway, breathing, and circulation.
- For opioid: naloxone 0.4 mg subcutaneous, intramuscular (IM), or IV (repeat if necessary); observe for 1–2 hours after naloxone administration.
- Transport to hospital.

Acute stimulant intoxication or overdose

Clinical features
- Dilated pupils.
- Excited, racing thoughts, disordered thinking, paranoia.
- Recent use of cocaine or other stimulants.
- Raised pulse and blood pressure.
- Aggressive, erratic, or violent behaviour.

Management
- Give diazepam in titrated doses until the person is calm and lightly sedated.
- If psychotic symptoms do not respond to benzodiazepines, consider short-term antipsychotics.
- Monitor blood pressure, pulse rate, respiratory rate, and temperature every 2–4 hours.
- Transport to hospital.
- Be alert for suicidal thoughts or actions (post-intoxication phase).

Acute opioid withdrawal state

Clinical features

- History of opioid dependence, recent heavy use ceasing in the last few days.
- Muscle aches and pains, abdominal cramps, headaches.
- Nausea, vomiting, diarrhoea.
- Dilated pupils.
- Raised pulse and blood pressure.
- Yawning, runny eyes and nose, piloerection.
- Anxiety, restlessness.

Management

- Treat specific symptoms as needed (diarrhoea, vomiting, muscle pain, insomnia).
- Consider starting opioid medication.

Psychosis

The hallmark of psychosis is the loss of contact with reality. Consequently, people with psychosis often do not realize that they have a mental disorder. Humanitarian emergencies may worsen chronic psychosis or precipitate acute psychosis because of rapidly changing environments, disruption of social networks, and disruption of medication supply.

Clinical features

- Delusions: fixed false beliefs that are firmly held.
- Hallucinations: hearing, seeing, or feeling things that are not there.
- Disorganized thoughts: absence of logical connections, speech that is difficult to follow.
- Unusual experiences of thought, belief, or speech (e.g. believing one's movements are directed by others).
- Abnormal behaviour: odd, eccentric, aimless, and agitated activity or maintaining an abnormal body posture or not moving at all.
- Less specific symptoms may be present, such as lack of energy or motivation, apathy and social withdrawal, poor personal care or neglect, and/or lack of emotional expressiveness.

Management

- General management principles (see ➲ Box 6.1 p. 107).
- Educate the person and the carers:
  - Psychosis can be treated and the person can recover.
  - Stress and substance abuse can worsen psychotic symptoms.
  - Do not argue if he or she expresses things that are not true.
  - Compliance with treatment is essential.
- Encourage participation in regular social, educational, and occupational activities and facilitate inclusion in the community.

Pharmacological treatment options for psychosis

- Haloperidol—adults: 1–2.5 mg daily (effective dose 4–10 mg/day; max. dose 20 mg).
- Chlorpromazine—adults: 50–75 mg daily (effective dose 75–300 mg/day).
- Risperidone: adults: 2 mg daily (effective dose 4–6 mg/day).

Common side effects

Extrapyramidal symptoms (such as Parkinsonism—combination of tremors, muscular rigidity and decreased body movements; or akathisia—inability to sit still), sedation, orthostatic hypotension, urinary hesitancy.

Additional notes

- Initiate only one antipsychotic, orally, at a time. Use for an adequate time at a typical effective dose before considering it ineffective.
- In case of significant acute extrapyramidal side effects: reduce or stop medication. If side effects persist, consider short-term use (4–8 weeks) of anticholinergics, e.g. biperiden 2 mg daily (effective dose 3–6 mg/day). Do not prescribe anticholinergic medication routinely for all patients on antipsychotic medication.

Bipolar disorder and manic episode

Bipolar disorder (also referred to as manic–depressive illness) is characterized by shifts between the two extremes of mood: elevated mood (or mania) and low mood (or depression). Typically the course is episodic: between episodes, mood is stable. Note that people who only experience elevated mood (manic episodes) are also classified as having bipolar disorder while people who only experience depressive episodes are not (classified as moderate–severe depressive disorder).

Clinical features of a manic episode

Several symptoms are present for >1 week, and cause considerable difficulty with daily functioning:

- Decreased need for sleep.
- Euphoric, expansive, or irritable mood.
- Racing thoughts and/or rapid speech.
- Distractibility.
- Increased activity or energy, restlessness, excitement.
- Impulsive or reckless behaviours such as excessive gambling or spending, making important decisions without adequate planning.
- Unrealistically inflated self-esteem.
- Loss of normal social inhibitions.
- Elevated sexual energy or sexual indiscretion.
- Psychotic symptoms including delusions (often grandiose or paranoid) and hallucinations may also be present.

Management

- General management principles (see ➜ Box 6.1 p. 107).
- Educate the person and the carers that bipolar disorder involves extreme moods, which should be monitored daily.
- Stress the importance of maintaining a regular sleep cycle.
- Alcohol and other psychoactive substances should be avoided.
- Provide pharmacological treatment. In many contexts, the use of lithium is not feasible due to lack of monitoring tools, and atypical antipsychotics are often not available. An acceptable alternative is to use an oral antipsychotic medication during the acute manic phase (see ➜ 'Psychosis' p. 120), and once mania is managed, introduce a mood stabilizer (i.e. valproate or carbamazepine)

Pharmacological treatment of psychosis in bipolar disorder

- Carbamazepine—adults: 200 mg/day (effective dose 400–600 mg/day to be given in two doses; max. dose 1400 mg/day).
  - Side effects: drowsiness, troubling walking, nausea.
- Valproate—adults: 400 mg/day (effective dose 1000–2000 mg/day to be given in two doses):
  - Side effects include lethargy, sedation, tremor, nausea, diarrhoea, weight gain, birth defects and developmental delays
  - *Do not* use sodium valproate in women of childbearing age or pregnant women. Carbamazepine should be used with caution.

Delirium

Clinical features

The major feature is impairment of consciousness, resulting in a reduced level of alertness, difficulties in sustaining attention, and diminished awareness of the environment (see Table 6.3).[4]

This is usually accompanied by:
- short-term memory problems
- emotional symptoms (emotional lability, often anxiety)
- perceptual disturbances (such as hallucinations)
- behavioural disturbances (inappropriate, impulsive, or violent behaviour; but in some cases, hypoactivity).

The onset of delirium is usually acute, and the symptoms occur within a few hours. The course is fluctuating, with periods in which the patient seems to be normal, and periods, particularly during the night, in which the patient is very confused and agitated. Patients with delirium often have disturbed sleep.

Delirium is common among hospitalized patients. Very sick, weak patients and young children and elderly people are more susceptible to delirium. Symptoms usually disappear within days if the underlying cause is treated. If the underlying cause remains untreated, death can result.

Causes

Delirium is always caused by underlying problems that need to be identified and treated. The list of causes is long. Major causes include:
- medications (e.g. opiates, anticholinergics, diuretics, digoxin, sedatives)
- medical conditions (septicaemia, metabolic changes, hyperglycaemia, hypoglycaemia)

Table 6.3 Differences between acute brief psychosis and delirium

Key features of acute or brief psychoses	Key features of delirium
• Severe behavioural disturbance such as restlessness and aggression	• Disorientation (the person does not know where he/she is or what time it is)
• Hearing voices or seeing things others cannot	• Fluctuating level of consciousness
• Bizarre beliefs	• Fever, excess sweating, raised pulse rate, and other physical signs
• Talking nonsense	• Poor memory
• Fearful emotional state or rapidly changing emotions (from tears to laughter)	• Disturbed sleep pattern
• Note: symptoms begin suddenly and last less than a month	• Visual hallucinations (seeing things others cannot)
	• Note: symptoms vary from hour to hour, with periods of apparent recovery alternating with periods of severe symptoms

- alcohol withdrawal (see ⟲ 'Substance use disorders' pp. 117–19).
- febrile illnesses (e.g. urinary tract infection)
- pulmonary infections
- intracranial causes (head injury, encephalitis, cerebral malaria)
- dehydration
- anaemia.

Management

- General management principles apply (see ⟲ Box 6.1 p. 107).
- Identify and treat the underlying cause.
- Check for causes and manage them if present:
  - Medical causes (e.g. metabolic abnormalities: correct them and ensure proper hydration and electrolyte balance).
  - Medication side effects (e.g. mefloquine or high dosages of corticosteroids). Identify and if possible stop medication that may have contributed to the delirium.
  - Alcohol or drug intoxication/withdrawal (see ⟲ p. 118).

Non-pharmacological management steps
- Protect the patient: remove potentially dangerous objects.
- If possible place the person in a quiet room.
- A trusted family member should be with the patient.
- Provide explanation to family members. Assure them that the condition is reversible and that the person is not going mad.
- Instruct family members and staff to provide 're-orientation cues' to the patient (tell the patient where they are, what the time and day is, etc.).

Pharmacological management
- Symptomatic treatment with antipsychotic medication (oral or IM), e.g. haloperidol 1 mg, repeat every 4–6 hours.
- Benzodiazepines should be avoided because they can increase the confusion.

Developmental disorders

Developmental disorder is an umbrella term covering disorders such as intellectual disability as well as pervasive developmental disorders including autism. These disorders usually have a childhood onset and have a steady course that persists into adulthood. People with developmental disorders are more vulnerable to physical and other mental health problems and to both neglect and abuse.

Intellectual disability

Characterized by impairment of skills across multiple developmental areas (i.e. cognitive, language, motor, and social) during the developmental period. Lower intelligence diminishes the ability to adapt to the daily demands of life.

Pervasive developmental disorders including autism

Features include impaired social behaviour, communication and language difficulties, and a narrow range of interests and activities that are both unique to the individual and carried out repetitively. Originating in infancy or early childhood, there is usually some degree of intellectual disability.

Assessment

Assess child's development using local developmental milestones or by comparing the child with other children of the same age in the same country (see Table 6.4). Look for the following:
- Oddities in communication (e.g. lack of social usage of language, lack of flexibility in language usage).
- Restricted, repetitive patterns of behaviour, interests, activities.
- The time, sequence, and course of these features.
- Loss of previously acquired skills.
- Family history of developmental disorder.
- Presence of visual and hearing impairment.
- Associated epilepsy.
- Associated signs of motor impairment or cerebral palsy.

Management

The goals of management are to support the person and protect them from abuse, enhance their developmental potential, and encourage a supportive and accepting environment.

General management principles
(See ➲ Box 6.1 p. 107.)
- Rule out other causes of developmental disorders such as medical problems or environmental issues.
- Educate the person and the carers (see ➲ next section (key education aspects)).
- Promote community-based inclusion in social activities.
- Be vigilant about issues of human rights and dignity (e.g. using informed consent; avoid institutionalization).
- Support carers (e.g. reduce stress, strengthen social support).
- Refer to a specialist for further assessment, if possible.

Key educational aspects for caregivers
- Accept and care for the child with a developmental disorder.
- Avoid institutionalization.

- Spend positive time with the child every day.
- Show love and affection.
- Learn what makes the child stressed and what makes them happy; what causes their problem behaviours and what prevents them; what are the child's strengths and weaknesses.
- Have a structured and scheduled day with times for eating, playing, learning, and sleeping.
- Keep them in a mainstream educational setting as far as possible.
- Be aware of general hygiene and train them in self-care.
- Give clear, simple, and short instructions on what the child should do (rather than what the child should not do).
- Reward good behaviour after the act (offer praise whenever the child is content and behaving well), and withhold rewards for problematic behaviour.
- Ignore problematic behaviour or use distraction when possible provided the child is not endangering themselves or others.
- *Do not* use threats or physical punishments.

Table 6.4 Possible indicators of developmental delay

By age 1 month	• Poor suckling at the breast or refusing to suckle • Little movement of arms and legs • Little or no reaction to loud sounds or bright lights • Crying for long periods for no apparent reason
By age 6 months	• Stiffness or difficulty moving limbs • Does not reach for objects • Does not make vowel sounds and little/no response to sounds, or familiar faces • Refusing the breast or other foods
By age 12 months	• Does not say single words • Does not look at objects that move • Listlessness and lack of response to the caregiver • Lack of appetite or refusal of food
By age 2 years	• Lack of response to others • Difficulty keeping balance while walking • Injuries and unexplained changes in behaviour • Doesn't know what to do with common things • Lack of appetite
By age 3 years	• Does not have interest in playing • Frequent falling • Difficulty manipulating small objects • Failure to understand simple messages • Inability to speak using several words • Little or no interest in food
By age 5 years	• Doesn't talk about experiences • Doesn't play a variety of games and activities • Can't wash hands, or get undressed without help

Behavioural disorders in adolescents

Clinical features

Common presentations of behavioural problems include repeated and persistent dissocial, aggressive, or defiant conduct (e.g. excessive levels of fighting or bullying, cruelty to other people, severe destructiveness to property, fire-setting, stealing, running away from home, frequent and severe temper tantrums, defiant provocative behaviour, and persistent severe disobedience).

Assessment

- Interview both the adolescent and the carers to assess for persistent or concerning behavioural problems.
- If the adolescent has a behaviour problem, ask further questions about extreme stressors in the adolescent's past or current life, parenting, and how the adolescent spends most of his or her time.
- Exclude alcohol and substance use problems, depressive disorder, and/or PTSD; if present, treat.

Management

- Provide basic psychosocial support as described in general management principles (see ➔ Box 6.1 p. 107).
- Take time to listen to the adolescent.
- Promote participation in formal and informal education, concrete, purposeful, common interest activities, and structured sports programmes.

Messages for the carers

- Adolescents need continuous care and support despite their behaviour.
- Make every effort to communicate with the adolescent.
- Try to identify positive, enjoyable activities that you can do together.
- Be consistent with respect to what the adolescent is allowed to do and not allowed to do.
- Praise or reward the adolescent for good behaviours and correct only the most problematic behaviours.
- Never use physical punishment.
- Confront the adolescent only when you are calm.

Messages for the adolescent

- Healthy ways to deal with boredom, stress, or anger include doing activities that are relaxing, being physically active, engaging in community activities.
- Talking to trusted people about feeling angry, bored, anxious, or sad can be helpful.
- Alcohol and other substance use can worsen feelings of anger and depression and should be avoided.

Dementia

Dementia is a chronic and progressive syndrome that produces changes in a person's mental ability, personality, and behaviour. It can easily be mistaken for psychosis or severe depression in the elderly.

Clinical features

Symptoms have been present for at least 6 months, are progressive in nature, and associated with a decline in intellectual functioning. It usually interferes with activities of daily living. Core symptoms are:
- memory loss/ forgetfulness
- disorientation
- cognitive impairment: decline in intellectual functioning and confusion.

Additional symptoms may include profound mistrust, making unfound accusations, transient psychotic symptoms (hallucinations, delusions), anxiety, depressed mood, deterioration in emotional control and social behaviour, loss of motivation, wandering; incontinence, difficulties with activities of daily living; lack of awareness of, or hiding, symptoms.

Assessment

Assess memory and cognitive functioning using any locally validated tool or through simple questions. Ask the person to:
- repeat three common words, then again 3–5 minutes later
- identify the time and location correctly
- name parts of the body
- explaining the function of a common item
- identify known people.

Confirm symptoms by interviewing a family member.

Management

- General management principles (see ➋ Box 6.1 p. 107).
- Provide psychoeducation to the carer to provide regular orientation information (e.g. large visible clock, calendar).
- Promote communication and stimulate memories; use simple, short sentences and minimize competing noises.
- Avoid changes to living situation or routine unless necessary.
- Promote regular physical activity and exercise.
- Manage concurrent medical conditions if present.
- Identify psychosocial impact on carers and address psychological distress. Provide carer with information about available resources (e.g. practical support).

Avoid the prescription of benzodiazepines as this may increase disorientation and forgetfulness. Avoid the use of antipsychotics unless patient has very disturbed behaviour, has not responded to psychosocial interventions, and there is a risk of imminent harm; use low-dose haloperidol for a short period starting at 0.5 mg, orally or IM and increasing *slowly* as required. Avoid IV haloperidol.

Medically unexplained somatic complaints

Physical symptoms that present in general healthcare settings frequently do not have an apparent organic cause and may be the somatic presentation of an underlying mental disorder, e.g. depression or anxiety disorder. In many cases, a clear cause remains elusive, in which case such symptoms are defined as a medically unexplained somatic complaints: somatic symptoms that do not have a known physical cause that fully explains the symptom. People with medically unexplained somatic complaints consume large amounts of medical time and medications and often cause frustration in both doctor and patient.

Clinical features

This category should only be applied:
- after conducting necessary physical examinations, *and*
- if the person is not positive for any other mental disorder *and*
- if the person is requesting help for the complaint.

Assessment

- Rule out physical conditions.
- Evaluate for psychological distress or mental disorder, such as depression, and for grief or acute stress.

Management

In addition to the general management principles (see ➲ Box 6.1 p. 107):
- *Do not* order more laboratory or other investigations unless there is a clear medical indication (e.g. abnormal vital signs):
  - Ordering unnecessary clinical investigations may reinforce the person's belief that there is a physical problem.
  - Clinical investigations can have adverse side effects.
- Inform the person that no serious organic disease has been found.
- Communicate the normal clinical and test findings and be honest if there is no need for any more tests.
- If the person insists on further investigations, explain that performing unnecessary investigations can be harmful because they can cause unnecessary worry and side effects.
- Acknowledge the reality of the symptoms and do not suggest that the patient is making it up or that the symptoms are imaginary. Emphasize the need to address symptoms that cause significant distress.
- Explore the person's own explanation for the cause of the symptoms. This may give clues as to the cause; help build a trusting relationship and increase adherence to management.
- Explain that emotional suffering and stress is often linked with bodily sensations (stomach ache, muscle tension, etc.). Discuss potential links between the person's emotions/stress and symptoms.
- Encourage continuation of/gradual return to daily activities.
- *Do not* prescribe medicines (unless advised by a specialist).
- *Do not* give vitamin injections or other ineffective treatments.

Psychological interventions

A number of brief evidence-based psychological interventions have been introduced into humanitarian settings in the last few years. In low-resource and humanitarian settings, the evidence of effectiveness is limited but promising. These interventions can be used if contextually well adapted and functionally integrated into sustainable systems of care, with training and supervision.

- *Psychological first aid*: provision of supportive care to people in distress who have recently been exposed to a crisis event. The care involves assessing immediate needs and concerns; ensuring that immediate basic physical needs are met; providing or mobilizing social support; and protecting from further harm.
- *Problem-solving counselling or therapy*: focuses on identifying key problem areas contributing to the person's mental health problems which can be broken down into specific, manageable tasks for problem-solving and coping.
- *Relaxation training*: involves training the person in techniques such as breathing exercises and progressive muscle relaxation to elicit the relaxation response.
- *Cognitive behavioural therapy*: involves active symptom and activity monitoring by the patient, with the goal to change thoughts and behavioural patterns that negatively affect symptoms (generally anxiety and depression).
- *Interpersonal therapy*: is a time-limited treatment which focuses on the 'links between the person's problems with functioning, mental health symptoms, and interpersonal crises'.
- *Acceptance and mindfulness-based behavioural therapies*: new forms of psychotherapy which incorporate elements of 'mindfulness' and 'acceptance and commitment' focusing on reduction of psychological distress.
- *Eye movement desensitization and reprocessing*: aims to reduce subjective distress and strengthen adaptive beliefs. It involves focusing simultaneously on (a) associations of traumatic images, thoughts, emotions, and bodily sensations; and (b) bilateral stimulation (repeated eye movements).

In high-income countries, these therapies are provided by a psychologist with advanced training. However, with good training and supervision, non-specialists, such as social workers or community health workers, can provide adapted versions of these treatments.

Social interventions

Humanitarian emergencies disrupt social networks and often undermine mutual support mechanisms. Social isolation is a key vulnerability factor in all the mental health problems identified above. The recreation of social networks, the fostering of social space, and reconnection of families are among the most important interventions for people with mental health problems. Health workers should support any community-initiated activities that foster reconnection, and should make an effort to liaise with and connect people to agencies and groups offering social interventions. Important elements are the use of participatory approaches and the promotion of community organization, ownership, and empowerment. An example of a community-based psychosocial intervention is shown in Box 6.3.

Box 6.3 Community-based sociotherapy

- This community-based group approach was introduced in Rwanda in 2005, to work on the consequences of the 1994 genocide, and was developed from then onwards.
- Groups of community members, with different personal histories of adversity and suffering share daily problems (e.g. family conflicts, fear, mistrust, gender-based violence, stigma, and poverty), gathered in weekly group meetings over 15 weeks.
- In this process, the group functions as a therapeutic medium and facilitates the development of peer support structures. The groups are guided by trained facilitators who aim to create a safe environment, where trust, care, and respect can be (re-)built and broken social relations are restored.

Additional resources

Additional details and available manuals for low-intensity interventions that can be applied in emergency settings are available:

- World Health Organization. Problem Management Plus (PM+): Individual Psychological Help for Adults Impaired by Distress in Communities Exposed to Adversity (Generic Field-Trial Version 1.0). Geneva: WHO; 2016 (℘ http://www.who.int/mental_health/ emergencies/problem_management_plus/en/).
- World Health Organization and Columbia University. Group Interpersonal Therapy (IPT) for Depression (WHO Generic Field-Trial Version 1.0). Geneva: WHO; 2016 (℘ http://www.who.int/mental_ health/mhgap/interpersonal_therapy/en/).

Building mental health services

Health providers in humanitarian settings are unlikely to be able to do all that is required for the establishment of robust mental health services in a humanitarian setting. This requires a multipronged approach. Collaboration with communities, intersectoral health partners, and mental health professionals will be essential.

This implies enhancing human resources with training and capacity building, which is likely to require direct collaboration with a mental health professional to aid with the training and supervision.

Assessment of needs and resources

Services should not be created without a prior assessment. MHPSS assessments aim to gain a better understanding of the humanitarian situation, identify the priority issues that need attention, and the resources available to start building a response. It is important that MHPSS assessments use an intersectoral approach that not only focuses on mental disorders but also on coping mechanisms and health-seeking behaviour. In humanitarian contexts, the use of non-validated, brief symptom-rating questionnaires for PTSD and depression is not advised for routine assessments because such instruments tend to conflate 'distress' with 'disorder' and may lead to grossly distorted prevalence estimates that are programmatically irrelevant. Instead, use the estimates in ➡ Table 6.1 p. 103 for planning purposes.[5]

Integration of mental healthcare

Globally, the number of mental health specialists is insufficient and mental health services are often unavailable and inaccessible to the vast majority of people. Integration of mental health interventions within primary care systems by training general healthcare providers has the advantage of making care more accessible, cost-effective, and less stigmatizing.[6] Moreover, many people with (undetected) mental disorders will initially visit general healthcare providers.

Often the only efficient way to provide mental health services to a large population is to build the local capacity of general health workers through training and supervision through *task shifting*.

Capacity building of general health staff serves to transfer essential knowledge, help them learn useful skills, and develop the right attitudes to help others. Training should include a balanced mix of both theory and practice. Financial pressure often prompts organizations to cut practical training and supervision but short theoretical training courses on their own achieve little and may on occasion do harm, because they do not allow a time or place for trainees to discuss case-specific variations, address the problem of treatment failure and drop out, or see any patient through to recovery. See online for further information on integration of mental healthcare.[5]

Levels of integration of mental healthcare

At national level
- Advocate for incorporation of mental health into health policy and legislative frameworks.
- Advocate for adequate resources dedicated to de-centralized care.

At primary healthcare clinic
- Establish mental healthcare services at logical points of access (including emergency rooms and antenatal care).
- Ensure that clinical services are organized in ways that allow sufficient time for clinicians to see persons with mental health problems.
- Ensure an adequate and sustainable supply of psychotropic medication.
- Ensure a continuum of care in which clinical mental health interventions are done in conjunction with social and community-based activities.
- Collaborate with indigenous healing systems.

At community level
- Engage communities in mental health through open dialogue.
- Include mental health aspects in awareness-raising activities for health and social work.
- Inform the population about the availability of mental healthcare.
- Provide information and support to carers of people with severe mental disorders.
- Promote social inclusion, engagement, and participation of people recovering from mental illness.
- Involve local community structures in the identification, support, and assistance of people with severe mental disorders.

References

1. WHO, UNHCR. mhGAP Humanitarian Intervention Guide (mhGAP-HIG): Clinical Management of Mental, Neurological and Substance Use Conditions in Humanitarian Emergencies (Version 1.0). Geneva: WHO; 2015.
2. IASC. IASC Guidelines on Mental Health and Psychosocial Support in Emergency Settings. Geneva: IASC; 2007.
3. UNHCR. Operational Guidance Mental Health & Psychosocial Support Programming for Refugee Operations. Geneva: UNHCR; 2013. http://www.unhcr.org/525f94479.pdf
4. Patel V., Hanlon C. Where There Is No Psychiatrist: A Mental Health Care Manual. London: RCPsych Publications a new version 2nd edition was published in 2018.
5. WHO, UNHCR. Assessing Mental Health and Psychosocial Needs and Resources: Toolkit for Major Humanitarian Settings. Geneva: World Health Organization; 2012. http://apps.who.int/iris/bitstream/10665/76796/1/9789241548533_eng.pdf
6. WHO, UNHCR. International Medical Corps (2018) *Toolkit for the integration of mental health into general healthcare systems in humanitarian settings.* Available at: http://www.mhinnovation.net/collaborations/IMC-Mental-Health-Integration-Toolkit.

Chapter 7

Epidemiology

P. Gregg Greenough and Andrew James Willis

Introduction

- With increasing complexity, humanitarian scenarios demand expert responders guided by data that measure the effectiveness of the humanitarian response. The phrase 'evidence-based approach' is common in all areas of medicine today, and is rightly becoming more prominent for humanitarian activities. At the onset of a crisis, data from rapid assessments determine population needs, identify who is doing what, and give responders a sense of the resources required to meet needs. For more sustained programmes, data identify priorities for action and gauge the adequacy of the response.
- Humanitarian stakeholders, led by the *UN OCHA as cluster lead for information management*, have demonstrated a commitment towards this evidence-driven decision-making, calling on policy and research leaders in all cluster sections to push for this common goal.[1] Although humanitarian work can often be overwhelming, clarifying the underlying issues and focusing efforts on areas of maximal impact can be of great benefit. The science of identifying public health trends in a population— epidemiology—has the potential to offer this clarification.
- The first step is considering: *what kinds of information address the health needs of the affected population in a humanitarian crisis?*
- To answer this question, the medical provider working in humanitarian crises must see health through a population lens and shift focus from individual patient care to population care, essentially public health.

This chapter aims to provide the reader with a basic understanding of how epidemiology can guide humanitarian health operations and programming. It examines the major forms in which epidemiology is practised in the field: basic data management, performing health assessments, managing surveillance systems, monitoring health indicators, and conducting field studies. In doing so it will give the reader the fundamentals necessary to understand, interpret, and use data in the humanitarian context.

Data management

Humanitarian aid increasingly relies on an ongoing collection of data to govern response priorities; however, the reality is that data in the humanitarian sphere may be less available, less reliable, and more difficult to collect. Especially during emergencies, keeping quality statistics about the response can be very difficult. Nevertheless, this information is vital to tracking the progression of a response, assessing services, informing resource allocation, and providing accountability.

Data usage classification in the humanitarian sector:
• *Internal data*: that which guides programme activities (e.g. audits for donors, monitored programme outputs or resources, and adherence to protocols).
• *External data*: that meant for the wider audience of stakeholders (e.g. advocacy campaigns, and sharing regional disease rates with other NGOs).

Types of data

• *Qualitative data* are not numeric values or simple true–false dichotomies. Qualitative data is useful for inquiries on perceptions and explanations, and generally obtained by open-ended questions.
• *Quantitative data* are numerically measured and allow one to draw conclusions between characteristics of a general population and health outcomes.

While this chapter deals largely with quantitative data, many of the principles can be applied to qualitative data as well. Qualitative information has an important role in humanitarian work because, while quantitative data can describe *what* is occurring, qualitative data can, if done correctly, portray an idea of *why* things are occurring. This type of data, in the form of stories, can represent a strong means of recounting the lives of peoples living in crisis. This is especially important for the purpose of advocacy, and efforts should be made to collect and share these stories.

Data collection

Recognizing the multiple demands in the field, it can be difficult for health providers to facilitate both healthcare provision and data collection at the same time. However, even in resource poor settings, efforts should be made to electronically collect data from written registries to ensure easier analysis, longevity, sharing, and security of the data in the case of evacuation.

It is important to identify the most critical indicators based on the programme needs and work, and aim to reliably capture this data. To facilitate this, it may be useful to *designate a staff member specifically trained for data management* to oversee the collection of data, including following up on incomplete data, and to enter written information into an electronic database.

What to collect

In a healthcare setting, some data are generally essential such as age, sex, and disease of patients, and dates and descriptions of activities for logistic health system support. Establish which additional pieces of information are necessary. Ensure that all variables can be useful for *informing programme decisions* as collecting extra data can add unnecessary time. Monitor this data collection and follow-up with those who collect or fill in data forms incorrectly.

One category of commonly missed data is resource consumption. Although it can be difficult to record what resources are used, especially during an emergency, this information can be essential for later planning or informing future interventions.

External sources of data

During circumstances that require external health structure support, epidemic management, or an emergency response, it may be necessary to regularly collect information from both internal programme sources as well as external sources, such as the MOH, or other NGOs. Be sure to consider the data quality of all sources, internal and external, and be wary of attributing equal weight to all evidence (see ➲ p. 136). Use of external data is discussed in further detail in the sections ➲ 'Health assessment' pp. 138–41 and ➲ 'Surveillance systems' pp. 142–4.

Data quality

Just as important as collecting data is assessing the *quality* of data. In the humanitarian setting, it can sometimes be difficult to gather reliable information. This does not mean this data cannot be factored into decision-making but rather that the limitations of the data must be understood.

In resource-poor settings, understanding the limitations of the data is as important as collecting it.

When collecting data internally, the best way to ensure data quality is to have standardized definitions and means of collecting the data.

In the humanitarian field, high staff turnover and changing programme priorities can make longitudinal analysis, the comparison of results over time, difficult. When collecting data make sure to take into account any change in data collection methods over the life of the programme as this may impact how results are compared to each other, as seen in Example 1.

Reporting

The most important data to report are often the most basic. Those deemed essential, as just discussed in the 'Data quality' section, should make up the basis of any report. Look for changes from one period to another or long-term trends.

Example 1: longitudinal malaria analysis

A project is assessing 10-year malaria incidence to determine long-term trends that could have implications for ordering drugs and advocacy. In the early years of the project, malnutrition and diarrhoeal diseases were of the utmost importance and malaria was considered an endemic disease and not the major concern. As such, a patient with a positive rapid test for malaria but also exhibiting malnutrition was classified as a case of malnutrition as opposed to malaria. This change in data collection may indicate a falsely lower incidence of malaria in earlier years, making current numbers seem excessively high in comparison.

Assessing trends

When providing some form of analysis, it is critical to keep in mind that not all increases are the same. Look at the changes in disease trends according to number and percentage. If cases increase from 10 to 15, it is 5 additional cases and a 50% increase.

Be wary of providing too much interpretation without deep understanding of the programme context and process. If widely unexpected data are found, check data quality and if the trends appear to be correct more information and perhaps a field assessment could be required.

Figures and tables

Charts are invaluable for describing findings and organizing them in a clear way. Bar and lines graphs, shown in Fig. 7.1, are easily understandable ways of visualizing trends.

Use of data

From a field perspective, the principle importance of maintaining data is to inform field decisions, this includes ordering drugs, identifying locations requiring assistance, and planning service delivery. At higher levels, data can be used for a variety of reasons including advocacy, accountability, and planning. Reporting often serves as a discussion tool and can inform any changes to the data collection process.

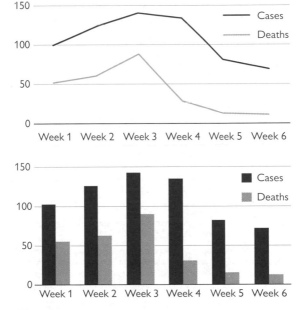

Fig. 7.1 Figures for representing data.

Health assessments

Before a programme can even be started, efforts must be made to understand the population being served. Health assessments help by characterizing the general population in a programme catchment area. This includes capturing predominantly quantitative data such as disease case numbers, vaccination rates, or household income as well as considerable qualitative information on the values of the population and their perception of the services rendered. This information is then used to guide the response. While essential prior to beginning a response, assessments should also be done throughout a response to ensure the programme is relevant and effective.

The most important part of performing an assessment is visiting the affected area. Information gathered from afar can be helpful but a site visit is necessary to provide the most useful and accurate information. Bring local partners who can translate local dialects and understand local culture.

Population estimates

Establishing population size is a necessary part of an assessment because it is used to establish a denominator from which rates and proportions can be derived to determine the extent of an issue. For example, the level of malnutrition within a population of children aged >5 years requires the total number of children in that age group at risk. This can be a challenge in the field due to unavailable or unreliable census data as well as continued population movement. Government census data, though not always entirely accurate, can provide some indications. Distribution lists or camp registration lists from WFP or UNHCR are helpful, especially in refugee settings. If feasible in size and relatively static, the population of interest can be counted manually using on-the-ground techniques or sampled using overhead images.

Rapid assessments

During an emergency, initial responders need to determine how early interventions should be targeted to provide the most benefit with the limited early resources, or whether indeed an intervention is warranted. Rapid assessments are performed to quickly identify:

- *who* is affected
- *how* they are affected (degree and causes of morbidity and mortality)
- *what* sector-specific needs they may have (shelter, water, sanitation, food, health, security)
- *where* the affected are located
- *impact* on infrastructure (transportation, communication, hospitals, power, and public services).

In the chaos of first response, there is often an overlap of efforts due to the legions of NGOs and multilateral organizations doing assessments. While not always well coordinated amongst responders, the aggregate information, managed by the OCHA, can provide a shared knowledge for all shareholders.

Multi-Cluster/Sector Initial Rapid Assessment (MIRA)

MIRA is a guidance document for the collection and management of rapid assessment data in crises. This framework, managed by UN OCHA, contains tools for data collection by all sectors in a response; these tools facilitate evaluation of the impact, scale, and severity of a sudden disaster. MIRA can be found here:

https://www.humanitarianresponse.info/en/programme-cycle/space/document/multi-sector-initial-rapid-assessment-guidance-revision-july-2015

Types of information needed

While the information needed is shaped by the type of response the organization is mounting, such as vaccination campaigns or water and sanitation, some general information should be collected to provide an overall picture of the communities visited.

Basic information that should be gathered on most health assessments includes:

- new diseases or changes in pattern
- new or different presentations of disease
- most common diseases and their trends
- proximity to clean water
- access to maternal health
- proximity to health structures
- access to affordable care and treatments
- economic stability
- principal sources of income
- previous emergencies
- relevant security concerns.

The local priority for a village may not align with the expertise of the visiting organization. Though the assessment leader may be involved in treating disease, the most important need could be water and hygiene. This can indicate a point where cooperation or information sharing with another NGO could be helpful.

Assessment of lead poisoning crisis

It is important not to become focused on any single indicator, as initial reports can sometimes be confused and the situation in the field could be very different than expected. This was demonstrated during the investigations into the largest incident of lead poisoning in history, in Zamfara, Nigeria, which was originally believed to be a severe local increase in malaria. The neurotoxic effects of lead were confused for similar neurological effects of severe malaria and reported to MSF surveillance as cerebral malaria. In this case, had an assessment focused solely on identifying positive rapid malaria detection tests at the local health post, it would have found only a moderate, seasonal elevation. Fortunately, by speaking with people in the village in a more thorough assessment, MSF confirmed reports of locally increased artisanal mining.

Community baseline

During emergencies it is necessary to focus not only on current events but also determine recent history as well. Attempt to judge a community's baseline health status as well as its resilience:

• Has the community encountered a similar problem in the past?
• How did they deal with it then?
• What common issues were present before the emergency?

While the emergency may indicate the most pressing current issue, a brief discussion of common diseases or seasonal issues (such as flooding) can indicate what to mitigate against.

Corroborating information

Verifying information is important when piecing together a confusing situation in an unfamiliar area. This ensures that the most important concerns are understood. Verification can be as simple as witnessing the effects of an event—a recently destroyed building or set of dug graves—which can help clarify the timeline or the impact.

For disease outbreaks, it is important to physically see patients whenever possible. This helps understand the disease presentation and affected population. Identifying sick individuals in the general population can indicate a bigger issue than isolated cases in health facilities so look for signs that point to the extent of a problem.

Sources of information

The most difficult aspect of assessments is finding accurate, credible, and timely sources of information. This is especially true for rapid assessments following emergencies where previously available information may have been destroyed.

Activities that generate important sources of information include:

• assessing infrastructure
• visiting health structures
• meeting community elders
• meeting police and emergency services
• collaborating with local NGOs
• visiting affected populations.

Key informants

While it may not always yield quantitative data, simply talking to people in the affected area often provides the most critical information. When on an assessment be sure to talk to key people in health facilities, in traditional and political leadership roles, as well as those most closely affected. Often it is necessary to seek out marginalized populations as they will have a less prominent voice.

Even if numerical data are not procured this way these discussions provide valuable context and may show an assessment team where to find numbers.

Community health facilities

In most community health facilities some form of registry is usually kept. Reviewing this can give an indication of common medical problems as well as dispensing practices. This information can be corroborated by talking to health workers as well as community members. Unfortunately, it is often difficult to ascertain longitudinal data that can point to changes in trends over time. However, health staff may be able to provide some perspective on previous trends.

Local partners

Other NGOs, including local organizations, can also provide valuable information. Local NGOs are often happy to partner with international organizations. In an emergency, it can be difficult to organize activities between NGOs but try to determine whether someone has already gathered reliable information from the area of concern that they will share.

Leaving the assessment area

When performing an assessment, it is important to be frank about the possible services the organization can provide. It can be difficult to visit villages that have endured lasting neglect but may, at the time, have less significant health concerns than another village. The population will no doubt desire some form of assistance so it is important to *acknowledge that the concerns of the village are real while also explaining the organization mandate* and how resources are allocated.

Surveillance systems

Surveillance is a continuous collection of specific data, tracked through a net-work, that is regularly analysed. While assessments attempt to determine the current health status of the population, *surveillance looks to monitor health status over time*. This data collection network functions as an early warning system to detect changes in health status and initiate a rapid response.

Establishing a surveillance mechanism is a top priority in emergency response activities to rapidly detect health issues, but is also useful for ongoing routine health monitoring of the affected population. As a mechanism of capacity building, surveillance systems can later provide a foundation for health information systems within a reconstructed, post-crisis public health infrastructure.

Types of surveillance

How data are recorded depends on if a surveillance system is active or passive and whether there is a need to capture every case (such as during outbreaks, emergency responses, or disease elimination campaigns) or if the emphasis is more on routine, non-outbreak monitoring.

- *Active systems:*
  - A central organization actively solicits information from a network of trained providers who record cases regularly.
  - Cases are reported to the centre at specified intervals.
  - This centre 'actively' solicits providers to send data and fill in missing fields; it also analyses data logs from surveillance sites regularly.
  - Most emergencies require an active system.
- *Passive systems:*
  - More common in pre- or post-crisis phases.
  - Depends on providers to record and send data as they become aware of them.
  - Passive systems are cheaper and less labour intensive to maintain, but provide less complete data than active systems and are thus less sensitive to changes in events when they occur.
  - System is generally more realistic in the long term.

Setting up surveillance systems

Establishing a functioning health surveillance system requires collaboration across a network of stakeholders who all understand the goals and roles of each part of the system. At its most basic levels, surveillance systems need a number of steps in place:

- *Recruitment of surveillance sites*: sites should be visited and have staff trained. As many sites should be recruited as resources allow.
- *Appropriate collection of data from primary sources*: log books, registries, or patient charts should be as complete as possible.
- *Aggregating data at health/provider structures*: data compilation is often done by data managers, heads of health centres, or government officials such as epidemiologists.
- *Transmission of data to central point*: transmission of data must be done regularly with a stable point of contact (active or passive).
- *Compiling data from multiple centres*: differences in population and data quality must be taken into account.
- *Analysis and interpretation*: some analysis may be needed before reporting, such as calculation of relative risk (RR) or rates.

Interpretation can require specific knowledge of the region, disease, and data limitations (see Box 7.1).

• *Sharing of data with partners:* results should be shared with all of the partners within the surveillance network.

The reliability of surveillance data is only as good as the weakest step. Excellent analysis can mean very little if collection of patient data is poor, just as poor interpretation of well-documented data can undermine the usefulness of the system.

Box 7.1 Thresholds

A threshold is a data point which, when exceeded, is used to indicate that an assessment is necessary. Establishing a threshold for specific diseases or indicators can take some of the need for interpretation out of surveillance data analysis. Thresholds should take into account global standards (such as for mortality rates) whenever possible but also adapt to the local context. Establishing appropriate thresholds requires good data, adequate understanding of the context, and good initial consultation. This is especially pertinent in surveillance to ensure timely responses if thresholds are exceeded.

Surveillance data

Establishing a surveillance system first requires determining which diseases or conditions are to be monitored. This can be targeted, such as during an outbreak, or be more general for overarching health monitoring. Every crisis context is unique and tracked diseases need to be tailored. In emergencies, mortality, nutritional states, and high-impact communicable disease are commonly tracked.

Simple early systems generally follow:

• mortality (crude and under age 5 years)
• causes of mortality
• Cases of lethal communicable diseases, including:
  • non-bloody diarrhoea (unspeciated)
  • bloody diarrhoea
  • meningitis (bacterial)
  • measles
  • acute respiratory infection
  • malaria.

Example 2: surveillance following the Haitian earthquake

Following the 2010 earthquake in Haiti, the international community worked with the Haitian MOH to establish a network of 51 health facilities across the country. Prior to the event, the Haitian MOH was tracking only six infectious diseases. After the earthquake, and with support from the US Centers for Disease Control and Prevention (CDC), the Haitian MOH expanded this list to 25, customizing it for the health effects of the earthquake and massive population displacement. For example, renal failure (from crush injuries), injuries, malaria, typhoid, and diarrhoeal illness were highlighted. This adapted surveillance network fortunately served to identify the first cases of cholera in October 2010, a disease which was not included in the former surveillance system.

Case definitions

After determining a list of desired health outcomes, use of standardized case definitions is critical. Since most health facilities lack point-of-care diagnostic testing in a crisis, syndromic case definitions, which rely primarily on symptoms rather than laboratory diagnostics, are generally used.

Examples of syndromic case definitions:
- Diarrhoeal illness: three or more loose or watery stools in a 24-hour period, with or without dehydration.
- Measles: a maculopapular rash and cough, coryza, or red eyes.

> The WHO Communicable Disease Control in Emergencies updated field manual lists common case definitions (and reporting forms) (see ℅ www. who.int/diseasecontrol_emergencies/publications/9241546166/en/).

Cases are generally identified as either:
- *'suspect'*: a case which meets the syndromic case definition
- *'probable'*: a suspect case also having other clinical or epidemiological evidence such as a link to another case, or
- *'confirmed'*: a case identified through laboratory tests.

Limitations of surveillance systems

Surveillance systems have a practical value as monitoring and early warning systems; however, there are limitations to their use.

Data limitation

Surveillance network data lack the sensitivity to capture every case and so do not reflect the true incidence or prevalence rates for a given disease. Further, most surveillance systems cannot inherently explain why changes in health outcomes occur over time or the reasons for improvements or failures in a given health programme.

Challenges in maintaining networks

Initial establishment of the system requires advanced coordination and training. Longer term, however, it can be difficult to maintain quality data while turnover and fatigue replace the initial enthusiasm for the system. This can be especially true of diseases that are infrequent. Regular follow-up in the field is often needed to maintain reliable data collection.

Health indicators

In humanitarian settings, there is a degree of standardization of key indicators which allow measurable outcomes and reflect the health of a population during crises. Various efforts have been made to guide which indicators are most important in a given situation. These include the following:

- UN OCHA: a source for sets of indicators specific to sector clusters that can be used to track a variety of activities and monitor the status of the populations in need (ℳ https://www.humanitarianresponse.info/node/24/indicators).
- The Sphere guidelines: a source of potential indicators that specifically identify basic living conditions that are especially useful during assessments (ℳ http://www.sphereproject.org).

Though indicators should be tailored to each programme, the following are types of indicators that are commonly seen in humanitarian operations.

Measures of proportion

Measures of proportion are most commonly expressed as percentages, but can also be expressed as a ratio (e.g. children are four times more likely to be out of school than in school, or 4:1). Though often used interchangeably, the terms proportion, percentage, ratio, and rate have some arithmetic and conceptual differences:

- *Proportion:* number of individuals with a characteristic as a share of total population, expressed as a fraction of a whole number, e.g. one-fifth of all deaths in a population due to violence.
- *Percentage:* a proportion expressed as per 100 people using 'per cent' or '%' instead of the denominator, e.g. 20% of the deaths in a population due to violence.
- *Ratio:* relative sizes of populations with and without a characteristic, e.g. 1 out of 5 deaths due to violence, would be a ratio of 1:4.
- *Rate:* number of events by unit of time, e.g. deaths due to violence in a village in a given month. Commonly used in humanitarian settings, mortality rates are expressed as number of deaths in a population over a specific time period.

Person time

Rates can be described by different units that include aspects of person and time. Often rates are described solely by the time frame, e.g. three cases/month. In this example, the person aspect is assumed to be the population in the area being monitored, meaning the rate is really three cases/month/area.

Another way of describing rates is in person days. This is a measure of time across a population. It allows comparison of rates between areas of different population sizes. Person days are calculated by multiplying the number of days in the observation period (30 days for a month) by the number of people in the data catchment area. The number of outcomes (e.g. deaths) are then divided by the number of person days and multiplied by 10,000 to give the number of outcomes that occur in 10,000 person days.

Mortality

Mortality rates are the most commonly used measures to quickly assess health status in an emergency. They can reflect death in the general population or a patient population.

- *Crude mortality rate (CMR)*: deaths/population size at risk during specific unit of time (e.g. region A has one death per 10,000 person days).
- *Age-specific mortality rate* (such as under-5 mortality rate (U5MR)): deaths in age group/population of specific age group at risk during specific period (e.g. two deaths in children under 5 years in 10,000 person days).
- *Group-specific mortality rate* (such as maternal mortality ratio (MMR)): deaths in sub-group/population of sub-group at risk during specific period (e.g. four maternal deaths in reproductive age women in 10,000 person days).
- *Cause-specific mortality rate* (especially violent vs non-violent): deaths due to specific disease or cause/population at risk during specific period (e.g. five cases of malaria deaths in the population per 10,000 person days).
- *Proportional mortality*: proportion of deaths due to specific cause/total number of deaths during specific period (e.g. 20% of deaths were due to violence of all deaths).
- *Case fatality rate (CFR)*: deaths due to specific cause/number of cases of cause in specific period (e.g. 50% of severe malaria cases died in period).

Morbidity

Morbidity can be presented as a prevalence or an incidence:

- *Prevalence*: the proportion of individuals in a population with a specific condition at a point in time (e.g. 50% of a village is suffering from symptoms of acute watery diarrhoea at time of assessment).
- *Incidence*: the number of new cases/or new presentations of a specific condition during a period of time (e.g. 40 people presented to the facility for symptoms of acute watery diarrhoea in the last month).

Many diseases have a specific form that indicates a more severe presentation (neurological symptoms with malaria, neuropathy with diabetes, infection with trauma). Seeing more cases of severe disease can suggest that something different is occurring. Reasons for more severe disease could include a new more virulent serotype, or a population reluctant to come to clinic. Both situations will require some form of follow-up.

Indication of the severity of illness may include:

- disease-specific admissions
- severe disease presentations
- per cent positivity (when rapid or other testing is available).

Nutritional status

Nutritional surveys are the best way to determine the burden of malnutrition on a population. This is commonly done by using coloured bands to measure the mid-upper arm circumference (MUAC) of children under the age of 5 years. Surveys will be discussed later in this chapter (see ➌ 'Field studies' pp. 149–54).

The two most commonly used measures of malnutrition:
- *Severe acute malnutrition (SAM)*: proportion of children age <5 years with weight-for-height ratio of <3 standard deviations (red on MUAC band)/total population children age <5 years.
- *Global acute malnutrition (GAM)*: proportion of children age <5 years with weight-for-height ratio of <2 standard deviations (red and orange on MUAC band)/total population children age <5 years.

Programme-specific measures

Programme-specific indicators are tailored to the information needs of the programme. A hospital, for example, may use length of stay or bed occupancy to measure its services, outbreak management will monitor the number of new contacts attached to each case, and a sanitation project may look at wells requiring repair.

Programme-specific indicators can be categorized as follows:
- *Resources*: resources invested in an initiative (e.g. financial and human). Tracking resources allows better planning.
- *Activities*: activities conducted in pursuit of objectives (e.g. a sanitation and hygiene sensitization public awareness session with 45 attendees).
- *Outcomes*: short- and medium-term results at population level (e.g. 40% increase in hand washing with soap before eating).
- *Impact*: long-term changes within the population due to the initiative (e.g. 80% decrease in under-five diarrhoeal disease incidence).

These indicators are generally used to describe programme performance and plan future decisions. In many cases, programme indicators serve as a benchmark for setting goals.

Measures of association

Measures of association, such as RRs (or risk ratios) and odds ratios (ORs), are less regularly used but nevertheless, provide powerful tools for understanding risk factors around a condition. The calculations, though fairly simple, are generally reserved for periodic analysis as opposed to regular reporting.

Uses for measures of associations can include the following:
- Outbreak settings: e.g. drinking from well A gives a ten times larger risk of diarrhoeal disease than well B, which would point to well A as the source of infection.
- Identifying problem areas: e.g. those in region A have a five times greater risk of experiencing violence than those in region B.
- Identifying those most vulnerable: e.g. females are three times more likely to suffer from sexual violence than males.

Relative risk

RR is the probability of developing a disease when having a specific exposure. It is often used to describe the size of an exposure's, or risk's, effect. A value of 1 means there is no change in disease frequency with exposure. With a value >1 the exposure increases the risk of disease while an exposure with a RR <1 is protective against the disease.

These calculations are easily made by dividing data into a four-by-four table (see Table 7.1) where

Table. 7.1 Four-by-four table		
	Disease	No disease
Exposed	A	B
Unexposed	C	D

$$RR = [A/(A+B)]/[C/(C+D)]$$

Odds ratio

Just as an RR identifies the risk, the OR describes the odds of getting a disease given a specific exposure compared to the odds of getting a disease without the exposure. This is more often used in academic studies than field settings. It best describes the strength of association.

Field studies

Sometimes a more detailed, in-depth, and narrow analysis is required than can be gleaned from common methods of data collection. This may require a field study, such as a survey. Studies involve more robust methods, such as population sampling size calculation and random sampling, and more thorough analysis, including statistical significance. Often this requires head-quarters (HQ) or epidemiologist support, nevertheless, an understanding of these concepts helps to recognize when and how field studies can support a project.

Key terms and concepts

Variable

An attribute of the population being studied such as age, gender, education level, access to healthcare, poverty, etc. Multiple variables can measure a characteristic in different ways. For example, wealth might be measured as household income (a number) or whether income is below a national poverty line (yes or no).

A variable is considered independent if it is known or presumed to cause a change in another dependent variable. For instance, sun exposure is an independent variable while sun burn is a related outcome, or dependent variable. Sun exposure is unaffected by a sun burn, but a sun burn is affected by sun exposure.

Confounding variable

A confounder is a variable not included in the analysis that is correlated with both the independent and dependent variables. At times, the confounding variable may not be obvious. For example, a disease may be more common in lowlands, but also where more slums are located; a study can conclude that the poor are more likely to contract the disease but in fact it is the geography that the poor inhabit not the poverty itself. Methods should be assessed so as to control for confounding variables and they should be accounted for in analyses.

Preparing for a study

Before beginning a study, it is important to establish a clear purpose. Why is this study necessary for the programme and how will it be used?

Designing a study question

A study's direction takes the form of a clear study question. *What does the study hope to assess?* A good study question is concise and, most importantly, achievable. A mortality study may, for example, want to identify the three most common causes of mortality in the catchment area, while a nutritional survey may attempt to assess the amount of severe acute malnutrition in a refugee camp.

Who will be studied?

The *study population* is the actual group being examined. Remember that study results are not necessarily *generalizable* outside of the study population; a study of children in Canada cannot necessarily be generalized to children in Angola.

- A population can be defined demographically (age, gender, ethnicity, etc.), geographically (urban, rural), or by other study-specific criteria.
- Segments within a population, such as a household or individuals, are the units of observation, and the basis for analysis.

When will the study take place?

It is important to ensure that results are not skewed by temporal events. For example, clinic registries may show fewer patients, which may be due to decreased access during the rainy season, rather than evidence of a healthier population. Finally, for planning purposes, study logistics can be affected by aspects such as rainfall, temperature, and road conditions.

Types of studies

- *Surveys* tend to be the most common form of humanitarian-based field study. They collect variables at a single point in time in the past. As such, they require only a single visit to each participant.
- *Cohort* studies follow a population for a period of time and assess the frequency and factors that affect a specific outcome.
- *Case–control* studies are generally used for interventions. They look at outcomes of those who received an intervention (cases) and compare them against controls that do not.

Sampling methods

Once the target population and timeline are established it is important to determine the methods through which data will be collected. Sampling refers to the systematic way data are gathered to ensure high data quality.

Probability sampling

Probability sampling uses random selection to try and reduce bias, so the study sample can be considered *representative* of the larger population.

- *Simple random sampling*: participants are randomly selected from a list, such as a registration list from a refugee camp.
- *Systematic random sampling*: participants are selected at specific intervals, i.e. every fifth name, from a population list beginning at a random point.
- *Cluster sampling*: when no sampling list is available, the population of interest is organized into clustered areas from which they can be randomly selected.

Example 3: random sampling

Suppose you wanted to know the degree of severe malnutrition within the community for which your organization provides therapeutic feeding. If only those presenting to clinics were sampled, you would miss those who were too ill to make it and subsequently died without accessing care, essentially 'under-representing' the true impact on the community. Random sampling minimizes this type of inherent bias by allowing everyone a chance to be chosen. It also allows you to apply statistics to the sample data in a way to estimate how close your sample outcome is to the true population figure and quantify how precise the results are.

- A field primer on how this is practically done is available online: ✍ http://odihpn.org/wp-content/uploads/2005/09/networkpaper052.pdf.

Non-probability sampling

A lack of randomization in non-probability-based samples means that respondents do not have equal chances of being selected. Such methods are employed for ease of access or for difficult-to-reach populations. Unfortunately, this type of sampling is not very representative of the general population.

- *Convenience sampling*: respondents are selected because they are easily accessed or readily available.
- *Snowball sampling*: referred by other respondents for reasons specific to the study objective.
- *Purposive sampling*: sought out for a specific reason based on the study objectives.

Sample size calculation

- For each probability-based survey, a sample size must be calculated to ensure the number of respondents necessary to detect whether findings are representative of the total population, or whether there is an actual difference between two populations. For example, sampling six people in Mexico City will not be representative of its other millions of inhabitants.
- Sample size calculation takes into account the estimated prevalence of the outcome of interest and the desired precision:
  - More precision or a rarer variable requires larger sample sizes.
  - The sample size should also account for possible non-response, those who choose not to participate, by adding another 10% to the calculated sample.
  - Sample size calculators can be found online such as the emergency nutrition assessment (ENA) tools found at: ✍ http://smartmethodology.org/.

Principles of study ethics

Similar standards to the informed consent process in clinical settings are used in public health research, with the caveat that humanitarian populations are uniquely vulnerable.

Valid informed consent

Valid informed consent contains three elements:

- Disclosure: researchers must explain the purposes of the study and provide the subject with clear information to allow the subject to make an informed decision.
- Capacity: subjects must be able to understand the information provided and draw a reasonable decision to participate based on that.
- Voluntariness: a subject's decision must not be subject to external forces, such as coercion or expectation of reward.

Special considerations

- In cases where the participant is illiterate, verbal consent that meets the above-mentioned criteria for valid informed consent may be acceptable.

- In most countries, the legal age for consent is 18 years.
- There are specific WHO recommendations for children >12 years of age that should be understood and followed.

In humanitarian crises, study respondents' participation in a study need to be assessed for any detrimental unintended consequences. For this reason, *review boards* may be organized at the local or national level for understanding the nuances of the population as well as an institutional board (an academic institution or an iNGO with an established research record). In general, no research should be done on displaced populations if it could be performed on non-displaced populations and if it is not likely to result in direct benefit to the population.

Ethical considerations
While the content of the informed consent process should be tailored to the study, certain information should be present in any informed consent script or process. The WHO Ethics Review Committee (ERC) has also created template informed consent and assent forms that may be adapted for specific studies, as well as other useful guidelines for planning and implementing informed consent protocols. These are available at:

⅋ http://www.who.int/rpc/research_ethics/informed_consent/en/.

Collecting data

Measurement tools are ways to collect data in an organized way. Often this tool is a questionnaire with a list of questions that are encoded into a database for storage and analysis but it could also include recording cases from a hospital. Traditionally, instruments have been paper based; however, new mobile technologies such as hand-held devices are becoming available to facilitate electronic data transfer, and increase data security.

Setting the tone
Before beginning a discussion on survey construction, a word about the importance of introducing oneself and the questionnaire. Politeness, respectfulness, and thoughtful explanations enhance good will and encourage higher participation and completion rates. Each section of the survey deserves its own preface. When embarking with a respondent on each new phase of inquiry, pause and relay to the respondent the next line of questioning. This encourages understanding, builds trust, improves survey reliability, and gives the participant an opportunity to opt out if they feel uncomfortable.

Choosing a questionnaire
- Using previously administered questionnaires has advantages since most have undergone scrutiny to ensure validity, reliability, availability, and ease of administration. A search of reports written by responders from previous humanitarian crises is a good place to start. Other formal and standardized examples include (but are not limited to):
  - the Multiple Indicator Cluster Survey (MICS) from UNICEF
    (⅋ https://www.unicef.org/statistics/index_24302.html)

- Demographic and Health Surveys (DHS) from USAID (✀ https://dhsprogram.com/)
- MSF surveys
- rapid health assessment surveys put forth by WHO
- the inter-agency Standardized Monitoring and Assessment of Relief in Transitions (SMART) surveys (✀ http://smartmethodology.org/)
- the US CDC National Health and Nutrition Examination Surveys (NHANES) (✀ https://www.cdc.gov/nchs/nhanes/).

- Survey questionnaires should be *piloted*, or tested, in focus groups to ensure clarity, understanding, and cultural appropriateness. Finally, select a small subset of the population to test the entire process with an eye to making changes with the feedback.

Asking a better question and getting a better answer
Once the question type is determined, the questions themselves can be refined to elicit good, reliable answers by reflecting on the nature of the respondent, time period for recall, and question construction.

Who answers the question?
- Ensure that questions are translated into local languages and subsequently back-translated to fully understand what is being asked.
- Where observable details may be culturally ambiguous, balance cultural appropriateness with what is acceptable/easy to discern.
- Whichever the chosen method, strive for consistency and reliability.

Choosing a recall period
- Asking respondents about events that happened in the past (retrospectively) requires recall.
- Aim for a viable recall period that is large enough to encapsulate relevant information but isn't so large that your respondent will have difficulty answering accurately.
- Use locally recognizable time-points such as holidays or seasonal activities to provide a reference point for a respondent.

Analysing and distributing data
Consider the ways in which an analysis of data will have meaning to those in the field who need to interpret and act on it. It is important to remember that an analysis outcome showing statistical significance does not mean the outcome has any practical purpose for the programme. Be sure to think back to the original study purpose when doing analysis.

Descriptive analytics
Descriptive analytics provide a description of the population in ways that are simple and relevant, such as the 'percentage of females under age 5 that are malnourished'. Examples include simple counts (five malnourished children), measures of proportion, or health indicators (discussed in ➜ 'Health indicators' pp. 145–8). Consider the ways in which the analysis can inform those in the field.

Inferential analytics
Inferential analytics are more complicated than descriptive analytics and relate the strength of association between independent variables and dependent ones. These are more complex analyses that may require specific software and technical expertise. The RR and OR (discussed in ➲ 'Health indicators' pp. 145–8), may serve as fairly simple forms of analysing associations between different study variables. Consider the example that a child attending school is 43% less likely to later live in poverty. This makes an association between school attendance (independent variable) and later poverty (dependent).

> *Example 4: using inferential analytics*
> A water and sanitation NGO develops a new sealed well that it believes will protect drinking water supplies from leeching flood water. But does it? To answer that question, a field study that measures the cases of watery diarrhoea (dependent variable) in one village with the new wells (independent variable) and another similar village without these wells could be done with the application of statistics to determine the likelihood of developing diarrhoea between the two villages, and make an inference whether the wells protect against developing diarrhoea in the greater population.

Correlation and causation
Be careful when interpreting data as correlation alone does not imply causation. For example, a rise in malaria cases may coincide with an increase in overall mortality. These additional deaths *could* be from malaria but, alternatively, the malaria season could also happen to occur when a conflict resumed in the area. In both cases, the malaria and deaths are correlated but only in the first case is the malaria causative of the deaths. Ensure that the data clearly supports any conclusions being made.

Sharing results
Most studies are done in partnership with local organizations and it is important to share findings back with them. Consider the audience when determining how findings and level of detail are presented and which format is best used; strongly consider sharing the findings with other groups, such as UN OCHA and the cluster system, as such analyses may be useful for planning or spur more research.

Reference
1. Foran MP, Greenough PG, Thow A, Gilman D, Schütz A, Chandran R, et al. Identification of current priorities for research in humanitarian action: proceedings of the First Annual UN OCHA Policy and Research Conference. Prehosp Disast Med 2012;27(3):260–6.

Understanding economic effects of humanitarian intervention

Dirk-Jan Omtzigt

Introduction

Humanitarians make a multitude of decisions that have both short- and long-term economic consequences for both the people that are assisting and the host community in which they operate. Humanitarians are guided by the *do no harm principle*, which finds its origin in medical ethics, but this principle should be applied beyond the medical realm, to the society at large and the economy in particular.

This chapter aims to provide economic context and considerations to assist the medical professional working in a complex emergency to apply the *do no harm principle* in economic terms. The early sections of the chapter provide a broad understanding of the economic context and the relationship between development, vulnerability, and aid. The second half of the chapter covers the implications of aid, including the practical application of economic principles for the field worker. While some of the content may not be directly actionable by all humanitarian providers, an understanding of these principles, especially by those who have input in shaping programming, is essential for ensuring the positive short- and long-term consequences of their interventions.

Core principles: economic development and vulnerability

Development economics is an academic discipline which deals with economic aspects of the development process in LIC. Within this broad topic, rather than an analysis of drivers of (under-) development, this chapter will provide an overview to allow an understanding of what economic development is and how humanitarian interventions impact this.

Economic development has been dramatically uneven and differences between countries are enormous. Illustrated by a comparison of growth trajectory between South Korea and the Democratic Republic of the Congo (DRC), after the Korean War, South Korea was one of the world's poorest countries with only $64 per capita income. In the early 1960s, it lagged behind DRC, which had a per capita income double that of South Korea. As of today, however, DRC has not seen any significant economic development since and currently ranks at the bottom of the UN Human Development Index. Meanwhile, South Korea has seen great development and has a per capita income 110 times as high as DRC.

Income disparities are growing

Income disparities have also grown over time. In 2014, gross domestic product (GDP; or income, in current USD) per capita in the US was >$54,629. In contrast, income per capita was $7757 in Botswana, $1650 in India, and a mere $253 in Malawi. (See Fig 8.1.) That means that the income per capita in the US is more than 200 times the income in Malawi, where the average person survives on $0.69 per day. Further, there is not just a high degree of income inequality between countries but also within countries Seven of the ten most unequal countries in the world are in Africa, most in southern Africa.[1]

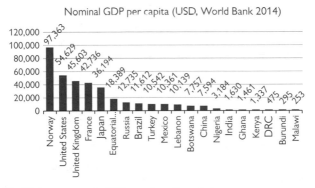

Nominal GDP per capita (USD, World Bank 2014)

Fig. 8.1 Income per capita. GDP, gross domestic product.

Global poverty is falling but is persistent in many places. (See Fig 8.2.) The number of people living in poverty has halved since 1990 and in 2015 there were 836 million people living on <$1.25 per day (primarily in Southern Asia and sub-Saharan Africa). In isolation, these figures can appear overly optimistic, as progress has been slower at higher (although still significant) poverty levels. The number of people living on <US $2 a day has declined only slightly since 1981, from 2.59 billion to 2.2 billion people in 2011.

Multidimensional impact of poverty

GDP per capita can be considered an incomplete measure of the situation, as poverty is multidimensional and economic growth alone does not constitute development. Poor people themselves define their poverty broadly to include lack of education, health, housing, empowerment, humiliation, employment, personal security, and more.

There is no single indicator, such as income, that can capture the multiple aspects of poverty.[2] Consider that there are 58 million out-of- school children of primary school age, and globally 781 million adults and 126 million youth worldwide lack basic literacy skills, >60% of them women. In 2012, 40 million births in developing regions were not attended by skilled health personnel, and >32 million of those births occurred in rural areas. According to the Oxford Poverty and Human Development Initiative (OPHI),* 1.6 billion people live in multidimensional poverty, which reduces resilience and makes them particularly vulnerable to shocks. (See Fig. 8.3.)

Substantial variability

Differences not only between, but within countries are large. People living in urban areas tend to be significantly better off than those residing in rural areas. A centre–periphery dynamic can be observed in many countries,

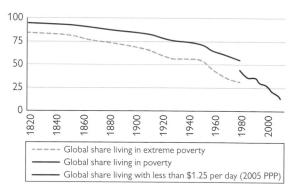

Fig. 8.2 Percentage of global population living in poverty. Source: World Bank and Bourguignon and Morrison (2002) and World Bank.

* OPHI has a public database of multi-dimensional poverty 101 countries, most also at sub-national level.

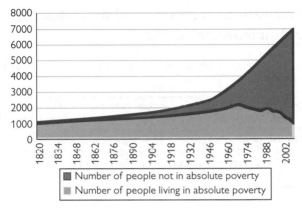

Fig. 8.3 Absolute number (in millions) of people living in in extreme poverty, 1820–2011.

e.g. poverty in Turkana (North Western rural Kenya) is 94% whereas only 22.5% of people in Nairobi are classified as poor. Similarly, in the Ugandan capital Kampala, 89% have access to electricity, whereas only 1.2% of the population in the rural region of Karamoja can turn on the lights.

Vulnerability to hazards

93% of people in extreme poverty live in places that are politically fragile, environmentally vulnerable, or both. Chronically vulnerable people exposed to hazards often leads to acute humanitarian need. Many households in South East Asia and sub-Saharan Africa are exposed to recurrent drought or flood, health risks such as malaria, animal disease such as food and mouth, commodity price fluctuations, political unrest, and violent conflict may push people from chronic vulnerability into acute humanitarian need.

A large part of development interventions is designed to reduce vulnerabilities and build resilience.[3]

> *Resilience* is the ability of an individual, community, or society exposed to hazards to resist, absorb, accommodate to, and recover from the effects of a hazard in a timely and efficient manner.

To increase people's resilience UNDP calls for:
- 'universal access to basic social services, especially health and education
- stronger social protection, including unemployment insurance and pensions
- a commitment to full employment, recognizing that the value of employment extends far beyond the income it generates.'

Overview of economics of development and humanitarian aid

Whereas progress has been made in terms of economic and social development, development and humanitarian action is still required in many parts of the world.

> Today, we recognize the millions of people who count on us for their very survival. The one billion people afflicted by hunger. The tens of millions forced to flee their homes because of disaster and conflict.
> The children who die from diseases we know how to cure. The women and girls who are brutalized by sexual violence. We need to tackle these problems at their root. But until we do, lives will hang in the balance. And the humanitarian community will be on the scene, rushing bravely towards danger, determined to help people in need.
>
> Secretary-General Ban Ki-moon
> Remarks to launch first World Humanitarian Day
> UN Headquarters, 19 August 2009.

Conceptually, aid professionals distinguish between acute and chronic crises, and the donor community tends to differentiate between humanitarian assistance and development assistance, and correspondingly aid flows are separated.

- *Humanitarian assistance* implies the immediately delivery of goods supplementing the existing capacity to delivery, bypassing the existing system and in some cases even weakening the existing system.
  This is non-permanent capacity, which ends when humanitarian assistance stops.
- *Development assistance* seeks to build a sustainable system that permanently increases the capacity to provide healthcare or provide food, which will continue to exist and function after the completion of the development intervention.

> People in fragile and conflict-affected states are more than twice as likely to be undernourished as those in other developing countries, more than three times as likely to be unable to send their children to school, twice as likely to see their children die before age five, and more than twice as likely to lack clean water. On average, a country that experienced major violence over the period from 1981 to 2005 has a poverty rate 21 percentage points higher than a country that saw no violence. A similar picture emerges for subnational areas affected by violence in richer and more stable countries.
>
> World Development Report, 2011.

Means of assistance

In 1970, the UN General Assembly (Resolution 2626) agreed that economically advanced countries would give 0.7% of their GNP (now gross national income (GNI)) as aid to the developing countries. Since the adoption of Resolution 2626, $3.62 trillion dollars in overseas development assistance (ODA) has been given by the OECD countries. Most countries, however, failed to live up to the agreed UN development assistance target; in 2014 only Denmark, Luxembourg, Norway, Sweden, and the UK continued to meet or exceed the target. In July 2015, countries recommitted to achieve the target of 0.7% of GNI for official development assistance, and 0.15–0.20% for least developed countries, in support of the Sustainable Development Goals.

Official versus non-official ODA

There are detailed and strict rules about what constitutes ODA[4] and other flows that contribute to humanitarian and development assistance are generally not captured in official ODA statistics. Two important sources are as follows:

Philanthropy: according to UNDP[5] in 2011, philanthropic North-South flows was >US$59 billion, including significant health sector donors, such as the Bill and Melinda Gates Foundation.

Remittances: although not captured in ODA statistics, research suggests that income transfer, or remittances, have significant effects on poverty reduction at the household level. In Somalia, for example, remittances are believed to amount to $1.2–1.6 billion and year, accounting for 20% of the country's GNI and upon which 40% of the populations relies for survival.

Progress on MDGs while humanitarian needs are growing

With concerted efforts by governments and development partners, sustained progress on the MGDs has been made:

- Globally, the number of people living in extreme poverty has declined by more than half, from 1.9 billion in 1990 to 836 million in 2015.
- The global under-five mortality rate has declined by more than half, from 90 to 43 deaths per 1000 live births between 1990 and 2015.
- Measles vaccination helped prevent nearly 15.6 million deaths from 2000 to 2013, with a 67% decline in measles cases reported globally.
- Since 1990, the maternal mortality ratio has declined by 45% worldwide.

Despite development progress, humanitarian needs have grown rapidly over the last few years. Worldwide displacement was at the highest level ever recorded by the middle of 2016 with >65 million people living in forced displacement, as a result of persecution, conflict, generalized violence, and human rights violations. Globally, one in every 122 humans is now either a refugee, internally displaced, or seeking asylum. If this were the population of a country, it would be the world's 24th biggest. In 2014, only 126,800 refugees were able to return to their home countries—the lowest number in 31 years and the average duration of displacement is now 17 years

Effects of climate change

In addition to conflict, climate change is also causing human displacement with an estimated 100 million people affected by natural disasters per year.

The July 2010 floods in Pakistan, for example, submerged one-fifth of the country and affected >20 million people. Natural disasters now cost >$100 billion in economic damages annually. It is estimated that by 2050, as many as 200 million people will be displaced by natural disasters and climate change.

The Intergovernmental Panel on Climate Change's 5th Assessment Report on Climate Change indicated that:
- climate-related extreme weather events such as floods and droughts are likely to be more frequent and intense in the coming years
- migration as an emergent risk and that 'human security will be progressively threatened as the climate changes' and that 'climate change is an important factor in threats to human security through […] increasing migration that people would rather have avoided'.[6,7]

Development and humanitarian assistance and funding

Overall humanitarian needs are increasingly rapidly, resulting in record financial requirements and logistical operations. In 2015, a record $19.1 billion was required to assist >114 million people in 35 countries. This is more than five times higher than in 2004. Further, currently >80% of humanitarian action takes place in protracted crises. However, funding modalities have not been adjusted accordingly, making planning difficult. (See Fig. 8.4.)

There is often a distinction made between humanitarian assistance and development assistance. While the principles of interventions which lead to strong and sustainable development are generally accepted by both, their focus of work and funding distinctions often translate to distinctions of perspective and priorities.

In the immediate emergency response, the emphasis is generally on life-saving approaches. In general, when a crisis moves from an acute to a chronic stage there is a more pronounced need to provide increasingly sustainable and economic solutions. This applies whether for the provision of clean water (see Box 8.1) or stronger health systems.

When feasible, the greatest impact of funding could be through the building of stronger, health systems. Building robust health systems that are more resilient to future crises is a much better and cheaper strategy than responding to a crisis, such as the Ebola epidemic, which cost an estimated

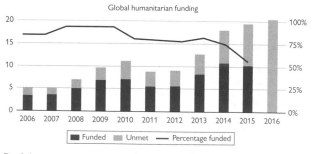

Fig. 8.4 Humanitarian funding needs.

Box 8.1 Economics of short- versus long-term solutions

In an emergency setting, transporting clean water via land is often used in the immediate situation, and Oxfam Ethiopia estimated that trucking 5 litres of water per day (basic survival quantity only) to 80,000 people in Harshin, Ethiopia for 5 months costs >US$3 million. This is compared with US$900,000 to rehabilitate all the non-operational local water schemes, necessary for sustainable development. This is equivalent to $38 per person for 5 months of water via trucking, as compared with $11 per beneficiary to rehabilitate water pumps, which have the additional benefit of supplying water beyond the crisis year.

$3.69 billion (almost equivalent to Sierra Leone's total economy). This is a complicated proposal, however, and depends on both funding sources and goals of the intervention.

Differences in funding recipients and 'ownership'
- Development assistance tends to focus on national-level and government ownership, which promotes stronger health systems in country. Funding allocations are often decided in consultation with the government and may go directly through existing line ministries.
- Humanitarian funding, however, is distinct in terms of recipient and primarily goes to UN agencies and iNGOs, or is self-funded. Of total international humanitarian assistance, only 0.2% went directly to local and national NGOs and 3.1% to the governments of affected states.[8]
- In South Sudan, 85% of health services are delivered by NGOs and UN Agencies This lack of government ownership means that the delivery of services can impede any long-term system planning and undermine the fragile social contract.

Funding cycles
- Unlike development funding, humanitarian funding is typically short term, making systems building and long-term planning difficult.
- The majority of international humanitarian assistance—66% in 2012—goes to long-term recipient countries. However, humanitarian appeals are generally short-term appeals with a 6–12-month horizon.
- Not all humanitarian funding goes to poor countries; vulnerability remains high in many MIC who now account for more than half the global humanitarian appeal.

Implications of aid

While there are no straightforward answers to the difficult quandaries humanitarians face in complex emergencies, this section identifies some of these dilemmas, and provides some guidance as to how to anticipate and judge the economic effects *and* how to mitigate them.

Considering 'do no harm'

It is well recognized that, despite the best of intentions, humanitarian assistance has a potential to disrupt the society in various ways:

- *Social order*: humanitarian assistance is valuable and can offer a substantial incentive to continue the status quo. Consider, does the provision or pattern of distribution of humanitarian assistance have the potential to cause or prolong conflict and suffering?
- *Social contract*: the provision of basic services is core to the social contract between the state and its citizens. To what extend does humanitarian assistance intervention undermine this contract?
- *Goods market*: the free provision of humanitarian aid in kind (food, water, medical care) impacts the local order. Consider, does provision of donations provide unfair competition for established commercial providers of these goods?
- *Jobs market*: humanitarian organizations often primarily employ local staff and tend to pay in excess of the market wage. How does this market force and wage discrepancy interfere with staffing at existing institutions?

What is the context you operate in and who benefits?

Understand the economy you operate in and the incentives or disincentive created by humanitarian action. Just as the normal functioning of society is disrupted by a conflict or natural disaster, the same is true for the economy. For example, transport links may have been cut as was the case in the aftermath of Typhoon Haiyan in the Philippines, leading to shortages. Further, import restrictions and conflict in Yemen have reduced imports to a small fraction of pre-crisis level (i.e. when 90% of food was imported), resulting in widespread shortages and spiking prices in basic supplies.

While many people suffer in these contexts, even in poorly functioning markets some people benefit from a complex emergency. Consider:

- Disruption creates scarcities, and the sole supplier of scarce commodities can make supra-normal profits with an aid effort.
- In a conflict setting, non-state armed actors can gain control over easily lootable natural resources (gold, diamonds).

Applying the 'do no harm' principle requires us as humanitarian actors to consider how our actions may benefit certain groups, such as particular ethnic groups or rebel groups, or individuals disproportionately benefit in such a way that it could create resentment or create incentives to perpetuate a conflict.

The relationship between aid and suffering

In conflict situations, aid has an economic impact on the local communities. Sometimes this economic impact can be positive, by injecting much-needed currency into the local community, not only with big ticket purchases, but also with smaller contributions such as buying vegetables, or employing a tailor. However, humanitarian funds can also, at times, prolong the conflict it is intended to alleviate. Consider the magnitude of the humanitarian response for the conflict in Darfur which prior to the expulsions was estimated at $1 billion per annum.

Arms purchases made possible by diverting aid tend to make conflicts drag on even longer. Another factor to be considered is the role of aid as a 'fig-leaf', a substitute for political action to resolve conflict. Those seeking to help the victims are caught in a trap: aid does help lower the level of violence—its fundamental role—but in the eyes of the political world that very fact minimizes the need to settle conflict, and thus actually prolongs it.

Conversely, aid can help shorten conflict, as the presence of the humanitarian personnel providing it tends to encourage a resumption of dialogue between the belligerents and to influence negotiations aimed at bringing about a cessation of hostilities.[9]

Pierre Perrin, International Review of the Red Cross, 1998.

Diversion of aid and looting

Hard data about the diversion of aid away from intended beneficiaries is scarce but there is ample anecdotal evidence of aid being redirected towards the warring factions through taxation or confiscation.

- Using the chaos of a humanitarian disaster, rebels and criminal elements routinely loot supplies. When the civil war broke out in South Sudan in December 2013, pre-positioned humanitarian supplies were looted. It is estimated that during the first 6 weeks of the conflict around 4700 tonnes of aid items—mostly food—were looted from UN warehouses.
- Sometimes local warlords don't steal humanitarian goods, but violate humanitarian principles and tax the transit of these goods.
  - In 2008 during its humanitarian assistance intervention in Darfur, the combined value of humanitarian goods stolen and fees paid to the government in Sudan amounted to 4.47% of MSF's budget.
  - ODI documented that at the height of the 2011 famine some agencies in Somalia gave into Al-Shabaab demands for payments as high as US$10,000.

We are unable to determine whether our aid helps or hinders one or more parties to the conflict ... it is clear that the losses—particularly looted assets—constitute a serious barrier to the efficient and effective provision of assistance, and can contribute to the war economy. This raises a serious challenge for the humanitarian community: can humanitarians be accused of fueling or prolonging the conflict in these two countries?[10]

Médecins Sans Frontières, Amsterdam.

Considerations

How to deal with these episodes is a source of controversy. When humanitarian actors enter into negotiations with armed groups, even in an attempt to lower tariffs or prevent looting, this confers some sort of legitimacy on these non-state armed actors. Meeting and negotiating with them, even to prevent looting, can offer them the perception of more power than they might normally be afforded. In unstable contexts, this can have serious implications.

Manipulating aid direction

Manipulation of humanitarian agencies in where to direct their aid is also a common problem. This can occur by:

- *Misconstruing where the highest need is.* Alex de Waal in his landmark book, *Famine Crimes* (p. 148), describes how during Operation Lifeline Sudan, 'both the government and the SPLA shifted from using starvation as a military tactic to strategic manipulation of aid, both to provision their forces and to protect key garrison. The structure of the aid programme has come to have an important influence over the structure of the military command.'

- *By targeting humanitarian aid workers.* Restricting humanitarian access can force aid delivery to be diverted by local agents to their chosen beneficiaries, providing power and legitimacy. Alternatively, cutting off aid can be a tactic of war.

  - Since 2000, 3000 aid workers have been killed, injured, or kidnapped since 2000 and in 2014, 190 major attacks against aid operations affecting 329 aid workers in 27 countries.

  - Examples include Al Qaeda bombing of UN headquarters in Iraq in 2003, and in October 2008, a suicide bomber struck the lobby of the Islamabad headquarters of the WFP, killing five UN humanitarian workers. On 20 April 2015, Al Shabaab militants killed four UNICEF workers in Garowe, Somalia. Similarly, in Islamic State of Iraq and ash-Sham (ISIS)-controlled territory in Syria and Iraq, humanitarian workers are targeted and humanitarian deliveries to Ar Raqqa and Deir ez Zor have been sporadic and minimal.

Considerations

The decision as to how to handle the situation can be complicated and there are no absolute truths how to negotiate with rebel groups and the government about the payment of fees. There are, however, (partial) solutions to reduce exposure to diversion of aid material, particularly if there is concern that aid serves to perpetuate a crisis. For example, in 2009, MSF took steps to reduce exposure to banditry by reducing the use of resources most valued by armed groups. They used donkeys and local trucks instead of vehicles and replaced valuable communications equipment with less attractive gear.

The 'who' and 'what' of aid

With the increasing number of international humanitarian responses, it is useful to consider what goods and services are being provided—and who, in the absence of humanitarian crisis, should provide them. For this, it is useful to categorize goods:

- *Public goods*: goods provided by the state and whose delivery is a crucial part of the social contract between the state and its citizens. Citizens pay tax and in return, public goods are provided which confer legitimacy on the state.
- *Private goods*: goods normally provided by a private company in a competitive market.
- *Mixed goods*: goods that are provided by both the public and the private sectors.

Collaboration or competition with existing providers

The ultimate aim of humanitarian assistance is to increase the supply of necessary public and private goods but not to displace the existing supply of those goods. If this balance is not met then international collaboration can amount to unfair competition with existing state and private providers, effectively crowding them out. For example, the provision of more free healthcare can in some circumstances undermine the private delivery of healthcare, or the delivery of food by WFP could be considered 'unfair competition' for the farmer who has tended his field.

Collaboration with the private sector

A 2012 article in the International Journal of Emergency Medicine examined the effect of the earthquake in Haiti on the workload of private and NGO providers, and concludes that '[F]ollowing the earthquake, public hospital and NGO providers reported a significant increase in their workload (15 of 17 and 22 of 26 respondents, respectively). Conversely, 12 of 16 private providers reported a significant decrease in workload. Although all groups reported working a similar number of hours prior to the earthquake (average 40 h/week), they reported working significantly different amounts following the earthquake. Public hospital and NGO providers averaged more than 50 h/week, and private providers averaged just over 33 h/week of employment.'[11] It would have been possible to buy in existing private sector capacity to assist with the response.

Considerations

If there is an acute crisis, humanitarians want to achieve speed and impact, and NGOs are often better at providing immediate assistance. It is, however, worth considering if existing providers can be subcontracted at a fee, such as what is being done for Syrian refugees. For example, WHO in Egypt has subcontracted specialized medical centres to serve 30,000 patients.

Acute crises frequently transform into chronic crises and there is no clear mechanism to overcome the humanitarian–development divide. Indeed, protracted conflicts lead to extended periods of displacement—refugees are, on average, displaced for 17 years. As humanitarian funding is often short term, often just 1-year planning cycles, when the immediate emergency phase has passed it is worth reaching out to developing partners, such as the World Bank, to ensure the long-term sustainability. Simple coordination of efforts is a good first step.

Free service provision

To allocate humanitarian goods, UN agencies and NGOs typically do not apply the market system but use rationing instead: every family receives the same package of food and non-food items, irrespective of their income and wealth. Similarly, nutrition support for children and medicine are provided free of charge to ensure there are no barriers to access. This sometimes leads to a misallocation of goods and a secondary market for surplus items, especially for non-food items, which often thrives in refugee camps.

Long-term effects

The provision of medicine for free can have negative medium- and longer-term consequences by changing the market demand dynamic seen commonly in both the health and agriculture sectors:

- Medicine availability: if health clinics supported by NGOs or humanitarian providers prescribe free medicine to patients, the demand for medicine on sale at local stores collapses and they go out of business. When the medical NGO eventually leaves, there may be no supply of medicine for the region anymore (even if people are willing to pay).
- Food provision: similarly, the provision of free food by NGOs or WFP can serve to change the local market demand and does not provide an incentive to farmers to plant and grow food. The entire supply chain may be disrupted from farmer to traders, and when the international community leaves, the local residents may see an absence of options which were previously plentiful.
- The long-terms effect can create dependency at the individual, household, or community levels where immediate basic needs cannot be met without external assistance.

Considerations

To minimize the local market disruption, *possible solutions to consider include the following:*

- Vouchers: instead of providing medicine in kind for free to the patient, humanitarian providers could consider introducing a voucher system on locally purchase goods which a beneficiary can use to collect their required medicine from the local pharmacist. The local pharmacist could, in turn can exchange the voucher with the NGO for payment. A word of caution: this may not be easily applicable for highly sensitive products such as medicine especially in regions with high counterfeit rates.
- Food for Work (FFW) Programmes can be an alternative way to ensure that food assistance does not create dependency. WFP in Mali established FFW that assisted in the construction of a small dam in Ouéléssébougou, in the Koulikoro region of Mali, which has contributed to the diversification of agricultural production.

- When feasible, food could be purchased locally instead of providing external food for free, which could inadvertently depress the local market for farmers producing crops. See Box 8.2.

Box 8.2 Utilizing the local market

In 2004, World Vision and the WFP set up a 'Joint Venture' in conflict-affected Southern Sudan, which served to buy up excess maize at market value. Organized through the local Yambio Farmers' Association, located in a fertile south western region of South Sudan, the excess maize was transported to deficit areas. The response was spectacular, with a substantial increase in production, illustrating that local farmers are often able and willing to respond to price signals and increased demand needs, if a system is in place for them to access. Further, stimulating the local market rather than shipping in grain from abroad, not only serves to meet the more immediate needs within the region, but potentially reduces the chance of a recurring famine.

Why not give cash?

The immediate reflex of humanitarians is to meet the need in kind; however, the provision of cash can empower people to make positive choices instead of being passive recipients of aid. Beneficiaries overwhelmingly state that it provides dignity. However, cash may not always be appropriate such as in contexts without a functioning market, or gender inequality (women who receive cash may not have agency to spend) or make them a target for robbery.

The decision tree in Fig. 8.5 from European Civil Protection and Humanitarian Aid Operations (ECHO) provides a useful guide for making an assessment, including the following:

- Selecting the beneficiary vulnerability criteria: this could be food for children under 5 years, pregnant and lactating mothers, and particular status groups—such as refugees.
- For private goods, such as food and shelter, consideration of whether the market is functioning—i.e. are there sellers and if demand increases as people are provided with cash, will there be a corresponding increase in supply or will it merely drive up the price?

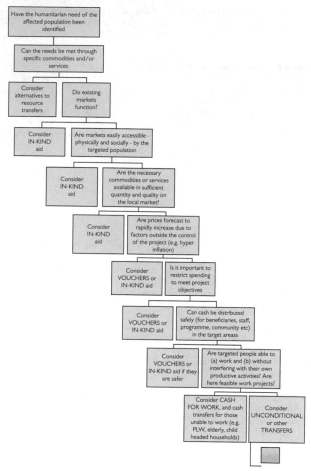

Fig. 8.5 Decision tree: cash or delivery in kind?[12]

Implications of staffing

Every aid operation relies on hiring of local staff, because they are better acquainted with the local conditions, know the local language, customs, and geography, and are generally more economical than 'importing' international staff. Recruiting local staff can also inject currency into the local economy, certainly a positive effect. However, the possible implications of recruiting staff from local public institutes into NGO employment must be considered in terms of the immediate *and* long-term implications for accessibility to care in the area.

Wage inflation and staffing

- While the influx of money from international and local staff can have benefits to the economy, it can also result in a distorted market and wage inflation, and have long-term implications.
  - Consider that many locations have a shortage of skilled local staff, and the increased demand for workers by newly arrived NGOs may serve to bid up wage rates of professionals.
- In fact, NGOs frequently bid up against each other, and the wage rate of the local NGO employee in some locations has been seen to be higher than that of a cabinet minister.
  - In South Sudan, civil servants were recruited to work for NGOs as advisors for the ministry they previously worked for at many times their original wage rate, effectively de-staffing the ministry.

Perceived benefits of NGO employment

- In locations where most professionals rely on public/governmental employment, NGOs may offer the opportunity of regular and dependable salaries, increased resources, and prestige.
- In some cases, the speed of promotion within NGOs far exceeds the rates which would be achieved in the public sector, particularly for clinical providers such as nurses and physicians.
- It is not uncommon to have the high-ranking national staff of NGOs be significantly younger than the more experienced public employees, which can cause tensions in the community.
- In addition, the pull towards working in the NGOs can cause a real staff shortage in the public sectors.

Consideration

To prevent a bidding war and wage inflation, NGOs should use the government wage structure as a good starting point, and when possible consult with local authorities for wage rates. NGOs could also coordinate wage rate structures for locally recruited doctors, nurses, drivers, and guards. To increase the supply of people with local knowledge without depleting the market, recruiting in the diaspora can be effective, particularly for countries such as South Sudan and Somalia, which have a sizable diaspora due to a long history of violence. When advertising for a local post, it would be advisable to also advertise this in diaspora population centres regionally or internationally. To mitigate the structural lack of staff supply, the NGOs should make the on-the-job training of local staff a priority.

References

1. Beegle K, Christiaensen L, Dabalen A, Gaddis I. Poverty in a Rising Africa. Washington, DC: World Bank; 2016.
2. Oxford Poverty & Human Development Initiative (OPHI). Multidimensional Poverty. ℘ http://www.ophi.org.uk/research/multidimensional-poverty/
3. UNDP. 2014 Human Development Report: Sustaining Progress: Reducing Vulnerabilities and Building Resilience. 2014. ℘ http://hdr.undp.org/sites/default/files/hdr14-report-en-1.pdf
4. OECD. What is ODA? OECD fact sheet, 2008. ℘ http://www.oecd.org/dac/stats/34086975.pdf
5. UNDP. Philanthropy as an Emerging Contributor to Development Cooperation. 2014. ℘ http://www.undp.org/content/dam/undp/documents/partners/civil_society/UNDP-CSO-philanthropy.pdf
6. Adger WN, Pulhin JM, Barnett J, Dabelko GD, Hovelsrud GK, Levy M, et al. Human security. In: IPCC, Climate Change 2014: Impacts, Adaptation, and Vulnerability. Part A: Global and Sectoral Aspects. Contribution of Working Group II to the Fifth Assessment Report of the Intergovernmental Panel on Climate Change. Cambridge: Cambridge University Press; 2014, pp. 755–91. ℘ https://www.ipcc.ch/pdf/assessment-report/ar5/wg2/WGIIAR5-Chap12_FINAL.pdf
7. Ruppel OC. Intergovernmental Panel on Climate Change (IPCC) Calls for More Attention on Human Mobility. OIM, 6 April 2014. ℘ http://weblog.iom.int/intergovernmental-panel-climate-change-ipcc-calls-more-attention-human-mobility#sthash.xUXXWuWp.dpuf
8. Development Initiatives. The 2015 Global Humanitarian Assistance Report. 2015. ℘ http://devinit.org/post/gha-report-2015/
9. Perrin P. The impact of humanitarian aid on conflict development. Int Rev Red Cross 1998;323:319–34.
10. Kahn C, Elena Lucchi E. Are humanitarians fuelling conflicts? Evidence from eastern Chad and Darfur. Humanitarian Exchange 2009;43:Art. 20.
11. Haar RJ, Naderi S, Acerra JR, Mathias M, Alagappan K. The livelihoods of Haitian health-care providers after the January 2010 earthquake: a pilot study of the economic and quality-of-life impact of emergency relief. Int J Emerg Med 2012;5:13.
12. European Commission. The Use of Cash and Vouchers in Humanitarian Crises; DG ECHO funding guidelines. March 2013. ℘ http://ec.europa.eu/echo/files/policies/sectoral/ECHO_Cash_Vouchers_Guidelines.pdf

International law for healthcare workers

Françoise Bouchet-Saulnier

Introduction

The international legal framework for healthcare and healthcare workers is contained in a variety of international treaties, regulations, and standards, which cover human rights and medical ethics to humanitarian law and criminal law. International humanitarian law (IHL) and medical ethics are in place to regulate the natural imbalance of power between doctors and their patients, further exacerbated in humanitarian activities when caring for victims of armed conflict or other forms of violence, vulnerable people, or unaccompanied minors. These rules underline the importance of healthcare, including humanitarian activities, and have been developed to safeguard the provision of care even in times of armed conflict, crisis, or violence. They are designed to preserve the autonomy of medical personnel, to protect them against security or military interference and ensure that healthcare is neither intentionally refused nor used as a weapon against groups.

International humanitarian law, also known as the *law of armed conflict* or *law of war*, imposes restrictions on all parties of an armed conflict and provides rights to humanitarian assistance to the victims. The origins of these laws are closely linked to the history of war, where leaders developed rules for military activities in order to maintain control, discipline, and efficiency of their military forces. By prohibiting acts of extermination and barbarism, these rules not only saved victims' lives but also preserved the humanity of the combatants and their ability to reintegrate into society. The codification of IHL occurred primarily in the nineteenth century, driven by non-governmental humanitarian initiatives and included diplomatic adaptation. IHL expanded steadily and covers today all situations of international (IAC) and non-international armed conflict (NIAC).

This chapter aims to provide healthcare providers with the information required to understand the rights and obligations accorded to the medical mission under international humanitarian law. It aims to clarify protections and provide the reader with the necessary frameworks to guide them in their work in complicated environments.[1–3]

From war law to humanitarian law

Humanitarian action takes place in many different contexts, including socioeconomically precarious situations, natural disaster, armed conflicts, and other situations of violence and insecurity. IHL has been designed specifically to cover situations of armed conflict including those with non-state armed groups (see Box 9.1). IHL outlines the duties of those engaged in armed conflict as well as the humanitarian organizations involved in relief operations. These laws balance the respect of state sovereignty with the right of independent organizations to develop humanitarian and medical actions based solely on the needs of the most vulnerable. The fundamental principles of humanitarian action (i.e. impartiality, neutrality, and independence) derive directly from humanitarian law.

The *International Committee for Relief to the Wounded* was created in 1863 in Geneva by Henri Dunant after witnessing the battlefield of Solferino: in a single day, 40,000 soldiers from both sides died or were left wounded on the field. On his own initiative, he set up care for the wounded and sick, organized the collection of the dead, and drafted international regulations authorizing such activities. In 1864, this became the first *Geneva Convention for the Amelioration of the Condition of the Wounded in Armies in the Field*. This established the concept of relief for the wounded without any distinction of nationality, defined the neutrality and independence of medical personnel on the battlefield, and created the distinctive emblem of the Red Cross (a red cross on a white background).

The four Geneva Conventions and Additional Protocols

The four Geneva Conventions of 1949 and two 1977 Additional Protocols (APs) (later joined by a third AP in 2005), constitute the heart of IHL. Adopted in reaction to the horror of World War II, the four Geneva Conventions clarify, codify, and extend towards the civilian population the various pre-existing rules of the laws of armed conflict.

- The *first*, *second*, and *third Geneva Conventions* apply to the wounded and sick members of the armed forces or prisoners of war.
- The *fourth Geneva Convention* established, for the first time in 1949, the rules protecting civilian victims of IACs.
  - The *Common article 3 of the fourth Geneva Convention* includes NIAC, and sets minimum guarantees for the protection of those who are not, or no longer, taking part in the hostilities: civilians, wounded and sick, and detainees.

In 1977, drawing from experiences of decolonization and civil war following World War II, two APs to the 1949 Geneva Conventions were adopted to strengthen protections for victims of both IACs (which involve two or more state forces,) contained in AP I, and NIACs (which involve non-state armed groups), in AP II. These conventions merged together the principles of military necessity and humanitarian imperatives by integrating the rights of protection and assistance for victims of conflicts within the rules for the conduct of hostilities.

Box 9.1 Defining terms

State: a geographic entity (nation or territory) considered as an organized political entity under one government. The term state in this text can also often refer to the governing body.

State actors: those directed by some form of recognized government.

Non-state actors: those which do not belong to or are not controlled by the government.

Customary international humanitarian law

International law recognizes 'international customary rules' which are those laws created by a state or arising from established state practices. This is very important to humanitarian law as the practice of negotiating on relief operations by the state and impartial relief organizations has created precedents (or *customary rules*) for the principles of humanitarian action.

In 2005, the ICRC published a set of 161 rules that have acquired the status of *customary international humanitarian law* (CIHL). These rules are binding on all state and non-state parties to conflict including those that have not ratified the Geneva Conventions *and* additional protocols.

The main IHL provisions are universally recognized in all types of armed conflicts and are summarized through the following five principles:

1. The principle of distinction

This principle dictates that the parties to a conflict must, at all times, distinguish between civilians and combatants, as well as between civilian objects and military objectives. The parties to the conflict may direct their operations only against military objectives.

In other words, civilian populations and objects cannot be lawfully targeted. If there is any doubt about whether a target is civilian or military, armed forces must presume civilian status and therefore refrain from attack. Civilian objects may only lose their protection from attack if they are used to commit acts harmful to the enemy.

Direct attack on civilians as well as indiscriminate attacks are prohibited by IHL at all times (AP I Article 48 and CIHL Rules 7, 11–13).

2. The principle of precaution, and proportionality in attack

The IHL principles of precaution and proportionality apply to any incidental damage to civilians and, particularly, medical services. Under IHL, when attacking a military target, commanders have the duty to take all feasible precautions in choosing the means and methods of attack to avoid or minimize incidental loss of civilian lives, injury to civilians, and damage to civilian objects that would be excessive to the direct military advantage anticipated. IHL stipulates that attacks expected to cause incidental civilian casualties and/or damage to civilian objects that would be excessive in relation to the concrete and direct military advantage anticipated, are unlawful and must not be carried out. It further clarifies that attacks cannot treat a number of clearly separated and distinct military objectives located in a city, town, village, or other areas with a similar concentration of civilians, as a single military objective. Such an attack would be considered as indiscriminate and disproportionate.

The requirement to calculate the proportionality of any attack in terms of military advantage versus civilian loss and damages entails the duty to take all precautions to avoid or minimize civilian loss and damages. This duty may lead to the cancellation or delay of an attack.

Attack on military objectives situated in the proximity of civilians must take precaution to avoid or limit the civilian loss and damage and to ensure that such loss and damage will be proportionate to the direct military advantage anticipated from the attack (AP I 51 and CIHL Rule 14, 15).

3. The principle of responsibility of parties to the conflict and commanders

The duty and responsibility that military commanders have for their orders and the actions of their subordinates are central to IHL. The law obligates all parties to the conflict, including non-state armed groups, to take all possible precautionary and proportional measures. This is reinforced by the possibility to bring charges of individual criminal responsibility for war crimes against commanders and at all levels of the chain of command, in front of national and international criminal tribunals.

Military commanders have duty and responsibility for their orders (AP I Articles 57 and 58, CIHL Rules 14–24).and the actions of their subordinates and can be held accountable for war crimes under Article 28 of the Rome Statutes of the International Criminal Court.

4. The right of protection and assistance for vulnerable people

Under IHL, the term protection refers to a specific legal status of 'protected persons' granted to different categories of people who are not taking part in the hostility or are out of combat. The different statuses of protection are designed to address the specific vulnerability of persons such as civilians, the wounded and sick, children and mothers of young children, women, and all persons deprived of liberty such as detainees and prisoners of war. It also covers medical personnel, relief and humanitarian personnel, and religious personnel.

IHL regulates three major categories of protection in humanitarian activities:

1. The general protection of the civilian population, including its rights to humanitarian relief. Goods essential for the survival belong to the category of 'protected goods' whose safe passage and access cannot be denied by any party to the conflict.
2. The protection of medical care for all wounded and sick without discrimination, including the special protection for healthcare facilities, personnel, transport, and supplies.
3. The protection of all persons deprived of liberty in conflict—including the mandatory right of visit for the ICRC—and the general rights to humanitarian relief for the civilians.

The wounded and sick, civilian population not taking part in the hostilities, and persons deprived of liberty are entitled to specific protection and access to humanitarian relief, such as medical care, evacuation, and supply of essential goods necessary to their survival.

5. The right of humanitarian initiative for impartial humanitarian organizations

IHL builds on the responsibility of all parties to fulfil their obligations towards populations and territories under their effective military control. IHL creates the unique *right of humanitarian initiative* for the ICRC and other impartial humanitarian organizations, which affords them the right and indeed, the responsibility, to propose services and activities to answer unmet vital needs and to alleviate the suffering of survivors of the conflict. Even if consent from the parties of the conflict is required, this consent cannot be arbitrarily refused when it comes to medical assistance or to responding to needs essential for the survival of the population. However, it is worth noting that under IHL, the rights of humanitarian action by private impartial organizations cannot justify interference with internal state affairs.

> The right of humanitarian initiative is established in IHL and is clearly referred to in the Geneva Conventions and APs. It entitles any humanitarian organization to offer its services and parties to the conflict must facilitate a rapid and unimpeded passage of relief material and personnel.

Law of weapons and law of war

IHL, as well as other international conventions, prohibit the use of some weapons due to their indiscriminate nature, their long-lasting effect on health and environment, or because they 'cause superfluous injury, unnecessary suffering' or excessively injurious effects.

In 1899 and 1907, the *Hague Conventions* were the first international treaties to prohibit certain weapons such as projectiles that disperse asphyxiating gas and bullets that expand or flatten easily in the human body. Since then, other treaties have been adopted to regulate the use of certain weapons, with some weapons authorized, except for certain uses (e.g. edged weapons, firearms, and incendiary weapons), and others strictly prohibited (e.g. biological and chemical weapons, and to some extent, landmines).

These treaties include the following:

- The *Convention on Cluster Munitions* adopted in Dublin in 2008 prohibits the use, stockpiling, production, and transfer of cluster munitions.
- The 'Convention on Prohibitions or Restrictions on the Use of Certain Conventional Weapons Which May be Deemed to Be Excessively Injurious or Have Indiscriminate Effects' (known as the *1980 Geneva Convention on Conventional Weapons*) is an important landmark on weapons use and restriction. It also has Aps on 'blinding lasers' (weapons which can cause injury via fragments undetectable by X-rays).
- CIHL Rules 73–85 regulate incendiary weapons, herbicides, and mines. They also prohibit chemical weapons, special antipersonnel bullets, or ammunitions in conflicts.

Medical practitioners who are confronted with patients exposed to or wounded by such weapons should be aware of the potential violations of international law.

Traditions of international law for healthcare

Preserving medical services in warzones and in crisis situations depends upon the triple protection of the wounded and sick, of the medical personnel and ethics, and of the medical facilities and transports.

Protection of the wounded and sick

As stated in IHL, maintaining neutrality of the wounded and sick and of medical personnel and units is the only way to protect and maintain vital medical services in war zones. It is impossible to maintain functional hospitals in war zones if there is a risk of attack for treating wounded affiliated with the 'enemy' or if medical personnel experience interference in the care of patients. Attacking medical services would amount to a war crime.

IHL stipulates the imperative to protect the wounded and sick. This includes the obligation to allow the collection, transport, and provision of care to the wounded by the fullest extent practical and with the least possible delay. This pertains to all parties in both IACs and NIACs and supports the rights of relief organizations to conduct impartial medical humanitarian activities upon negotiations with the parties to the conflict.

No discrimination is allowed among the wounded and sick, regardless of the circumstances of the wounds or illness, their potential participation in the conflict, or their affiliation to any armed groups. This provision is crucial, especially in NIACs where combatants affiliated with non-state armed groups are often considered as criminals under domestic law. Still, they are protected from attack/arrest until the end of their medical treatment, and medical staff cannot be punished for providing medical treatment. Any military or security influence on the care of patients would violate medical ethics by attempting to discriminate between patients on a basis other than medical considerations.

On a practical side, the protection of the wounded and sick stops as soon as their treatment is over. At such time, they return to their previous status and may be arrested or targeted if considered as combatants or criminals. This must be taken into account when transferring patients to medical facilities across front lines as although the transfer itself cannot be subjected to military interference, it may not be possible to return the person to their previous location after recovery.

Protection of medical personnel and medical ethics

IHL requires that humanitarian personnel[4] engaged in medical duties must be protected in all circumstances. Medical personnel are obligated by IHL to treat all patients without discrimination and are protected to ensure that they are able to resist military interference and can act with independence and autonomy. This fundamental principle means that patients cannot be registered according to their ethnicity, politics, religion, or participation in the hostilities. Medical personnel must maintain and control the ethical, neutral, and impartial nature of medical structures and activities.

While the law outlines that this protection can be lost if medical personnel commit, outside their medical and humanitarian function, an act harmful to the enemy, this shall not be used as a mechanism to intimidate medical providers or restrict their provision of healthcare. Indeed, such loss of protection refers only to activities amounting to direct participation in the hostilities and clearly excludes the treatment of patients considered 'criminals' or 'enemies' that is mandatory under IHL and medical ethics.

Respect of medical ethics of health workers

In situations of conflict, there may be tension between the IHL duty to provide neutral medical care and confidentiality[5] and domestic laws (i.e. those which may require reporting victims of violence to the police). To resolve such tensions, IHL mandates that medical confidentiality and the patient's best interest prevail over domestic law. IHL also clarifies that medical personnel cannot be punished or prosecuted under domestic law for providing medical care compatible with medical ethics, to any wounded and sick patient, whatever the circumstances.

> Medical personnel cannot be punished for giving medical care to enemy wounded and for not reporting their name to the state authority.

Principles of medical ethics are essential for managing the various legal issues raised by humanitarian activities. For example, securing medical confidentiality and informed consent from patients requires vigilance and, particularly in unstable situations, sharing medical data for public health concerns must meet the highest criteria of anonymity and non-identification of patients. In such contexts, the principles of medical ethics (including medical confidentiality) supersede other duties to report individual cases of violence to authorities.

Additional standards for medical providers have been adopted, including by the World Medical Association, which outline ethical principles in armed conflict and pertaining to torture, detention, and medical research.

> Foreign medical practitioners in humanitarian activities must be both registered for such practice in their country of origin and have an agreement in a Memorandum of Understanding (MoU) with the MOH and/or medical board of the country of operation. Depending on the situation and the nature of the medical activities, the MoU can set conditions regarding rights and conditions to practise medicine, professional insurance, and the management of data.

Protection of medical facilities and precaution in any attack

Medical facilities and transports must be protected at all times and cannot be attacked.[6] Medical facilities have both general civilian protection and special protection; warring parties must ensure that staff and facilities are not attacked or suffer indirect collateral damage.

Medical facilities (including vehicles) are allowed to use the medical protective emblem of the Geneva Convention (a red cross, red crescent, or red crystal); however, they remain protected from attack as a civilian object even if they do not display this specific emblem.[7]

Any deliberate attack on a protected hospital is a war crime under the statute of the International Criminal Court. It is difficult to prove intentionality, however, and so IHL and most domestic criminal law agree on a broader definition. An attack on a medical facility is a violation of IHL and may constitute a war crime if it was either intentional or due to negligence by not properly verifying the military or civilian nature of the target, if disproportionate force was used, or if prior warning of an imminent attack failed to be provided.

Although medical facilities can lose their protection under certain circumstances stipulated in the Geneva Conventions, IHL expressly stipulates that there is *no* loss of protection even if wounded or sick combatants affiliated with the enemy or illegal armed groups are inside the medical facility (see Box 9.2) The same applies to the presence of weapons collected from the wounded and sick inside the facility, which is often a regular practice to maintain neutrality and protection of the facility.

Box 9.2 Loss of protection of medical units

Under IHL, medical units may only lose their protection if they are used to commit, outside of their humanitarian function, an act harmful to the enemy. This is an extreme situation upon which strict conditions have been placed. IHL does not give concrete examples of what constitutes acts harmful to the enemy, leaving dangerous room for potential exploitation by warring parties. That a hospital may lose its protection on allegation of being used as a command and control centre or as shelter for military meetings or un-armed combatant is commonly argued. This raises grave concerns and should stir the vigilance of healthcare facility managers as to the rules they set in place for visits, communication, and of course, for a no-weapons policy inside hospitals.

However, even where a medical facility loses its protected status, immediate attack is not allowed. Protection of the hospital can only cease after due warning has been given, setting a reasonable time for the evacuation of the patients or to remedy the harmful situation. This rule is mandatory in both IACs and NIACs. In case of attack, the use of force must fulfil the duty of precaution and proportionality, i.e. a gunman firing from a hospital would permit a response against the gunman only after warning remains unheeded, but cannot justify destruction of the entire hospital.

International crimes, sanctions, and humanitarian medical action

The prohibition of torture, war crimes, crimes against humanity, and geno-cide form part of contemporary international criminal law, and can lead to international prosecution. These crimes affect the function of medical personnel, who can be caught between caring for their patients and being called to appear in court nationally or internationally to attest to the medical findings of the mistreated individuals. Doctors should be able to identify the medical and psychological impacts of such criminal practices and to draft appropriate medical certification.

Defining torture and ill treatment

The prohibition of torture is one of the few absolute obligations of international law recognized and accepted by states. The prohibition applies in times of peace as well as in armed conflict, on the basis of various international conventions.

Definition

The various definitions of torture revolve around three main concepts:
1. The intentional infliction of severe physical or psychological pain.
2. This pain is inflicted with one or several specific objectives, including to obtain confessions or information, to obliterate the personality of the victim, or to diminish his physical and/or mental capacities.
3. These acts are performed by agents of the state, under its control or with its consent.

With regards to the above definition:
- International conventions against torture are not limited to pain, but also extend the prohibition to other cruel, inhuman, or degrading acts.
- The threshold of pain required to qualify as torture is often subject to interpretations by states, and so international court cases are establishing landmarks to define these thresholds.
- In situations of armed conflict, it is not conditional that the definition of the torturer be limited to state agents only. The IHL widening of this definition is intended to cover abuses committed by all actors involved in detention and interrogations, including non-state armed groups and other non-state and non-official authorities.

The prohibition of torture is accompanied by an international system of criminal sanctions known under the name of 'universal jurisdiction', allowing prosecution in any country regardless of the nationality of the perpetrator or the country where it occurred. (This is demonstrated by the indictment of Augusto Pinochet by a Spanish court in 2000 after his arrest in the UK in October 1998.)

Humanitarian involvement in torture and ill treatment

Humanitarian medical personnel rarely face the dilemma of directly participating in the torture of detainees (which is a concern primarily for military and prison doctors); however, humanitarians may be requested to give medical care to detainees near their facilities.

If requested to provide medical care for detainees, humanitarian providers should:

- record the patient's identity, the name of the detaining power, the place of detention, and should inform the ICRC
- aim to ensure, as a minimum guarantee, that the patient will not be taken back to detention or interrogation against medical advice before the end of the medical treatment
- ensure that access to medical care for the detainees is not bargained or delayed as a means of pressure.

If a patient is taken back to detention or interrogation against medical advice and/or later brought back with new signs of violence, healthcare personnel should stop their activity to prevent complicity. In such cases, healthcare providers must relay such concerns to the various authorities and hierarchies involved. If there is no change in the situation, it can be made public, including being brought to the attention of the medical board of the country. For example, in January 2012, MSF decided to stop its work in detention centres in Misrata, Libya, after staff were requested to patch up detainees mid-way through torture sessions. MSF raised the issue with the authorities but no action was taken and MSF took the decision to withdraw and speak out.

Finally, medical personnel and humanitarian organizations should ensure and secure the good medical documentation of each patient and keep it available for any later action of the patient.

> Medical and humanitarian actors have an important role in the prevention of torture through their involvement in the assistance of detained and ex-detained persons. When confronted with an ex-detainee who has suffered ill treatment, medical personnel should—in addition to providing medical treatment and a medical certificate—enquire where and with whom this person was detained. This will enable them to know if and where other persons may still be in danger. Managing this information must respect the principles of confidentiality and 'do no harm'. The ICRC is the international organization mandated to deal with such information under agreed international legal and ethical frameworks.

Prevention of torture
The prevention of torture is linked to the guarantees covered by human rights and humanitarian law relating to conditions of detention and interrogation. While detention is usually justified by judicial reasons, it may also take the form of 'administrative detention' based on security reasons in some situations of crisis or conflict. The goal is then no longer to judge but to extract information, screen, and control certain individuals. The prevention of torture currently focuses on strengthening judicial and legal guarantees of detention, and on the right to effective remedies for people deprived of their liberty, whatever their specific legal status.

Obligations of medical actors for preventing and documenting torture
Since torture is linked to situations of detention, medical providers have a protective role to play, including raising awareness and alerting the various

security forces, state agents, and bodies involved in case of ill treatment of individuals. Several international regulations have agreed to define better medical practice in detention and to navigate the multiple professional and ethical dilemmas entailed with such activity. This includes reaffirming the principles of medical ethics to ensure that they always act in the best interest of their patients.

The Standard Minimum Rules for the Treatment of Prisoners

In 1977, the United Nations adopted the Standard Minimum Rules for the Treatment of Prisoners[8] which established that every detainee must have a medical examination when entering a detention centre. This allows for the distinguishing of violence occurring at the time of arrest and interrogation before entering the detention centre, and that occurring during the detention. In 1982, this was complemented by the adoption of the Principles of Medical Ethics relevant to the Role of Health Personnel, particularly Physicians, in the Protection of Prisoners and Detainees against Torture and Other Cruel, Inhuman or Degrading Treatment or Punishment.[9]

These principles go beyond those established by the Nuremberg Code of 1947, which was limited to medical experiments on prisoners. They reinforce the rules of medical action and ethics for the treatment of prisoners and add to medical duties spelt out by IHL. Through six core principles, this document supports non-discrimination and the provision of equal medical treatment for those detained, such as: 'health personnel, particularly physicians, charged with the medical care of prisoners and detainees have a duty to provide protection of their physical and mental health and treatment of the same quality and standard as is afforded to those who are not imprisoned or detained.' It also specifies circumstances under which medical practices constitute a violation of medical ethics, including passive complicity of ill treatment, which occurs when healthcare personnel pursue a goal other than to evaluate, protect, or improve the physical and mental health of the person concerned.

Istanbul Protocol

In 2004, a Manual on the Effective Investigation and Documentation of Torture and Other Cruel, Inhuman or Degrading Treatment or Punishment, known as the Istanbul Protocol, was adopted by the UN High Commissioner for Human Rights. The Istanbul Protocol clarifies the obligations of physicians in documenting torture and ill treatment, and their prohibition of any participation in these practices.

Medical activities which constitute participation and complicity in torture include:

- evaluating an individual's capacity to withstand ill treatment
- being present at, supervising, or inflicting maltreatment
- resuscitating individuals for the purpose of further maltreatment or providing medical treatment immediately before, during, or after torture on the instructions of those likely to be responsible for it
- providing professional knowledge or individuals' personal health information to torturers
- intentionally neglecting to provide evidence and falsifying reports, such as autopsy reports and death certificates.[10]

Ethical management of dual obligations

The *Istanbul Protocol* recognizes that physicians must balance the sometimes contradictory obligations of caring for patients and other legal and ethical obligations, including 'dual obligations'. See Box 9.3.

Box 9.3 Dual obligations

Dual obligations occur for medical practitioners caught between obligations incompatible with the respect of medical ethics. This is the case, for instance, with the duty to provide care to victims of torture and the duty not to participate in ill treatment. There can also be conflict between the duty to respect confidentiality and the consent of the patient and the duty to report cases of violence and certain medical information to the authorities for security or judicial reasons. This dual obligation is heightened in cases where the authorities are involved in the violence. In such cases, disclosing information can result in more harm and less medical care for the patient.[11]

The Istanbul Protocol acknowledges the issue of dual legal obligations and sets rules and ethical principles to be followed, including the:
- absolute prohibition of doing harm to the patient
- obligation for the physician to inform the patient, in every circumstance, of the nature of their medical mission and any external pressures or constraints
- obligation to obtain the patient's consent for all acts, and obligation to respect medical confidentiality in case of doubt.

The *Istanbul Protocol* also provides guidance on how to visit places of detention to ensure quality of care and avoid putting survivors and witnesses at risk.[12] It offers guidelines for the medical evaluation of torture and ill treatment[13] including templates for physical and psychological medical examinations to document torture and ill treatment.[14]

Genocide, war crimes, and crimes against humanity

Humanitarian relief providers are often at the forefront of violence. They can be key witnesses with the ability to uncover broader criminal practices such as the use of chemical weapons, mass rape, or war-related injuries on civilians. When patients (and providers) are killed because of their ethnicity, the pattern is not one of an armed conflict but rather of extermination, as was experienced in an extreme way during the genocide in Rwanda in 1994.

Rome Convention and International Criminal Court

In 1998, the adoption of the Rome Convention and the creation of the International Criminal Court provided common definitions of crimes such as genocide, war crimes, and crimes against humanity.

Genocide

The definition of genocide under article 6 of the Rome Statute includes any of the following acts committed with intent to destroy, in whole or in part, a national, ethnical, racial, or religious group:
- Killing members of the group.
- Causing serious bodily or mental harm to members of the group.

- Deliberately inflicting on the group conditions of life calculated to bring about its physical destruction in whole or in part.
- Imposing measures intended to prevent births within the group.
- Forcibly transferring children of the group to another group.

War crimes

The definition of a war crime under article 8 of the Rome Statute includes:
- the use of weapons prohibited by IHL
- various forms of violence directed against a person not taking direct part in the hostilities or who are out of combat, in particular murder, mutilation, cruel treatment and torture, and gender-based sexual violence
- the use of starvation against civilians as a war crime in IAC
- the recruitment of children under 15 to a participate in hostilities
- the intentional directing of attacks against:
  - buildings, material, medical units and transport, and personnel using the distinctive emblem of the Geneva Conventions
  - buildings dedicated to religion, education, art, and charitable purposes; historic monuments; hospitals and places where the sick and wounded are gathered
- medical activities violating medical ethics.

Crimes against humanity

The definition of crimes against humanity under article 7 of the Rome Statute includes any of the following acts when committed as part of a widespread or systematic attack directed against any civilian population, with knowledge of the attack:
- Murder.
- Extermination.
- Enslavement.
- Deportation or forcible transfer of population; imprisonment or other severe deprivation of physical liberty in violation of fundamental rules of international law.
- Torture.
- Rape, sexual slavery, enforced prostitution, forced pregnancy, enforced sterilization, or any other form of sexual violence of comparable gravity.
- Persecution against any identifiable group or collectivity on political, racial, national, ethnic, cultural, religious, gender as defined in paragraph 3, or other grounds that are universally recognized as impermissible under international law, in connection with any act referred to in this paragraph or any crime within the jurisdiction of the Court.
- Enforced disappearance of persons.
- The crime of apartheid.
- Other inhumane acts of a similar character intentionally causing great suffering, or serious injury to body or to mental or physical health.

Sexual violence

For the first time, gender-based sexual violence was included as a potential component of both war crimes and crimes against humanity and also of genocide under specific circumstances. This includes the internationally agreed definition and prosecution of rape, sexual slavery, forced prostitution, forced pregnancy, forced sterilization, or any other forms of sexual violence of a comparable gravity. To be considered a crime against humanity, sexual violence has to be perpetrated in addition to other forms of violence against individuals such as murder, extermination, enslavement, deportation or forcible transfer, illegal imprisonment or severe deprivation of physical liberty, torture, persecution, enforced disappearance, apartheid or other inhuman acts causing great suffering or serious injury to body or mind.

See➲ Chapter 5 for more information on background and clinical management.

Medico-legal care for survivors of violence

The medical care of survivors of violence (including sexual violence) involves specific responsibility for medical actors including:

- providing medical treatment to the survivors and providing a medico-legal certificate
- understanding the nature and causes of the assault, and assessing the risk of recurrence
- taking steps to place the victim out of danger, if necessary and possible
- providing specific care and protection for minors who are survivors of sexual violence.

This care assumes coordination with other social actors: the police, the legal and judicial systems, protection organizations such as ICRC, UNICEF, UNHCR, civil society organizations, etc. However, in most contexts of humanitarian action, the availability of social and protection networks is ineffective or very limited. Therefore the medical provider must make decisions by reflecting on the reality of the protection environment, the best interests of the patient, and the fundamental medical principle of 'do no harm' rather than on theoretical legal standards.[15]

The development of international criminal justice puts new emphasis on the role of medical practitioners treating survivors of violence, including sexual violence. Medical practitioners face a double role of providing medical care to survivors and securing the material element and physical evidence of potential criminal activities.

Various comprehensive international protocols are available; however, practitioners are typically confronted with three main challenges:

1. To keep protocols as simple as possible to allow its implementation in precarious and insecure contexts.
2. To ensure that the medical care and safety of survivors and doctors are not jeopardized.
3. To ensure that medical confidentiality and patient consent prevail over external judicial pressure and any other legal duty to report the crime (see ➔ 'Ethical management of dual obligations' p. 185).

Fighting for justice should not occur through exposing survivors without their informed consent. These risks and dilemmas were illustrated in 2013 during the Minova trial in the Democratic Republic of Congo, where lists of rape survivors were collected by military and human rights investigators in medical facilities without the consent of the survivors and in violation of medical confidentiality. As a consequence, most rape victims were frightened and refused to confirm the facts. Of the 39 state officers brought to trial, only 25 officers were convicted of pillage and only two of rape.

The medical certificate

It is important that the medical practitioner who examines the victim draws up the medical certificate as early as possible. *Countries often have standard templates of medical certificates; they need to be available within the health facilities.* The drafting of medico-legal certificates is regulated in most countries and typically falls to doctors or forensic medicine experts. In humanitarian situations, however, medical case management is often provided by NGOs and their medical staff typically deliver the certification. This is often the first and only document that a victim will have to use at a later stage. With no statutory limitation applicable to the prosecution of war crimes and crimes against humanity, prosecution could possibly take place at a much later date, often up to 10 years or more. Not drafting these certificates eliminates the initial medical record of such assaults. The medical certificate cannot in itself prove a crime but is an element necessary in the legal determination by a judge of the circumstances of the event. There are verified accounts of MSF certificates issued to survivors of violence being admitted as valid documents in domestic or international courts.

Completing medical certificates

The question of whether an incident of rape/sexual assault/torture occurred is a legal issue and not a medical diagnosis. Consequently, medical certificates should record only the findings of the medical examination. The patient's account of the circumstances of the assault should be included stating his/her own words. The certificate may include optional conclusions with regard to the compatibility of medical findings with the victim's account or the absence of findings. The latter is often the case in sexually active people or when there is a long delay between the event and the medical consultation, and it does not invalidate the patient's claim of rape.

Confidentiality of certificates

The medical certificate is a document covered by medical confidentiality. It must only be given to the victim. Doctors or health structures may receive a request from the police, the judiciary, UN agencies, other organizations, or authorities to provide information or medical certificates for patients who have been treated for sexual violence. In such cases, doctors should obtain the express consent of the patient before sharing the medical certificate or any information covered by medical confidentiality.

Maintaining medical confidentiality

Reporting cases of violence—notably violence on minors—is a legal requirement in most countries. UN Security Council Resolution 1888 calls on the UN, government agencies, and NGOs to 'support improved monitoring, documentation and reporting of crimes of sexual violence'. To support this, the *International Protocol on the Documentation and Investigation of Sexual Violence in Conflict* was launched in 2014.[16] However, when facing such decisions, it must not be forgotten that individual information on patients always remains protected by the fundamental principles of medical confidentiality and 'do no harm'. Providers must always and only act with the patient's informed consent and in the patient's best interest, such principles prevailing over any other legal duty.

Assessing the nature and pattern of violence

In cases of violence, medical care should include questions to assess if the victim is still in danger. Understanding the circumstances that resulted in the physical injuries enables the individual case to be addressed and to identify possible systematic patterns of violence. This issue is a greater challenge in crises or armed conflicts where most humanitarian activities take place and where the referral to dedicated state institutions and procedures is no longer an option.

To assess the risk of recurrence, it is important that the victim gives an account of the circumstances of the assault which should be included in the medical file. While medical practitioners are not responsible for the security of a patient outside the medical facility, it is their responsibility in the direct aftermath of a physical assault to work with the survivor to identify the immediate protection solutions available.

Depending on the context, specific security measures can be adopted in medical facilities:

• In armed conflict, special attention must be given to patients under arrest or detention brought to medical facilities. They should be admitted under a special medical procedure to ensure that they cannot be taken away before the end of their medical treatment and that their detention situation can be referred, with their consent, for follow-up to the ICRC or an alternative organization.

• Specific attention should also be given to survivors of violence when the victim lives with or in the vicinity of a known perpetrator. Survivors identified as isolated and vulnerable may remain under the constant threat of repeated violence.

• Protection of minors requires particular attention. The most frequent issue in humanitarian contexts is the lack of solutions to protect minors from their abusive environment and to prevent direct contact with the perpetrator. This is of particular importance when taking care of survivors of sexual violence in precarious settings such as camps or slums. See Box 9.4.

• Removing someone from danger involves working with the survivor to find the most appropriate solution given the context and the available resources. Several solutions can be considered including keeping the patient for a few nights at the hospital, distancing the person from the danger or relocating him/her, and helping the survivor's return to his/her home.[17]

Care and protection of minors who are survivors of (sexual) violence

Medical teams face complicated decisions when treating minors who are alone or isolated, including issues related to consent and protection. Indeed, some isolated minors may have fled violence, either within the family or in their immediate surroundings. Referring to the law and ethics does not provide all the answers and conclusions are rarely concrete. Medical practitioners therefore have to take into account the minor's situation, medical emergency, and the context, then arbitrate to act in the child's best interest.

Box 9.4 Protection of minors

A large number, if not the majority, of survivors of sexual violence are minors. For example, in the MSF clinic treating patients of sexual violence in Mathare (Nairobi, Kenya), half of the survivors admitted are minors and 63% of the minors admitted in 2014 knew the perpetuator of their assault. There is a specific medical duty to protect children from parental/family mistreatment and/or negligence in protecting the minor from violence by others. This also requires specific attention by the medical practitioners caring for minors who are survivors of violence.

Care for minors
- Emergency medical care for minors should never be delayed in the absence of a responsible adult.
- The interview and medical examination of a minor must not be done unaccompanied, and a third person should always be present.
- The medical practitioner should record who the adult accompanying the minor is and ensure that there is a reliable connection between the minor and the accompanying adult, and assess the adult's ability to act in the best interests of the child.
- The medical practitioner should discuss with the minor without the person accompanying her/him being present in order to achieve an unrestricted and unbiased gathering of the child's account of events. There may be some elements that the minor would not disclose in the presence of his/her close relatives, etc.
- The full account from both the minor and the accompanying person must be recorded in the patient's medical file and on the medical certificate (even if contradictory).
- Doctors can also take into account the age and maturity of the patient when it can influence medical recommendations/decisions. Indeed, the situation and considerations for a minor aged 12 years will not be comparable with that of a minor aged 17 regarding, for example, continuing a pregnancy.

In parallel, medical teams need to examine the situation of minors who are alone or isolated to understand why the family is not present and if a responsible adult can be identified and called upon or a temporary adapted shelter found *before discharging the minor from the medical facility.*

Right to health and legal advocacy

The right to health and to healthcare is a fundamental human right in all situations of peace or conflict. However, it falls short of being applied concretely to many patients around the world due to individual states' health policies and financial commitments to affordable medical care and an international context where the price of drugs is an obstacle for numerous LIC or MIC.

Further, in situations of war, despite prohibitions by IHL, attacks on the wounded and sick, healthcare facilities, and personnel are occurring at an increasingly alarming rate. Whether or not they are dismissed as a mistake, 'justified' by the loss of protected status or committed with the intention to spread terror, they lead to practical deprivation of healthcare to the population.

The health workers in developing countries may fear retribution for speaking out on the injustices faced by their patients, so human rights organizations and iNGOs therefore can play a key role in giving voice to healthcare workers' and patients' demands.

If there is a medical intervention that is not accessible or suboptimal for a given population, simply raising awareness about the need for change may not be enough. Medical advocacy includes using testimonies and data to create strong arguments for change.

Medical advocacy

Medical advocacy can be a tool to address seemingly uncompromising medical challenges and has developed in many ways. Organizations, such as Physicians for Human Rights (PHR), use medicine and science to document and draw attention to mass atrocities and severe human rights violations, focusing on the protection of medical institutions and health professionals working on the frontline.

Another approach has been the Health Care in Danger Project, an initiative from the ICRC and Red Crescent Movement aimed at increasing awareness and addressing the issue of violence against patients and healthcare workers, facilities, and vehicles, and ensuring safe access to healthcare in armed conflict. See ➔ Chapter 11 for more information.

In 2000, the UN Committee on Economic, Social and Cultural Rights affirmed health as a fundamental human right indispensable for the exercise of other human rights. The UN Human Rights Council appointed a special rapporteur for the right to health who reports on state practices and contributes to joint publications from the Office of the High Commission on Human Rights and the WHO on the right to health, such as *Human Rights Guidelines to Pharmaceutical Companies in Relation to Access to Medicines.*

See ➔ Chapter 3 for more information about advocacy.

References

1. Bouchet-Saulnier F. The Practical Guide to Humanitarian Law. Lanham, MD: Roman & Littlefield; 2014. ⅋ http://guide-humanitarian-law.org/content/index/
2. ICRC Health Care in Danger campaign launched in 2011. ⅋ http://healthcareindanger.org/hcid-project/
3. MSF Medical Care Under Fire campaign launched in 2013. ⅋ http://www.msf.org/en/article/medical-care-under-fire

4. International Humanitarian Law Arts 24–27, 28–30 and 32, GC I Arts 36 and 37, GC II Art. 20 GC IV Arts 15 and 16, AP I Arts 9 and 10, AP II Rules 25 and 26, Customary IHL Study International Human Rights Law ICCPR ECHR ACHR ACHPR.
5. AP I, Art. 16, AP II Art. 10, CIHL Rule 26. World Medical Association (WMA) Ethical principles of Health care in Times of Armed Conflict and other emergency, 2014.
6. International Humanitarian Law Arts 19–23 and 33–37, GC I Arts 21–35 and 38–40, GC II Arts 18,19, 21, 22, and 57, GC IV Arts 12–14 and 21–31, AP I Art. 11, AP II Rules 28 and 29, Customary IHL Study International Human Rights Law CESCR, General Comment No. 14.
7. International Humanitarian Law Arts 36, 38–44, 53, and 54, GC I Arts 39, 41, and 43–45, GC II Arts 18 and 20–22, GC IV Arts 8, 18, 23, 38, and 85, AP I Annex 1, AP I Art. 12, AP II AP III Rules 30, 59 and 60, Customary International Humanitarian Law Study Regulations on the Use of the Emblem of the Red Cross or the Red Crescent by the National Societies.
8. Resolution 2076 [LXII] adopted by the First UN Congress on the Prevention of Crime and the Treatment of Offenders and approved by the Economic and Social Council, 13 May 1977.
9. Resolution 37/194 of UN General Assembly on 18 December 1982.
10. Office of the High Commissioner for Human Rights (OHCHR). Manual of the Effective Investigation and Documentation of Torture and Other Cruel, Inhuman or Degrading Treatment or Punishment ("Istanbul Protocol"). OHCHR, 2004, para. 53.
11. Ibid, paras. 66–73.
12. Ibid, paras.74–119; 120–160.
13. Ibid, Annexe IV.
14. Ibid, paras. 161–233; 234–315.
15. ICRC. Professional Standards for the Protection Work: Carried Out by Humanitarian and Human Rights Actors in Armed Conflict and Other Situations of Violence. 3rd ed. ICRC; 2018. ☞https://www.icrc.org/en/publication/0999-professional-standards-protection-work-carried-out-humanitarian-and-human-rights
16. International Protocol on the Documentation and Investigation of Sexual Violence in Conflict Basic Standards of Best Practice on the Documentation of Sexual Violence as a Crime under International Law. June 2014. ☞ https://www.gov.uk/government/uploads/system/uploads/attachment_data/file/319054/PSVI_protocol_web.pdf
17. Inter-Agency Standing Committee (IASC). Guidelines for Integrating Gender-based Violence Interventions in Humanitarian Action. IASC; 2015. Child protection, p. 73; Protection, p. 241. ☞ https://interagencystandingcommittee.org/system/files/2015-iasc-gender-based-violence-guidelines_full-res.pdf

Security

Norman Sheehan and Chris Houston

Introduction

Since the end of the Cold War, the face of geopolitics has changed, and with these changes so too have the institutional and operational challenges faced by the humanitarian agencies. Among those challenges, safety and security have rapidly become more and more of a concern for international organizations. In the past, aid workers could feel sufficiently comfortable with the protection afforded to them by international humanitarian law (i.e. the Geneva Conventions), knowing that combatants would respect their presence and neutrality. This is no longer the case. Over the past 15 years, the environment surrounding humanitarian operations has become increasingly dangerous. Aid workers are frequently targeted, attacked, and killed. Serious incidents are on the rise. At times, humanitarian workers are viewed as political targets, putting them more at risk for serious injuries. Gone are the days where conflict was between two clearly identified law-abiding armies. We live in times where child soldiers, fighters high on narcotics, insurgents, and bandits are present. We live in times when global superpowers bomb hospitals.

Security guidance such as this cannot provide advice for every situation, and a single document cannot serve as the sole source of security and safety information. This chapter provides general precautions and guidance based on sound practices, but each situation is different. Always use your own best judgement and common sense to determine the best course of action.

The responsibility to ensure the safety and security of yourself and your colleagues is a legal, moral, and ethical issue. You should never think that you can take a risk with your own safety, as an incident in which you are injured will have an effect on the organization's ability to deliver assistance to others, will divert resources to resolving any problem you created, and could even shut down the whole project.

This chapter will discuss procedures and protection measures, but it will also discuss the critically important issues of acceptance. Humanitarian workers are most safe when the communities that they serve trust the foreign medics, benefit from the programmes, and have a mutual respect for each other. Your compound might have a high wall around it, but you'd better be inviting in some local stakeholders for some tea if you want to be accepted and protected by the community that you wish to serve.

Humanitarian security overview

Definitions and data

Security is the protection of assets (buildings, stock, people) from harm caused by violence. Safety is the protection of people from all causes of injury. This chapter focuses on security, but touches on a couple of non-security hazards that are closely relevant such as fire safety and vehicle safety.

Between 1997 and 2015:
- 1440 humanitarian workers were killed.
- 1329 humanitarian workers were wounded.
- 1064 humanitarian workers were kidnapped in security incidents (source: ℘ http://www.aidworkersecurity.org).

Recent years have seen a significant increase in security incidents affecting humanitarian workers, a 66% rise in incidents was seen between 2012 and 2013.

National and international staff

The majority of security incidents affect national staff—this is unsurprising, as the majority of medical humanitarian staff are national staff. Statistically, both groups are approximately equally affected by incidents, but their risk profile varies:
- In the event of a crisis, international staff are more able to leave.
- International staff tend to have chosen their humanitarian career from many different opportunities, national staff may have fewer employment options and their acceptance of the risks may vary.
- The families of international staff tend to be safely in a different country, the families of the national staff are nearby, possibly suffering from the crisis being addressed.
- Their proximity can leave some national staff vulnerable to extortion.
- Although increasingly international staff refers to more third country nationals, Western mainstream media will generally cover tragedies that befall staff from the global north quicker than tragedies that affect those from poorer nations.
- Those from the global north might enjoy higher levels of protection from their home government than staff from developing nations.

Understanding security theory

The three strategies used to reduce security risks are:

Acceptance
- Acceptance is gained from the local population and needs to be won and maintained. If you are delivering medical humanitarian aid, acceptance will likely be your primary security strategy.
- For the medical humanitarian agency, think of it like this: people will help protect you because they benefit from your medical facilities and services.

Protection

Locks, fences, and walls provide barriers between you and threats. Undoubtedly you will use physical barriers, but without acceptance, they will simply be a delaying tactic.

Deterrence

- The presence of guards with firearms is the most overt form of deterrence and typically humanitarian agencies avoid the use of weapons. Other types of threats are more common—e.g. the threat to close the medical programmes if there is insecurity.
- Field coordinators working in insecure settings will often remind key stakeholders that any harm or threat to the staff or projects will swiftly be followed by project suspension or closure.

There will generally be a mix of strategies, different agencies use different mixes—but for medical humanitarians, acceptance will most likely be the key strategy.

Planning ahead

Humanitarian agencies must prevent, recognize, and if necessary, effectively respond to a security crisis situation that affects them. Those who have prepared and trained in advance cope much better and manage the situations in a more comprehensive and smooth manner that lead to more successful outcomes for the organization and for individuals affected by the crisis. To do so, organizations must set the groundwork in advance, by developing management and response plans. These include a crises management plan, developed from the HQ level in order to respond to emergency situations, as well as country-specific plans which detail standard operating procedures to use on a day-to-day basis.

Although field workers may not be the ones responsible for developing such plans, having an understanding of the fundamentals of their development and implementation is an essential step in security. There will probably be organization-, country-, and project-specific plans for your agency. Good plans will be comprehensive in nature and it is advised to read them in advance of departure.

Public relations and information security

Frequently, humanitarian agencies are good at public and media relations in the countries where donors reside and where they have HQs. Often, the need to explain programming, motivations, and strategies to beneficiaries, host communities, and governments is given a lower priority. To neglect to explain oneself to those around the agency can be a security weakness. A lack of engagement with local communities, media, and neighbours can leave a void that might be filled with rumours, speculation, and misunderstandings that can lead to security problems. Be transparent to those around you.

That said, some information should be kept secure. Details that would help potential abductors or thieves should be guarded. Most security incidents happen in transit, so in contexts where such risks are real, good information security practices and robust journey management practices include the following:

- Sharing information on trip/movement plans only with those who need to know. In highly insecure contexts, even those on the trip and the drivers might not know the route or the return time until the last moment.
- Randomizing journey routes and times. This might even include deliberately making plans and changing them.
- Avoiding sharing information about visits of international staff who might be at a higher risk of abduction (i.e. if their status in the organization or their nationality makes them a particularly attractive target).
- Invariably, local knowledge is critical. Learn who is trustworthy and who can provide local security updates and analysis. Subscribe to specialist security monitoring services for humanitarian agencies. Monitor local and social media and triangulate information.
- Discreetly seek advice from a range of sources. Share information with other agencies and solicit their advice. Do not rely only on the advice of

expats; local people invariably know the context better. But also, trust probably has to be built in both directions before people will openly share information.

Avoid getting too caught up in the details of what types of military forces, weapon, vehicles, or manoeuvres surround you. You need to find the balance between knowing what is necessary to stay safe without feeding the common misunderstanding that humanitarian agencies are spies for donor governments. Don't pry into the affairs of militaries or document their actions beyond what is necessary for staying safe.

Recognizing danger in your working environment

Identifying potential danger is crucial to maintaining a secure working environment. A key to keeping safe and reducing vulnerability is to be aware of the overall environment, your immediate surroundings, and how you and your agency are perceived.

- If you are driving around in a new vehicle, don't be surprised if people assume you are exceptionally wealthy. Take the time to consider the likely assumptions that local people might have about you and your organization. Are you rich? Are you a tool of a donor government? Are you profiting from poverty? In many places your social life will be relevant—do male and female staff cohabit, do you consume alcohol, do you have parties? You may be judged by standards that differ from your home country.
- Be careful how you dress. Avoid military styles, colours, or emblems that may be fashion trends, but can look highly suspicious in many contexts.
- Be aware of your own actions, limitations, habits, and strengths.
- Make attempts to understand the local political and cultural scenes, and the timing of any major events, i.e. elections and religious holidays.
- Know when and where civil unrest, crime, road hazards, and driving dangers typically occur and if it is safe to use public transportation.

Field communications

All operational areas, especially higher-risk contexts, need adequate communication systems. Some communications equipment, including radios, mobile phones, and satellite phones might require host government approval/licensing to use or import.

Communications systems or equipment should have these general characteristics:

- Redundancy: a communications systems must have back-up if the primary methods fail.
- Reliable/easy to operate: the equipment should require little maintenance, be easily operated, must work during emergencies, and have the ability to make contact outside of the country.
- Adaptable/scalable: all systems should be easily adapted to a variety of uses and environments.
- Cost-planned: the cost for equipment, training, and maintenance should be anticipated and be included in proposals for projects.
- Compatible: equipment should be compatible with other organizations' communication systems. Where there is no humanitarian aid radio network or countrywide emergency notification system, other organizations, such as the UN and embassies, likely have systems that can be used during emergencies.

Organizational contacts and communication procedures

Teams should have written communication procedures and standards. Contact lists should be kept up to date. As part of the security procedures, communication procedures should be established in advance. This should include:

- having important contact numbers of staff, HQ, air evacuation insurance company, police, hospitals, local authorities, and international contacts distributed to staff and implementation of a project 'telephone tree' for staff to follow in emergencies
- ensuring that phone numbers and radiofrequencies are posted in the office and periodically verified
- printing contact details on small cards that all staff can carry and that can be placed in all vehicles and residences.

Radio usage and basic communications in remote areas

- In many locations, radio networks are typically used as a more dependable source of communication.
- Be aware that these sources of communication are not secure, and conversations are easily intercepted.
- Most radio networks used in the field operate on two main types of frequencies, termed high frequency (HF) or very high frequency (VHF).

High frequency

- HF radios are a preferred option for communication in remote areas and are ideal for long-distance communication, and in ideal environmental conditions, can transmit up to several hundred miles by using waves along the ground or reflections of waves off the atmosphere.

- While HF radios can communicate over long distances, ranges and receptions are highly dependent on atmospherics, i.e. time of day, electrical storm activity, sunspot interference, etc.
- HF radios require a large antenna and base stations, but they can also operate in areas without electricity. Stationary HF units can be powered by a standard car battery, which can be charged through solar panels or through a standby generator.

Very high frequency and ultra-high frequency

- VHF and ultra-high frequency (UHF) radios are generally used by staff in the field especially in refugee camp settings and humanitarian emergency response operations. VHF works best with base units, and staff communicate through hand-held units. VHF and UHF radio waves travel in a short-range, line-of-sight manner.
- Radio-to-radio range will vary depending on obstructions and in good open conditions can reach 5–10 miles (8–16 km) or less. If transmission is difficult, it can often be improved by moving slightly by a short distance or to a higher location (e.g. it is usually better to broadcast from the upper floor of a building than the ground floor).
- When a repeater is used, this automatically receives and transmits messages, and will extend the range to a radius of 10–20 miles (16–32 km) of the repeater location.
- Keep in mind also that the condition of the radio's battery can also affect the quality of the transmission and the distance at which messages can be received.

Radio procedures

- Speak clearly and succinctly.
- Do regular checks to verify that equipment is functioning.
- Learn the phonetic alphabet (see Table 10.1).
- If you are nervous or inexperienced about using a radio, plan what you will say in advance.

Table 10.1 Radio (phonetic) alphabet

A = Alpha	H = Hotel	O = Oscar	V = Victor
B = Bravo	I = India	P = Papa	W = Whiskey
C = Charlie	J = Juliet	Q = Quebec	X = X-ray
D = Delta	K = Kilo	R = Romeo	Y = Yankee
E = Echo	L = Lima	S = Sierra	Z = Zulu
F = Foxtrot	M = Mike	T = Tango	
G = Golf	N = November	U = Uniform	

Site safety and security management

Security guards

You agency might use contracted security guards or it might employ security guards. There are advantages and disadvantages with both.

Their responsibilities include ensuring security and protection of the organization's property and staff, as well as supporting the evacuation plan in the event of emergency and/or insecurity. It is important that your guards are able to explain the mandate of your organization and talk about the medical projects that your agency provides. The use of unarmed or armed guard service will very much depend on the mandate of the organization and the risk level in the country you are working in.

In general, NGOs do not use armed guards in the vast majority of the places where they work. NGOs are neutral parties, and provide services to people regardless of political or ethnic affiliations. Having no tolerance for weapons in compounds or vehicles reduces the threat of armed conflict from the population. There are exceptions to this though, most notably, Somalia and Afghanistan.

If armed guards are to be considered, ask: what approaches are other NGOs taking? What is the government policy and procedures on armed guard services and what is professionally available? What are the local or national procedures for vetting, training, and management, of guards?

Assuming acceptance to be the key strategy of your agency, the focus should be on building trust and relations with key stakeholders in the area.

General precautions

In addition to security guards, the following should be in place in all offices, warehouses, and service points:
- Install adequate lighting.
- Clear bushes/overhanging tree branches around perimeter.
- Ensure that all staff wear a visible photo ID when on office premises. The ID should be collected upon termination of contract/employment.
- Require that all visitors show identification and leave it with reception or the security guard. Visitors should be issued with a visitor pass that is collected when they leave. All staff should be clear that no visitors are allowed in unless there is an explicit authorization from the person they want to see or who agrees to see them and is escorted by a staff member.
- Ensure that emergency procedures are reviewed and known.
- Certify relevant staff in basic first aid training.
- Ensure that first aid kits are placed in accessible locations in all facilities and vehicles.

The above list probably seems simplistic, intuitive, or common sense, but frequently these basics are overlooked in the field. Security audits done only at daytime can easily miss consideration of the importance of good lighting. The pressure of an acute humanitarian crisis can also distract humanitarian workers from sufficient reflection on these issues.

Entry points

- Keep household keys separate from vehicle keys. Monitor who has keys.
- Change locks if the keys are lost.
- Keep doors and windows locked.
- Have good illumination around entry points.
- After dark, keep curtains or blinds closed.

Fire precautions

Standard fire precautions:
- Good building choice, concrete or brick is better than thatched or lightweight construction types—this is more important for buildings where cooking, storage, or engineering tasks occur.
- Regularly checked smoke detectors near all cooking and heating sources and by the main electrical box.
- Ensuring an adequate number of appropriate fire extinguishers for all buildings—one per floor at least.
- Proper maintenance of firefighting equipment.
- Locate and mark the electrical circuit breaker for all offices and residences. They should be kept free from obstruction and never be in a locked space.
- Flashlights should be easily accessible to all staff.
- In remote locations with large warehouses, fire stations of fire buckets filled with sand and shovels should be established.

Become familiar with the routes to approved hospitals/clinics and to airstrips. Know how to exit the residence in the event of an emergency, even in the event of a power outage. Know which windows are the safest to exit from.

Operational guidelines

In-country travel journey management

- Know the locations and contact details of the nearest police stations.
- Keep your phone charged at all times. Consider carrying a backup phone on a different network.
- Plan the exact route you will take, and leave your itinerary with a colleague.
- Carry a list of the reputable hotels, NGOs, and UN stations which are along your route.

Document safeguarding

- Carry a copy of your passport at all times, or other key documents and keep the originals in the hotel or the office. If you must carry your original passport, consider disguising it with a plain, slip-on cover.
- Keep a copy of your passport at the office. This will make it easier to replace your passport if it is lost or stolen. Email a scanned copy to yourself.

Hotels

- Use hotels pre-approved by the country office. If your organization does not have a presence, then contact other NGOs/UN, the appropriate embassy, or consulate for recommendations on hotels' general security and evacuation information for that location.
- Ensure colleagues have your hotel location, room number, and the hotel telephone number.
- Take note of the evacuation route in case of fire or emergency. Use the stairways at least once to become familiarized.
- Keep a flashlight by your bed.
- Always secure doors when inside the room with locks and security chains, or a simple wedge jammed under the door. Push a chair or rubbish bin in front of the door so that there will be a noise if the door opens.
- Never sleep with ear plugs in.
- Keep the room curtains closed when it is dark outside.
- Don't open the door to visitors (including hotel staff) unless you can positively identify them.
- Hotel staff seeking to enter the room in the evening should be requested to return in the morning.
- When not in the room, consider leaving on the light, TV, or radio.

Road safety

Vehicle collisions are especially prevalent in developing countries; >90% of the 1.2 million people who are killed in traffic accidents every year live in LIC and MIC, which are home to just half of the world's vehicles. Unlike Western countries, road safety rules are usually lax and even non-existent in some countries where humanitarians work. As car ownership rises, even more lives will be lost on the roads: WHO has estimated that between 2000 and 2020, the number of road deaths in sub-Saharan Africa will rise by 80%.

To mitigate risk associated with collisions, robust rules for vehicular usage are critical. Key recommendations include the following:
- Safety rules reinforced, including:
  - mandatory seatbelt use for all staff in front, rear, and bench seats
  - no mobile phone use or texting while driving
  - speed limits are strictly adhered to
  - motorcycles helmets are mandatory.
- Passengers restrictions: must be employees or are engaged in agency work (or family/friends if policy allows).
- Vehicle maintenance and reporting:
  - Ensure appropriate documentation and maintenance requirements (generally ~5000 miles (~8000 km), or as-needed basis).
  - Collisions reporting procedures include information about when, where, who was involved, injuries and treatment, police report, and any other actions.
  - These accident and police reports are required for insurance claims and can also be used to analyse trends.
- All extended road travel should include an individualized journey management plan, including points for assistance, medical facilities, and safe accommodation.
- Extended road travel should only take place with a first aid kit, water, and self-rescue equipment (where appropriate). Consider sending a first aid-certified employee and a mechanic on arduous trips.
- Trip plans should be kept confidential to only those that are travelling and transport or logistics manager or other appropriate staff.
- Screening requirements for drivers including a valid licence, basic medical and vision testing, vehicle maintenance requirement, and training in safe driving.
- Managing procedures at checkpoints: approach checkpoints slowly with headlights off (sidelights on) and with the interior lights on, during the evening. Take sunglasses off, turn off communications equipment to avoid unexpected noises, have documentation available, don't make sudden movements, permit searches, explain your mandate, and use the opportunity to promote the agency if information is requested. Don't offer bribes.

Choosing a vehicle

The type of vehicle which is ultimately used depends on various factors including the sociopolitical environment, and will be an individualized decision. In some conflict-prevalent environments, high-profile vehicles may be valuable to differentiate your organization from the local population, and thus promote neutrality. In other environments, having new or distinguished vehicles can cause additional security risks. In most contexts, the need for a robust and reliable vehicle trumps other considerations. Most larger agencies tend to use Toyota Land Cruisers® or, less commonly, Land Rover Defenders®. Throughout the world, the widespread use of the Land Cruiser® by humanitarian agencies and others has resulted in common availability of spare parts, and greater likelihood of repair and maintenance skills.

Assessing travel risks

Always seek local advice and triangulate advice between different groups from different backgrounds.

Trained drivers will be aware of exactly what action to take in the event of an abduction attempt, whereas most drivers will probably forget the rules and instinct will take over. Rather than detail all actions for all scenarios, for the most part, it is better to concentrate on the critical principles. In the event of a carjacking:

- Give up the vehicle and valuables as instructed.
- Avoid displays of anger, rudeness, or aggression.
- In general, any robber will be watchful for anything that signals resistance and be nervous about delays so keep your hands visible and make no sudden moves.

The key message is: never put your life at risk by resisting armed robbery as no vehicle or amount of money is worth your life.

Kidnaping and hostage-taking

In recent years, there has been a rise in the number of abductions of humanitarian workers. The likelihood of any individual worker being targeted is low, but the consequences for the individual, the programme, and the agency are very high. Knowing how to act and deal with such a scenario will improve anyone's chances of survival and might make a traumatic experience slightly less horrific.

Awareness of targeting

Kidnappers and hostage-takers almost always choose their targets after careful surveillance. Potential targets are those with visible assets or a clear affiliation with a certain group. Humanitarian organizations are generally perceived as well funded, so holding aid workers for ransom could be seen as a source of income for some groups. Overall, kidnapping humanitarian staff or taking them hostage is still rare, but increasing. If a staff member is abducted, the organization is the senior authority and must be contacted immediately by the field office. HQ will coordinate hostage release efforts.

Conduct recommendations

If abducted

The first hour after the abduction is the most dangerous. The captors are nervous, the victim might not realize what is happening, and the situation can be very volatile. If you are abducted:

- Remain as calm and composed as possible, particularly when being transported somewhere by the captors.
- Talk to the captors if it does not make them more nervous. Establishing a basic rapport can help captors to see you as an individual person and may help your situation.
- Explain everything you have on your person. This will ensure that the captures do not think you are hiding anything, and will hopefully prevent strip searching.
- Do not consider escape except in very rare circumstances when you are absolutely certain you will succeed. You could be injured or killed if you try to escape.
- Accept that you must obey the abductors' orders, taking steps to preserve a sense of self-esteem and personal dignity as the situation allows.

During captivity

- Remain calm. Your only task is survival.
- Maintain your mental health with positive thinking and the knowledge that efforts are certainly being made on your behalf for your release. Focus your thoughts on the future and freedom.
- Always remember that the organization is working to safely secure your release, and do not interfere with this process. Except in some special cases, victims should not negotiate for their own release or discuss what action their organization might take. Such discussions could compromise the negotiations.

- Develop a rapport with the captors if possible and try to earn their respect. It might be helpful to inform them about the organization's work in their area. Do not adopt a belligerent, hostile, or sullen attitude. Do not discuss controversial subjects, such as politics or religious beliefs.
- Inform the captors about any necessary medical treatment.
- Plan and stick with a daily programme of activity, and exercise if possible, and try to keep an accurate record of time.
- To maintain physical health, eat food that is given, even if it is unpalatable.
- Keep as clean as circumstances permit. Ask for adequate washing and toilet facilities and basic personal hygiene items. If appropriate, gradually ask for more personal hygiene items.
- Take advantage of any comforts or privileges the captors offer, such as books, newspapers, writing materials, or access to a radio. If not offered, ask for them. If appropriate, gradually, ask for more such items or privileges.
- Be discreetly sceptical towards any information the captors give you.
- If there is a rescue attempt, drop quickly to the floor and seek cover. Keep your hands over your head. Do not move or try to run. When appropriate, identify yourself.

Release

The time of release also could pose risks for the victim. When the time for release comes, victims should proceed with great care.

Specifically:

- Listen to captors' orders and obey them exactly.
- Do not make sudden or unexpected moves.
- Stay alert. Be prepared to act quickly if things go wrong.
- Be prepared for delays and disappointments.

Post-release reactions

A former captive's emotional reactions do not always appear immediately and recovering from the incident is a slow process requiring patience and understanding. Request a post-traumatic stress debriefing. As soon as the former captive realizes that he or she is a normal person having a normal reaction to an abnormal situation, the healing process can begin.

Sexual harassment and assault

Sexual assault is probably one of the most under-reported security issues in the humanitarian sphere. Stigma towards victims and patriarchy reduce the likelihood of survivors coming forward. Humanitarian agencies and workers ethically and legally must make maximum efforts to eliminate any forms of sexual assaults or abuse. Recent allegations of abuse of children by UN Peacekeepers grab headlines and damage the reputation of the whole industry, but also we must not be blind to sexual gender-based violence in any form towards any person.

Avoiding sexual harassment

Professional responsibilities or cultural sensitivities must never require you to submit to behaviours that invade your personal boundaries, or make you feel unsafe or uncomfortable. If a situation feels inappropriate or makes you uneasy, remove yourself from the situation. Never sacrifice yourself or your sense of safety for the sake of professional responsibilities or cultural sensitivities. The following tips are offered:

- Listen to your instincts. If your instincts indicate that something isn't right, remove yourself from the situation as quickly as possible.
- Personal boundaries (privacy, personal space) are different everywhere. Don't assume that your personal boundaries are the same as those of people in another country. Try to figure out what is the common cultural understanding of personal boundaries and find where you can feel comfortable. Follow the cues of local women and men.
- Be careful with smiling and eye contact, which can mean different things in different countries. They can be viewed as an invitation that you don't mean to offer.
- Dress with respect for the culture. In most places, you're already likely to stand out. By dressing appropriately, you can minimize potential hostilities.
- Receive all guests, even those you know, somewhere outside your home, such as at the door, on the porch, or in the compound. Once someone is in your house, you're much more vulnerable.
- If someone harasses you, responding to harassment can escalate the situation. In some situations, it can be more effective to ignore the harassment; pretend ignorance, confusion, or lack of understanding of the situation or language; move away from the harasser; or remove yourself from the situation.
- Keep your personal information personal. You might feel pressured into divulging personal information such as your hotel name, address, or your mobile phone number. This puts you at risk. Instead, give the office information, especially the telephone number and location, since there are protections in place there for you. You also could offer to take the person's contact information, be vague, or lie if necessary.
- If you're being harassed by a colleague, inform your supervisor or someone you trust. Or contact the human resources department.

Sexual assault

Globally, sexual assault is the most under-reported violent crime and all ages, ethnicities, and economic groups are at risk. Understanding the local environment and culture and avoiding situations or locations where an assault could occur can significantly reduce the risk of sexual assault. But despite best efforts, these crimes can still occur.

There is no single best way to respond when threatened with sexual assault. Use your best judgement for the specific circumstances. Consider these options:

- Passive resistance: talk to the attacker to try to change his mind or discourage him from pursuing sexual contact.
- Active resistance: fight off the attacker. Scream, shout for help, run away, or fight back, such as with a knee to the attacker's groin. The weakest areas of a potential attacker may be the eyes or the Adam's apple.
- Carrying a whistle or personal alarm might also help deter an opportunist attack. If in a vehicle, use the car horn or shout 'Help' or 'Fire,' as people are more likely to respond.
- Comply: if there is no way out, and you feel your life is in danger, focus on survival. Remember: life cannot be replaced.

Medical humanitarian NGOs tend to have a kit available for care to rape survivors. This will tend to include post-exposure prophylaxis, emergency oral contraception, and treatment for STIs. Make sure your location has these supplies available.

Political instability and war

Landmines and unexploded ordnances

Any area that has experienced conflict and war could be contaminated with landmines or unexploded ordnances. General principles are that where it is known that landlines or other unexploded ordnances exist:
- Humanitarian workers should take care to receive and follow local advice.
- Do not stray into any areas with warning signs; know the local customary way of marking dangerous locations.
- Do not stray off paths.
- Specific training for all staff working in such areas is necessary.
- For more information, visit ℘ http://www.mineaction.org.

Riots, mobs, and civil unrest

In some settings, crowds can turn menacing or violent such as during civil unrest, ethnic or communal violence, and disorder around relief distribution:

Measures for risk reduction
Anticipating crowd and mob violence needs to be considered as part of your ongoing situational analysis at both the general national and the local operational levels.

Assess your vulnerability
- What is the cause of the tensions, and at whom is the resentment directed?
- Are foreigners, or aid agencies, a target?
- Can local authorities, or traditional/religious leaders, deflect resentment directed at them onto foreigners or aid agencies?
- Are some of your local staff more at risk because of their ethnic or social identity?
- Is there a pattern that could repeat itself?

Exchange information
- There is a greater risk that collective frustration and anger will be directed against your organization when there is misinformation.
- To prevent this, communication should be managed proactively and having open communication with those outside of your organization can help to mitigate resentment and potential danger. See ➔ 'Public relations and information security' pp. 199–200.

Crowd control measures
- Anticipate the expectations of the local populations with regard to your organization and don't encourage a crowd to gather unless you are confident that you can meet those expectations.
- If there are events such as meetings or distributions where large groups are gathering, organize them carefully in advance, and with cooperation from local representatives.
- If distributing supplies/equipment, have multiple distribution points and schedule distributions throughout the day for different sections of the population.

- In advance of any distributions:
  - Work out procedures to minimize uncontrolled crowd movements, long queues, and waiting times.
  - Create waiting areas with shade and water and areas to sit down; ensure that there are designated crowd control staff to assist with information and movement procedures; physically channel people into a manageable queue/through small avenues; and arrange for an exit route away from the entry points.

Increased security measures

During times of unrest

- Increase the number of guards around your compound.
- Consider asking local authorities for protection, but also be aware that this might jeopardize your independence. The rules of engagement that will be used to protect you should be established in advance.

Negotiation

When confronted with an angry crowd at your office, try to defuse the anger, but simultaneously prepare to protect yourself if the situation deteriorates. Key tactics are the following:

- Seek advice from local staff who can understand the local languages and culture and can provide insight into the controlling and driving forces.
- Trusted local staff can function as key advisors, and can help determine if the crowds are representative of the overall community or not, and may be able to contact the key community leaders and request their presence to help defuse the situation.
- Designate one person to immediately alert other agencies who might be at similar risk and/or who could assist with negotiating and defusing the conflict.
- Negotiate with the demonstrators though a small number of their representatives:
  - Hold these talks in the compound, but not in the heart of the building. Adopt an anger-defusing negotiation strategy. Talks over tea early and frequently can avoid getting to this stage. Listen attentively and respectfully; avoid making quick promises, rather that you are willing to pursue the discussion further but not under threat or duress.
- All employees should prepare for evacuation. Lock the doors of all rooms that are vacated; exit the compound at a place where the crowd has not yet gathered and where you are not visible to it.
- A site should have a separate emergency exit not visible from the main entry/exit point, and back routes should be familiar in advance.

Following such an event, make sure to maintain a heightened security alert for some days and more. Consider very carefully your public relations position and messages and if the perception is negative towards your organization, you may wish to review your approach. Uphold promises: you will need to re-establish relationships and perhaps repair your 'acceptance' in your environment; hold talks, even if you now have increased protection. Don't only have talks with the formal authorities but communicate with a wider environment of ordinary people, religious/cultural leaders, women's groups, and youth groups.

Surviving looting

Looting, of warehouses, convoys, offices, and residences, is not an infrequent occurrence. Key principles to bear in mind are as follows:

- The highest priorities are to protect your life, to protect vulnerable staff, and to try to maintain communications.
- Don't resist, and try to prevent aggression against staff members by allowing the looters to take what they want.
- Remain calm and try to defuse the anger. Don't show fear: signs of high vulnerability may give some looters the confidence to turn on you.
- In general, it is advisable to leave the place being looted, if possible, in case the situation escalates. This may not always be possible; it could be even more dangerous outside. In those cases, try to hide, and retain a means of communication.

Evacuation procedures and protocols

An evacuation can occur for medical or security reasons. Decision-making is often fast, and so to ensure smooth operations, planning must be done in advance and staff need be aware of the concepts and procedures.

Having the necessary information available and plans in place for every field site is key to being able to respond immediately should a medical emergency occur. Having this knowledge and plans pre-arranged can be the difference between life and death.

Medical evacuation

Be aware that medical facilities and treatment options vary widely from country to country. While many developing countries do have strong medical services available (often in the capital), this is not universally the case.

- All international staff need valid medical evacuation insurance in place, and with cards in hand prior to travel.
- National staff are usually covered under a local in-country health policy for treatment within the country.
- Be aware what emergency medical services are available from nearby medical agencies such as MSF or ICRC.

Security evacuation

Circumstances that might require security evacuation of international staff and/or their families or consultants to a site outside the country include mounting terrorist activities and threats, insurrection and other civil disorder, or a natural disaster or other sudden crises. Security evacuations are usually considered a last resort, occurring after official efforts to resolve or mitigate potential threats are unsuccessful.

Evacuation basics

Evacuation phases and pre-planning

Evacuations typically have four phases, and agencies have their own methods for designating these phases, such as letters or colours. Staff should be aware of these phases, and make sure that they have performed their own individual preparations in advance.

Advance decision-making

Within each organization, make sure there:

- is a clear delegation of authority protocols to ensure all safety concerns regarding local staff and assets are secure
- are details on who assumes financial responsibility and remains in close communication and coordination with HQ
- is a clear line of authority and detailed responsibilities for anyone not evacuating.

If you plan to leave national staff behind to run the project or to suspend it, consider who will protect the assets, how staff will be paid, and how staff left behind will communicate with HQ. The circumstances in which you depart will heavily influence your ability to ever return. Be ready to give more autonomy to local staff.

Pre-planning
- Each project office should have a current list of fixed assets (office furniture and equipment), which should be on file with the home office.
- A local staff member should be designated to serve as custodian of project property.
- The home office also should have copies of all important project documents, such as the financial commitment report, leases, insurance policies, and project contracts.
- Know in advance what paper files you will destroy/shred and which you will take.

Be aware that an evacuation can be an emotional event as the departure of international aid agencies can have a variety of meanings to the local population, including the removal of a symbolic safety barrier. Evacuations must be properly planned and executed with great care.

Evacuations can often have unintended or unexpected consequences, particularly for the local population who may be already under stress from a conflict situation and confused about how to interpret a sudden evacuation of international staff. At times, an iNGO security evacuation has been interpreted as abandonment by the local population, more typically in situations lacking a pre-established evacuation plan and with a sudden departure without sufficient delegation of responsibility or informing local authorities. In some situations, such as in South Sudan during the conflict, there was an assumption that the international staff knew of a pending disaster, resulting in panic among the locals, many of whom fled into hiding. In this case, weeks later, after no military activity or military advance materialized, the iNGO team attempted to return but were met with sentiments of abandonment. Ultimately, due to hostility, they were unable to resume services.

Human resources

It is not possible to talk about security without talking about people management.

- Disgruntled, divided, or poorly motivated employees are a potential source of insecurity.
- Problems can be avoided by having fair and transparent recruitment and human resource management.
- International supervisors must invest in good working relationships with their national peers.

Simple things such as thanking people, giving positive feedback when possible, updating everyone on the progress of the programme, and spending time with all of the staff are all necessary. Small gestures such as asking about a person's family, making someone a cup of tea, or sharing a meal are valuable investments in personal relationship building. No emergency is so acute that there isn't time for basic manners.

If you ever need to terminate someone's employment, do it in a respectful manner. Don't forget that this may be a cause of great shame for them. It is important that the terminated employee saves as much face as possible. Never raise your voice, always treat people with respect, and let others see you treating them with respect. Staff in developing countries might be supporting a wide extended family with their income. Even if their performance doesn't warrant a letter of recommendation to future employers, it is normal to provide a certificate confirming the time worked and some notice period paid to terminated employees.

All security policies, guidance, and best practices implemented and practised by development agencies, donors, and the UN are drawn from decades of shared experience of many programme implementers and security experts in the NGO community and are mutually shared in the interest of everyone's safety and security.

Further reading

Humanitarian Outcomes. Aid Worker Security Database. ℜ http://www.aidworkersecurity.org
Lloyd Roberts D. Staying Alive: Safety and Security Guidelines for Humanitarian Volunteers in Conflict Areas. ICRC; 2006. ℜ https://www.icrc.org/en/publication/0717-staying-alive-safety-and-security-guidelines-humanitarian-volunteers-conflict-areas

Chapter 11

Medical care under fire: a perspective from the international medical organization Médecins Sans Frontières

Camille Michel, Kenneth Lavelle, and Thomas Nierle

Introduction

On 3 October 2015, patients and staff were killed in the US-NATO (North Atlantic Treaty Organization) aerial bombing of the MSF hospital in Kunduz, northern Afghanistan. As President of MSF International, Joanne Liu, said in a speech delivered at the UN in Geneva a few days later, they 'joined the countless number of people who have been killed around the world in conflict zones and referred to as "collateral damage" or as an "inevitable consequence of war" '. This tragic attack is, indeed, neither a new phenomenon nor an isolated one.

Similar events include, but are not limited to the following:
• In autumn 1981, four of the 12 hospitals supported by MSF were deliberately bombed by Soviet planes in Afghanistan.[1]
• In August 2009, an Afghan governmental clinic in the Paktika province of Afghanistan was bombed by NATO and Afghan forces.[2]
• In 2012, an explosion inside the compound of a maternity clinic run by MSF in Khost, Afghanistan, injured seven people, including one child.
• On 28 October 2015, a hospital supported by MSF in Saada, Yemen, was bombed by the Saudi-led coalition.
• On 28 November 2015, a barrel bombing on an MSF-supported hospital in northern Homs, Syria, caused seven deaths, the partial destruction of the hospital, and an influx of 47 wounded patients needing to be transferred to nearby field hospitals, some of whom died en route.

While these types of attacks are not new, the reporting of them has increased, primarily due to the improved coordination and professionalism in the humanitarian sector, improved methods of communication, and an increase in media coverage and visibility. Each time a medical facility, staff, and patients are attacked, the very core of humanitarian action is endangered. In war contexts where healthcare structures are targeted deliberately and systematically (such as recently in Syria and Yemen), meaningful humanitarian action simply becomes impossible.

Addressing violence against healthcare

Violence against healthcare is a major humanitarian concern, which impacts the ability of medical NGOs to deliver quality healthcare and adversely affects the safety of staff and access to care for patients. This violence unfortunately has a consistent outcome: the deprivation of healthcare for the civilian population.

Various initiatives have been launched to address this issue of violence against healthcare, including the ICRC 'Health Care in Danger' project in 2011, which examined the tangible impact on the delivery of healthcare, and the development of the 'Safeguarding Health in Conflict' coalition, a group of iNGOs working to protect health workers, services, and infrastructure. Around this time, in 2012, WHO was mandated by its Assembly to work on this topic from a global public health perspective.

In 2013, MSF launched the 'Medical Care under Fire' project, which following the Kunduz attack in 2015, adopted a more proactive approach with the launch of the '#Not a Target' campaign. This campaign aimed to ensure that (1) attacks on health facilities were prevented, and that (2) if such attacks *did* occur, that they resulted in the highest possible political cost with substantial public mobilization and visibility. Using momentum from key multilateral fora, increased public pressure then led to the adoption on 3 May 2016 of the UN Security Council resolution on the Protection of the Medical Mission (S/RES/2286).

Legal and ethical principles

As outlined in ➜ Chapter 9, under international humanitarian law (IHL) dating back to the nineteenth century, medical facilities, personnel, and patients are protected from indiscriminate attacks. This is a core principle of humanitarian medicine, and according to the Geneva Conventions of 1949, 'the wounded and the sick' must be treated humanely 'without any adverse distinction founded on race, colour, religion or faith, sex, birth or wealth, or any other similar criteria'. It is outlined that any party engaged in a conflict is obliged to conduct warfare in a way that civilian casualties are prevented and that medical personnel give priority to patients on medical grounds alone. In today's reality, these are principles that need to be actively maintained and constantly negotiated, but they remain essential for the foundations of humanitarian medical responses. See ➜ Chapter 9 for further information.

Classification

Work into the violence seen against healthcare has shown a diversity of victims, perpetrators, and causes of violence. While the violence is difficult to generalize due to a lack of clear patterns and a complex variety of victims, perpetrators, and motivations, a non-exhaustive classification is as follows:

Perpetrators

Can be non-state armed actors, regular armies, international forces, patients and relatives of patients, medical personnel or civilians. Further, perpetrators can be victims—subsequently or simultaneously.

Victims

Can be patients, families of patients, civilians seeking refuge in medical structures, but also medical and paramedical personnel and all the support staff working in medical structures.

Types of attacks

Can include violence against the wounded and sick (violence, threats, blocking access, discrimination, violation of confidentiality), violence against personnel (violence, threats, kidnappings, coercion, abuse, killing), and violence against infrastructure and vehicles (armed intrusions, shootings, lootings, bombings).

Motivations

Can be military strategy, political strategy (discrimination based on religion or other), accusation of partiality, real or perceived grievance (preferential treatment, bad quality of care), theft and economic gains, and reprisals.

Consequences

Can include deprivation of healthcare for civilians, insecurity and movement of personal, closure of programmes or stopping of activities, reorganization of hospital wards, reduction of admissions, and suspicion towards medical structures.

Causes of violence significant enough to lead to the restriction of humanitarian space, are diverse, but the increase in occurrence is considered by some to be due to the growing presence of asymmetric warfare or new wars,[3] which are notably characterized by a multiplication of non-state armed groups with weak chains of command and a poor understanding of IHL.[4]

Risks and dangers faced on the field

Despite legal protections, violence against medical structures, personnel, and patients has become increasingly common and systematic, and is associated with the politicization, and criminalization, of healthcare.

Politicization of healthcare

The lines between military and humanitarian action have been increasingly blurred because of the large-scale financial involvement of governments and intergovernmental organizations in healthcare programmes (e.g. the UN in Afghanistan). The extent of politicization of healthcare is substantial and widespread, and examples include Bahrain, where in April 2011, government forces used medical facilities to arrest protesters or in Pakistan, where the US used a fake vaccination campaign to approach Osama Bin Laden (leading to suspicion of immunization programmes in the region[5]). To investigate alleged violations of international human rights law in Syria, the UN established the Independent International Commission of Inquiry on the Syrian Arab Republic in August of 2011. Their report found that 'health care has become militarized to the extent that many in need prefer not to seek medical assistance in hospitals for fear of arrest, detention, torture or death'.

> Healthcare is *criminalized* when the basic impartial provision of medical care becomes a crime in the eyes of a government. For example, Syria issued antiterrorism laws on 2 July 2012 which criminalized medical aid to the opposition.[6]

Polymorphous violence

Direct attacks on health facilities may be the most visible form of danger, but violence against the medical mission takes multiple forms. The international media generally give accounts of the attacks against medical personnel, particularly international practitioners, but available data shows that the majority of victims are local staff, patients, and civilians.[7] Apart from isolated acts against staff or patients, there is also regular harassment and obstruction to care, and some contexts are characterized by continuous violence and threats and a system that discriminates against patients on ethnic or religious grounds.

Risks for the staff

In the field, staff face many risks, including direct physical aggression and threats, for a variety of reasons. In some cases, medical staff can be accused of treating the 'enemy', raising the tension and risk for both patients and providers. This was demonstrated when a mob of Rakhine women physically blocked MSF international medical staff from bringing Rohingya patients into Sittwe General Hospital in Eastern Rakhine State, Myanmar, in 2013. Further, in Leer and Bentiu, South Sudan, SPLA soldiers targeted health workers in January and April 2014, respectively, in an attempt to block the provision of healthcare to the Nuer population that had fled into the bush.

At times, medical staff may face aggression by patients or relatives of patients themselves. This can be linked to the perception of the quality of the care provided, such as when patients believe that others receive better care or that they are being discriminated against, or when treatment has been ineffective and patients may presume medical error. Even personal feuds, and their manifestation in various cultures, can endanger medical staff. For example, in a MSF-supported emergency room in Yemen, one patient was summarily shot and executed, out of revenge by another murdered man's son.

Risks for patients

Patients can also be at risk of physical assault for ethnic, tribal, political, or religious reasons. Regularly, and in varying contexts (Central African Republic, South Sudan, Lebanon, etc.), patients face the risk of being arrested in medical structures and refused appropriate medical care because they are former combatants or even simply for belonging to a specific tribe/religion. During the armed conflict in December 2013 in Central African Republic, there was a recurrent intrusion of armed actors in a MSF-supported hospital and medical staff had to physically restrain and prevent entry to Séléka members who were looking for anti-Balaka patients to abduct and execute. In some countries, medical teams have had to reorganize wards, separating patients according to clans and tribes to prevent intra-facility violence, causing significant disruption. Discrimination can be common in other ways, such as Myanmar, where in the Rakhine State, local medical staff extort or even refuse treatment to Rohingya patients.

Violence against facilities

Medical facilities are often a target of violence, including being looted, destroyed, or bombed in the context of armed conflict or violence, or for political or economic reasons. The resultant reduction of activities or closure of the medical facility deprives the population of healthcare. Further, the targeting of facilities often appears systematic, aimed to prevent a specific population or armed group from accessing healthcare. In Masisi, for example, a province of the Democratic Republic of Congo, looting of health centres was frequent; patients reported that this was intentional, and believed to be intended to prevent the opposing side of the conflict from being able to access care there.

Consequences

With multifaceted perpetrators and limited international condemnation, these attacks, have not abated. Recent attacks captured by the MSF Medical Care under Fire project in 2014 and 2015—in just three countries—include:
- South Sudan:
  - two occurrences of hospitals run by MSF damaged during aerial strikes in South Kordofan
  - hospital looted in the town of Leer
  - 22 civilians seeking refuge killed in Bentiu State Hospital
  - 11 patients killed in Malakal hospital.
- Syria:
  - at least five occurrences of hospitals damaged by air strikes, killing patients and staff (Idlib, August 2015) and destroying the equipment and pharmacy.
- Iraq:
  - a MSF-supported clinic and a hospital in Tikrit were shelled in June 2014, by unknown perpetrators.

With these types of risks and dangers currently being experienced in many humanitarian settings, the end result for patients and civilians is the deprivation of health services.

Whether it be because:
- medical structures are destroyed and looted
- patients fear retaliation if they present to a hospital or they consider the hospital itself a dangerous place
- medical personnel are forced to flee
- healthcare structures are relocated or shut down
- working conditions for medical personnel are intolerable, the end result is a reduction in humanitarian space which poses serious challenges for all organizations working in these contexts and ultimately weakens the entire healthcare system.

The consequences of this are clear and dire—medical space is endangered and its access is restricted both for patients and medical staff.

When violence hampers the possibility for humanitarian organizations to access populations in need and hinders the safe access to care for patients, the basic principles of humanitarian law are violated.

Learning to prevent attacks

The continued violence against healthcare underlines the necessity of putting on the political agenda the issue of the protection of health facilities, staff, and patients and, in a wider sense, the protection of civilians, so that humanitarian organizations can continue to provide assistance to people in need. There are no straightforward solutions, but there are several lessons learned from the experiences that can help to mitigate risks.

• Medical services need be adapted to the needs of the population. The provision of quality medical services, consistent communication with patients, and the strict respect of medical ethics are paramount to win the trust of patients and communities.

• Ensure transparent human resources policies and hospital management rules. Consistent and impartial patient flow and organization of wards is essential for the smooth hospital functioning and avoids patient perceptions of preferential treatments.

• Although challenging for humanitarian actors, it is important to maintain a consistent dialogue with all armed actors and authorities. This is necessary not only to inform them about medical needs, but also to improve their awareness on medical ethics and humanitarian principles. This contributes to preserving working space and safeguards the protection of medical structures, personnel, and patients.

• To ensure the respect of medical facilities as conflict-free zones, medical NGOs have to be visible and transparent about their activities and operational principles. All stakeholders have to understand the principles of impartiality, neutrality, and independence followed by international humanitarian organizations, so that they are not confused with political actors that may be parties to the conflict.

References

1. Malhuret, C. Report from Afghanistan. Foreign Affairs 1983/84;62(2):426–35. ℘ https://www.foreignaffairs.com/articles/afghanistan/1983-12-01/report-afghanistan
2. Amnesty International. Afghanistan: Kandahar bombing and NATO clinic attack, highlight increasing danger to civilians. 27 August 2009. ℘ https://www.amnesty.org/en/press-releases/2009/08/afghanistan-kandahar-bombing-and-nato-clinic-attack highlight-increasing/
3. Kaldor M. In defence of new wars. Stability 2013;2(1):1–16.
4. Cone J, Duroch F. Don't shoot the ambulance: medicine in the crossfire. World Policy J 2013;30(3):Fall.
5. McNeil DG Jr. C.I.A. Vaccine Ruse May Have Harmed the War on Polio. N Y Times 9 July 2012. ℘ http://www.nytimes.com/2012/07/10/health/cia-vaccine-ruse-in-pakistan-may-have-harmed-polio-fight.html?pagewanted=all&_r=0
6. Darronsoro G. Afghanistan: pourquoi les humanitaires sont une cible de l'armée américaine. Libération 5 October 2015. ℘ http://www.liberation.fr/debats/2015/10/05/afghanistan-pourquoi-les-humanitaires-sont-une-cible-de-l-armee-americaine_1397491
7. Australian Red Cross. Health care in danger. IHL Magazine 2013;1.

Further reading

Abu Sa'Da C, Duroch F, Taithe B. Attacks on medical missions: overview of a polymorphous reality: the case of Médecins Sans Frontières. Int Rev Red Cross 2013;95(890):309–30. ॐ https://www.icrc.org/eng/assets/files/review/2013/irrc-890-sada-duroch-taithe.pdf

Cone J, Duroch F. Don't shoot the ambulance: medicine in the crossfire. World Policy J 2013;30(3):Fall.

ICRC. Violence Against Health Care, Part I: the problem and the law. Int Rev Red Cross 2013;95(889):1– 250. ॐ https://www.icrc.org/spa/resources/international-review/review-890-violence-against-health-care-2/review-890-all.pdf

United Nations. Security Council Adopts Resolution 2286 (2016), Strongly Condemning Attacks against Medical Facilities, Personnel in Conflict Situations. 3 May 2016. ॐ http://www.un.org/press/en/2016/sc12347.doc.htm

The authors wish to thank Dr. Françoise Duroch for her precious guidance, suggestions and commentaries, and Dr. Maude Montani for her attentive rereading and editing of the text.

Medical logistics in humanitarian settings

Bernard Chomilier and Christine Chomilier

Introduction

Logistics means ensuring that supply meets the demand. The role of a logistician is to make sure that the goods (including food, shelter, medicines, etc.) arrive on time to the people in need. To achieve this goal, the role of the logistician will be *managing the supply chain*, which means to procure, transport, store, and often distribute the goods.

The nature of the humanitarian work makes the supply chain often more complex than a commercial supply chain. The suddenness of some events, including natural disasters, (earthquake, floods, typhoon, etc.), and the uncertainty of the environment (war, civil unrest, etc.) oblige humanitarian logisticians to create a supply chain more agile and adaptable than a commercial one. To assist this, humanitarian organizations have joined efforts and expertise to develop medical logistics reference materials under the UN Logistics Cluster for broad programming benefit.

In some cases, the medical providers in the field have a role in the procurement of supplies, particularly of medicines, whereas in other cases, they may work directly with a logistician. In either case, it is important for the providers in the field to have a firm grasp of logistics, and what is required to ensure continued availability of essential supplies. Collaborative planning and understanding the logistical principles and contextual constraints are essential for a well-functioning programme.

Logistics in humanitarian medical context

The logistician

The medical logistician acts in support to humanitarian intervention and manages the supply of products, including pharmaceuticals, medical supplies, equipment, nutrition, and sanitation, which allow healthcare systems and care providers to function properly.

Humanitarian operational context

- The specific setting determines the constraints that the logistics officers face, and these are particularly relevant in humanitarian settings. Political stability (or conflict) and local recourses (including cold chain, road conditions, or even season) influence the choice of supply routes and modes of transport, the selection of service providers, and the type of contract issued.
- When assessing the operational context, consider the following elements.

External environmental factors

- This refers to external factors which are beyond the control of the organization, including geography, climate, infrastructure, security situation, and economic considerations.
- These factors have a more pronounced effect on operations in humanitarian settings than they do in a standard Western setting. For example, rainy seasons can block access to certain areas for a period of time, or political instability or fighting can restrict access to areas normally accessible which can impact many aspects of planning, including the cost of operation.

Internal operational requirements

- These refer to elements determined by programme requirements.
- This can include the location of the final delivery points, volume, frequency, and time of the deliveries.

The supply, transport, and storage markets

- The local market and the actual capacity of service providers can impact planning. This can include the overall relationship between suppliers and customers (i.e. supply and demand), and the organization's position and leverage in the market.
- There are also specific cultural considerations and local practices which need be considered in humanitarian contexts. In some settings, the operational context will be influenced by the setting, which may limit work on specific days and or holidays.

Delivery principles

Ensuring that a logistics network functions appropriately will depend upon the specific focus of the programme and the needs for delivery frequency and location. From the logistics planning perspective, the delivery mechanisms to supply the goods need to consider the delivery type, frequency, and location.

Delivery type: who is receiving the distribution?

- There are two principal categories for the type of delivery:
  - *Direct delivery*: when supplies are delivered directly to beneficiaries, e.g. shelter supplies.
  - *Service delivery*: when services are provided to specific beneficiaries, e.g. provision of health services or social counselling.
- Most humanitarian medical programmes are predominantly for service delivery, that is, supplies delivered to the team or health facility which medical providers then dispense to the beneficiaries.

Delivery frequency: when does the product need to be delivered?

- There are two principal categories for the delivery frequency:
  - *Pipeline*: describes supplies which are required and provided on a regular basis, which encompasses the notion of recurrence.
  - *One-off*: describes supplies which are distributed on a one-time basis to the beneficiaries, common in acute emergencies (e.g. providing shelter, blankets, etc.)

Delivery location: where does the product need to reach?

The site where supplies must reach is as varied as humanitarian interventions themselves. Location will fundamentally affect the lead time of the order (from days to even months in remote areas) as well as the modes of transport to be used.

Classifications of supplies

- As opposed to non-medical supplies, medical items are subject to specific considerations to guarantee the quality of the product through the entire supply chain from production to administration to the beneficiary for safety reasons.
- Strict rules must be followed along the entire supply chain to optimize quality of the products and effectiveness. Some products have special additional concerns and could be considered hazardous, under regulation, or sensitive to temperature control through the entire supply chain.
- The items commonly procured in humanitarian interventions include a broad range of products, typically categorized as below:

Drug family

- The term 'drug family' reflects broad categories of medications, such as oral drugs, injectable drugs, infusions, vaccines, etc.
- Commonly used among humanitarian organizations, drug families are reflected in logistics medical items catalogues.

Essential drugs

- Refers to the generic products that can be exported/imported with regular regulation rules and medical supplies transport.
- These drugs are commonly used in the majority of countries; however, specific drugs such as narcotics and psychotropics are outside this list because they are highly regulated.

WHO Model Lists of Essential Medicines

- The WHO Model List of Essential Medicines is an important tool as it serves as a guide for the development of national and institutional essential medicine lists. This document is at the disposal of the national MOH and as such, humanitarian organizations are generally required to follow the national drug list when running medical programmes in a country.
- Since 1977, this list has been updated and revised every 2 years by the WHO Expert Committee on Selection and Use of Medicines. The current versions are the 20th WHO Essential Medicines List and the 6th WHO Essential Medicines List for Children updated in March 2017 (℗ http://www.who.int/medicines/publications/essentialmedicines/en/).

National drugs list

- Each country has a National Drug List, approved by the MOH, often based on the WHO Model List of Essential Medicines.
- The list includes safe, effective, and affordable medicines needed to address the priority health problems defined in the national health strategies of the MOH.

Renewable medical supplies

- In addition to the drugs, all programming will require the procurement of 'renewable medical supplies'. These include single-use and sterile

products as well as safety equipment for both the patient and the providers.
• Like non-renewable supplies, all these items have a manufacturing and expiration date and a batch number.

Medical equipment
• This term refers to the range of supplies used by the medical provider, designed to support the diagnosis, monitoring, and treatment of patients.
• There are special considerations to obtaining these items, as they can be heavy and bulky to transport.

Laboratory family
• Includes diagnostic tests, reagents, lab supplies, and equipment.
• Be aware that some of these products are 'dangerous goods' and will need specific packaging for transportation, with specific requirements for exportation/importation.

Medical kits
• 'Medical kits' containing essential supplies have been developed by various organizations with the intention to improve standardization and allow a rapid response at the onset of an emergency.
• Several medical kits are available, some of which are recognized and approved by the WHO.

The supply chain concept

To ensure the supply chain meets the needs of the intervention, the logistician needs to understand the requirements of the medical programme and likewise, the programme officers to understand the constraints of the logistics components, which can affect the delivery lead time and/or the cost. A joint assessment by medical and logistics experts working closely together from the earliest stages of any intervention is essential.

Assessment

The assessment is the process determining operational capacity by gathering, analysing, and disseminating logistics-related data, which will vary between countries.

Logistics Capacity Assessment

- Useful information regarding in-country logistics infrastructure and services is available the Logistics Capacity Assessment (LCA) by WFP Logistics, under the Logistics Cluster leadership.
- These LCAs are regularly updated and provide standardized logistical information and country capacity which is shared with the humanitarian community globally.
- LCAs exist for many countries and can be found at ℘ http://www.logcluster.org/tools/lca.

Emergency assessment

- These rapid assessments are done to determine the post-disaster logistics infrastructure, and possible logistics bottlenecks. Performed on site, it typically examines the existing capacity of airports, ports, railways, waterways, road networks, warehousing, local supply, fuel, customs, truck transporters, freight forwarding agents, telecommunications, etc.
- While large organizations have their own assessment forms and templates, smaller organizations can utilize standardized emergency assessment template documents available through the Logistics Cluster website (℘ http://www.logcluster.org/rapid-assessment-toolkit).
- Small organizations can also gather information from recognized agencies/NGOs such as the UN (the UNDAC team, for example), Logistics Cluster, Red Cross, MSF, and others.

Planning

Any logistics operational plan must define the following factors:
- *Logistics set-up*: this refers to where logistics hubs, warehouses, and important bases will be established.
- *Human resources*: consider what profiles for personnel you need, where they would be based, and for how long. General requirements often include a coordinator, warehouse experts ± potentially port experts, aviation experts, and fleet managers.
- *Transport*: this includes the means of transport that will be needed (air, ship, road, rail, multimodal), which will have an impact on the overall set-up and budget. In sudden-onset emergencies, the use of an air operation is often a necessary but very expensive solution, but should be used for a minimum period of time.

- *Sourcing*: this includes where supplies will be procured (international, regional, local).
- *Warehousing*: consider the need for transshipment hub and field warehouses.
- *Fleet needs*: this refers to the needs of the medical teams for transportation, including how many and which types of light vehicles are required to support the medical team work,
- *Reporting*: logistics generally reports to the head of operations, but it is very important that medical teams and operations personnel have a clear picture of the overall supply chain for better planning.
- *Budget*: all planned expenses should be budgeted for, including costs of procurement, transportation, and relevant programme and operational expenses (e.g. fuel consumption, rental costs, etc.).

Sourcing

Identifying where supplies can be obtained to meet the organization's requirements will depend on the situation and the time available. Price, availability, and quality are core considerations. In general, sourcing can usually come from three main options: procurement, existing stocks, and in-kind donation, outlined as follows:

Procurement

Procurement refers to obtaining goods from outside sources. The procurement of medical items follows the same basic principles of any other goods including having a standardized, fair process.

Counterfeit drugs

A specific note about procurement of drugs is knowledge about the risk of counterfeit drugs. Production of counterfeit drugs is a relatively common practice and extremely difficult to control. The best way to avoid the purchase of counterfeit drugs is to use recognized suppliers with a good manufacturing practice (GMP) certificate (see ➔ 'Procurement of drugs' pp. 245–7). For more details on counterfeit drugs issue, see the WHO guidelines: ℜ http://whqlibdoc.who.int/hq/1999/WHO_EDM_QSM_99.1.pdf?ua=1.

Existing stocks

- For a quick response in emergency situations, some organizations have their own pre-stocked supplies which can be sent directly.
- To prepare for a rapid response, organizations often have their stocks located in different strategic areas around the world.

Drugs donation

- A donation of drugs is an idea which seems rooted in good will, but is, however, racked by many perils. To maintain appropriate standards, drugs donation should follow four strict principles developed by the WHO:
  1. Donations of medicines should benefit the recipient to the maximum extent possible. All donations should be based on an expressed need. Unsolicited medicine donations are to be discouraged.

2. Donations should be given with due respect for the wishes and authority of the recipient, and in conformity with the government policies and administrative arrangements of the recipient country.
3. There should be effective coordination and collaboration between the donor and the recipient, with all donations made according to a plan formulated by both parties.
4. There should be no double standard in quality. If the quality of an item is unacceptable in the donor country, it is also unacceptable as a donation.

More detailed information on drug donations guidelines are available at ℘ http://www.who.int/medicines/publications/med_donationsguide2011/en/.

Delivery

Once sourced, consideration needs to be given to the total transport process, from procurement until the items reach the destination. This includes analysing the transportation time and mode(s) needed to make sure the products will not spoil during transport.

Transport

- Each mode of transport requires contracting and it is important to find a reliable partner, through a fair competitive process.
- Different modes of transport each have distinct rules, regulations, and procedures

See Table 12.1 for the benefits and drawbacks of the main modes of transport.

Customs

Customs clearance procedures need to be considered from the earliest stages to prevent delays with importation. The customs procedures and the requirements for importation and clearance can vary between countries, but the process is similar (see Fig. 12.1):

- To import any commodity from another country, an importer will need a clearing agent/company, that is duly registered and licensed by the customs authorities to process the import documentation through customs. Normally the customs authorities in each country will have a list of licensed clearing agents on their website database who are authorized to conduct the business of a customs agency.
- Humanitarian organizations can get tax exemption from local authorities. In sudden-onset emergency operations, the government will guarantee tax exemption to humanitarian organizations, but this will require procedures to be followed.
- For more information on customs and tax exemption, see ℘ http://log.logcluster.org/response/customs/index.html.

Table 12.1 Advantages and disadvantages of the four main means of transport[a]

Mode criteria	Road	Rail	Sea	Air
Relative speed	Moderate	Moderate	Slow	Very high
Reliability	Good	Good	Limited	Very good
Cost per tonne/km	Medium	Low/medium	Low/very low	High
Flexibility	High	Low	Low	Medium
Other considerations	Extensive network	Limited and fixed infrastructure	Restricted network	Limited network
	Short and medium distances, e.g. Europe/middle East. From a neighbouring country to operation site. Internal transport; short/medium distance	Large consignments. From port of discharge to inland operation site (warehouse). Ecological	Large quantities; less urgent; prepositioning phase; second phase; long distance with no time constraint	Emergency phase; expensive goods; cold chain; no alternative option; small shipments; e.g. diplomatic pouch; long distance with time constraints
Advantages	Relatively fast; no transhipment; direct delivery; flexible; cost	Economical; large loading capacity; range and speed (in most countries)	Economical; large loading capacity; no restriction on loading capacity; cheap	Fast; reliable; limited losses; direct; easy tracking and tracing
Disadvantages	Road may be dangerous (land mines) or blocked (rainy season); sometimes, driver's nationality or vehicles registration not acceptable	Difficulty finding freight cars; delays; transhipment; inflexible; tracking	Slow; transhipment at ports; use as a second means of transport for large volumes; higher theft risk in the port; not flexible	Expensive; restricted to journeys between airports; restricted loading capacity (dangerous goods, size of shipment, weight, fuel, size of packages, etc.)

[a] Humanitarian Logistics Certification—Fritz Institute.

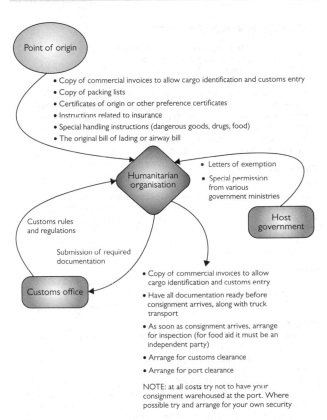

Point of origin

- Copy of commercial invoices to allow cargo identification and customs entry
- Copy of packing lists
- Certificates of origin or other preference certificates
- Instructions related to insurance
- Special handling instructions (dangerous goods, drugs, food)
- The original bill of lading or airway bill

Humanitarian organisation

- Letters of exemption
- Special permission from various government ministries

Host government

Customs rules and regulations

Submission of required documentation

Customs office

- Copy of commercial invoices to allow cargo identification and customs entry
- Have all documentation ready before consignment arrives, along with truck transport
- As soon as consignment arrives, arrange for inspection (for food aid it must be an independent party)
- Arrange for customs clearance
- Arrange for port clearance

NOTE: at all costs try not to have your consignment warehoused at the port. Where possible try and arrange for your own security

Fig. 12.1 Documentation flow for customs clearance (Logistics Cluster—Logistics Operation Guide).

Emergency operations

- Humanitarian crisis response requires three elements:
  - Staff trained for emergency operations.
  - Emergency stock strategically located.
  - Emergency procedures.
- Emergency situations often require different approaches to allow an immediate response which emphasizes speed and flexibility. A fast response can start with incomplete information, and is equivalent to the idea of 'launching a missile first and then guiding it'. Most organizations use a 'push–pull' strategy, including the use of prepositioned kits in their warehouses to start an operation.

Push–pull strategy

Push
- At the start of a crisis response, a rapid assessment can be done to allow an organization to estimate what goods are needed.
- These goods are then 'pushed' towards the crisis from stock.
- During this initial response, a team typically conducts a more thorough needs assessment, while other members of the team are providing services and distributing necessary supplies.

Pull
- As the initial response finishes (about 2–3 weeks), improved needs assessments allow the team to clearly determine needs.
- They then order, or 'pull' the goods towards them as needed.

Staging areas

- The arrival of goods into an operating area is a particular logistical constraint in many emergency operations. Airports are often congested and disorganized, and can be avoided by using 'staging areas' outside of the immediate emergency zone.
- This was demonstrated during the Haiti earthquake in 2010, when a staging area was created in the Dominican Republic. In this case, there is an intermediate step called 'call forward' which exists between the push and the pull. Some goods are pushed to the staging area and then pulled to the operation when needed.

Use of kits

- Experience has shown the benefit of pre-packed and stockpiled kits, ready for rapid deployment to an emergency operation.
- There are a range of standard kits, and most have been developed jointly by the main organizations involved in humanitarian response such as WHO, UNICEF, MSF, Save the Children (SCF) IFRC, and ICRC.
- Kits can also be sub-divided into modules or supplementary kits which can be purchased from UN agencies (e.g. WHO, UNICEF), NGOs (e.g. MSF, SCF), or through the manufacturer (e.g. IDA).
- Commonly used kits are the Emergency Health Kit, First Aid Kit, Resuscitation Kit, Diagnosis Test Kit, and Obstetric Surgical Kit.
- To look at the composition of kits in more in detail, see the Emergency items catalogue, RC Volume 2 (http://www.ifrc.org/emergency-items).

Storage of medical supplies

Temperature

- All programmes need to consider the safe and controlled storage of supplies, including:
    - *quality control*: this includes considering sensitivity to heat, cold, and humidity during the supply chain and storage.
    - *item turn-over*: medical items have an expiration date. Goods should always be dispatched following the FEFO system (first expired, first out) rule to avoid waste.
    - *design of the storage space*: a good medical warehouse is planned/designed in advance, considering the items to be stored.
- Depending upon the requirements of the items, the supplies may be stored either at room temperature, under cold chain conditions, on palettes, or in racks.

Standard storage temperature

Temperature control is essential to keep medical products in the right condition (Fig. 12.2).

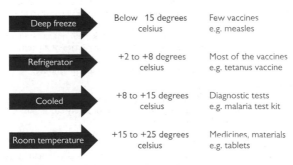

Deep freeze	Below 15 degrees celsius	Few vaccines e.g. measles
Refrigerator	+2 to +8 degrees celsius	Most of the vaccines e.g. tetanus vaccine
Cooled	+8 to +15 degrees celsius	Diagnostic tests e.g. malaria test kit
Room temperature	+15 to +25 degrees celsius	Medicines, materials e.g. tablets

Fig. 12.2 Typical temperature requirements according to product/category. (For further information on the cold chain, see 'Cold chain/vaccination' pp. 248–9.)

Inventory management

- Cost-effective and efficient supply chain management requires accurate information regarding what goods are in stock, what goods are coming, and what goods should be sent.
- This is not always straightforward, as effective planning requires knowledge of quantity required (including safety stock), supplier stock availability, seasonal demand, the production lead time (how long it takes to make the product), and the transport lead time (how long it takes for the product to be transported).

Stock planning

Stock monitoring

Without accurate monitoring of stock levels, an effective supply chain will be impossible. This can be done through the following:

- *Stock card or stock ledger:*
  - Serves as a record of all supply movement in the warehouse.
  - May be a physical piece of paper or a file in a computerized system, administered by the warehouse manager.
- *Bin card:*
  - Serves as a document as to the status of a particular material/item held in one stack in the warehouse, placed physically next to the item in the storage area.
  - Relates one specific batch of an item in stock, with one created for each new purchase order, batch, or new expiry date of an item.
- *Stock reports:*
  - Weekly/monthly stock status of all items in the warehouse.

Safety stock

- As the level of demand for medical items needed for a programme is rarely known with absolute certainty, a buffer or safety stock must be incorporated into the inventory.
- As a general guide, this is usually a 1-month consumption to absorb any seasonal distortion or unexpected event.
- As much accuracy as possible is necessary as overstocking could cause items to be in the warehouse too long, with the risk of expiry whereas understocking could cause a risk of stock outs.

Free stock

- Free stock is the amount of stock available for use. Physical stock in the warehouse is not the same as 'free stock'.
- *Free stock = physical stock on hand + stock on order from suppliers + stock in transit − stock allocated to consignments − stock reserved for special purposes.*

Reordering process

The reordering process is the time between deciding to reorder and the delivery to the warehouse. This includes the lead time (the internal process to place the order and the delivery time). There are two main methods of inventory reordering which can be used depending upon the needs of the programme, termed the reorder level policy and the reorder cycle policy.

Reorder level policy
- Refers to when an order is placed when the stock has reached a certain level.
- The reorder point (ROP) is the lower level of inventory which triggers the action to replenish that particular inventory stock.
- The ROP is normally calculated as the forecast usage (according to historical data) during the replenishment lead time plus safety stock. See Box 12.1.
- This is a flexible ordering system, but could lead to numerous ad hoc orders for replenishment

Box 12.1 Reorder level policy

For example:
- Lead time: 3 months.
- Monthly consumption: 100 vials.
- Safety stock: 150 vials.

Reordering point: $(100 \times 3) + 150 = 450$ vials.

This item should be ordered when the stock level reaches 450.

The quantity which should be ordered would be decided according to the forecasting of the medical team.

Reorder cycle policy
- Refers to the placement of an order on a regular basis, called a review period (e.g. every 3 months).
- This system is best in stable environments, when large orders can be placed at once.
- There are two main methods when using the reorder cycle policy: the minimum stock system and the maximum stock system.
- For both systems, do not wait until the end of the review period to check the stock availability. Stock checks must occur regularly and urgent orders placed if consumption exceeds forecasting.

Minimum stock system
- The minimum stock system is best used when the usage rate is low compared to the order quantities, which means that orders will not be placed at every review period. See Box 12.2.

Box 12.2 Reorder cycle policy: minimum stock system

For example:
- Safety stock: 1 month of stock = 50 vials.
- Review period: 3 months.
- Average demand: 50 vials/ month.
- Average review period consumption: 150 vials.

Therefore, minimum stock level: $50 + (50 \times (3+2)) = 300$ vials.

Lead time: 2 months.

Ordering quantity: $50 + (150 \times 2) = 350$ vials (confirmed with medical teams).

- *Minimum stock level = safety stock + average demand × (review period + lead time)*.
- Minimum stock ordering process:
  1. Determine ordering action:
     - If your free stock is less than the minimum stock level, an order is placed.
     - If your free stock is more than the minimum stock level, no further action is taken.
  2. Ordering quantity:
     - *Ordering quantity = safety stock + review period average consumption × lead time*.

Maximum stock or top-up system
- The top-up system is best used when the usage rate of the items is high compared to the order quantities, which means that orders will need to be placed at every review period.
- In the top-up system, a maximum stock level is defined.
- At the review point, the order quantity is calculated by subtracting the free stock from the maximum stock level.
- The maximum stock level is calculated by adding the average amount of stock, which is used during the review period, plus the lead time to the safety stock level i.e.
- *Maximum stock level = safety stock + average demand × (review period + lead time)*.

Procurement of drugs

General rules and regulations

- The aim of procurement is to ensure that the right items are supplied at the right quality, at the right quantity, at the right place, at the right time (to buy and deliver), at the right cost, from the right source: commonly known as the 'Six Rights'.
- Procurement principles are transparency (process fair and documented), accountability (funding through donation and proper use of the money provided), and efficiency (no waste of money).

Generic items

In medicine, 'generic' applies mainly to drugs marketed under their chemical, non-proprietary name, but which:

- are comparable to a brand/reference listed drug product in dosage form, strength, quality and characteristics, and intended use
- contain the same active ingredients as the original formulation.

Generic products generally become available once the patent protection for the original developer has expired, and the market competition often leads to substantially lower prices for the generic forms (such as with anti-retroviral drugs, leading to increased access to treatment).

Specificities on drugs procurement

When purchasing drugs it is important to consider the following areas to make sure the drugs will have the right quality:

Shelf life and manufacture/expiration date

- Drugs and sterile, renewable laboratory products have a date of manufacture and expiration date that is clearly shown on packaging.
- Their shelf life, the length of time that the product may be stored without becoming unfit for use or consumption, is monitored with high care from manufacturer until extended delivery point.
- Procurement should consider the maximum shelf life, expiration date, transport, and field storage, and generally a minimum of 2 years is used as a guideline.

Good manufacturing practice

- GMP indicates the minimum standard that a medicines manufacturer must meet in their production processes to have their products be of consistent high quality, appropriate to their intended use, and meet the requirements of the marketing authorization or product specification (℅ http://www.gov.uk/guidance/good-manufacturing-practice).
- It covers the production of the product from the raw materials to final product including the manufacturing processes and procedures used for each batch. In addition, it also tests the documentation procedures as well as the personal hygiene of staff.
- When selecting a pharmaceutical company, *only* consider those with a GMP certificate.

Good manufacturing practice (GMP) is that part of quality assurance which ensures that products are consistently produced and controlled to the quality standards appropriate to their intended use and as required by the marketing authorization. GMP is aimed primarily at diminishing the risks inherent in any pharmaceutical production, broadly including cross contamination/mix-ups and false labelling. Above all, manufacturers must not place patients at risk due to inadequate safety, quality or efficacy; for this reason, risk assessment has come to play an important role in WHO quality assurance guidelines.

WHO, 'Essential Medicines and Health Products'[1]

Batch number
- Pharmaceuticals require a continuous focus on quality control, including batch laboratory testing from raw material to final product. A certificate of analysis is issued for each batch by the manufacturer as necessary documentation for the import process.
- These batch numbers are linked to a quantity of material from a single manufacturer and mentioned on the packaging. It enables tracing along the production chain, recording during storage, and recall in case of problem.

Exportation and importation of medical goods
- There are agreements, regulations, and international and national regulations, which determine the requirements for transporting medical goods which also involve the country customs as well as the MOH.
- It is generally recommended to use a clearing agent to assist with this process. It has a cost, but will be cheaper and faster than doing it yourself!

Medical goods documentation
There are specific documents for transporting medical items required by the legal authorities:
- Certificate of Analysis: issued by the manufacturer for each drug and each batch, which certifies quality testing and conformity to requirements. This includes the certificate of origin (evidence of the country of manufacture of an item) and the release certificate (evidence that a specific batch has been checked by the legal regulatory authority in the producing country).
- Dangerous Goods Declaration: description and nature of the goods being moved according to the specific means of transport. A 'dangerous good' label must be made visible on shipping boxes.
- Import licence: provided by recipient countries to authorize the import of drugs and issued by the MOH or the National Drug Regulatory Authority. The clearing agent generally does this duty, with the customs and respective country authorities.
- Export licence: provided by the country of origin to authorize release of controlled substances to the recipient country. As with the import licence, a clearing agent is generally responsible.

Import/export of controlled substances
- Controlled substances, which include narcotics and certain psychotropic drugs, are under additional and very strict international control conventions signed and implemented by governments in order to track and register any movement.
- Special consideration into legal requirements is necessary when purchasing, transporting, or storing controlled substances.
- In each country, the MOH is the ultimate owner and will transfer this responsibility to another country MOH when exported/imported with specific documentation.
- Special export and import licences are needed to move controlled substances which are more difficult to obtain than for standard medicines.
  - *Export licence*: one document issued by the exporting country to authorize the drugs or substances to leave the country and to be taken over by the receiving country. This is also called the 'transfer of responsibility'.
  - *Import licence*: another document issued by the importing country to the country to import. Also known as permit, certificate, or authorization. It means that the receiving country accepts to endorse the responsibility regarding the product and becomes responsible for its follow-up on the territory.
- Controlled substances must also be stored in a 'bonded warehouse', adding another layer of complexity to their transport

Labelling and packaging
- Packaging of medical items requires particular attention to avoid damage during transport and warehousing.
- Information required on the packaging includes the contents, manufacturer information and batch number, manufacture/expiry dates, and any specific characteristics such as temperature stability.
- All this information needs to be seen at any time when transporting and/or storing and this could influence the packaging requirement.

Cold chain/vaccinations

Cold chain

- The cold chain is mainly concerned with vaccines but is also used for other medical products with temperature sensitivity such as some diagnostic tests or laboratory reagents.
- Cold chains require close monitoring, timely transportation, and appropriate storage to minimize risk of exposure.
- Many humanitarian operations have a vaccination component, and vaccines are highly temperature sensitive, requiring stable temperatures from manufacturer to beneficiary.
- From shipment and storage, all vaccines must be kept at +2°C to +8°C (+35°F to +50°F).
- A few vaccines such as measles or oral polio (OPV), are kept under slightly colder temperatures, −15°C to −25°C (+35°F to −13°F).
- Be aware that the cold chain needs attention in both hot *and* cold environments. (Cold climates also need careful monitoring due to fluctuations in ambient temperatures and variations from the acceptable range for the products.)

Equipment

- Insulated shipping containers are used to ship from the manufacturer, which guarantee the cold chain generally via dry ice.
- In-country, refrigerators or freezers are used, which depending upon the resources available, can run on various source of energy: electric/solar (compression equipment) or kerosene/gas (absorption equipment).
- As the level of service goes from more urban to rural areas, the equipment available will generally vary from cold stores/freezers → refrigerators → cold boxes/ vaccine carriers.

Temperature monitoring

- Monitoring temperature is of fundamental importance to ensure there are no temperature fluctuations to interrupt the cold chain and impact the efficacy of the vaccines.
- Temperature monitoring with data recording must be done at least twice a day. Any temperature change requires immediate attention, whether due to human error or equipment dysfunction.
- Vaccine-specific equipment (freezer or refrigerator) includes:

Vaccines vial monitor (VVM)

- The VVM is a heat sensitive label (a circle with a small square inside) placed on a vaccine vial to register cumulative heat exposure over time.
- The combined effects of time and temperature cause the inner square of the VVM to darken, gradually and irreversibly.
- A direct relationship exists between the rate of colour change and temperature: the lower the temperature, the slower the colour change; the higher the temperature, the faster the colour change.

Vaccine cold chain monitor cards
- Monitor cards are used for long-distance shipments with control at arrival point.
- Any problem is reported as it means that the vaccine efficiency has been affected and vaccines are not to be used.

Shipping and customs

In addition to the procedures for drug importation, vaccinations additionally have specific requirements:
- The shipping box with documents must be clearly labelled with the words 'Containing vaccine shipping document'.
- National Regular Authorities or the Head of Customs must be informed prior to the flight arrival to facilitate the customs clearing process and safely accommodate the shipment to a cold storage.
- The cold chain monitor (VVM) has to be checked to confirm that the vaccines arrived in good condition at the airport without breakdowns in the cold chain.

Information management

Humanitarian situations are liable to have rapid changes, and to guide decision-making, essential information related to the supply chain must always be known. This information includes not only the quantity of drugs ordered, but where they are in the supply chain process and what products are held in each location.

The main documentation which should be organized and available through the different steps of the overall supply chain includes:

Procurement
- Request order: internal request to initiate the procurement.
- Request for quotation: bidding process with approved suppliers.
- Purchase order or contract between the organization and suppliers.
- Goods received note: acknowledgement of the receipt of the goods.

Transport
- Waybill: for road transport.
- Airway bill: for air transport.
- Bill of landing: for sea transport.

Warehouse
- Goods received note.
- Release note/dispatch requisition: order to dispatch from a warehouse.

See templates of commonly used documents at ✆ http://log.logcluster.org/response/warehouse-management/annexes.html#sample-template.

Reference

1. World Health Organization. Essential Medicines and Health Products. ✆ http://www.who.int/medicines/areas/quality_safety/quality_assurance/production/en/

Further reading

Logistics Cluster. Logistics Operations Guide. ✆ http://log.logcluster.org/

Mc Guire G. Handbook of Humanitarian Health Care Logistics. 3rd ed. 2015. ✆ http://www.humanitarianhealthcarelogistics.com/handbook.htm

Médecins Sans Frontières. Essential Drugs – Practical Guidelines. 2016. ✆ http://refbooks.msf.org/msf_docs/en/essential_drugs/ed_en.pdf

MedLog Fritz Institute. Certification in Humanitarian Medical Logistics Practices (Medlog) Program [On-line Training]. ✆ http://fritzinstitute.org/PDFs/Course%20Information/MedLog%20Overview-letter.pdf

World Food Programme. Managing the Supply Chain of Specialized Nutritious Foods. 2013. ✆ http://documents.wfp.org/stellent/groups/public/documents/manual_guide_proced/wfp259937.pdf

WHO Model Lists of Essential Medicines. ✆ http://www.who.int/medicines/publications/essentialmedicines/en/

Chapter 13

Working for international organizations

Rod Volway

Introduction

Heading off into the field for the first time, it can be really difficult to know what to expect and how to prepare. Being flexible is key as the unexpected can be common and often aid workers will depart on extremely short notice—especially at the onset of an emergency.

There are many points to consider when preparing to depart for a mission, including the fundamentals of the post (durations, salary). If your assignment is temporary—perhaps to gain international experience to see if it fits—you will need to consider your home situation: do you rent out your house? If not, is there someone who can help look after it? In order to prepare, you will want to know living standards (shared apartments/compounds/own housing), what you can resource locally, and availability of communications. This chapter is intended to help someone prepare and better understand what to expect. You will want to understand the humanitarian operation you plan to join; some research should take place prior to the job interview and be more in-depth once you have accepted an offer.

Aligning expectations

Information gathering

Where you go, who you work with, and what your role is are three inter-connected keys that have a crucial impact on how your assignment unfolds. Before you accept an assignment with an organization, research the agency itself, and make sure that it operates in a manner which is consistent with your own belief system and technical focus.

For research into the country of assignment, there are many resources available to better understand the agency's involvement, sectors represented, and to provide historical context. The two OCHA-operated websites are a great start:

- OCHA: ℰ https://www.unocha.org/.
- Reliefweb: ℰ https://reliefweb.int/ (operated by OCHA, contains some job openings as well as country information).
- BBC News country profiles: ℰ http://news.bbc.co.uk/1/hi/country_profiles/default.stm.
- Central Intelligence Agency (CIA)—The World Factbook, especially for statistics: ℰ https://www.cia.gov/library/publications/the-world-factbook/.
- WHO provides data, statistics, and public health news: ℰ http://www.who.int/.

Check the website of your new employer—though sometimes dated, this still can be a good source of context and history. From the site, one can access information from briefings/reports from field sites to agency press releases, as well as understand what other agencies are working in that area. While the realities on the ground will often differ from what might be presented on a website, you should nonetheless be able to obtain fairly reliable information.

Understand your agency's goals

Some agencies focus on maternal and child health and public health only: others focus on emergency/trauma with a short-term mandate to hand over to the government. In certain contexts, agencies operate 'outside' of their mandate due to needs: a shorter-term agency may consider a longer mandate when they don't feel local partners have capacity, or an agency focused on public health may recruit midwives to practise as well as train local women.

As a health professional, you may be called upon to help shape your agency's mandate. This will require understanding, the ability to rapidly assess needs and resources (of the agency you work with—both at a local level as well as a global one), and diplomacy. Decisions may be made by non-medical 'generalists' who ideally, but not necessarily, always work in consultation with health professionals. It can be challenging when field providers recognize unmet need that the agency does not feel it has the capacity to assist. In these cases, it can sometimes be useful to consider engaging other organizations who may have more specialized mandates in specific areas.

Anticipate operational differences

All organizations operate with their own systems and policies. There are key differences between how organizations direct their field operations, including the amount of autonomy given to the field teams. Additionally, some organization feel a stronger mandate while operating in an insecure operation and as a result, may want staff to remain in a field site when other agencies have decided to evacuate. This can have important implications for the field workers' comfort levels.

For someone heading out on one of their first missions, it is important to consider such operational differences and make sure that they are aligned with your own belief system. This often informal information is admittedly difficult to obtain, but the best source would be other field workers, from both the agency which you are exploring working for, as well as those who work for other organizations (most seasoned workers have a sense of how other organizations operate).

Consider obligations in your home country

Going on assignment can be a stressful endeavour. To minimize unnecessary distractions, before leaving, attempt to minimize obligations at home. Don't assume that you will be able to remotely manage known obligations. For example, setting up direct debits for bills can be a big help. If you are a home-owner, consider if you want to rent out your house or if there someone who can help look after it. You might consider hiring a property manager—there is no sense in worrying about broken window screens at home as you are attempting to set up and manage a cholera treatment clinic.

Anticipate the cultural context

Prior to leaving on any mission, it is important to carefully consider the cultural and society norms of the country in which you will be working. This can include the following:

- Do you speak the language or will you be operating through a translator? In certain countries, English is widely taught in schools and understood. In other missions, finding an English speaker may be daunting. You might want to obtain a phrasebook before you go.
- What are women's traditional roles and positions in society, and for female field workers, how might this impact your perceptions and behaviours? Is it necessary for women to adjust their daily behaviour, and if so, is this something you would be comfortable with?
- Religious freedom varies from country to country. Some countries are strictly aligned to one belief system but allow the practice of other religions, yet laws could be strict regarding 'evangelism'. Those who practise a different faith must consider scrutiny of personal belongings (could the amount of materials you are bringing be construed as for more than for your own use?); also consider how casual discussions with your colleagues might be seen in light of laws forbidding conversion. It needs to be understood that violation of any laws may lead to jail time and can have a severe impact on your agency's operations.
- The beliefs regarding sexual orientation, including laws. How might this impact you and is this an environment in which you would be comfortable? Marriages or civil unions recognized in your home country

might not be valid—or even be illegal. Primary concerns are safety as well as acceptance—two common-law individuals might not be able to reside together—let alone the implications for a homosexual relationship. Even if your mission is 'accompanied', your agency will only be able to secure visas based upon relationships recognized in that country.

- Make sure that your own personal belief system is considered and is congruent with the areas in which you will be living and working.

It is also very important to remember that to work effectively, a field worker must be accepted and respected by the local community. This not only allows the person to do their job, but also typically affords them co-operation, appreciation, and a level of protection which is only possible through local support. In an effort to demonstrate respect for local beliefs, it is reasonable for field workers to sometimes make concessions when in the field, including more minor adjustments such as not discussing politics or in some cases male physicians deferring examinations of women to female colleagues. When local culture conflicts with the field worker's own belief system, there may be a limit to the concessions which one is comfortable giving. In such cases, it is important to discuss it with your HQ or supervisor as early as possible to find a solution.

Consider your own individual situation, and alignment with the society and culture in which you would be working, and ultimately, if the adjustments of concessions which you may need to make to work effectively will be acceptable to you.

Practical considerations

Your agency should provide you direction and information regarding visas for your mission but it never hurts to independently check as there can be misconceptions about visa needs and so on. The British Airways website provides good information on visa details.

Allow plenty of time—you may need to courier your passport and you may need to work through an external service. It is worthwhile to know the visa requirements in surrounding countries. In the event of security issues, you may be required to relocate on short notice thus you should know if you require a visa ahead of time—or in rare cases there might be restrictions on entry for your nationality. Note that this might be different for your colleagues of other nationalities, hence it is good to check.

Finances

- Understand the access to money in your new posting. Some agencies provide cash advances in the field whereby you can receive money on a monthly basis as deducted off your salary—inquire in advance as to if your agency provides this option—otherwise you will need to plan accordingly.
- Even if cash advances are provided, you still need to bring sufficient funds to last around 5 weeks as cash advances generally are only provided from earned salaries and not advanced.
- Be aware that with debit cards, although ATMs are virtually everywhere these days, even ones which accept major bank or credit cards do not always accept all foreign cards.
- Consider bringing credit cards from two different institutions. Check the terms and conditions of the credit cards you plan to bring, as some offer quite steep surcharges for international use, while others levy no fees for the same. Having a backup card will go a long way if there are problems with the main card or issuing bank.
- Store your cards separately and securely.
- Some banks give more favourable exchange rates to credit cards over the regular bank cards as the credit card network is stronger—and they assume that they'll make a good profit on the daily rate charged on cash advances. Hence, some savvy travellers overpay their credit card by the amount that they plan to withdraw the following day.

What to pack

There is no simple 'one-size-fits-all' checklist and so it is difficult to paint a precise and detailed picture for a 'what-to-pack' checklist. This topic, however, outlines considerations as you devise your own checklist.

- Almost certainly you will be issued with a laptop computer dedicated for your use. Not all agencies permit VOI applications such as Skype to be used on their computers. Ask before departure, and if in doubt, you might consider bringing a laptop/netbook or tablet. If the latter, consider getting SIM-ready—a number of 'developing' countries are far more liberal with cellular technology than 'developed' countries and data packages can be quite affordable.

- Most electronics especially laptops and other mobile devices are 110/ 220 V but if yours is not, bring a voltage converter/transformer, in addition to an adapter plug. Ensure you know what adapters you require—and when available, purchase equipment that works across systems. Technology has made travel simpler. There is no need to carry CDs thanks to iPods; and books, especially those hardcover journals, have largely been replaced by e-book readers (though verify that your e-reader content provider will deliver in the location you are headed to: some will not push content outside US/Europe etc.)
- Consider local purchase. Understanding what you can get overseas makes a huge difference as you pack:
  - You should attempt to bring a 6-month supply of anything you *must* have: whether prescription/non-prescription medications, special dietary needs, or other. Within that period you will almost certainly find local arrangements. Even if items cost a bit more, you carry less with you and support the local market in your new home.
- As you pack, consider using a robust semi-hard shelled, wheeled suitcase. While some people prefer backpacks over wheeled luggage, these are rarely required unless working in a very remote region.

Other items to consider

Items that frequent the inside of a humanitarian aid worker's suitcase include:

- a lifestraw (ℜ http://en.wikipedia.org/wiki/LifeStraw) or similar device to filter poor water to be able to drink water in the event of emergencies
- re-useable water bottle—or two
- a flashlight, head-lights in particular are useful
- a multi-purpose knife/tool is always useful
- yoga mat: great for exercise as well as a cushion for sitting or sleeping
- batteries—specifically AA or AAA: ones that recharge via USB are golden when travelling
- solar charging—especially for any electronics you are bringing: eliminate the need for adapters and other chargers while conserving energy
- some culinary delights for your new co-workers—nothing ensures a warmer welcome for a new team member than chocolate or cookies for your new colleagues.

Professional considerations

Every mission will offer challenges, including working in a new environment that has varying resources and staffing. This is something which the field worker should be prepared for as it may involve adjusting their standards. Humanitarian work may require extreme hours, performing duties which they otherwise might have assistants to help with, without optimal resources—often under stressful settings. Work hours might not be standard and being 'on-call' 24/7 is common.

> Try to adapt to the new environment to the best of your ability and work to find ways in which you might be able to improve a situation. Is there any way to task-shift or defer responsibilities to others who might have capacity to do so? Really focus on maintaining a good working relationship with colleagues, help them when possible, and avoid complaining. When things are done differently from what you might be familiar with, ask why—often you will learn something and it will serve in your own best interest.

Working in a team

Humanitarian work, especially when performed in emergency settings, is stressful and exhausting. There is really no more challenging an environment than being thrown into a team with people who you don't know, trying to assess the needs, figuring out roles on the team in terms of proposal writers, budget developers, and operational support, all the time being in an potentially remote location and without optimal food/water—while sharing bedrooms and showers with others.

- A cohesive team can make a huge difference to the quality of work and personal satisfaction. It is crucial that a team works efficiently and there is no larger cause of breakdown than those stemming from misunderstandings or confusion over roles.
- A strong team *assumes positive intent* and does not interpret something said as negative (despite how it might sound) and does not keep lists of grievances.
- Humour goes a long way. It can lighten the mood and also show colleagues your 'human' side.
- Help out your colleagues. They are likely also tired and frustrated, and offering a helping hand or sympathetic ear would be appreciated, and likely reciprocated at another time.
- Strong teams also learn to know one another outside of work. Too strong a focus on the challenges at hand does not help alleviate them but rather 'fuels the fire'. Teams should have dinners, go for drinks, and/ or play sports together. And, of course, you will develop some long-lasting relationships.

See ➲ Chapter 14 for more information.

Working via translators

When deployed in a country where you don't speak the local language, you will find that you must give up a good degree of control over any situation, and rely heavily on the translator for essential information.

- Many will want to learn the local language. Should you want to learn a second language for professional development, you might consider focusing on one of the *other* five UN languages: Arabic, French, Mandarin Chinese, Russian, or Spanish.
- Be aware, however, that local dialects often rule and a single country can have numerous regional languages.
- In most settings, the reality is that you will at some point, and to some extent, be working with translators which will require patience and skills in order to ensure the correct message gets through.
- Confidentiality is a professional requirement for all translators. (See Box 13.1.)
- Be aware of the loss of sociocultural nuances and subtleties which you are accustomed to in your home country, which is especially important in areas which have security concerns.

Translator skills

- Generally an agency will recruit translators who, ideally, are overseen after a brief probation period by a senior staff member fluent in the language to evaluate linguistic ability in the two languages.
- Translators should translate precisely—without summary. Their role is to facilitate a conversation between two parties, not to provide responses.
- In some cases, the translator may notice something irregular about what they are to translate—they should still translate but might add their comments *provided they clearly articulate to you* that this is their own observation.
- For those new with using translators, watch out for:
  - translators who summarize: the third party speaks a few paragraphs worth then only a few words are translated back to you
  - translators who respond to the third party without consulting you.

Box 13.1 Confidentiality

Ensuring confidentially with the translator is critical, no matter with whom you are having the dialogue, or how insignificant the information may appear. Translators should be aware that everything must be held in the strictest confidence, that they cannot discuss things even 'anonymously' with family/friends etc. Likewise, the person being interviewed must be reassured of this confidentiality. The translator should be comfortable with sensitive matters (e.g. gender-sensitive or sexual orientation issues) and without fear of backlash (primarily in cases of ethnic/tribal matters). Sociocultural aspects needs be considered, and both the translator and the patient should be comfortable with regard to gender, ethnicity, etc. Especially when working with non-regular translators, it should be clear that they are free to turn down the request without fear of reprisal.

Administrative roles

Humanitarian workers will be faced with new challenges beyond 'just' their provision of care in low-resource and stressful contexts. Most health providers in home countries have a cadre of support staff, who assist with various administrative and operational tasks. This is often not the case in the field, and all members of the team often find themselves with responsibilities which may be new or previously part of an administrator's role.

Human resource management

Depending on your specific role as well as the structure of your organization, you may be responsible for the oversight of multiple staff.

Strong agencies value their human resource leadership as strategic members of the senior management team, no longer just the watchdog—at HQ, in the country office, and in the field. As such, you may be required to work with all three different levels: the field and country offices for matters pertaining to nationals, and HQ for your own/other internationals.

- You are encouraged to obtain a copy of the host country's labour laws and read up. These laws can have broad implications for the management of the local staff, including disciplinary matters and due process requirements. Labour laws will vary from country to country, but many are geared towards the workers' rights—some even with a bias against international agencies.
- For disciplinary matters, make a clear effort to flag concerns around performance and encourage correction: generally through letters. A strong human resource department will support you. Most legal systems will insist on seeing a clear chain of communication.
- Considering identifying a local labour lawyer in advance of any issues, in order to consult if questions or concerns arise.
- Most humanitarian agencies have systems to measure performance of staff on an annual basis. To effectively conduct a performance review, each manager should share the report with each staff member, and then discuss the findings. There should be no surprises—feedback should occur throughout the year, not just at the end of it.
- A supervisor should not rely only on these evaluations for disciplinary actions or to terminate someone's employment—rather, in cases of problematic employees, there should be a demonstration of regular attempts to help an employee identify weaknesses and of corrective actions constantly taken.
- When disciplinary action is taken, make sure to establish a follow-up plan. This could include a probation period, supervision, or other appropriate measures.
- Ensure a reasonable 'statute of limitations' is in place: a driver who was caught speeding should not have a warning letter retained in their file forever.

Media and public relations

Each humanitarian agency will have their own policies regarding how they manage external communications. Traditionally, while most agencies have been fairly conservative, limiting media engagement to the senior-most person people or HQ, there is still a need to prepare staff should they be contacted by a journalist.

Interacting with journalists
- If contacted by a journalist, don't agree to an interview without first discussing it with the head of mission and/or HQ. Your agency may have a preference for journalistic contact and may have much more background information to understand prior to any interviews.
- In matters where a colleague has been seriously injured or killed, sensitivity to the family is of the upmost concern: no one should learn that a loved one has been hurt or become a casualty from the media.
- Keep in mind that the media also has an important impact on promoting the work which humanitarians do. Thus the role of the media in humanitarian work should not be disregarded or viewed as an interruption to our work, but rather, when appropriate, as an opportunity to build a partnership that can mutually benefit both agencies.
- Know that there is never such a thing as 'off the record': whether travelling to the site of an interview or enjoying a cold drink at the end of the day—assume that the 'recorder' is still on.

Social media
- Social media provides nearly as many challenges as benefits. While an agency might restrict formal interviews with journalists, it is not practical to dictate who staff can have as a contact on social media.
- Staff should be reminded that *any* communications—written or spoken—must follow protocol and should be considered 'on the record'.
- When posting on social media, remember that your individual behaviour reflects on the organization with whom you are affiliated. Consider the broader cultural and social environment—pictures or comments may not be intended to be offensive but can be, and it is important to consider cultural sensitives.

Photography
- Many agencies will have specific guidelines around the photographing of project beneficiaries—especially children—but in general, one should ensure that adults consent to any photos predominantly of them or their children (but if it is a 'wider' shot of a group of people, generally one might be able to take photos without expressed permission).
- Some cultures prohibit photos of women or in general—your employer/colleagues are best to advise on this.

Budgeting
Managing a budget is something which many medical officers or team members are expected to do on a regular basis—but the reality is that many have no prior experience of how this is done. Understanding how budgets work is critical and although each agency will have unique titles and particularities, the following is some general advice to help in the orientation.

Budget allocations by donors generally take public (government) or private funds and allocate according to the needs in the proposal. Most donors allow 5–15% overheads at the HQ level while others can be higher than 20% on top of direct programme (in-country) costs. The operational funds are generally allocated on a 1-year timeframe but can be up to 3 or even 5 years in some cases—especially in a more development-focused mission.

- The finance department of each agency will provide codes for a budget, generally in pre-existing categories such as 'National staff', 'In-country travel' and programme-specific costs such as 'Medical equipment' or 'Pharmaceuticals'.
- Your project might be funded by multiple donors, so you may need to work off of more than one budget. It may be possible to roll several budgets into one 'master' budget, especially at a sector level.
- Be aware of the role of currency exchanges—e.g. a donor government in Europe might fund via an American agency to a country in Africa.
- While one would always advocate careful and thoughtful spending of resources, one should be aware of the realities associated with non-use of anticipated funds:
  - Once returned, pre-allocated funds cannot always be re-allocated as donors tend to earmark funds by committing to an agency—preventing use by another agency.
  - Many organizations' operational budgets have a gross total which includes a percentage for 'overhead' allocations. If allocated resources are not used, this can have a significant change to expected operational resources. Discuss with your organization to understand how to manage these issues.
- Managing budgets considering 'life of a grant' is to consider the individual monthly budgets as opposed to averaging expenses evenly across each month. Some projects anticipate much higher spending at the beginning of the programme, perhaps due to start-up costs or procurement, while others may anticipate much heavier spending later in the project. Having an understanding of this will allow you to anticipate the expected burn rate, (which can fluctuate monthly) and to more accurately forecast monthly spending.
- Most finance teams prepare monthly spending-versus-budget reports which should be reviewed for accuracy and expectations. Finance teams are reliant upon others to produce these reports: generally they need to wait for the global HQ to close books before the country office then field site. Collaborate with them, and build these reviews into your schedule.

Personal well-being

Humanitarian work can be physically and emotionally exhausting. When entering a new environment, one must be prepared for having a range of emotions. Due to the nature of the job, humanitarian aid workers are often living in unstable environments. Additionally, it can seem incongruent psychologically that aid workers can live relatively comfortably when the vulnerable people we are trying to assist live in squalid/dangerous conditions not far away. There will be an interest in you as a foreigner, and although there is usually no ill intent, this can lead to a sense of lack of privacy and the impression of living in a 'fishbowl'. Ensuring your own personal well-being must be a priority.

Stress management

Effective stress management will vary based on a person's culture, gender, personality, identity, and many other factors. Each person experiences stress differently and must manage it in her/his own way. For stress management to be effective, it must be consistent and include the techniques that work best for the individual.

Switch off

Learning how to mentally 'switch off' work at the end of the day is a very important skill. It allows you to leave work at the office so that it does not interfere with home life. Make this a conscious process; talk yourself through the steps you take to switch off. Develop rituals that help you switch on and off as you start and stop work. Some people prefer to finish up work at home, others prefer to stay later at the office and complete work there as opposed to taking it home. Each person is unique so learn what works best for you.

Maintain a personal life

- Working in an environment where your work can easily take priority over a personal life, it is important to socialize, both inside and outside of your agency. A tendency to lean too far one way or the other is not healthy.
- Whether socializing with or without colleagues, it is important to manage the amount of discussions around work: too much griping about challenges does not allow for 'processing' and moving on. Further, it can cause increasing resentment among colleagues who may have different sources of reference.
- Even too much discussion around work in general—daily matters, positive aspects—can make our minds 'typecast' and limit one's mindset.
- Make an effort to learn one personal thing about each aid worker you socialize with: such as their family situation, hobbies, or what they did before they entered this field of work.
- When living and working together, you will discover odd peculiarities of your colleagues. Try to have some level of acceptance. Don't forget that your colleagues are also discovering your eccentric traits!

What to avoid when coping with stress

Of note, there are also stress-relieving outlets which are unhealthy and can worsen the problem. These include alcohol and drug use: these may appear as 'no-brainers' but they do deserve a mention.

Consumption varies between settings—from being a culturally acceptable and even expected method of socializing to those countries in which alcohol is strictly prohibited. Often working in a 'dry' country can result in binge-drinking. You will need to make your own judgements about this topic, but do be aware that drunkenness is never a good thing, and can impact local perceptions and negatively affect both you and your organization's work.

It should go without saying—especially by health professionals who know the risks and addictive tendencies—but beware of the trap of prescription/ non-prescription drugs in many settings. Proximity and access to pharmaceutical supplies make these surprisingly easy to access, and has resulted in team members becoming reliant on sleeping pills and painkillers that, even if used for pain or an acute accident, can quickly lead to dependence. Also, in many counties recreational drugs are fairly widely available—not necessarily legally. Although it may seem obvious, you should be aware that you are subject to the laws of the countries in which you work—some of which are extremely harsh.

Returning home and reintegration

A return home is a mixed bag of excitement and potential awkwardness. We delight at meeting family and friends and describing our 'adventures'. However, some stories will just not relate and over time one learns the stories to avoid.

Expect to return home different and to need some adjustment time. After especially difficult missions, it is often difficult to relate to the seemingly excesses in your home country. Things such as the cost of a coffee being equal to someone's daily wage elsewhere can be difficult to rectify in your mind. Be prepared to have some mixed emotions when you return, and allow yourself some time to gradually adjust and reintegrate. When you return home, you may be surprised at the physical and emotional fatigue you feel after an intense mission, which can be exacerbated by jetlag. Consider keeping your schedule free for a few weeks when you return, and a basic calculation might be 1 week for every 6 months out—especially when early in one's career. Though it is in our nature to want to begin the next chapter of our lives immediately, it is far simpler to take a break in between chapters than during. Consider using this time to slowly attend to personal issues—e.g. renewal of your driver's licence, medical/dental check-ups, housing matters, and of course people to 'catch up' with.

Part II

Approach to clinical humanitarian medicine

Chapter 14

Approach to clinical care in humanitarian contexts

Raghu Venugopal

Introduction to clinical care in humanitarian contexts

Clinical care in humanitarian contexts must be recognized as a challenging endeavour to both the novice and experienced clinician. There may be language barriers, differing cultural norms such as the need to obtain consent from not only the patient but also family members, and the austere conditions of the ward. Resources will be limited, referral and advanced testing often impossible, and you may find yourself working outside of your comfort zone. Local colleagues may have a different medical practice that you can learn from or may disagree with, and this will need to be approached with diplomacy and medical evidence. You will need to rely on your clinical skills more than ever before to make the best diagnosis you can, be resourceful, and be a wise steward of the limited resources around you. Nonetheless, working with patients facing poverty and crisis is rewarding and the gratitude of your patients will be something you remember for a lifetime. The following are some points to consider as you undertake your work.

On the treatment of patients

- Above all else, do no harm. Even if your patient has a ruptured ectopic pregnancy, but you have never done a laparotomy—this is not the time to experiment. Try to temporize the situation with a blood transfusion and seek means to evacuate the patient to a surgeon.
- Quality matters. Humanitarian settings are no excuse for sub-standard care (e.g. expired medications and faulty equipment):
  - If you are not qualified to perform a procedure in your home country, you are not qualified to perform it in a humanitarian setting.
  - Surgical interventions should reflect the WHO surgical safety guidelines.[1]
  - Know your limits. Avoid medical misadventures. Don't experiment.
- Treat patients with respect and dignity at all times, and prompt all staff to do the same. As they say in the Central African Republic, 'Zo kwe zo'—'each human is a person'. Your colleagues may be watching how you treat patients, and you can be a positive role model.
- Ensure patient and staff safety. The medical facility should be neutral and respected by all parties to any conflict. This may require asking combatants not to wear uniforms or bring weapons into the medical facility. Facilitate the process by having spare clothes to change into.
- Promote respect for patient privacy as you would like it to be in your home environment. Even in the most challenging environment, sensitive information should be shared on a need-to-know basis.
- Access to healthcare is a basic human right for which vulnerable groups may need additional efforts to ensure access. Consider the needs of the elderly, minorities, sex trade workers, women, homosexuals, etc., and how to ensure privacy and reduce stigma.
- Not all patients can be cured in austere humanitarian environments. Cure as much as you can and comfort always.
- Even though you will see lots of patients in difficult settings, such as under a tree, overcrowded wards, or in the back of a Toyota Land Cruiser®, it's important to apply standard safety and hygiene procedures. Practise good universal precautions so that you, your team, and your patients remain healthy. Nosocomial infections can be especially deadly among the immunocompromised, newborn, and malnourished patients.
- Obtain informed consent in a culturally appropriate manner. Explain the illness, treatment, side effects, and options in a way patients will understand. Enlisting a family member or friend is crucial when the treatment may be long, painful, and difficult or when adherence is important. Consent also extends to photos and use on social media.

Self-conduct in the field

Strive to be humble. Your local team members with less formal training should be respected for their local knowledge and experience. They can teach you a lot. Your nurses may show you how to keep insulin cool underground in earthenware pots. Your local colleagues can often tell you if diseases such as leishmaniasis, schistosomiasis, or sleeping sickness are prevalent. You will not know the solution to every problem and you are likely not the first clinician to face this problem, so remember to ask your colleagues, especially your local ones.

When you first arrive, observe and listen. Learn as much as you can about the local environment and culture. Watch the entire process of the patient experience, from admission and triage through to consultation and treatment. To promote the best experiences in the field:

- Find a way to get along with others. Team dynamics can be challenging at times and accept that there will be differences between your experience and expertise compared to your colleagues.
- Be flexible, diplomatic, and put the patient first while not ignoring that you work within a system and community where there are limits and realities.
- Adapt yourself to the local rules and conduct, not the opposite. You are a guest of the host nation. However, do not completely abandon your moral compass if you see something is grossly wrong or negligent.
- Realize you will be in this context for a short period of time—people have come before you and will come after you. Don't think you need to change all that seems wrong. Local staff will get frustrated if things continue to change with every new expatriate arrival.
- Avoid overtly criticizing, as that can undermine the sense of team unity and be culturally offensive. Instead, try to understand the reason why things were set up the way they were and offer constructive feedback at the right time, and with the right tone.
- The entire team dynamic should be viewed as supportive and with collective accountability.
- It is important not to be seen to contradict local clinicians in front of their colleagues and patients, as this will cause divisions within the team, and undermine trust. Instead, it is advisable to:
  • quietly pull a clinician aside and speak to them in a confidential manner about your observations
  • have a team meeting and speak about broad observations in a way that does not assign blame on any particular person
  • be seen to be identifying your own learning opportunities, and thank the local staff for their efforts to teach you as well
  • certain actions which are grossly negligent may need a formal warning in coordination with your human resources manager.
- Even in a crisis, try to remain calm.
- Be ready to adapt. Working conditions are almost never perfect and you often have to make do with less than ideal resources. Don't let best get in the way of good.

On local realities

Recognize the importance of context
- Always reflect on what the population wants and needs and don't impose what you think are their needs. Creating medical programmes to suit donors' wishes is to be avoided.
- Search for approaches to prevent disease and improve patient and population health. Better water sources or bucket chlorination may prevent cholera. A bed net distribution may reduce malaria transmission. Thinking 'upstream' can reduce morbidity and mortality.
- Try to find local solutions and community resources, where possible, to address health problems. For example, a 'walking blood bank' created by rallying local community members, may be longer lasting and sustainable than bringing blood from the capital and investing in unsustainable refrigeration.
- Look beyond temporary solutions to the root causes of problems. Community education efforts on hand washing and safe birthing can complement clinical care. Advocating for more primary care by community health workers or a local ambulance service as well may be useful to meet wider population needs.

Work with local authorities and staff
- Whenever possible, work cooperatively with the relevant health authorities. Remember that local authorities have the greatest responsibility for the health of the population even if they may be unable or unwilling to bear this responsibility. When possible and not compromising clinical care, try to follow national guidelines and protocols.
- In an effort to increase local capacity, teach best practices as much as you can. Empower your local staff with as much knowledge, skill, and confidence as possible so that when you leave, you will have left the local healthcare system stronger. Regular teaching sessions and performing medical rounds as a group on the most challenging and longest admitted patients is useful.
- From the moment the intervention begins, have a handover and exit plan. The deeper you plant your flag, the harder it is to pull it out. This cannot be done without the cooperation of local leaders and providers who should be your main collaborators. It takes more energy sometimes to work with local healthcare providers than managing things on your own, but collaboration is better in the long run for the population in many situations.
- Know where you can refer patients. If you don't have an operating room in your project, learn where the nearest one is before someone who needs emergency surgery arrives.

Protecting limited resources
In humanitarian settings, providers must be aware of the finite resources and consider their own resource utilization. Further, in some places where a population earns a subsistence wage, NGOs are erroneously viewed as

seeming to have unlimited resources, with the ability to bring in any additional supplies which are needed. In this context, be aware that theft does occur. Taking some of these resources home for their families or the community's use does not always have a negative connotation to some, and at times can be exceedingly difficult to prevent. Address this reality by the following:

• Speaking with the staff and making it clear that the resources are not inexhaustible.
• Ensuring resources are secure. You have to find co-workers you trust and create systems that make theft difficult. Regular inventories can aid with noticing if items are missing or being used at a high rate that is unjustified medically.
• Identifying one person responsible for assisting with the control of the various resources. This person can be responsible for monitoring the inventory, and allocating supplies, which can be verified by a supervisor weekly during spot checks. Be up front about spot checks, and put a positive spin on them; propose that the checks are in place to make sure that if there are minor discrepancies, or if anyone else is tampering with the inventory, it will be caught early.
• Medical supply is one of the most difficult and most costly aspects of the work. It is everyone's business, including clinicians, coordinators, and logisticians.
• Medications and diagnostic tests can be ruined due to improper storage, so make sure resources are stored appropriately.
• Find a balance between ruptures/stock-outs and materials expiration. Work with a pharmacist if possible, and keep an inventory so that you know when to replenish stocks. See ➲ Chapter 12 for further information.

Advocacy

Medical care in humanitarian assistance is primarily at the bedside and you can amplify your efforts if you can undertake advocacy for the struggles the population is facing. In coordination with the organization, consider recording your experiences (e.g. blogging, speaking to reporters in coordination with your manager) and sharing the stories of those you assist in a respectful and honest manner when you return home or from the field. Ensuring patient privacy should be respected as one might do in your home society. This endeavour can be a satisfying manner to express your frustrations, observations and successes. Some examples can be found at ℘ http://blogs.msf.org.

For more information regarding media relations see ➲ Chapter 13.

When things go wrong

Don't forget to remember the successes of your work such as the patients you saved, as many others will die in crises and austere settings. Remember you cannot do it all. You will not leave for home totally satisfied.

- Even if your patient cannot be saved, understand that your solidarity and accompaniment of those facing conflict, crisis, and disaster is singularly important.
- Take time to speak to the patient's family in a manner that is locally acceptable. If you can explain that you did everything possible and consulted on all resources available, it may bring some comfort to the family. In some settings, the family will not expect to hear this from the doctor, and could suggest doubt, so do balance your approach to the context.
- Analyse poor patient outcomes for systemic problems (i.e. mortality and morbidity review). It is crucial to analyse the deaths and adverse outcomes to find practical ways to avoid them in the future. This can be held once per week and should include not only the input of doctors, but nurses and other health providers as well.
- Analyse your programme outputs such as mortality rates. High rates should prompt improved resources, training, staff, or triage. Low mortality rates may mean you are missing the most vulnerable population.
- Have different means to de-stress and debrief. You are human too. Remember that local staff also need ways to de-stress and debrief (consider support groups particularly for staff working with traumatized populations such as sexual violence survivors or where there is high mortality).
- Learn to reflect and improve upon your own shortcomings. Think about gaps in your skills, and reach out to your manager and organization to improve upon them.
- Know who your backup is and use them. Other people in your organization may have experience and can suggest solutions.

Reference

1. World Health Organization. WHO Surgical Safety Checklist. 2009. ℞ http://www.who.int/patientsafety/safesurgery/tools_resources/en/index.html

Chapter 15

Mass casualty triage

Christos Giannou and Jennifer Turnbull

Introduction to mass casualty triage

Historical perspective: triage as military practice

Historically, triage comes out of military practice during the Napoleonic Wars and concerned the sorting of mass casualties that occurred after major battles when the means for treatment were limited. Not all wounded could be treated given the level of medical knowledge; even those for whom treatment was available could not fully benefit because of the large numbers. The logic was to 'do the best possible for the largest number'.

It is not only the military that have had to adopt this logic: civilian institutions and humanitarian agencies faced with major disasters have had to embrace it as well.

It is vital that humanitarian workers have an understanding of the concept of mass casualty triage, not only because these incidents may strike at any time but because, in fact, the deployment of international humanitarian personnel often is a consequence of mass casualty events. Field workers should prepare themselves for a wide range of conditions for which large numbers of patients may present for care. This can include natural disasters, civil violence, population displacements, and events unrelated to disaster or war directly, such as a motor vehicle collision involving a bus packed with people.

The logic of mass casualty triage

The triage of large numbers of patients involves a *rationing of medical care* according to a determination of priority for treatment. In addition, one must accept that not all patients can be treated.

Mass casualty triage represents a paradigm shift in the provision of medical care from 'doing everything possible for every patient' to 'doing the best possible for as many patients as possible'.

Mass casualty triage is a balance between needs (number of patients and type of pathology) and the resources available (material and human). The precise definition of a mass casualty situation, and when to implement a mass casualty disaster plan, which reorganizes the functioning of the hospital or health system to meet the extra demand, should be decided at the field level based on the material and human resources available. Mass casualty triage and a mass casualty plan are inseparable and used when the casualty burden to the system challenges the resources available.

Mass casualty clarified

Differences: medical triage versus mass casualty triage

Triage for mass casualties differs greatly from the triage experienced in a typical medical practice, where the greatest medical need is the determinant factor in deciding priority of care. The modern, everyday concept of hospital triage is often a simple dispatching of patients to various clinical areas for medical care; priority for treatment is then determined within the dispatched department according to severity (mangled limb compared to a simple fracture). In a situation requiring mass casualty triage, there is a rationing of care according to categories that define the urgency of treatment compatible with the best possible outcome for the greatest number of patients; or, in some cases, no treatment apart from simple palliative measures. It is perhaps unfortunate that the same term is used for two very different circumstances and can lead to misunderstanding.

Compensated multiple casualty versus uncompensated mass casualties

A distinction must be made between the compensated event, usually termed a *multiple-casualty incident*, where hospital resources are stretched but all patients can still be managed, and the uncompensated event, the *true mass casualty* situation, where the hospital is overwhelmed.

A multiple-casualty incident
- Does not incapacitate local resources.
- For example: ten war-wounded patients—three severely injured, seven less so—arrive simultaneously at a hospital with three operating rooms and three surgeons. The principles of triage and priority for care still apply: who will go to operation first (severely injured) and who will wait for their operation (seven less severely injured).
- In this compensated, multiple-casualty incident, all patients still receive the best care possible under the circumstances.

A mass casualty situation
- When the need exceeds the capacity of the resources.
- For example, ten war-wounded patients—five severely injured in the same hospital with capacity to operate only on three. The decision of which three to operate first may well imply leaving the other two to die; their injuries are so severe that they would not survive the time necessary to operate the first three, and they might not survive even if they had been the first operated. This would be futile care for the most severely injured and meanwhile the salvageable patients may well die. This requires a triage 'balancing act'.
- The definition of futile care will change between the two scenarios.
- Unless otherwise specified, the rest of this chapter pertains specifically to uncompensated mass casualty events.

Yet further distinctions: one-off versus continuous events

For mass casualty planning and operations, a further distinction is made between a one-off event—an earthquake, or isolated act of terrorism such as a bomb explosion—and major armed conflict.

- After the *one-off event*, most casualties are evacuated to the hospital at one time; and the patient flow then ceases.
- During *continuous events*, such as armed conflict, casualties arrive at hospital the next day, and the next, and so on; the patient flow stops only with the cessation of hostilities.

This distinction has a great impact on hospital organization, especially on the personnel roster. With the one-off event, all hospital personnel are usually available and work to exhaustion to treat all the life-threatening injuries. With the continuous flow of casualties from sustained combat, exhausted hospital personnel will not be capable of caring for the patient load indefinitely and a different schedule is required which can influence triage decisions if the competent staff are not available 24 hours a day.

The stress of a wartime scenario on a medical system was demonstrated in a West African capital city which had only one major surgical facility and few national surgeons. The first humanitarian surgical team initially worked 48 hours straight and then collapsed, incapable of continuing to operate. A replacement surgical team then worked an 18-hour operating day with 6 hours of compulsory rest. This schedule was maintained for weeks at a time. Severely injured patients who arrived during the 6-hour rest period underwent 'automatic triage': they were either still alive when the surgical team returned to work, or they were not. Given enough surgical personnel and nursing staff, a 24-hour operating schedule could be implemented but this is not always the case and requires a balance between needs and resources available.

The ethical dilemmas of triage

This rationing of medical care has obvious ethical implications: it is one thing to do 'everything for everybody' and quite another to do 'the best possible for the greatest number'. This paradigm shift is often difficult to accept for medical personnel whose training and everyday work is exactly the opposite. What happens to those severely injured patients for whom little can be done under the circumstances? What are the criteria? Who decides? Do any patients—children—have an innate priority over others—the elderly? The best possible outcome for the greatest number implies that some patients will be left to 'die in peace and with dignity'.

Any mass casualty disaster plan should consider local and interpersonal beliefs among team members and ethical standards that can have an impact on priorities for care. Such beliefs and standards should be discussed but should not alter the inherent medical neutrality of triage: patients are treated only according to medical need *and* as a function of the resources available. Context, rather than dogma, imposes the working criteria, and an understanding of the logic of triage determines what can and what cannot be done for any single patient.

Triage models and organization

- Many different triage models are used globally which organize the infrastructure, equipment and supplies, and human resources into a system that differs from everyday practice.
- Categorizations in triage also vary, and include both military and civilian-humanitarian options, which respond to different tactical and logistic constraints. Colours are often used to facilitate the identification of triage categories: red, yellow, green, and black.
- Patients are triaged under a two-stage process: 'sift and sort'. This two-phase process is the key element in the determination of the proper priority for treatment of mass casualties. (See Fig. 15.1.)
- Some patients will require care that exceeds the local capabilities or would be considered futile due to the high likelihood of mortality, i.e. severe penetrating head injury or not breathing. These patients are identified quickly and provided with comfort care in a quiet and peaceful environment. They are allowed to die in peace and with dignity.

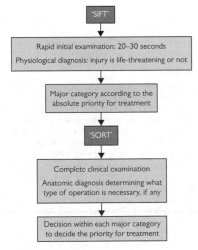

Fig. 15.1 Sift and sort algorithm.

Triage teams

All models define triage teams with distinct roles but the actual composition of such teams is very context specific and depends on the availability of qualified personnel. Depending on the staffing of a specific hospital, these necessary functions are distributed or accumulated among a number of key persons. In a small hospital, one person may have several functions.

Triage team leader

- This is the main coordinator, and responsible for activating the triage plan—an event that cannot be taken lightly, as it will disrupt the normal functioning of the health facility.
- This person is also responsible for contacts with the 'outside world' including police and military authorities (if necessary), civilian authorities, other hospitals, and the 'media' etc. Many duties can, and should, be delegated, but the team leader retains overall coordination.
- He/she is often the hospital director.

Head nurse/matron

- Chief organizer, responsible for changing nursing and paramedical staff rosters, emptying hospital beds to make room for new arrivals, and mobilizing extra non-medical resources (kitchen, laundry etc.) in conjunction with the hospital administrator.

Clinical triage officer

- The person charged with the actual clinical triage of patients and usually with the most clinical experience. Whether they are a surgeon, anaesthetist, or nurse is of less importance than the confidence the rest of the staff has in this person; everyone has to live with the triage decisions made. Consequently, it is often emotionally easier for a foreign international humanitarian worker to perform triage than a national colleague who may have friends and family among the casualties, although mass casualty triage is *never* an emotionally easy task.
- Depending on the size of the hospital, the same person may perform the *sift* as well as the *sort* phases of triage, or a different person may perform the second-phase sorting of the first-priority patients while the chief clinical triage officer (CTO) is continuing with the first-phase sift.
- The CTO should not be involved in patient care during actual triage, with one exception: putting a comatose patient in the lateral security position to prevent vomiting and aspiration, or asphyxia.

Resuscitation teams

- Designated teams of doctors and nurses responsible for the resuscitation of first-priority patients in preparation for operation.
- The second-phase sorting of patients occurs within these teams, either by the CTO or by a second triage officer.

Follow-up teams

- Designated doctors and nurses who complete a full examination of those patients awaiting operations, or who can be discharged from the hospital, and implement treatment protocols as necessary.
- The continued observation of patients allows for the identification of those who change their original triage category because of deterioration, or improvement, of their condition while waiting.
- The second-phase sorting of patients also occurs within these teams, either by the CTO or by a second triage officer.

Triage algorithms

In mass casualty events, triage occurs at several points within the health system, as well as at each level of the transport process. It is repeated again and again in the hospital environment: a succession of triage decisions that reflect the evolution of a patient's condition, if appropriate.

ICRC hospital triage categories

There are several systems of triage categories in use around the world. In the humanitarian context, that of the International Committee of the Red Cross (ICRC) has proven to be simple and easy to use. The categories are for a hospital with surgical capabilities, but can be adapted to the prehospital context. The dead and uninjured are removed from consideration.

The categories progress according to priority of treatment from urgent to untreatable, assessed via the following considerations:
1. ABCDE assessment to determine the physiological insult.
2. The anatomic site of injury.
3. The mechanism of injury: burns can have delayed effects, particularly inhalation injury; blunt trauma is more difficult to diagnose than penetrating projectile wounds.
4. The time since injury: a patient in shock shortly after injury probably has severe haemorrhage; hypotension several hours later, following only slight blood loss, may be due to simple dehydration.

Category I: serious wounds requiring resuscitation and immediate surgery (RED)

This category consists of patients suffering life-threatening injuries that require immediate surgery *and* who have a high likelihood of survival. They usually account for 5–10% of patients after a mass casualty event. According to the standard ABCDE assessment paradigm, examples include:
- airway: head and neck injuries, including burns, affecting the airway with need for tracheostomy
- breathing: tension pneumothorax or significant haemothorax
- circulation: traumatic amputation, internal haemorrhage including haemothorax
- disability: closed head trauma with lateralizing signs of conization.

Category II: second priority wounds—require surgery but can wait (YELLOW)

These patients have relatively serious wounds that require surgical treatment, but are not immediately life-threatening and, therefore, can wait for surgery, especially in a hospital context where they receive antibiotics, analgesics, and intravenous fluids. Category II patients usually comprise a quarter to a third of mass casualties. Examples of such injuries include:
- breathing: minor pneumo- or haemothorax
- circulation: haemodynamically stable with penetrating abdominal injury
- disability: head injury with stable airway and Glasgow Coma Scale (GCS) score >8
- disability: paraplegic patient even if surgery is not contemplated
- extremities: compound fractures
- extremities: major soft tissue injuries.

Category III: superficial wounds—ambulatory management (GREEN)
This category comprises a surprisingly large percentage of mass casualties: 50–60%. The sheer numbers create a problem of patient-flow management.
- Wounds that are superficial and do not require surgery or intervention beyond wound care/suturing under local anaesthesia and/or dressing.
- Simple closed fractures requiring splinting or casting.

Category IV: severe wounds—supportive treatment (BLACK)
These injuries are the most severe; so severe that survival is unlikely given the skill and/or resource limitations. Attempts at curative procedures for these patients are usually at the expense of others who are more likely to survive with an 'acceptable' outcome. Time, effort, and resources cannot be spent on what may be considered futile care.
- Head injury with GCS score <8.
- Tetraplegia.
- Second- and/or third-degree burns covering >50% of body surface area.
- Massive blood loss and no blood or plasma expanders available.

Note: category IV patients are not abandoned and 'left to die'. They should receive full supportive care including analgesia and wound care. Patients who do survive delay to surgery can be taken to the operating theatre once category I and severe category II patients are treated. In multiple-casualty incidents that do not overwhelm hospital capabilities, category IV should only be applied to patients who are not spontaneously breathing (unless advanced airway techniques and ventilation are available).

Prehospital triage
The same basic triage categories apply in the prehospital context with a distinction made between *priority for evacuation* versus *priority for treatment*.

Priority for evacuation
- Distance, means of transport, and time to evacuation, as well as the security of transport—very important in a war zone—must all be taken into consideration in deciding which patients to transfer first.
- A patient with severe internal haemorrhage has priority for evacuation if the receiving hospital is a short time away, such as in an urban context. In a rural area, hours away from a surgical hospital, this patient will probably die en route; the patient does not have evacuation priority.

Priority for treatment
- An algorithm based on the ABCDE paradigm can be applied (Fig. 15.2).
- The first competent person on the scene should begin triage:
  - The triage officer—often a firefighter or police officer—calls out: 'all those who can walk, stand up and come with me'. These ambulatory patients are separated from those unable to move, and who are presumed to be more seriously injured.
  - The dead are removed to one side and efforts are then concentrated on the remaining unable to move.
  - Most ambulatory patients have relatively minor injuries, but not all: the ambulatory must therefore undergo a secondary triage.

- In an urban environment, patients will 'self-evacuate': private means are used to transfer patients without waiting for ambulances and triage, a common occurrence; especially in low-income countries due to a lack of prehospital services.

Prehospital triage algorithm: ABCDs

The algorithm in Fig. 15.2 is scientifically based but the reality of triage is more pragmatic.

- If patients can speak their name in response to a question, then the airway is clear (A) and they are lucid (D).
- Rather than count breaths per minute, the patient is *observed* to have either a 'normal' breathing pattern or obvious dyspnoea, with laboured or rapid respiration (B).

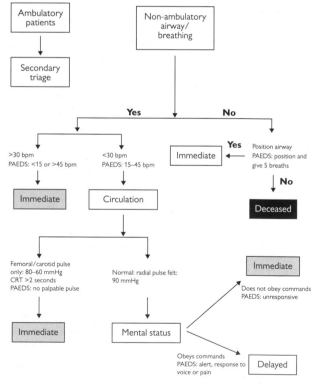

Fig. 15.2 ABCD prehospital triage algorithm. CRT, capillary refill time; PAEDS, paediatric patients, bpm, breaths per minute.

- Capillary refilling time can be difficult to determine: cold, darkness. The peripheral pulses should be felt (C): the radial pulse means a systolic pressure of at least 90 mmHg; the femoral, 70–80 mmHg; and the carotid pulse indicates a pressure of at least 60 mmHg.
- The mental status (D) is best described by the AVPU system: Alert; responsive to Voice; responsive to Pain; Unresponsive. (The GCS is a hospital-based system.)
- Obvious major fractures and soft tissue injuries (E) are easily observed.

Note: paediatric respiratory rates cited are approximations and judgement should be used based on the child's age.

Note: for major penetrating trauma, particularly war wounds, the paradigm changes to C-ABCDE: catastrophic haemorrhage comes first. For acceleration/deceleration injuries (car crashes, fall from a height), the paradigm is A(C)BCDE: airway, (cervical spine), breathing etc.

In both the prehospital and hospital setting, provision should be made for keeping patients warm. Injured patients lose body heat, even in a tropical climate. Hypothermia in the injured patient leads to coagulopathy with fatal results.

Preparation for mass casualty triage

Mass casualty triage is far more than algorithms and planning; training and review are key to implementation. All levels of personnel (medical and non-medical) should be involved in the preparation of a disaster plan.

Community-based first responders

One of the most efficient forms of disaster response is community-based first aid, a programme developed by many National Red Cross/Red Crescent Societies. Every family has at least one member trained in first-aid; schools and neighbourhood sports clubs are a prime focus. Firefighters and police are usually trained in first aid. Such community members are 'on the spot' when a catastrophe, such as an earthquake, strikes and constitute the very first responders. Often, non-medical staff such as guards, drivers, or community workers or ordinary citizens are among the first to signal a mass casualty event or to encounter the injured.

Components of a hospital mass casualty disaster plan

The reception of a mass influx of casualties is always chaotic, even in the best of health systems or hospitals. A hospital disaster plan re-organizes the space and infrastructure; equipment and supplies; and the personnel: medical, paramedical, and non-medical. In a hospital facility, it is the paramedical staff—stretcher and trolley bearers—who best know the bottlenecks of a hospital and impediments to patient flow; their input is crucial. This creates a *system* that makes analysis of what is necessary a systemic one.

Situation analysis
This is a series of questions: the answers determine the context and how preparation should proceed:
- What are the scenarios that might lead to a mass casualty event?
- How is the health system structured in the community: prehospital services; number of health centres; number and type of hospitals; possibility of transferring patients to other hospitals in-country or abroad?
- What is the role of the health facility in the community; will the health structure serve other functions (e.g. shelter of non-injured but displaced people) in case of a major event?

Roles and responsibilities
- Assignment of roles within the triage teams with clear job descriptions.
- Identification of a team responsible for managing the administrative functioning of regular services in the health facility during the event.

Communication
- How is the alarm triggered and what is the communication method within the hospital and with prehospital services?
- Is there any method of contacting hospital personnel who are off-duty?
  - In most humanitarian settings, there are only a few staff with VHF radio communication. A communication tree, based on the proximity of staff to each other both at night (i.e. in their community) and during the day, is a helpful tool.
- Communication with family and friends presenting to the hospital in search of their kin is essential.

Site planning
- Separate hospital areas should be designated for the triage area and for the different triage categories. This usually involves an entire reorganization of the internal hospital departments.
- Take into account large numbers of non-injured but psychologically traumatized people; they need a separate area away from patients.
- Management of fatalities in a culturally appropriate manner to be determined in consultation with national colleagues.
- Staff will be required for stretcher or trolley patient transfer internally.
- Security: crowd control is absolutely key, particularly in a war zone when the 'curious' include men with guns. Consider mechanisms for crowd control, including police. Various forms of an 'obligatory passage', permitting only a single stretcher to pass through, have been deployed in an attempt to control access to the triage area.

Supplies
- Separate stock of essential medications and supplies for the resuscitation area according to the clinical protocols of the hospital. The quantities will depend on the capacity of the hospital and the expected events. The stock should include analgesics, antibiotics, tetanus vaccine and serum, IV fluids and perfusion sets, dressings, burn kits, chest tube kits, minor surgery kits, syringes, and needles; blood bank preparation, if applicable.
- This reserve stock must be prepared beforehand and managed properly with easy accessibility and up-to-date stock.
- Maintenance of critical equipment, such as suction pumps, oxygen supply, and ventilators if available, is also essential.
- Pre-prepare special medical charts (at least 100) to be used in mass casualty events. A simple patient chart with essential information and a homunculus drawing is useful (see Fig. 15.3).

Training
- Train all personnel, including non-medical and paramedical, on the principles of triage and the current plan. Everyone in the hospital should know what they have to do, and how this may differ from their everyday work.
- Simulation exercises to be conducted, preferably every 6 months, in order to test hospital preparedness.
- Revision and updating of the plan on a regular basis to take into account personnel changes and difficulties encountered during the simulation exercises.

Triage Number:

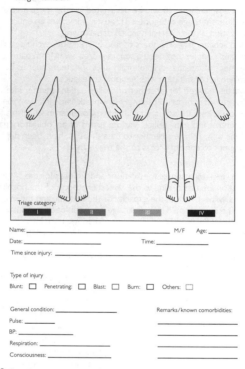

Triage category:

| I | II | III | IV |

Name: _____ M/F Age: _____

Date: _____ Time: _____

Time since injury: _____

Type of injury

Blunt: ☐ Penetrating: ☐ Blast: ☐ Burn: ☐ Others: ☐

General condition: _____   Remarks/known comorbidities:

Pulse: _____   _____

BP: _____   _____

Respiration: _____   _____

Consciousness: _____   _____

Fig. 15.3 Sample patient triage card.

Further reading

Giannou C, Baldan, M. War Surgery: Working with Limited Resources in Armed Conflict and other Situations of Violence, Vol. 1. Geneva: International Committee of the Red Cross; 2009, pp. 189–208.

Russell R, Hodgetts TJ, Mahoney PF, Castle N. Disaster Rules. Oxford: Wiley-Blackwell, BMJ Books; 2011.

Sztajnkrycer MD, Madsen BE, Alejandro Báez A. Unstable ethical plateaus and disaster triage. Emerg Med Clin North Am 2006;24(3):749–68.

The Sphere Project. Humanitarian Charter and Minimum Standards in Disaster response. 2011. ℘ http://www.sphereproject.org/handbook/

World Health Organization. Mass Casualty Management Systems: Strategies and Guidelines for Building Health Sector Capacity. Geneva: WHO; April 2007. ℘ http://apps.who.int/iris/handle/10665/43804

Chapter 16

Medical triage

Peter Moons

Introduction to medical triage

Medical emergency triage is a process of rapidly sorting patients into groups based on the urgency of their condition. The main objective of triage is to make sure that the most appropriate patients get treatment first to avoid late identification of a critically ill patient and possibly a harmful delay in their care. Initial triage does not include a full evaluation of the patient, but rather serves to categorize patients and to distinguish those who need immediate medical attention from those who can wait to be seen.

The concept of general medical triage should be distinguished from mass casualty triage. Medical triage is used in the day-to-day care of patients, whereas mass casualty triage is a process put in place following an incident that overwhelms the local resources (see ➜ Chapter 15).

Triage in humanitarian settings

In certain humanitarian settings, the volume of patients can be very heavy and vulnerable or seriously ill patients may end up at the end of a long line of patients. *Be aware that the quietest patient may be the sickest.*

There are several advantages of effective triage in a humanitarian medical setting, as the process facilitates:

• timely recognition of the sickest patients,
• identification of patients in need of isolation due to the possibility of epidemic disease (e.g. a patient presenting with a weak or absent pulse with watery diarrhoea in a region known for cholera),
• timely organization of the evacuation of patients requiring a higher level of care.

The last thing one wants to do at the end of a long day with curfew approaching, is to need to return to the healthcare clinic for a sick patient who was not timely identified during a triage process.

Mechanisms for triage

While several triage systems have been developed and validated for well-resourced settings, there are only a few which have been externally validated for low-resource settings. The triage process used most commonly in resource-poor settings was developed by WHO as part of its *Emergency Triage, Assessment, and Treatment* (ETAT) course. ETAT is developed and validated for triage of children and although it has not been specifically validated for use in an adult population, it has been adapted in several places with additional criteria for use among adult patients. ETAT uses a minimal number of clinical signs that are easily taught and recognized, it requires minimal equipment and is very effective as it can be done in as little as 30 seconds. A full training package for ETAT is available online.[1]

Emergency triage, assessment, and treatment: methodology

Patients are classified as having:
- emergency signs that require immediate treatment,
- priority signs that require early assessment,
- non-urgent signs which can wait.

Recognizing emergency signs

Emergencies can be identified by using the *ABCD* system where A stands for Airway, B for Breathing, C for Circulation, Coma, and Convulsions, and D for Dehydration (severe). *When any of the ABCD signs are present, the patient should be considered an emergency and treated immediately.*

A: Airway
- Is the patient breathing?
- Is the airway obstructed?

Look, listen, and feel for air movement. Obstructed breathing can be due to blockage by the tongue, a foreign body, swelling around the upper airway, or severe croup, which may present with abnormal sounds such as stridor.

B: Breathing
- Does the patient have severe respiratory distress?
- Is the patient blue at the lips or under the tongue (centrally cyanosed)?
- Is the patient breathing very fast and getting tired and/or is there severe chest in-drawing or use of accessory respiratory muscles?
- Look for difficulty talking or in infants, difficulty with breastfeeding.

C_1: Circulation (shock)
- Does the patient have warm hands?
- If not, is the capillary refill time >3 seconds?
  - Note: in some cold climates, capillary refill may best be checked at the sternum area on the chest.
- If so, is the pulse weak and fast?

C_2: Coma
- A rapid assessment of conscious level (using AVPU-score A for Alert, V for response to Voice, P for response to Pain, U for Unresponsive).
- A patient that does not respond to voice is considered an emergency.

C_3: Convulsions
- Generalized tonic–clonic movements of the limbs and body but also look for partial seizures (e.g. subtle movements in the face and mouth or eye twitching) at the time of triage.

D: Dehydration
Does the patient have diarrhoea and/or two or more of the following signs?
- The patient is lethargic or unconscious.
- The patient has sunken eyes.
- The patient has dry mucous membranes.
- The skin pinch goes back very slowly.

A summary overview of the triage process is displayed in Fig. 16.1.

Recognizing priority signs

When ABCD has been completed and there are no emergency signs, continue to assess the priority signs. These signs can be remembered with the symbols 3(TPR)–MOB.

When priority signs are found, a patient should be moved to the front of the waiting line where some supportive treatments can be started.

Local context

The list of priority signs previously described was developed for use in children. This can be altered to include adult pathology and/or locally relevant conditions.

Examples of additional priority signs are:
- pregnant women with potential complications (e.g. in labour, with vaginal bleeding, STI or fever),
- victim of sexual violence,
- danger to others or self (e.g. violent patient),
- bites and stings,
- symptoms or signs of active pulmonary TB.

3(TPR)–MOB
- Tiny baby: any sick child aged <2 months. These children are difficult to assess and are also vulnerable to infection.
- Temperature: patient is very hot or cold.*
- Trauma or other urgent surgical condition.
- Pallor (severe).
- Poisoning.
- Pain (severe).
- Respiratory distress (see ➲ Chapter 37 for more details).
- Restless, continuously irritable or lethargic.
- Referral from another health centre for a serious problem (urgent).
- Malnutrition: visible severe wasting.
- Oedema of both feet.
- Burns (major).

* Note: formal temperature recording is typically done later when other measurements such as anthropometry are performed (so as to not slow down the triage process).

Recognizing non-urgent patients
- Patient whose ABCD assessment is negative and pass without any priority signs (3(TPR)-MOB) are generally considered 'non-urgent'.
- It can be useful to triage them in subcategories to facilitate patient flow to, for example, specialized clinics (e.g. vaccination clinic or family planning).

TRIAGE

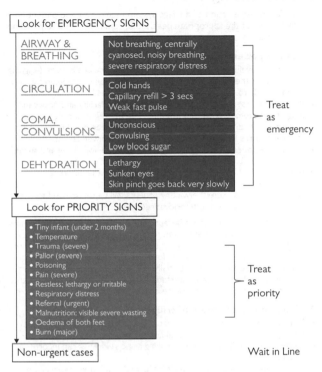

Look for EMERGENCY SIGNS

AIRWAY & BREATHING	Not breathing, centrally cyanosed, noisy breathing, severe respiratory distress
CIRCULATION	Cold hands Capillary refill > 3 secs Weak fast pulse
COMA, CONVULSIONS	Unconscious Convulsing Low blood sugar
DEHYDRATION	Lethargy Sunken eyes Skin pinch goes back very slowly

Treat as emergency

Look for PRIORITY SIGNS

• Tiny infant (under 2 months)
• Temperature
• Trauma (severe)
• Pallor (severe)
• Poisoning
• Pain (severe)
• Restless; lethargy or irritable
• Respiratory distress
• Referral (urgent)
• Malnutrition: visible severe wasting
• Oedema of both feet
• Burn (major)

Treat as priority

Non-urgent cases   Wait in Line

Fig. 16.1 Overview of the triage process.

Need for re-assessment

- Remember that patients triaged as 'priority' or 'non-urgent' may deteriorate.
- Quick reassessment should be carried out regularly based on local resources and should begin with an assessment of the airway and continue through the ABCD system described in ➲ 'Recognizing emergency signs' pp. 291–2.

Implementing triage

Successful implementation of a triage system requires a good patient flow design, training of the appropriate health staff, community involvement and patient education.

Design of patient flow

It is helpful to evaluate patient flow in the current practice before designing a flow chart for the situation after the implementation of triage. In this process, one needs to consider the following issues:

- What is the first point of contact with the health facility and how can triage be implemented at that point (e.g. before registration)?
- Where are children with emergency conditions seen now? Is this room easily accessible from the triage area? Is this room well equipped?
- Where are patients waiting? Is there enough room for sitting and shade? Is there access to drinking water and latrines?
- After triage, is there a system to clearly recognize the different categories of patients (priority vs non-urgent)?
- How can we make sure the waiting patients will be re-assessed to check that their condition is not deteriorating?

Having a system in which the different patient category groups are clearly recognised is essential for the system to function properly. Having separate waiting rooms is not feasible in most settings, but using different coloured patient cards and separate benches for each group of patients is one possible solution (see Fig. 16.2). Especially in the early stages of triage implementation, people may not understand where to sit or why they need to wait. Crowd control and reassurance is key.

Training in the concepts of triage

- Train a core group of staff to conduct the first triage with mentorship and regular team meetings to evaluate the process.
- Triage involves difficult decision-making as no guidelines can incorporate all unique situations.
- When staff are unsure, they must 'up-triage' to a higher, more acute category or consult a senior colleague.
- The ABCD signs should be explained in a simple manner to non-healthcare staff who may actually be the first contact with a patient (i.e. drivers, security guards or janitors). Non-healthcare staff should be encouraged to immediately seek a healthcare professional when a patient with emergency signs arrives.

Triage, by definition, is supposed to be inherently neutral and impartial to politics, sex, religion and ethnicity; however, the triage officer may be challenged based on these criteria. Even if the community understands and accepts the triage process, the triage officer may still be faced with considerable stress, and even danger, to prioritize culturally or politically important persons or certain groups (e.g. armed actors).

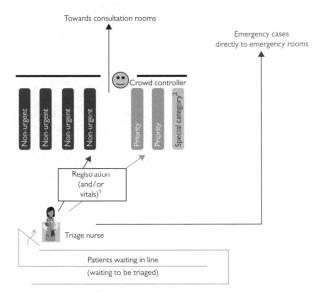

Fig. 16.2 An example of triage set-up and patient flow.

[1] After triage, registration can be done. The time that patients are waiting in the waiting area can also be used to measure weight, height, temperature, etc.

[2] According to local need, an extra bench can be created for special categories (e.g. scheduled clinic visits).

Community involvement and patient education

For the successful implementation of triage, it is essential that the community be educated on the goals and processes of triage.

- Community leaders and members should be consulted and outreach teams employed to educate the population as well as those waiting to be seen at the health centre.
- The general population should understand that patients triaged as non-urgent will still be attended to.

Reference

1. World Health Organization. Emergency Triage Assessment and Treatment (ETAT). WHO; 2005. http://www.who.int/maternal_child_adolescent/documents/9241546875/en/

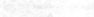

Approach to paediatric care

Daniel Martinez Garcia, Laurent Hiffler, and Jaap Karsten

Introduction to paediatric care

When joining a team for a humanitarian mission, providers may enter a highly stressful, chaotic, or low-resource environment—and in many cases, this can include the additional task of suddenly being presented with paediatric patients. For the non-paediatrician, this can be extremely challenging, as many will have to reach back to the recesses of their minds to medical school, which for some, was the last time they had experience with this population group.

Recent figures demonstrate that we must be better prepared for treating newborns, infants, children, and teenagers in humanitarian, conflict, or disaster settings. According to UNICEF, more than one in nine children are currently living in areas of conflict. An additional half a billion children are living in areas where floods are extremely common and nearly 160 million are living in high or extremely high drought severity zones. Furthermore, children represent almost half of all people living in extreme poverty although they only make up an estimated one-third of the world's population.

Although children represent a large proportion of patients in emergency settings, many healthcare providers are often underprepared to deal with high volumes of ill children. Being faced with a large paediatric patient population can be daunting, but a systematic and structured approach to assessment, triage, and treatment is essential. The more a provider prepares beforehand, the better clinical care they will provide. While paediatric textbooks can provide basic information, the evidence base for paediatric care in humanitarian settings is evolving. Providers should attempt to stay abreast of developments and use up-to-date evidence-based guidelines to guide paediatric patient care. Further, there are paediatric-centred approaches, such as the Integrated Management of Childhood Illness (IMCI) strategy,[1] which promote the use of resources in the most cost-effective way towards reducing child mortality.

In such an evolving and challenging discipline, this chapter does not intend to replace paediatric training, but aims to highlight the approaches to paediatric care, and provide key insights and guidance to help the practitioner with clinical judgement and decision-making.

Approach to paediatric assessment

Children will present for care in a variety of settings, whether it is under the makeshift tent of a mobile clinic, or in the hospital setting where more detailed assessment of vital signs may be possible. Regardless of where the child is first encountered, a rapid decision can be made as to whether this child is 'sick' or 'not sick'. The Paediatric Assessment Triangle (PAT) can be used to assess a child, without even placing a hand on them (see Fig. 17.1).

- 'Appearance' looks at the child's tone, how they are interacting with their environment, whether they are consolable by the parent/caregiver, their gaze, and their speech or cry.
- 'Work of breathing' is a rapid assessment of whether the breathing appears too fast or too slow, whether there are abnormal breath sounds, or increased work of breathing based on a quick look.
- 'Circulation' refers to the child's colour and the presence of any pallor, mottling, cyanosis, as well as active bleeding.

Children determined to have abnormalities based on the PAT should be rapidly assessed in more detail.

All children presenting for care should be triaged, and emergency conditions treated using the ETAT system developed by WHO. See ➔ Chapter 16 for further details. PAT is done usually before triage in a regular base.

Integrated Management of Childhood Illness

IMCI is a strategy created by WHO and UNICEF which focuses on the prevention and treatment of the top five causes of mortality in children under 5 years old: acute respiratory infections, diarrhoeal diseases, measles, malaria, and malnutrition.[1] Its strategies aim to reduce under-five child morbidity and mortality in countries with poor health infrastructures through improved management of childhood illnesses, proper nutrition, and immunization. The management guidelines improve quality of care by promoting a continuum of care from the community level to the hospital and include preventative interventions.

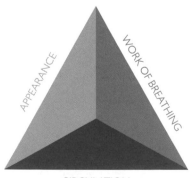

CIRCULATION

Fig. 17.1. Paediatric Assessment Triangle.

At the *community level*, IMCI promotes early interventions at home and care-seeking behaviour by identifying danger signs (see Box 17.1); it encourages improved nutrition and prevention of major diseases. In *health structures*, the IMCI strategy promotes proper and early identification of childhood illnesses using the Assess, Classify, Treat, Support (the mother), and Follow-up model. After triage assessment, general danger signs are sought and treated. Children are then assessed based on presenting symptoms, classified based on signs, and then treated with the appropriate algorithm.[1]

> ### Box 17.1 IMCI general danger signs
> - Is the child able to drink or breastfeed?
> - Does the child vomit everything?
> - Is there a history of convulsion?
> - Is the child lethargic or unconscious?

The impact of IMCI implementation can be profound. In the aftermath of a disaster or in a refugee setting, a public health team familiar with IMCI will likely save more lives with fewer resources than a team of paediatric intensive care specialists. When providers are familiar with both preventive and curative strategies to improve child health, there is a real opportunity to improve child health in humanitarian settings. Non-paediatricians need not shy away from IMCI—it is easily understood and can be incorporated into daily clinical routines. Implementation of IMCI depends heavily on community health workers who might have basic literacy or clinical training, therefore ongoing capacity building is of underlying importance.

Paediatric and neonatal Early Warning Scoring systems

Signs and symptoms of critical illness can be more subtle in children, and decompensation occurs late in the disease process. Once the more obvious signs of decompensation are apparent (e.g. hypotension in shock), it is often too late and outcomes may be poor. Efforts should therefore be focused at early detection and treatment. Early Warning Scoring (EWS) systems have been developed to detect these subtle changes and allow for early treatment that saves lives (See Fig. 17.2 for an example of a neonatal EWS.)

EWSs reinforce timely detection of imminent life-threatening conditions, and encourage action before they advance to the critical stage. While most EWSs have been developed for high-resource settings, they have been increasingly adopted in humanitarian contexts with good outcomes and are pending more formal validation. Although there can be challenges, these tools increase awareness of early detection, empower the nursing staff, and facilitate communication within the medical team. Implementation of an EWS can be challenging in low-resource settings, but can be a prudent step to improve health outcomes for paediatric populations.

Surname:

First name:

Date of birth:

Time of the birth:

Hospital:

Maternity unit □ Neonatal unit □

Date:

Term □ Preterm □ GA:

Weight: ≥2500g □ <2500g □ <1500g □

Meconium □ Urine □

Time	8	10																			

Temperature °C

≥38																					RED ZONE
37.5–37.9																					ORANGE ZONE
36–37.4		•																			GREEN ZONE
35.1–35.9																					ORANGE ZONE
≤35																					RED ZONE

Respiratory rate

≥80																					RED ZONE
60–79																					ORANGE ZONE
31–59		•																			GREEN ZONE
26–30																					ORANGE ZONE
≤25																					RED ZONE

Grunting

																					RED ZONE

Heart rate

≥190																					RED ZONE
150–189																					ORANGE ZONE
100–149		•																			GREEN ZONE
80–99																					ORANGE ZONE
≤79																					RED ZONE

SpO₂	≥ 94% Pink		GREEN ZONE
	90–94%		ORANGE ZONE
Colour	≤90% Dusky		RED ZONE

Neurology	Alert—Active—Awake to feed		GREEN ZONE
	Irritable—jittery		ORANGE ZONE
	Poor feeding		
	Floppy—difficult to awaken		RED ZONE
	Seizure		
	Tetanic spasms		

| | Glucose ≥45mg/dL | | GREEN ZONE |
| | Glucose ≤45mg/dL | | RED ZONE |

Others:

Score	GREEN	6	4
	Orange	0	2
	Red	0	0

Response	All observations in GREEN ZONE: continue observations as determined by doctor or midwife
	1 observation in ORANGE ZONE: Contact doctor or midwife. Management plan and review discussed. Repeat observation in 30–60 minutes
	≥2 observations in ORANGE ZONE: IMMEDIATELY contact doctor or midwife
	Any observation in the RED ZONE: IMMEDIATELY contact doctor or midwife

Example:
Baby in the maternity unit.
At 8.00 am all the observations are in the green zone and we continue with the monitoring.
At 10.00 am the baby starts to be irritable and refuse to breastfeed. In this case there are two observation in the orange zone, four in the green zone, and none in the red zone. The nurse calls immediately the doctor.

Fig. 17.2. Example of a neonatal Early Warning Score system.

Guidance for the care of paediatric patients

It is not possible to cover in a brief chapter what clinicians will learn during a 3–9-year residency training. Once children are assessed and classified based on a detailed history and complete physical exam, high-quality guidelines, such as those found in ➜ 'Further reading' p. 306, should be used to treat them. While evidence-based paediatric medicine, particularly in the humanitarian settings, is sometimes in evolution, the most up-to-date guidelines from your organization should be used. The following sections are intended to be useful notes for clinicians treating ill children in resource-limited settings.

Rely on clinical skills and keep your differential broad

- An often striking reality of working in a humanitarian setting can be the lack of advanced diagnostic options to help guide decision-making. Our ears, eyes, nose, hands, and brains will have to search deep into our memories to revive old clinical skills.
- Perform a complete physical examination and make sure you undress the child to look for the otherwise unnoticed rash or subtle increased work of breathing.
- Look for ear, throat, or urinary tract infections before you classify the child's illness as 'fever of unknown origin' or as malaria.
- Keep a broad differential in mind—what is a rare disease in England might be a common condition in Niger. Narrowing the differential runs the risk of missing an important diagnosis.
- Many sick children are unvaccinated. This adds additional pathologies you may never have seen to common tropical conditions (e.g. tetanus in a child recovering from burn wounds).
- Patients living in harsh conditions have a higher chance of having a more severe condition, arriving later to care and having multiple pathologies at the same time.
- You're not alone: the nurse standing next to you may have years of experience with many of these bewildering presentations. He or she may not volunteer this information out of respect for the new doctor or nurse from overseas, but you will never regret asking.
- Get assistance from telemedicine if available. Telemedicine does not exclude the need for clinical acumen in the field, but can be of great support in managing complex children (e.g. ℘ https://collegiumtelemedicus.org).

Strive for cultural understanding

A child is not the same child everywhere. Biology apart, sociocultural and legal definitions of children differ, which impact macro determinants such as social status, rights, and societal value of the life of that child, and patient variables such as pain or suffering quantification and stress.

Strive to understand the sociocultural context which impacts caregivers' understanding of their condition and treatments. Nonetheless, cultural understanding does not mean blind acceptance of tradition and cultural norms. If you discover a child being abused in a setting where no legislation exists nor protects them, or where it is not socially considered a problem, your ethical duty to protect your patient remains, but needs to be pragmatic, sensitive, and compassionate.

You might conceptually struggle with situations such as very young teenagers fraught with the responsibility of taking care of their own prematurely born babies, male and female genital mutilation, or suspicion of physical abuse, as what you might consider as inappropriate, illegal, or immoral may not be so in other cultural settings. Follow the same considerations regarding patient safety, dignity, respect, and protection of confidentiality as you would do in any other professional medical setting.

Be attuned to advances in evidence-based management

Be aware that despite years of experience, there remains lack of consensus on some of the fundamentals of paediatric management in humanitarian settings, including fluid resuscitation (colloids vs crystalloids, amount, and rates), fluid maintenance choices, transfusions, and inotropes (see Box 17.2).

Further, there is now further research and rethinking of the management guidelines for severely acute malnourished (SAM) children with discussions ranging from the pathophysiology of kwashiorkor, to the role of some micronutrients such as thiamine and magnesium, and even the safety of ReSoMal.

While it might be unfeasible for the non-paediatrician to question the guidance put forth by international regulatory bodies, it is important to be aware that these standards are not considered definitive, but rather, are continually evolving and being updated.

Consider population-level impact

Doctors are trained to focus on the medical needs of individual patients and are used to spending disproportionally more time on taking care of the critically ill. It feels gratifying to save a child's life by timely placement of an intraosseous needle and treatment of shock, as compared to preventing disease by ensuring all children get vaccinated before they leave the ward. But the reality is that resources are often limited and difficult decisions have to be made. This also means sometimes sending a patient home with a condition for which there is a cure (e.g. childhood cancer) but which would

Box 17.2 Controversies in fluid management

The FEAST trial drew attention to possible shortcomings in the current approach of administering IV fluid boluses to children in resource-limited settings.[2] This study found a completely unexpected excess mortality in septic children treated according to standard international guidelines for fluid resuscitation. These findings precipitated heavy medical debate that continues to date, and currently there is no consensus as many potential sources of bias were identified (anaemia level, comorbidities, oxygen needs, definition of sepsis and shock). More research is required and clinicians treating children with sepsis in resource-limited settings should cautiously administer IV fluids with active surveillance. The study was also a reminder of the importance of treating critically ill children in a bundle of care (e.g. treating hypoglycaemia, anaemia, providing oxygen and warmth, and increase monitoring) and not focusing on a single intervention.

be unattainable in a given setting, or establishing restrictive admission criteria to newborn units based on weight or gestational age or into paediatric wards only up to age 5 or 10 years. While a lot of lives will be saved, not all will be. There is little that compares to the horrible and often long-lasting feeling one will have knowing that the battle against a treatable condition has been lost due to lack of awareness of the severity of the condition, staff, drugs, protocols, basic hospital infrastructure, appropriate referral system, equipment, and/or simply available time.

References

1. World Health Organization. Integrated Management of Childhood Illness Chart Booklet 2014. Geneva: WHO; March 2014. ℘ http://apps.who.int/iris/bitstream/handle/10665/104772/9789241506823_Chartbook_eng.pdf

2. Maitland K, Kiguli S, Opoka RO, Engoru C, Olupot-Olupot P, Akech SO, et al. Mortality after fluid bolus in African children with severe infection. N Engl J Med 2011;364(26):2483–95.

Further reading

Hospital Care for Children. Randomised Trials in Child Health in Developing Countries. [Latest edition July 2016–June 2017]. ℘ http://www.ichrc.org/evidence-0

Mehta NM, Jaksic T. The critically ill child. In: Duggan C, Watkins JB, Walker WA, eds. Nutrition in Pediatrics. 4th ed. Hamilton, ON: BC Decker Inc; 2008, pp. 663–73.

World Health Organization. Pocket Book of Hospital Care For Children: Guidelines for the Management of Common Childhood Illnesses. 2nd ed. Geneva: WHO; 2013. ℘ http://www.who.int/maternal_child_adolescent/documents/child_hospital_care/en/

World Health Organization. WHO Recommendations on the Management of Diarrhoea and Pneumonia in HIV-Infected Infants and Children: Integrated Management of Childhood Illness (IMCI). Geneva: WHO; 2010. ℘ https://www.ncbi.nlm.nih.gov/books/NBK305342/

Part III

Syndromic management

Chapter 18

Shock

Laura Hawryluck and Miroslav Stavel

Context of shock

When working in humanitarian settings, one important presentation which should never be missed is shock. An often misunderstood term, shock refers to a state of inadequate tissue perfusion, usually one of haemodynamic instability. If uncorrected, shock can lead to widespread microcirculation damage in organs and tissues, which then leads to further release of inflammatory mediators, a spiralling decline in organ function, and ultimately death if not corrected quickly. Shock is one of the leading causes of death worldwide and, in LIC, it is implicated in just under half of the mortality in children <5 years (related to infection).[1] About 90% of worldwide deaths due to pneumonia, meningitis, and other infections occur in low-resource countries.[2]

Challenges in humanitarian settings

The presentation of shock in humanitarian settings can have some important differences from that seen in the developed world:

- Causes may be more traumatic in nature if working in areas of conflict.
- Septic causes may be due to illnesses that the providers have rarely or never previously seen outside of a textbook.
- Severe burns as a cause of shock are more frequent.
- Patients may be undernourished or suffering from untreated chronic illnesses and have delayed presentations to health centres.
- Greater prevalence of multidrug-resistant bacteria.
- Reliance on traditional or faith healers which can cause patients to have delayed, or more complicated presentations.
- Lack of routine awareness of shock states, Advanced Trauma Life Support® (ATLS®) principles in trauma and advanced cardiovascular life support (ACLS) and paediatric advanced life support (PALS) principles.

Further, diagnosis and management is challenging in low-resource and humanitarian settings which often lack diagnostic tests, and require reliance on history and physical signs to diagnose the cause(s), assess the severity of shock, monitor the effectiveness of resuscitation, and determine treatment of the underlying cause(s). The presentation of shock, however, can be recognized rapidly by the experienced provider and any causes of shock are readily treatable even in resource-constrained humanitarian settings, so rapid recognition and response is essential. This chapter aims to provide practical guidance to make sure that all workers are able to perform rapid assessment, crucial re-assessments, and implement corrective measures.

Note: research shows that the amount of fluid resuscitation routinely used in septic shock algorithms in developed countries may in fact be detrimental and worsen outcomes in humanitarian settings due, possibly, to rapid reversal of the patient's compensatory vasoconstrictor response or through an increased severity of reperfusion injury—leading to worsening shock and organ failure. Conversely, in some situations more fluid resuscitation may be needed than providers expect in conditions such as gastroenteritis (to give one example) due to its different aetiologies (e.g. cholera), often greater severity, and resulting in more profound volume loss. What remains clear and unchanged is the need for tailored resuscitation and frequent re-evaluations of response to treatment.

Clinical assessment: recognition of the patient in shock

Initial clinical assessment

- The patients most at risk for shock are often not ones in obvious distress.
- Initially, compensatory mechanisms may be deceptive and a patient may present without typical signs yet still be in shock with organ underperfusion. Remember, blood pressure doesn't always equal blood flow.
- Younger patients in particular have a robust ability to compensate and enough physiological reserve to mask the true severity of their illness—right until the point they suffer a respiratory and/or cardiac arrest.
- Actively look for the pale, sweaty, anxious, or limp-looking adults or children as the sickest patient is often the quietest and may be hidden at the end of a long line of patients waiting to be seen.

Triage: ABCD sequence

- For systematic assessment and timely recognition, the 'ABCD' sequence (defined in Table 18.1) triage system should be in place at all levels of care to recognize emergency and priority signs.
- If any emergency sign is found, then an immediate response is to be initiated to stabilize that sign—before proceeding to the next sign.

Table 18.1 ABCD triage system for shock

Airway and Breathing	• *Is there evidence of airway obstruction? Is the patient spontaneously breathing? Is there tachypnoea, signs of severe respiratory distress, or cyanosis?*
	• *Do you have reason to anticipate imminent loss of airway?* Think of head and neck trauma, facial / neck burns, high spinal cord injuries. You may want to consider early control of the airway or early transfer if feasible in the field
	• *Do you have reason to anticipate a difficult airway?* Consider early control of airway (even with a simple oral airway device) and calling for help if available
Circulation	• *Are there signs of instability, mottling, and weak peripheral pulses or delayed capillary refill?*
	• *Any signs of chest or abdominal trauma or bleeding?*
Disability/Coma	• Use 'AVPU' (acronym for 'alert, voice, pain, unresponsive') rapid assessment scale of conscious level
	• *Could there be traumatic brain injury and rapid deterioration of level of consciousness? Could there be a high spinal cord injury?* Anticipate airway issues
	• *Could there be a spinal cord injury?* Place the patient in precautions
Dehydration	• *Is there a history of severe diarrhoea and vomiting?*

- The sequence is also useful during treatment when ongoing reassessment is vital but not always done in humanitarian settings.
- Specific details on triage systems used in adults and children (e.g. the ETAT approach for children) can be found in ➋ Chapter 16. For full details, see ➋ Chapter 16.

Signs and symptoms of shock

- Shock is a state of evolving deterioration and patients who may initially be alert and with stable vital signs can rapidly become confused and drowsy.
- Continued close monitoring is essential and in low-resource settings, clinical assessment rather than advanced investigative methods is the cornerstone for recognizing clinical changes for the patient.
- Trends over time may be more important than single values.

The specific signs and symptoms which the clinician should monitor are as follows:

Mental status
- Anxiety, confusion, agitation, apathy, or otherwise altered level of consciousness.

Vital signs
- Weak, thready, or absent peripheral pulses.
- Tachypnoea (often overlooked and inaccurately reported).
- Low or undetectable blood pressure and narrow pulse pressure (these are late signs).
- Tachycardia (or bradycardia as a very late sign).

Hydration status
- Dry mucous membranes.
- Skin tenting (due to decreased skin turgor).
- Low or no urine output.

Extremities and skin
- Cold hands and feet.
- Prolonged central capillary refill time (>3 seconds).
- Pallor, mottled skin, and sweating.
- Warm and flushed extremities (may be present in septic or anaphylactic shock due to vasodilation).

Musculoskeletal
- Hypotonia.
- Inability to walk or move (patients are often on the ground—when first arriving at a health clinic, ensure all those on the ground are seen early).

Traumatic injuries: symptoms and signs
- Neck pain—cervical spine injuries.
- Unilaterally decreased breath sounds and an asymmetrical chest—tension pneumothorax.
- Diminished heart sounds and distended neck veins—cardiac tamponade.
- Penetrating injuries:
  - Peritonitis (may signal internal abdominal bleeding).
  - Bony pain (a tender extended thigh may indicate a femur fracture).

Types of shock and their presentation

Classifications of shock

Shock can present due to a variety of factors, but generally falls into one of five categories:

Category 1: hypovolaemic shock.
Category 2: distributive shock.
Category 3: cardiogenic shock.
Category 4: obstructive shock.
Category 5: mixed shock (two or more of the above occurring together).

The recognition and management of each of these will be covered in more detail below, highlighting those conditions more common in humanitarian settings.

Hypovolaemic shock

Definition:
An actual loss of circulating volume—either whole blood (haemorrhage) or plasma component (e.g. severe dehydration or burns) to the extent that it no longer supports adequate circulation in the body.

Common causes in humanitarian settings
- Dehydration: e.g. secondary to gastrointestinal infections, poor oral intake, or losses following burns.
- Bleeding: e.g. due to trauma, surgery, or obstetric complications.

Presentation
Dehydration
- Severe dehydration due to gastrointestinal losses generally occurs gradually, as the body has various compensation mechanisms but there is a tipping point where shock can present with a rapid onset.
- The most extreme example is cholera where large amount of fluids can be lost in a matter of hours.

Bleeding
- In addition to more obvious causes of bleeding, internal bleeding is often not clearly apparent and requires a high level of suspicion based on history and clinical presentation.
- Paracentesis, culdocentesis, and bedside portable ultrasound can aid in making a diagnosis of intra-abdominal haemorrhage.

Clinical cautions
- It is important to evaluate fluid status carefully as shock may not be apparent until >40% of circulating volume is lost.
- For management decisions, use the clinical signs mentioned previously. *Do not* rely on blood pressure to diagnose, as systolic blood pressure may remain unchanged until 30–50% of circulating volume is lost. This is true especially in children where blood pressure doesn't change until shock is in advanced stages.

Distributive shock

Definition:

failure of vascular regulatory mechanisms leading to disproportionate vaso-dilation and capillary leak resulting in loss of intravascular volume.

Common causes in humanitarian settings

- Septic shock, burns.

Less common causes

- Anaphylactic shock, neurogenic shock.

Presentation

Septic shock

- This is the most common case of distributive shock, particularly in regions where routine vaccination may be incomplete, nutrition and sanitation are poor, and where immunocompromising conditions such as malnutrition and HIV are prevalent.
- Although total body fluid content remains unchanged, toxins released by infective agents cause vasodilation and capillary leak, leading to intravascular depletion.
- Signs and symptoms may be similar to ones seen in hypovolaemic shock but without a history of diarrhoea, vomiting, and associated weight loss.
- Fever may not always be present, especially among malnourished population, neonates, and those who are HIV positive. Hypothermia may be the leading and even more worrisome sign.
- Management is with IV fluids and vasopressors if available (see
  ➋ p. 305).
- A new bedside clinical score, the quick Sepsis-related Organ Failure Assessment (qSOFA), can be used to identify patients at greater risk of poor outcomes who need early treatment and frequent re-evaluation. The qSOFA in adults consists of: respiratory rate ≥22/min, changed mentation, or systolic blood pressure ≤100 mmHg.[3]

Burns

- Burns are common in humanitarian settings and can present as hypovolaemic or distributive shock (due to inflammatory mediator release) or as a mixed picture of both.
- Delays in treatment and some traditional local treatments that sometimes get applied to burns may result in sepsis which will worsen distributive shock from the burn itself
- See ➋ Chapter 51 for more details.

Anaphylactic shock

- Anaphylaxis is rare in low-income settings due to factors such as less apparent drug and food allergies but can follow stings from arthropod insects or bites by animals such as snakes.
- Anaphylaxis presents with respiratory, cardiovascular, gastrointestinal, and cutaneous signs. In severe cases, these may be accompanied by angio-oedema, bronchospasm, hypotension, and syncope.

- The most important treatment modality is rapid and correct administration of epinephrine (adrenaline) *intramuscularly* (use 1:1000 (1 mg/mL) solution: adults 0.3 mL, children 15–30 kg 0.15 mL, children <15 kg 0.01 mL/kg, this can be repeated every 5–15 min for 3–4 doses), with steroids, antihistamines, and IV fluids. Ensure the correct concentration and dose is used as this is prone to potentially serious medication error.

Neurogenic shock
- This follows a traumatic spinal cord injury, typically above the T1 vertebral level, which disrupts sympathetic nerve function, resulting in unopposed vagal stimulation.
- Patients will have the triad of hypotension, bradycardia, and vasodilation.
- This is a diagnosis of exclusion, after more common causes of hypotension in trauma have been excluded.
- Management is with IV fluids, parenteral atropine, epinephrine (adrenaline), and avoiding hypothermia.

Cardiogenic shock

Definition:
failure of the heart as a pump as a result of right-sided heart failure, left-sided failure, or both, resulting in low cardiac output. This can occur with conditions such as myocarditis, myocardial infarction, cardiomyopathies, acute valvular disease, or prolonged arrhythmias.

Common causes in humanitarian settings
- Myocardial infarction, myocarditis, heart failure (i.e. decompensated valvular heart disease due to rheumatic fever), ischaemic cardiomyopathy, or dilated cardiomyopathy.
- Infantile beriberi (vitamin B1 deficiency).

Presentation
- Patients will have distended neck veins, will be severely short of breath with accessory muscle use, may have a productive cough of blood-tinged sputum, show signs of cyanosis, mottling with cold extremities, and decreased peripheral pulses.
- They may be complaining of severe abdominal pain due to decreased perfusion and development of ischaemic gut.

Clinical cautions
- Cardiogenic shock is rare in paediatric populations; however, severe thiamine (vitamin B1) deficiency in children, particularly those who are malnourished, can cause shock and heart failure.
- This is also seen among malnourished children with severe bacterial infections, malaria, and during refeeding.
- Bedside ultrasound if available is an invaluable tool in evaluating these patients.
- Diagnosis and management in low-resource settings is challenging as diagnostic possibilities and access to intensive care are limited.

Obstructive shock

Definition:

occurs when there is an obstruction to the circulation resulting in inadequate venous return and cardiac output.

Common causes in humanitarian settings
- Cardiac tamponade secondary to TB, other infections, penetrating trauma, malignancy, or autoimmune diseases.
- Tension pneumothorax.
- Rarely, massive pulmonary embolism.

Presentation
- Patients will present with distended neck veins, peripheral oedema, signs of decreased cardiac output and respiratory distress in the case of tension pneumothorax, and pulmonary embolism.

Clinical cautions
- Prognosis for survival will depend on the stage at which shock is first managed as early recognition and treatment improve the outcome. Tension pneumothorax and tamponade are relatively easy to treat in the humanitarian settings as a well-placed needle can serve to decompress and surgical skills are often available.
- Massive pulmonary embolism and resulting right-sided heart failure is challenging and may be impossible to stabilize depending on resources.

Mixed shock

Shock due to severe malaria for example
- Severe malaria (usually caused by *Plasmodium falciparum*) may lead to shock because of acute massive haemolysis causing acute severe anaemia, failure of oxygen delivery, and multiorgan failure.
- Shock is often mixed—of distributive and hypovolaemic nature.

Clinical cautions
- Watch for hypoglycaemia and rapid decrease of level of consciousness.
- Urgent blood transfusion will be required—prepare to transfuse or transfer early.
- Fluid resuscitation needs to be carefully titrated as administering rapid IV fluid boluses may lead to further dilutional anaemia, worsening reperfusion injury, pulmonary oedema, and cardiac failure.
- See → Chapter 29 for further management.

Management guidelines for shock

Management of the different types of shock will depend upon quickly identifying the condition and offering specific and rapid interventions. General information about shock and its management can be found in many mainstream publications, and so we will concentrate mainly on situations commonly experienced or specific for humanitarian settings.

General principles

The over-arching aim is to restore balance between oxygen and energy requirements and supply. The initial management principles are the same regardless of the cause as this may not be obvious at that time.

The main principles include:

• Place the patient in a warm and draft-free environment—keep dry and cover with blanket, place out of direct sun.
• Fix any obvious ongoing cause of shock (e.g. stop acute bleeding, look for source of sepsis).
• Follow the ABCD sequence (Table 18.2)—this way you are less likely to miss something.

Specific considerations for paediatric populations

Nutritional status is a very important consideration in resource-limited settings as it will have direct repercussions on treatment choices and expected outcomes. Recognition and management of shock in malnourished children is particularly challenging and bears a high mortality rate. The WHO paediatric ETAT guideline is a very useful reference for caring for critically ill infants and children.[2]

Management in children without malnutrition

Hypovolaemic shock

• Give bolus of 10–20 mL/kg of normal saline or Ringer's lactate over 30–60 min. Reassess afterwards. Giving boluses in smaller aliquots (i.e. 10+10 mL/kg) and frequent re-evaluations of response may be a better strategy.

Special note

The 'Surviving Sepsis' campaign raised awareness of sepsis and septic shock in high-income countries (HIC). It recommends rapid IV resuscitation and early goal-directed therapy aimed at normalizing central venous blood pressure, arterial blood pressure, urine output, and central venous oxygen saturation by using rapid fluid boluses, inotropes, and blood transfusions.

However, the paediatric FEAST trial[4] published in 2011—a study across Uganda, Kenya, and Tanzania with >3000 children—challenges this approach in sub-Saharan Africa. It showed that fluid resuscitation in children presenting with febrile illness and impaired perfusion due to malaria or severe bacterial infection did not save lives and giving children fluids more slowly to maintain normal levels, rather than rapid fluid resuscitation, is safer and more effective in aiding recovery. This trial did not include malnourished children. With this information in mind, from only one well-performed trial, caution needs to be exercised in ordering IV fluid boluses in septic children in low-income settings, particularly in sub-Saharan Africa

Table 18.2 ABCD management principles

A+B	• Give oxygen if available—remember that shock means there is lack of oxygen and nutrient delivery to tissues and end organs. Oxygen concentrators, a commonly used source of oxygen in humanitarian settings, are able to generate 5–10 litres per minute of oxygen. Higher flows from cylinders may deplete quite rapidly • Remember the importance of positioning if decreased level of consciousness results in airway obstruction • If available—and they commonly are not—consider intubation and/or surgical airway if needed. (Note: if these are needed, and are not available, and positioning manoeuvres do not help, providers need to be prepared to palliate the patient.) • If concern exists regarding a spinal cord injury: stabilize the neck—if no collars are available, tape the head to rolled towels placed on either side of the neck and log roll the patient
C	• Obtain IV access with two large-bore IV catheters. If this is not possible, proceed rapidly to intraosseous access if available. In basic settings, you may attempt rehydration via a nasogastric tube • Take blood for emergency blood tests—blood glucose and haemoglobin if available • Note: if hypotension persists after fluid resuscitation (20–30 mL/kg is still a reasonable initial target as long as reassessments are frequent), epinephrine is usually on essential drug lists and while it can be given as 10 mcg dose IV which may be repeated every 3–5 min prn, an infusion of 1 mg epinephrine in 250 mL D5W (5% glucose in water) or normal saline (concentration of 4 mcg/mL) can be run at rates between 2 and 20 mcg/min (30–300 mL/hour). Be careful to avoid extravasation as it will cause a third-degree burn. Such drugs require careful monitoring and need to be used with caution in humanitarian settings

D	• If hypoglycaemia is present or suspected—treat immediately:
	  • Children: glucose 10%: 5 mL/kg (less irritant)
	  • Adults: glucose 50%: 1 mL/kg (used rarely in children when dilution not possible)

• If signs of shock persist, repeat the bolus at 10 mL/kg.[2]
• If the child has a haemoglobin level <5 g/dL or haematocrit value <15%, transfuse as soon as possible and minimize IV fluids to maintain hydration. Transfusion should be considered once estimated blood loss reaches >40% or haematocrit drops to <20%.
• In hypovolaemic shock, the patient should show rapid improvement with better colour and perfusion, and a stronger and slower peripheral pulse.
• If the response to the treatment is not as expected, reconsider your diagnosis—sepsis or malaria may be responsible for the clinical findings in which case fluid boluses may not be beneficial.
• Beware of fluid overloading, as most likely you will not have the means of managing associated complications.
• Ensure appropriate fluid management after the shock is resolved.

Management in malnourished children

Shock is notoriously difficult to diagnose and to manage in this population.

Diagnostic challenges

- Septic shock is responsible for the majority of shock presentations in this fragile population.
- Children often present as hypothermic and their respiratory and heart rates are unreliable indicators of severity of condition—slow respiratory and heart rates are often worse than fast ones as they may indicate a lack of capacity to compensate and impeding demise.
- Baseline abnormalities can lead to an overdiagnosis of shock and overestimation of its severity:
  - Capillary refill time may be already prolonged (and/or pallor may be present.
  - Skin turgor may be decreased as a result of malnutrition.
  - Loose stools, common in this population, are often associated with poor nutrition rather than acute infection and may not be indicative of acute dehydration.
- Marasmic children (wasted without oedema) get overdiagnosed with severe dehydration and in children with kwashiorkor (malnutrition with oedema) intravascular depletion may go unnoticed.
- Despite the best management choices children presenting with a combination of marasmus and kwashiorkor have very poor prognosis due to a high risk of cardiac failure and pulmonary oedema.
- See ➜ Chapter 28 for more information on management of shock in this population.

Caution: in a malnourished population, IV fluids are reserved only for the treatment of shock and are not recommended for the general management of malnourished children. While the malnourished may appear severely volume depleted, less experienced clinicians should resist the temptation of administering IV boluses and the systematic use of IV fluids. There is a high risk of cardiac failure and pulmonary oedema associated with this type of treatment; this is especially true in kwashiorkor, which suffers high mortality.

Specific considerations for adult populations

- Think and act together. Begin treatment based on your first best instinct of the nature of the problem, and at the same time, refine your diagnosis.
- Most adult patients in shock present with either dehydration, sepsis, blood loss, or cardiac failure. In a minority, however, the picture is mixed, which means treating more than one pathology at the same time.
- When faced with a patient in shock, first, get them to the highest, most appropriate level of care (e.g. organize transfer from peripheral health post to hospital), while starting treatment at the same time.
- Anticipate patient transfer and notify the logistical team and coordination team so that non-medical preparations can be made ahead of time. Don't forget to budget for space in a vehicle for a family member if possible.

Follow the ABCD sequence—this way you are less likely to miss something (Table 18.3).

Table 18.3 ABCD sequence: specific considerations for adults

A+B	• Oxygen is important especially in heart failure, sepsis, and anaemia • If you can measure oxygen saturation, and it is >95% you may wish to not use oxygen and spare your limited resources

C	• Open two reliable IV lines
	• Trendelenburg position (legs elevated) can briefly temporize low blood pressure
	• Ensure complete vital signs are reliably and frequently recorded
	• Unless the patient shows evidence of cardiogenic shock with heart failure (crepitations bilaterally on lung auscultation; limb oedema; and an elevated jugular venous pressure) begin with 1–2 litres of either Ringer's lactate or normal saline
	  • Vital signs should generally improve unless you have mixed cardiogenic shock with pulmonary oedema
	  • Patients with cholera, septic shock, or severe burns may easily need 10–20 or more litres of fluid in the course of their treatment
	  • After the first 2 litres, continue to give fluid quickly until vital signs and clinical status improve
	• In an elderly patient or someone you suspect has cardiac insufficiency, give fluids more carefully, auscultating the lungs and monitoring respiratory effort frequently to prevent pulmonary oedema
	• In haemorrhagic shock, be aware that transfusion of fresh whole blood should be initiated as soon as possible. packed red blood cells, platelets, and plasma should be used if whole blood is not available. While arranging for blood products, IV crystalloid resuscitation should be initiated. However, note that aggressive crystalloid resuscitation alone will result in dilution of haemoglobin, clotting factors, and platelets. 'Permissive hypotension' (i.e. systolic blood pressure 90 mmHg) should be entertained to potentially diminish ongoing bleeding (from an uncontrolled source). This approach seeks to avoid 'driving' blood flow to the uncontrolled bleeding area while balancing flow to other vital organs. Efforts *must* be made to avoid or reverse hypothermia, acidosis, and hypocalcaemia or the clotting factors will not function and the haemorrhaging will not stop
	• While fluid may temporarily support the blood pressure, patients with acute, severe anaemia due to bleeding or malaria need blood transfusion

D	• Re-evaluate level of consciousness frequently and if spinal cord injury is suspected, the ability to move arms/legs and feel touch/pain
	• Watch for hypoglycaemia which may occur in all shock states, often due to adrenal dysfunction
	• Whoever is monitoring the patient needs to be aware of signs of impending danger:
	  • General signs: worsening level of consciousness, vital signs, urine output, increased mottling
	  • Specific signs: talk to your team—what are signs of trouble with this specific patient that you want to be notified of immediately?

For suspected septic shock
- Do not delay antibiotics at this stage of illness. Consider empirical treatment—an imperfect, rapid diagnosis with a patient surviving is better than a perfect, delayed diagnosis with a dead patient:
  - Suspected sepsis: broad-spectrum antibiotics, typically in combination (i.e. ampicillin + gentamicin or ceftriaxone ± gentamicin), IV fluids (see ➜ p. 320), and source control.
  - Suspected malaria: antimalarials (in order of preference: artesunate, artemether, or quinine IV/IM), IV fluids, and blood.
- All the antibiotics in the world cannot replace good source control—e.g. laparotomy to treat colonic perforation or abscess formation.

The Global Intensive Care Working Group of the European Society of Intensive Care Medicine suggests the steps in Fig. 18.1 in the management of sepsis and septic shock.

For cardiogenic shock
- Consider IV dopamine, IV digoxin, or judicious IV epinephrine depending on local resources. This requires advanced medical skills and teams should weigh possible benefits against possible harm caused. Note the epinephrine dose would be similar to that outlined earlier.
- If pulmonary oedema is present, keep the patient sitting up. Furosemide is a slow treatment when a person is in shock. Careful administration of morphine may be used for its venodilating effects and symptomatic relief of dyspnoea. Nitrates work quickly but a systolic blood pressure of >100 mmHg is needed.
- Watch for arrhythmias as a cause of further deterioration and need for cardioversion.

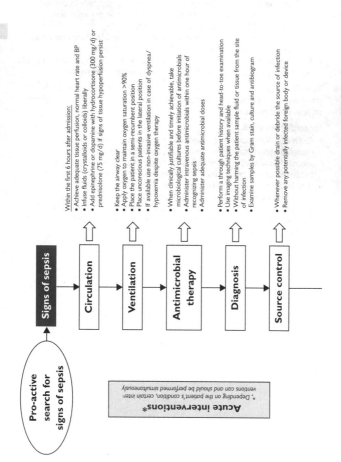

Acute interventions*

*. Depending on the patient's condition, certain interventions can and should be performed simultaneously

Pro-active search for signs of sepsis → Signs of sepsis

Circulation

Within the first 6 hours after admission:
- Achieve adequate tissue perfusion, normal heart rate and BP
- Infuse fluids (crystalloids or colloids) liberally
- Add epinephrine or dopamine with hydrocortisone (300 mg/d) or prednisolone (75 mg/d) if signs of tissue hypoperfusion persist

Ventilation
- Keep the airway clear
- Apply oxygen to maintain oxygen saturation >90%
- Place the patient in a semi-recumbent position
- Place unconscious patients in the lateral position
- If available use non-invasive ventilation in case of dyspnea/hypoxemia despite oxygen therapy

Antimicrobial therapy
- When clinically justifiable and timely achievable, take microbiological cultures before initiation of antimicrobials
- Administer intravenous antimicrobials within one hour of recognizing sepsis
- Administer adequate antimicrobial doses

Diagnosis
- Perform a through patient history and head-to-toe examination
- Use imaging techniques when available
- Without harming the patient sample fluid or tissue from the site of infection
- Examine samples by Gram stain, culture and antibiogram

Source control
- Whenever possible drain or debride the source of infection
- Remove any potentially infected foreign body or device

Post-acute interventions

Antimicrobial therapy:
- Reassess the effectiveness of antimicrobial therapy regularly
- Administer antimicrobials for an adequate but not prolonged time

Glucose control:
- Whenever possible check blood glucose levels
- Maintain blood glucose >70 mg/dL (4 mmol/L)

Deep vein thrombosis:
- Use prophylactic heparin or apply elastic bandages on both legs
- No deep vein thrombosis prophylaxis in pre-pubertal children

Enteral nutrition and stress ulcer prophylaxis:
- Allow the patient to eat and drink small amounts once she/he is fully resuscitated and awake

Sedation and pain relief:
- Use opioids to relief pain but be cautious in unstable patients
- Only sedate the agitated and uncooperative patient
- Encourage mobilization as soon as the patient is stable

Wean invasive support:
- Remember that every therapy and intervention has the potential to harm the patient
- As soon as the patient is improving, try to actively wen the extent of invasive support

DO NOT use hypotonic fluids for fluid resuscitation; DO NOT use fluid balance as a guide for fluid therapy; DO NOT use high dose steroids; DO NOT use muscle relaxants (except for endotracheal intubation); DO NOT use succinylcholine in immobilized patients; DO NOT use furosemide unless hypervolemia, hyperkalemia and/or acidosis are present; DO NOT use dopamine for renal indications; DO NOT use sodium bicarbonate; DO NOT use non-steroidal anti-inflammatory drugs; DO NOT use sodium bicarbonate; DO NOT restrict oxygen; DO NOT diagnose "ever of unknown origin"; DO NOT use insulin if blood glucose cannot be measured regularly.

Fig. 18.1 Management of sepsis and septic shock. Reproduced under creative commons licence from Dunser, M.W., et al, Recommendations for sepsis management in resource limited settings, Intensive Care Med. 2012 Apr; 38(4): 557–574, Springer (www.ncbi.nlm.nih.gov/pmc/articles/PMC3307996/).

Prevention of shock

- To prevent shock, the aim would be to recognize patients at risk early and not let them progress to advanced stages of shock. For the clinician in a healthcare structure, there are two main areas to concentrate on:
  - Make sure patients at risk of progressing to shock (those with unstable vital signs without organ dysfunction) or those in an actual state of shock are identified during triage or the admission process.
  - Patients already admitted to healthcare structures need to be monitored appropriately to recognize deterioration and allow intervention prior to the development of critical condition and shock.
  - If the shock is haemorrhagic in nature, direct pressure, the appropriate use of tourniquets (with diligent surveillance), prevention of hypothermia, acidosis, and hypocalcaemia, consideration of administration of rapid clot-forming preparations, and frequent re-evaluations of re-bleeding are important.
- At the end, the best healthcare provider is not the one whose patients are saved at the brink of death but the one whose patients don't get to that stage.

Palliation for patients in shock

The reality in the humanitarian context is that shock may not be survivable due to the late presentation, severity of multisystem organ failure, and availability of resources. Providers working in the humanitarian setting need to understand the limits of what they can achieve and be prepared to change the treatment goals to palliative ones if the patient is too critically ill to survive and if resources are simply not available to cure or stabilize them. This is a very difficult decision to make and one that can haunt the provider who knows the patient would likely or even certainly have survived if he/she had been in a different environment.

As difficult as these situations may be, providers working in humanitarian settings need to be prepared to provide palliative care—sometimes very quickly upon assessing the patient in shock. Sometimes it is important to remember that alleviating pain and suffering is at the heart of medicine and humanitarian work. For more, see ➔ Chapter 47.

References

1. Dünser MW, Festic E, Dondorp A, Kissoon N, Ganbat T, Kwizera A, Haniffa R, Baker T, Schultz MJ; Global Intensive Care Working Group of European Society of Intensive Care Medicine. Recommendations for sepsis management in resource-limited settings. Intensive Care Med 2012;38(4):557–74. Erratum in Intensive Care Med 2012; 38(4):575–6.
2. World Health Organization. Guideline: Updates on Paediatric Emergency Triage, Assessment and Treatment: Care of Critically-Ill Children. Geneva: WHO; 2016. ✍http://www.who.int/iris/handle/10665/204463
3. Singer M, Deutschman CS, Seymour CW, Shankar-Hari M, Annane D, Bauer M, et al. The Third International Consensus Definitions for Sepsis and Septic Shock (Sepsis-3). JAMA 2016;315:801–10.
4. Maitland K, Kiguli S, Opoka RO, Engoru C, Olupot-Olupot P, Akech SO, et al. Mortality after fluid bolus in African children with severe infection. N Engl J Med 2011;364(26):2483–95.

Chapter 19

Fever

Laura Sauve and Kevin Chan

Context of fever: why the epidemiology matters

Fever is one of the most common presentations to healthcare providers and it is important to remember that fever is a sign, and not a diagnosis. While most causes of fever are benign, many others could be life-threatening including infections, malignancies, rheumatological conditions, and inflammatory conditions, and in humanitarian conditions, could lead to significant mortality and morbidity.

Patients will present with fever at all levels of medical care, at all ages, and in varying degrees of acuity. While basic history, physical examination, and diagnostic approaches don't change from one context to the next, the local epidemiology must guide the approach to the febrile patient particularly when working in a resource-constrained setting. The prevalence—or even existence—of particular causes of illness in a geographic region and in a patient population will affect your approach and differential. Additionally, in the humanitarian aid context, the overlay of malnutrition makes fever both less likely but also more ominous.

It is critical to be aware of infectious disease prevalence in the region of work, as well as current outbreak situations. Even within countries, there are areas where malaria needs to be at the front and centre of one's approach to fever. HIV prevalence in the region also alters how one looks particularly at prolonged fevers. Outbreaks can change one's approach, including management and isolation of patients.

Keep in mind, however, that a lack of high fever does not exclude serious illness as not all patients will mount a fever, especially in newborns, and HIV+ve, malnourished, and elderly populations.

Clinical assessment of fever

In all cases of fever, a careful history and physical examination can guide the diagnostic approach. Key elements of the febrile patient's history include:
• duration of illness
• accompanying signs/symptoms
• consideration of local epidemiology/outbreaks
• ill contacts (e.g. with measles, Ebola virus disease, cholera, TB, HIV in the mother or a sexual partner).
• if possible, also consider immunization status as well.

Recognizing the patient who is becoming septic and providing prompt supportive care, particularly providing oxygen, fluid resuscitation, and empiric antibiotics or antimalarials as appropriate, is a critical step.

> ### Fever in severe malnutrition
> Patients with severe malnutrition who have a serious bacterial infection or malaria are much less likely to mount a high fever than well-nourished adults or children. Early empiric therapy and cautious fluid resuscitation is critical.
>   See ➔ Chapter 18 for more information.

Fever in infants and young children
Infants and children are unable to describe symptoms, and tend to deteriorate quite quickly. The fevers can mask serious illness and rapid deterioration, and the aetiologies of disease are very different from adults. Newborns <1 month of age may not mount much fever at all, and conversely, a febrile newborn is much more likely to have a serious bacterial infection (meningitis, sepsis).

Danger signs in febrile children
Children maintain their blood pressure until very late in an illness; pay attention to much earlier signs of severe illness:
• Signs of severe respiratory distress: grunting, nasal flaring, head bob.
• Shock: cool extremities (may be warm in septic children), prolonged capillary refill (>3 seconds).
• Lethargy—infant is unable to even breastfeed.
• Bulging fontanelle in an infant or stiff neck in an older child

Approach to patients with fever

In humanitarian settings, the causes of fever can be due to both common causes seen in Western settings, as well as those causes specific for the context. Additionally, increasing displacement leads to humanitarian responses which involve patients who may have a combination of possible presentations. Due to this broad differential, and often a lack of diagnostic resources, it is useful for providers to approach fever with a syndromic approach. The differential diagnosis of febrile patients can be guided by the age of the patient, duration of the fever, and of course localizing signs/symptoms. Guidance for identifying the cause of the fever based on these parameters is provided in this chapter.

Special considerations

There are special considerations which must be kept in mind when evaluating patients with fever in humanitarian settings.

Vaccine-preventable diseases

Healthcare workers (especially expatriate) should be attentive to vaccine-preventable infections that are now rare in resource-rich countries, such as *Streptococcus pneumoniae, Haemophilus influenzae* type B, and even *Neisseria meningitidis* because few LIC and MIC have those bacterial conjugate vaccines, especially in the context of humanitarian emergencies.

Diseases which require urgent intervention

Certain diseases which are common in humanitarian settings can progress rapidly and require urgent management to prevent morbidity and mortality. These include:

- malaria—in areas with malaria
- sepsis (bacteraemia/meningitis)—including:
  - meningococcal meningitis or sepsis—presents as a septic patient with palpable purpura, especially in the context of an outbreak
  - neonatal sepsis/meningitis.

Diseases which may require isolation to prevent epidemic/nosocomial transmission potential

These are diseases infrequently seen in Western settings which have the potential to cause outbreaks, especially in close quarters and refugee settings. For any suspected case, if possible, isolate from other patients following local infection control protocols. See Box 19.1.

- Measles (and chicken pox).
- Viral haemorrhagic fever (Ebola virus disease).
- Clusters of severe respiratory infection (Middle East respiratory syndrome (MERS), severe acute respiratory syndrome (SARS)), possibly TB.
- Meningococcal meningitis or sepsis.

Differential diagnosis of fever of short duration (<7 days)

Even in the tropics, common diseases account for the majority of fevers. Consider common diseases first: viral respiratory tract infections, otitis media, pneumonia, gastroenteritis, and urinary tract infections. Based on local epidemiology, tropical diseases should also be considered. Additionally, rare diseases with outbreak potential/public health importance should be considered.

In any acutely ill febrile patient, sepsis should be considered as a diagnostic possibility which can be caused by infection from a wide variety of organisms including bacteria, viruses, parasites, and even fungi. The best possible supportive care given the resources available (see ➋ 'Management of fever' p. 337) is critical, regardless of the underlying cause of sepsis.

Fever without localizing signs (and no rash)

Malaria

- Presents with anaemia, splenomegaly, and altered level of consciousness. In children especially, can present with vomiting.
- Any febrile patient in a malaria endemic area should be tested; can be rapidly fatal especially in young children and pregnant women.
- See ➋ Chapter 29 for further details.

Enteric fever (typhoid)

- Often no localizing signs but may have gastrointestinal symptoms, abdominal tenderness, fatigue, and increasing fever.
- May also present with headache, malaise and anorexia, diarrhoea or constipation. May present with a maculopapular rash, 'rose spots'.
- Fever tends to be lowest in the morning and increases through late afternoon/early evening; patients have normal heart rates despite fever.

Urinary tract infections

- Common in all settings.
- May have smelly urine, dysuria, or crying with voiding, costovertebral angle tenderness.
- Often with no localizing signs in children; may lead to sepsis and even meningitis in neonates.

Bacteraemia

- Sepsis may be caused by many organisms, often with localizing signs. However, these bacterial agents can cause fever without a clear source.
- Neonates: group B *Streptococcus*, *Escherichia coli*, *Klebsiella* species, *Listeria*—assume meningitis unless you can prove otherwise.
- Older infants, children, and adults: *Streptococcus pneumoniae*, *Staphylococcus aureus*, *Haemophilus influenzae* type B, *Neisseria meningitidis* (meningococcus), *Salmonella* species, other Gram-negative infections.

Non-infectious causes

Thyroid storm: primarily an adult condition, is often associated with tremors, tachycardia, restlessness/agitation, or diarrhoea.

Fever with localizing signs (no rash)

Ear/nose/throat

Respiratory tract infections are some of the most common causes of fever in all settings, and range from minor to life-threatening. Causes include the following:

- Viral upper respiratory tract infection, otitis media.
- Mastoiditis: a complication of otitis media, presents with tender swelling behind ear.
- Sinusitis: facial tenderness on percussion and possibly foul-smelling nasal discharge.
- Epiglottitis:
  - Often *Haemophilus influenzae* type B; uncommon with universal vaccination.
  - Very ill appearing, with fever, difficulty swallowing, drooling, hoarse voice and/or stridor.
  - Patients often sit in a tripod position (head forward, leaning on their hands, and shallow breathing).
  - Early intubation of the child is required to protect the airway. Use an endotracheal tube size 1 mm in diameter smaller than typical.
- Strep throat, pharyngeal abscess.

Respiratory/difficulty breathing

Bacterial pneumonia, bronchiolitis, and pertussis (in infants) are common. See ➲ Chapter 37 for further details.

Abdominal pain/diarrhoea

Common in all age groups
- Dysentery and enteric fever.
- Amoebic liver abscess.

Particularly in children
- Appendicitis.
- Young children localize pain poorly; urinary tract infection, pneumonia and even malaria may present as fever with abdominal pain.

Particularly in adults
- Ascending cholangitis:
  - May present with Charcot's triad: fever, jaundice, and right upper quadrant abdominal pain; or
  - Reynolds' pentad: Charcot's triad with septic shock and mental confusion.
- Bowel perforation.
- Cholecystitis: generally presents with right upper quadrant abdominal pain or epigastrium, constant and severe (which may refer to right scapula), nausea, and vomiting and diarrhoea, high fever, shock, and jaundice.

Bone and joint pain

Localized
- Consider if the child may have sickle cell disease especially if there is painful swelling of hands/feet (dactylitis), with anaemia, or jaundice/scleral icterus.
- Septic arthritis: joint hot, red, tender, and swollen.

- Osteomyelitis: local tenderness, warmth, and possibly swelling with functional limitation of the involved bone (e.g. refusal to weight bear); most often haematogenous source but can be secondary to direct inoculation after an injury or contiguous spread from a nearby infection.
- Acute rheumatic fever: acute arthritis (may be monoarthritis but typically polyarthritis) may be a presentation of acute rheumatic fever. To fulfil the Jones criteria, patients should have two major manifestations or two minor and one major; major manifestations include carditis, polyarthritis, chorea, erythema marginatum, and subcutaneous nodules. Minor criteria include arthralgia, fever, elevated acute phase reactants, and prolonged PR interval on an electrocardiogram.

Generalized
- Arboviruses (dengue, chikungunya, Zika) are common sources in the tropics. Check local epidemiology.
- Dengue fever: known as 'breakbone fever' for a reason, dengue often presents with fever and prominent bone and joint pain, conjunctivitis/conjunctival suffusion, often maculopapular rash. Watch for warning signs of severe disease: severe abdominal pain, persistent vomiting, mucosal bleed, liver enlargement, fluid accumulation, etc.

CNS signs
Coma, altered level of consciousness, and seizures suggest a CNS source.
- Meningitis: may be bacterial or viral.
- Encephalitis: this is often viral, but can be caused by other organisms.
- Cerebral malaria: see ➜ Chapter 29 for further details.

Jaundice
- Yellow fever: most cases of yellow fever have subclinical infection. About 15% develop fever, jaundice, renal failure and haemorrhage, disseminated intravascular coagulation (DIC), coma, and death.
- Viral hepatitis, especially hepatitis A and hepatitis E.
- Other illnesses, such as malaria and leptospirosis may also present with jaundice and fever.

Genitourinary symptoms (adolescents and adults)
The differential is broad but includes:
- Fournier's gangrene—necrotizing infection of the perineum
- Prostatitis—inflammation of the prostate gland
- Tubo-ovarian abscess/pelvic inflammatory disease
- Pregnancy related—infected retained products of conception, septic abortion.

Ocular symptoms
- Bacterial orbital/periorbital cellulitis: often presents with swelling and protrusion of the eye.
- Conjunctival suffusion/ocular pain: in these cases, consider leptospirosis, also dengue fever, chikungunya virus, and Zika virus.
- Leptospirosis: presents as an acute febrile illness with fever, myalgia, headaches, epistaxis, diarrhoea, nausea, and abdominal pain. Ocular manifestation including conjunctival suffusion and uveitis, retro-orbital pain, and photophobia. Immune phase (> 7 days) associated with fever, meningitis, and uveitis. About 5–10% develop an icteric phase with jaundice, renal failure, haemorrhage, cardiac arrhythmia, pneumonitis, and myocarditis.

Fever with rash

Approach fever with rash with careful attention. Several potentially fatal illnesses can be heralded by fever with petechiae or purpura (non-blanching, purplish macules), including meningococcemia/septicaemia, severe malaria, severe dengue fever, or even haemorrhagic fever; some, especially measles and meningococcal disease, have outbreak potential (see Box 19.1).

- Measles: classical presentation—head-to-toe maculopapular rash, fever, 3 Cs and a K: coryza, conjunctivitis, cough, and Koplik spots (white spots in the buccal mucosa).
- Meningococcal disease:
  - >50% will present with meningitis—headache, fever, stiff neck/bulging fontanelle.
  - 20% develop meningococcemia with fever and petechial/purpuric rash, which may progress into hypotension, acute adrenal haemorrhage, and multiorgan failure.
- Both measles and meningococcal disease have outbreak potential and isolation and infection control protocols must be followed in suspected cases. See Box 19.1.
- Rickettsia: transmitted by ticks or lice, rickettsial infections are highly limited geographically and some forms have increased prevalence where extreme poverty and migration coexist. Depending on the infection, it may be life-threatening. While rash is most common, some present as fever without localizing signs. Headache and myalgia are common.
- Typhus: louse-borne disease in areas with poor hygiene. Severe but non-specific febrile illness with abdominal pain. 50% have a dull red rash that spreads. May have a dry cough, headache, arthritis and myalgia, nausea, and vomiting. Only occurs in limited geographic areas.
- Arboviruses—dengue, chikungunya, and Zika: (see ➲ p. 331 for details).
- Acute HIV infection.

Box 19.1 Prevention: isolation/infection control

Patients who may have transmissible illnesses (especially measles, viral haemorrhagic fever, TB, and meningococcal diseases) should be treated in a separate space from those without infections. Healthcare workers should also consider their own health, and consider if protective equipment is needed (particularly haemorrhagic fevers, but also TB and meningococcal diseases).

Immunization is a critical part of prevention of infectious diseases; measles vaccination is particularly critical in humanitarian emergencies.

Sickle cell disease and fever

Sickle cell disease is a group of red blood cell disorders that lead to abnormal haemoglobin and affects approximately 1 in 400 people of African origin. It is common in areas where malaria is common (sub-Saharan Africa, South Asia). Affected patients may present with painful swelling of the hands and feet (dactylitis), fatigue or fuzziness from anaemia, jaundice, or scleral icterus. As patients with sickle cell disease are functionally asplenic, they are at high risk of sepsis, particularly from encapsulated bacteria (such as *Salmonella, Pneumococcus*, and meningococcus). Give IV ceftriaxone if a patient with sickle cell disease has fever.

Differential diagnosis of fever of medium duration (7–21 days)

A few specific infections have a more subacute course. Consider:

- Leptospirosis: can present in the immune phase (≥7 days) with fever, meningitis, and uveitis. (See ➲ 'Fever with localizing signs, ocular symptoms' pp. 330–1.)
- Viral haemorrhagic fevers (includes Ebola, Lassa, dengue, and yellow fever (see ➲ Chapter 32)—present with fever but the minority have bleeding. Other symptoms include flushing of the face and chest, petechiae, frank bleeding, oedema, hypotension and shock, malaise, myalgia, headache, vomiting, and diarrhoea.
- African trypanosomiasis—endemic in sub-Saharan Africa in rural, densely vegetated areas. Presents with fever, headache, malaise, myalgia, facial oedema, pruritus, lymphadenopathy, and weight loss. CNS involvement takes weeks to months and includes headaches, mood disorders, behaviour change, focal deficits, and somnolence.
- Typhoid fever and paratyphoid fever.
- Typhus and other rickettsia.
- Malaria—think *Plasmodium vivax* and *P. ovale* (more indolent courses than *P. falciparum* which would nearly always present acutely).
- Acute rheumatic fever (see ➲ pp. 330–1).

Differential diagnosis of prolonged fever (>21 days)

Prolonged fevers tend to be less acutely life-threatening but may still be extremely serious. TB, syphilis, and opportunistic infections associated with HIV can have protean manifestations and could occur on each of these lists.

Prolonged fever without localizing signs (no rash)

- Malaria—see ➲ Chapter 29.
- TB—while the most common manifestation of TB is prolonged cough, it can present in any body system:
  - Miliary/disseminated TB: children, especially <5 years, may present with simply prolonged fever but may have pneumonia, meningitis, or other symptoms.
  - TB in the setting of HIV infection may also present as prolonged fever even in adults.
- Syphilis (fever without rash or genital lesion would be an unusual manifestation).
- Viral—Cytomegalovirus (CMV) and Epstein–Barr virus (EBV) are very common causes of prolonged fever though infrequently diagnosed acutely due to the less acute presentation; they may also present with sore throat, malaise, and hepatosplenomegaly.
- Brucellosis—Associated with contaminated food (unpasteurized dairy or undercooked meat) or close contact with infected animals, 2–4-week incubation period, presents with fever, muscle aches, fatigues, headache, and night sweats.

Prolonged fever with localizing signs (no rash)

Ear, nose, and throat
Sinusitis.

Abdominal pain
Abscesses including amoebic liver abscess—abdominal pain, fever and chills, malaise, jaundice, joint pain, anorexia, and weight loss.

Limb/bone/joint pain
- Untreated classic bacterial osteomyelitis, tuberculous osteomyelitis, or joint infection.
- Brucellosis (typically back pain).
- Filariasis (caused by *Wuchereria bancrofti, Brugia malayi* and *B. timori*, and ultimately lead to elephantiasis)—three main presentations:
  1. Acute adenolymphangitis (ADL)—sudden onset of painful lymph-adenopathy with an associated fever. Characterized by a retrograde lymphangitis. May look like elephantiasis (significantly swollen limb).
  2. Filarial fever: fever without the adenitis.
  3. Topical pulmonary eosinophilia—dry cough, wheezing, dyspnoea, anorexia, malaise, and weight loss. Most cases are asymptomatic, but splenic destruction may occur due to acute and chronic granulomas. May develop chyluria (milk-like urine).

CNS
- African trypanosomiasis (see ➲ p. 333).
- Cryptococcal meningitis in HIV.

Jaundice
- Viral hepatitis.
- Leptospirosis (see ➲ p. 331).

Splenomegaly
- Visceral or systemic leishmaniasis: subacute/chronic fever, weight loss, hepatosplenomegaly, and pancytopenia (geographically limited to parts of South America, the Mediterranean, parts of Africa, parts of Asia) (see ➲ Chapter 30).
- Schistosomiasis (Katayama fever): fever, chills, lymph node enlargement, and liver and spleen enlargement. May get bloody diarrhoea and abdominal pain, frequency, dysuria, and haematuria (geographically limited to Africa, South America) (see ➲ Chapter 30).

Fever and facial swelling
American trypanosomiasis/Chagas disease: presents a week after exposure and lasts for 60 days. Fever, malaise, and swelling around the bite. Most are asymptomatic. Long-term effects in about 30% can include constipation and abdominal pain, heart failure and palpitations, swallowing difficulties, cardiomyopathy, tachycardia and arrhythmia, lymphadenopathy, and hepatosplenomegaly. Occurs only in Latin America.

Fever with rash
Syphilis.

Non-infectious causes of prolonged fever to consider
- Malignancy.
- Collagen vascular disease.
- Autoimmune diseases:
  - Rheumatoid arthritis, (including systemic juvenile idiopathic arthritis) which can present with prolonged arthralgia or arthritis, fever, salmon-pink rash, and leucocytosis (white blood cell count of >10,000 mm^3). Lymphadenopathy, hepatosplenomegaly, sore throat, abnormal aspartate transaminase (AST)/alanine transaminase (ALT) are often seen.
  - Inflammatory bowel disease.
  - Systemic lupus erythematosus.
- Periodic fever syndrome.
- Drug-induced fever (erythromycin, heparin, isoniazid, pethidine (meperidine), nifedipine, penicillin, phenytoin, quinidine).
- Chronic hepatitis.
- Cirrhosis.
- Deep vein thrombosis.

Investigations for fever

Investigations must be driven both by the clinical presentation/differential diagnosis and the resources available. Higher-level hospitals may have specific diagnostic testing available for many of the conditions discussed on ➲ pp. 329–32 and p. 335. In particular, fever without localizing signs can be difficult to diagnosis in the absence of laboratory testing.

When available testing is minimal, high priority testing should be for:
• HIV testing
• malaria smear/rapid test
• haematocrit or complete (full) blood count if available—to determine presence of neutrophilia or neutropenia
• lumbar puncture (all newborns with fever, older children/adults with meningitis signs or altered level of consciousness)
• CXR (if respiratory complaints)
• specific bacteriology tests which can be useful (if available), as guided by the history and physical examination:
  • urinalysis/urine culture
  • blood culture
  • stool culture
  • sputum or other samples for mycobacterial smear/culture.

Is all fever really malaria?

The 2015 guidelines for the treatment of malaria released by WHO (➾ http://www.who.int/malaria/publications/atoz/9789241549127/en/) recommend that malaria testing be routine for all cases of suspect malaria. The risks of not doing so include potentially missing an important alternative diagnosis, contributing to antimalarial resistance, and giving unnecessary treatment.

Management of fever

The ultimate management of febrile patients depends on the most likely diagnosis. If the patient has danger signs of sepsis, however, initial management should include provision of oxygen, acquiring IV access and starting fluid resuscitation (cautiously in the setting of severe malnutrition), and providing empiric antibiotics and antimalarials if appropriate.

Empiric treatment of any febrile patient must be guided by their age, clinical setting, and local epidemiology (especially malaria prevalence, HIV prevalence, and ongoing outbreaks) as the treatment is ultimately based on the diagnosis (with the exception of paracetamol or ibuprofen for comfort).

Children

For the child who appears febrile, septic, and unwell with an unknown source of fever—treat with paracetamol, and provide broad-spectrum antibiotics, such as IV ceftriaxone and antimalarials if appropriate. If the temperature normalizes but the vital signs remain abnormal (tachycardic/tachypnoeic), the patient is more likely sicker than you suspect. Be more vigilant! See Fig. 19.1 for emergency management.

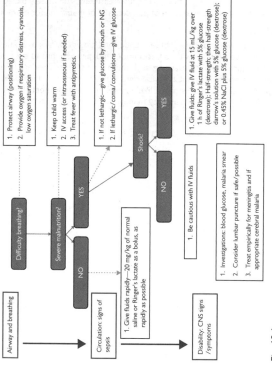

Fig. 19.1 Emergency management of a febrile child.
(Adapted from the Pocket Book of Hospital Care for Children).

Anaemia

**Margaret Salmon, Lily Muldoon,
and Max Ritzenberg**

Context of anaemia

Anaemia is a condition in which the number of red blood cells (RBCs) or their oxygen-carrying capacity is insufficient to meet physiological needs. The causes of anaemia worldwide are multifactorial but can generally be categorized by three syndromes: iron deficiency (iron deficiency anaemia, hookworm, and schistosomiasis), malaria, and haemoglobinopathies (sickle cell disorders and thalassemia).

Anaemia is a public health issue affecting LIC, MIC, and HIC but it is the poor and least educated who are most susceptible to the profound consequences on social and economic advancement. For example, children with anaemia, especially iron deficiency anaemia (IDA), can suffer significant cognitive and physical development delay affecting physical and psychological health, education, and future employment. Women of childbearing years can suffer lost productivity and lower quality of life due to anaemia-related fatigue and other effects on their health. In addition, maternal IDA can influence maternal and neonatal outcomes such as birth weight and duration of gestation which itself affects long-term child outcomes. It may also lead to increased child and maternal mortality and may predispose to infection and heart failure. Pregnant women with anaemia exacerbate the condition with blood loss from childbirth and through lactation. Although studies have largely been of IDA, detrimental findings are found also with those with non-IDA, supporting a primary role for anaemia as a risk factor for poor outcomes.

Global anaemia prevalence in 2010 was 32.9%, causing approximately 68.4 million years lived with disability (8.8% of total for all conditions). The scope of anaemia in humanitarian settings is enormous. Health providers should expect, on average, 42% of pregnant women, 30% of non-pregnant women (age 15–50 years), 47 % of preschool children (ages 0–5 years), and 12.7% of men >15 years to be anaemic at baseline due to IDA alone.

Anaemia defined

- Criteria for anaemia, based on haemoglobin (Hb) levels, are specific for age, sex, and stage of pregnancy.
- Haematocrit (Hct) is another measure of anaemia status using volume percentage of RBCs in blood. (See Table 20.1.)
- Anaemia levels are affected by altitude (≥ 900 metres) and cigarette smoking, both of which cause a generalized upward shift in concentrations.

Epidemiology

- Two billion people, or nearly one-third of the world's population, are anaemic.
- IDA makes up one-half of this group, followed by anaemia due to helminth disease and malaria.
- Groups most at risk are women of reproductive age (because of menstruation), pregnancy, lactating women, and children from 6 months to 2 years of age (because of rapid growth).
- Pregnant women have increased iron needs as a result of the dual requirement of their growth and that of the fetus (especially true in pregnant adolescents). Severe anaemia during pregnancy is an important contributor to maternal mortality.
- Africa and Asia are the most heavily affected regions (85% of burden) with Africa having the highest prevalence.
- Anaemia represents a complex interaction between nutrition, infectious diseases, and other factors which presents a challenge to effectively address both individual and population determinants. (See Table 20.2.)
- See Table 20.3 for aetiologies of anaemia.

Table 20.1. Haemoglobin and haematocrit thresholds used to define anaemia

Age or sex group	Hb (g/L)	Hct mmol/L	%
Children (6–59 months)	110	6.83	33
Children (5–11 years)	115	7.13	34
Children (12–14 years)	120	7.45	36
Non-pregnant women (≥15 years)	120	7.45	36
Pregnant women	110	6.83	33
Men (≥15 years of age)	130	8.07	39

Table 20.2 Determinants of anaemia in the public heath context

Classification	Causes	Examples
Immediate determinants	Nutritional iron intake	Iron content of food and availability
	Infectious disease	Malaria Helminth infection TB HIV/AIDS
	Blood loss	Helminth infection (hookworm) Schistosomiasis Trauma
	Other nutritional deficiencies	Vitamin B12, vitamin A, folate
	Chronic inflammation	Helminth infection Cancer Rheumatoid arthritis
	Inherited disorders	Thalassemia and sickle cell disease Haemolytic anaemia
Secondary determinants	Food availability	Food security and fortification Household income
	Healthcare	Healthcare access Knowledge of health workers Sanitation and hygiene
Underlying social and political determinants	Agricultural output	Crop yields and livestock
	Economic circumstances	Regional and local wealth Education Equity and equality
	Health policy	Anaemia control programmes Fortification policies

Based in part on model presented in Pasricha S, Drakesmith H, Black J, Hipgrave D, Biggs B. Control of iron deficiency anemia in low- and middle-income countries. Blood 2013;121:2607–17.

Table 20.3 Aetiologies of anaemia in the clinical context

Underproduction	Destruction	Loss
Viral infection	Infection	Acute blood loss
Nutritional deficiencies	Drugs	Chronic blood loss
Bone marrow failure	Autoimmune	
Renal failure	DIC, HUS, TTP	
Chronic illness	Other haemolytic disease	

DIC, disseminated intravascular coagulation, HUS, haemolytic uremic syndrome, TTP, thrombotic thrombocytopenic purpura.

Evaluation of anaemia

Patient history

Nutritional history, recent infections or infectious symptoms, HIV risk or exposure, obstetric/gynaecological history, recent blood loss, ethnicity, autoimmune disorders, bleeding (gums, epistaxis, purpura), and melena. (See Table 20.4.)

Table 20.4 General symptoms and signs of anaemia

General symptoms	General signs
Shortness of breath and/or dyspnoea on exertion	Pallor (conjunctiva, palms, nail beds)
Fatigue/energy loss	Tachypnoea and/or tachycardia
Dizziness, lightheadedness, or syncope	Elevated jugular venous distension, murmurs, or oedema
Headache	Bounding pulses
	Altered mental status/lethargy (signs of severe anaemia)

Symptoms specifically associated with IDA include:
• pica: unusual cravings for non-nutritive substances, e.g. paper, ice, or dirt.
• koilonychias: upward curvature of the nails.
• angular cheilitis: soreness of the mouth with cracks at the corner.

Anaemia detection methods

There are a variety of haematocrit and haemoglobin detection methods:
• Cyanmethaemoglobin system: most accurate and reliable, however, is expensive and dependent on laboratories and electrical power.
• HemoCue®: portable system but requires disposable cuvettes and battery power.
• Colour-based point-of-care assay: portable, inexpensive, and rapid but is the least reliable.
• Centrifuge method (measures haematocrit): is portable and inexpensive but needs further study of effectiveness in clinical setting.

Determining aetiology

• Check blood Hb, stool for helminth disease and occult blood, malaria smear or rapid test, check pregnancy status if female of childbearing age.
• When available, check RBC count, RBC indices, white blood cell (WBC) count, platelet count, coagulation studies, and reticulocyte count. Also check iron studies (serum ferritin, total iron binding capacity, serum total iron and transferrin % saturation), peripheral blood smear (if automated blood analyser is not available), and serum B12 level.
• Check the mean corpuscular volume (MCV) to help determine the aetiology of the anaemia. (See Fig 20.1.)

Anaemia testing

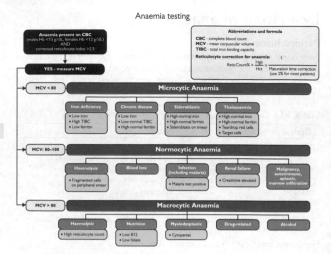

Fig. 20.1 Anaemia aetiology using mean corpuscular volume (MCV). CBC, complete blood count.

Treatment options for anaemia

Iron supplementation
- 80 mg of oral iron supplementation daily is the recommended WHO dose for endemic areas with anaemia >40%. Ferrous sulfate is the cheapest but difficult to tolerate due to gastric upset so compliance is an issue.
- Iron micronutrient powders, also called MNPs or sprinkles, are in single-dose sachets and added to meals at point of care. Trials show comparable efficacy to liquid, but limitations are cost and availability.

Transfusion
- Simple anaemia is not an indication to transfuse.
- If you suspect bleeding as the source of anaemia; stop bleeding at site if possible and transfuse as clinically indicated based on signs of shock.

Infection treatment
- If positive for malaria (see following 'Special considerations' section).
- If you suspect anaemia is helminth related: albendazole (400 mg PO × 1) or mebendazole (500 mg PO × 1 or 100 mg PO twice daily for 3 days).

Special considerations
Malaria
- Severe malaria can manifest as severe anaemia, among other things. Severe anaemia in the setting of malaria is associated with lower mortality rates than other syndromes associated with severe malaria.
- Thresholds for transfusion are somewhat controversial. Suggestions are:
  - In high malaria transmission areas: Hb <50 g/L or a Hct <15%.
  - In low malaria transmission areas: Hb <70 g/L and Hct <20%.
- When treated with artesunate, clinicians must be aware of the potential for delayed haemolysis and late-onset anaemia in parasitaemic patients.
- Malaria in pregnant women is especially complicated as they are more susceptible to severe anaemia.
- Though less common, *Plasmodium vivax* can also cause progressive anaemia.

Human immunodeficiency virus (HIV)
Anaemia can result from opportunistic infections, antiretroviral (ARV) treatment or HIV itself.
- Zidovudine (AZT)-related anaemia: most often occurs within 4–12 weeks of starting AZT (though can be earlier). Severe anaemia is rare but possible.
  - If Hb <70 g/L or 25% from patient's baseline, change to different ARV.
  - If baseline Hb <80 g/L, don't start AZT.

Post disaster
In post-earthquake data in Japan, more than 20% of the elderly and children under 5 years of age had lower haemoglobin levels after the earthquake compared to before the earthquake. Check MCV.

Pain

Joseph O'Neill

Introduction to pain

Patients often will not volunteer a complaint of pain. Some who have been living with chronic pain may not necessarily even demonstrate objective signs. It is essential, therefore, to make asking about pain a habitual element of all patient interviews.

'Do you have pain? Where is it located? What is it like? What makes it better? Worse? Is there more than one pain? How long has it been present?' You may want your patient to rate the severity of pain on a scale (1 to 10 is most commonly used) so that the impact of treatment can be followed and disease progression tracked.

Diagnostic clues for pain

- Care should always be taken to find reversible causes of pain (urinary tract, meningeal infectious, oral or genital disease, etc.).
- A careful physical examination can be helpful in making a diagnosis. Nuchal rigidity or photophobia in the setting of headache pain or urinary urgency and frequency in the context of adnominal pain should, for example, lead the clinician to consider definitive treatment for an underlying CNS or urinary infection. Similarly, abdominal pain with rebound tenderness should prompt consideration of surgical intervention.
- Finally, it is always important to determine if constipation is present, as pain from constipation can be made worse by use of opiates.

Treatment of pain

When effective medicines are not available and the cause of the pain is not reversible, the clinician must rely on non-pharmacological approaches bearing in mind that:

• emotional and spiritual components of pain can be powerful contributors and should be explored
• time spent listening, recruitment of religious and cultural practices, positioning of the patient or stabilization of a joint or limb in the most comfortable way, distraction, massage, rocking, hot/cold compresses, breathing exercises, meditation, and music all have potential benefit.

When effective pain drugs are available, the WHO recommends a three-step analgesic ladder approach to pain.[1] See Table 21.1.

Step 1: use non-opioids
• This category includes aspirin, paracetamol/acetaminophen, and a host of non-steroidal anti-inflammatory drugs (NSAIDs).
• Care should be taken with NSAIDs in the setting of dehydration as they can cause renal injury.

Step 2: add weak opiates
• If pain is not controlled with non-opiates, weak opioids, such as codeine or tramadol, or low doses of strong opiates should be added.
• 5–10% of patients cannot metabolize codeine so a trial dose is worthwhile before relying on codeine for pain control.

Step 3: use strong opiates
• If more analgesia is required and they are available, strong opiates should be used (generally in conjunction with an adjuvant non-opioid analgesic).
• Oral morphine is typically the cheapest and most readily available strong opiate in developing world settings.
• Other opiates with different potencies, routes of administration, and pharmacokinetic properties may be available as well. If they are, good resources are available to guide the clinician in their use.[2]

Morphine
• Oral morphine is usually dosed every 4 hours. Modified- or sustained-release morphine tablets are given every 12 hours. In an adult patient who has not used opiates before, a starting dose of 5–15 mg is reasonable.
• The analgesic effect can be expected to begin 30 minutes after oral administration and typically lasts for 4 hours. If there is consistent 'end-of-interval' pain, it can be given every 3 hours.
• Morphine has no ceiling dose and should be titrated to achieve the lowest pain with the fewest side effects. Patients typically do not notice an analgesic effect of increases less than 25% so increases should be 25–50% irrespective of the starting dose.
• Although it is uncommon and sedation usually occurs first,[3] care should be taken to watch for respiratory depression, especially in naïve patients and particularly when naloxone is not available as may be the case in a humanitarian relief setting.

Table 21.1 Pain medications chart

WHO Step 1	Route	Adult dose (mg)	Frequency	Notes
Paracetamol/ acetaminophen	By mouth	325–1000	4–6 hours	Not to exceed 1 g/6 hours or 3–4 g/day
Ibuprofen	By mouth	300–600	3–4 times a day	Caution if dehydration, elderly, renal disease

WHO Step 2	Route	Adult starting dose (mg)	Frequency (hours)	Notes	Oral morphine equivalency
Codeine	By mouth	15–60	3–4	#	6.6 mg = 1 mg oral morphine
Tramadol	By mouth	50–100	4–6	#	10 mg = 1 mg oral morphine

WHO Step 3	Route	Adult starting dose* (mg)	Frequency (hours)	Notes	Oral morphine equivalency
Morphine	By mouth	5–15	3–4	#	1 mg = 1 mg
Morphine	Parenteral	2.5–5	3–4	#	1 mg parenteral = 3 mg oral morphine
Oxycodone	By mouth	5–10	3–4	#	1 mg = 1.5 mg oral morphine
Hydrocodone	By mouth	5	3–4	#	1 mg = 1 mg oral morphine
Hydromorphone	By mouth	1–2	3–4	#	1 mg = 4 mg oral morphine
Hydromorphone	Parenteral	0.2–0.6	3–4	#	1 mg = 20 mg oral morphine
Methadone	By mouth	1.25–5	Every 8–12	#	Variable—consult expert advice
Methadone	Parenteral	0.5–2.5	Every 8–12	#	Variable—consult expert advice

* Opiate naive.
# When converting from one opiate to another the final equianalgesic dose should be reduced by one-third to account for incomplete tolerance.

- Once an effective regimen is determined, opiates should be prescribed around the clock. PRN doses for 'breakthrough pain' should also be made available as a back-up. These are generally 10–20% of the total 24-hour dose of the around-the-clock schedule given every hour. The total of all breakthrough doses in a 24-hour period are factored in to determine the next day's around-the-clock schedule.
- If a long-acting morphine formulation is available, the around-the-clock dose can be administered on an every 12-hour basis. In this case, short-acting morphine is still used for breakthrough pain.
- Opiates must be used judiciously, especially in patients who have never taken them before. It is best to start with low doses and titrate upwards, watching for respiratory depression, decreased consciousness, or toxicity. Care should also be taken if other sedating medications or alcohol are being used.
- Naloxone is a potent opiate antagonist that can reverse opiate effects and can be lifesaving in the situation of opiate overdose. It must be used carefully with opiate-dependent patients and those in pain that is being managed with opiates so as not to precipitate withdrawal or pain crises.

Side effects and cautions

- Common side effects of opiate use are constipation, nausea and vomiting, and neurotoxicity (usually presenting as confusion or drowsiness). Laxatives should always be given (unless diarrhoea is present) when opiates are prescribed to prevent constipation.
- Opiates, if they have been used for over a week, should not be stopped abruptly. Tapering the dose will prevent a withdrawal syndrome.
- Specific pain syndromes that may respond better to drugs other than opiates are addressed in the WPCA Palliative Toolkit,[4] and discussed in ➔ 'Some specific presentations' p. 353.

Some specific presentations

Neuropathic pain

Caused by direct injury to a nerve and is typically described as 'shooting' or 'electric' sensations, often in the legs and feet.

- This type of pain is frequently encountered in regions where HIV and/or TB are prevalent as some of the commonly used medications for these conditions cause neuropathic pain. Isoniazid, if not given with pyridoxine, is a common example.
- There are many other causes of neuropathic pain as well, including advanced diabetes, trauma, nerve compression, post-herpetic neuralgia, and HIV.

Treatment of neuropathic pain with tricyclic antidepressants (amitriptyline is a common choice) or anticonvulsants (gabapentin, valproate, phenytoin, etc.) is often more helpful than use of opiates.

Inflammation, distention, and space-occupying lesions

Pain from an engorged liver, tumour in a confined space (e.g. the brain or spinal cord), or swollen joints can be, at least temporarily, reduced by the judicious use of steroids.

Colicky abdominal pain

Is sharp, localized and paroxysmal and should prompt consideration of a fully or partially obstructed hollow structure (gut, biliary duct, or urinary tract). Agents that increase gut motility (e.g. erythromycin, metoclopramide) are contraindicated in the setting of full or partial bowel obstruction. Anticholinergics (hyoscine/scopolamine) can, however, be helpful in reducing pain in this situation as can placement of a nasogastric tube.

Pain resulting from muscle spasms

(Often secondary to muscle injury or splinting.) Can be improved with benzodiazepines and/or baclofen.

References

1. World Health Organization. WHO's Cancer Pain Ladder for Adults. ℘ http://www.who.int/cancer/palliative/painladder/en/
2. National Cancer Institute. Cancer Pain (PDQ®)—Health Professional Version. 2017. ℘ http://www.cancer.gov/cancertopics/pdq/supportivecare/pain/HealthProfessional
3. Pattinson KT. Opioids and the control of respiration. Br J Anaesth 2008;100(6):747–58.
4. Worldwide Hospice Palliative Care Alliance (WHPCA). Palliative Care Toolkit: Improving Care in Resource Poor Settings. 2015. ℘ http://www.thewhpca.org/resources/palliative-care-toolkit

Jaundice

Michelle Tubman

Introduction to jaundice

At all levels of humanitarian intervention, jaundice is a surprisingly common presenting complaint. In this context, it is often due to an infectious cause, and endemic diseases, including malaria and yellow fever, are often the culprit. Some epidemic diseases, such as hepatitis E, have occurred in refugee and internally displaced persons camps, largely due to poor hygiene and contaminated water supplies.

In addition, public health emergencies, including viral haemorrhagic fevers, may include jaundice in their constellation of symptoms. Non-infectious causes, such as glucose-6-phosphate dehydrogenase (G6PD) deficiency, are not uncommon in Africa and South East Asia, and surgical causes, including cholecystitis, may also be encountered. Depending on the diagnosis, there may be specific treatments available, but for some pathologies, the treatment is largely supportive or palliative. In addition, when lab testing is unavailable and the aetiology cannot be determined, syndromic management of jaundice becomes important.

History and examination of jaundice

Local context

- Understanding the epidemiology and clinical presentation of diseases endemic to the country you are working in is essential.
- Common endemic infections that may present with jaundice include malaria, yellow fever, dengue, and amoebiasis.
- Epidemic infections, including hepatitis A and E, may occur in areas where there is overcrowding and limited access to potable water, proper sanitation, and hygiene.
  - If a hepatitis E outbreak is suspected, inquire about pregnancy or recent delivery as this is associated with high mortality.
- Being aware of local cultural behaviours, including the use of alcohol, recreational drugs (including khat), or traditional remedies is important and should guide history-taking if appropriate.
- G6PD deficiency is very common in Africa and the Mediterranean, and is also present in some areas of South East Asia. Inquiring about prior episodes of jaundice, or a family history of jaundice, may guide you towards this diagnosis.
- Inquiring about fever, abdominal pain, and other concomitant symptoms; bed net use, sources of drinking water, and family members with similar symptoms, may be useful.

Physical exam

The physical examination of patients with jaundice should focus first on signs of liver disease, with the goal of determining whether the patient has an acute or chronic jaundice syndrome.

- Jaundice in dark-skinned patients may appear as yellow staining in the sclera, hard palate, and palmar or plantar surfaces of the hands and feet.
- Signs of chronic liver disease may include spider angiomas, gynaecomastia, testicular atrophy, palmar erythema, and ascites.
- The presence of hepatomegaly or splenomegaly may suggest a more acute infectious cause of jaundice, as does the presence of fever.
- If there are mental status changes in the context of jaundice, this is concerning for hepatic encephalopathy.

Investigations for jaundice

- Jaundice is classically defined as a serum bilirubin level >2.5–3 mg/dL (42.8–51.3 μmol/L), accompanied by yellow skin and sclera.
- In a well-resourced setting, investigations to consider would include the following:
  - Complete blood count, peripheral smear, and reticulocyte count (anaemia and elevated reticulocytes may indicate haemolytic jaundice; look for malarial parasites on peripheral smear if rapid testing not available).
  - Serum bilirubin (both total and direct), AST, ALT, alkaline phosphatase (ALP), lipase, amylase (may see elevated ALP, lipase and amylase in obstructive jaundice and elevated transaminases in hepatitis).
  - Urinalysis (primarily for urine bilirubin, correlate with serum bilirubin which is likely to be elevated if this is present).
  - Liver function tests (albumin, glucose, coagulation studies), primarily to determine the severity of liver disease.
  - Infectious hepatitis serology.
  - Abdominal ultrasound, particularly if hepatic or obstructive causes of jaundice are suspected.
- Obtaining a diagnosis in resource-poor settings can be difficult. In these cases, it may be more prudent to use the investigations you have available to guide treatment. In malaria or yellow fever endemic areas, the use of rapid diagnostic tests may be an important first step. Obtaining a haemoglobin measurement may also be important. If there is concern for a hepatitis E outbreak, doing a pregnancy test in women of childbearing age would also be crucial.

Management of jaundice

Jaundice can be caused by a wide variety of benign and life-threatening conditions, and patients may be asymptomatic, or they may present with signs of infection, anaemia, or other signs of liver disease. Use a systematic approach to investigate patients presenting with jaundice, especially to look for treatable conditions. The differential diagnosis is typically organized by the phases of bilirubin metabolism: pre-hepatic, intra-hepatic, and post-hepatic. However, in settings with limited diagnostic testing available, it is more useful to consider aetiologies based on their syndromic presentation:

- Acute jaundice with fever.
- Haemolytic jaundice.
- Hepatic jaundice.
- Obstructive jaundice.
- Neonatal Jaundice (see ⊃ Chapter 43 for more information).

Acute jaundice with fever

Consider the following infectious causes in endemic areas:

Viral hepatitis

Jaundice preceded by acute flu-like illness with malaise, nausea, vomiting, anorexia, right upper quadrant pain. Treatment is supportive. Higher morbidity and mortality in pregnant and postpartum women.

Dengue fever

Can present similarly to viral hepatitis. Treatment is supportive. Avoid NSAIDs. Blood transfusion may be required.

Yellow fever

Typically causes a self-limited flu-like illness, but 15% will experience a toxic second phase 24 hours after remission with jaundice and haemorrhagic shock. Treatment is supportive.

Malaria

Can present as haemolytic jaundice due to intravascular haemolysis. Jaundice is rarely seen, but signifies more severe disease. See ⊃ Chapter 29 for more information.

Urgent considerations

- Hepatitis E carries high morbidity and mortality in pregnant and postpartum women; consider admission for observation.
- Jaundice in malaria cases usually signifies severe *Plasmodium falciparum* infection.
- Screen all patients for encephalopathy, indicated by mental status changes, and admit all for treatment.
- Viral haemorrhagic fevers may also present with jaundice.

Other diagnostic considerations

- Sepsis can cause jaundice due to hypoperfusion of the liver, and some bacteria produce endotoxins that affect the liver. Antibiotics and fluid therapy should be aggressively used if sepsis is suspected.
- Acute cholangitis may present with Charcot's triad of fever, jaundice, and abdominal pain. It is usually secondary to choledocholithiasis or malignancy of the biliary tree. Antibiotics and biliary drainage are the main therapies.

- Liver abscess usually presents with right upper quadrant abdominal pain and fever, as well as non-specific constitutional symptoms. Patients may also present with jaundice. Treatment should include antibiotics, and possible surgical drainage.

Prevention strategies
- Clean water and latrines reduce the risk of hepatitis A and E.
- Malaria prevention strategies, including bed nets, reduce the risk of malaria, yellow fever, and dengue.

Haemolytic jaundice

Consider the following causes of haemolytic jaundice, which are all common in malaria-endemic areas. Clues to a haemolytic cause of jaundice include dark urine, hepatosplenomegaly, and signs of anaemia (paleness of skin, fatigue, lightheadedness, dyspnoea, and tachycardia).

G6PD deficiency
Genetic disorder resulting in acute episodes of haemolysis. Common triggers include infection, fava beans, antimalarial medications (most commonly primaquine), and NSAIDs. Treatment is supportive; transfuse if needed.

Sickle cell disease
May present with acute haemolysis, acute sequestration in the spleen, or aplastic crisis. Folic acid supplementation and transfusion are treatment options.

HELLP syndrome
Pregnant women in their third trimester or postpartum with severe pre-eclampsia may develop haemolysis, elevated liver enzymes, and low platelets (HELLP). Prompt delivery of the baby is the treatment.

Other diagnostic considerations
Late trimester pregnancies may also be rarely complicated by acute fatty liver of pregnancy and may present with jaundice. It is also treated by acute delivery of the baby.

Prevention strategies
Acute haemolytic crises in G6PD deficiency are prevented by avoidance of common triggers; patient education is key.

Hepatic jaundice

Hepatic jaundice occurs when a pathological process renders the liver unable to conjugate or excrete bilirubin. Viral hepatitis would also be included here, as described previously.

Drug hepatitis
Consider exposure to medications, herbal remedies, and hepatotoxic herbicides or pesticides. Treatment is supportive and includes identification and discontinuation of exposure to toxin.

Alcoholic hepatitis
Often presents acutely, similar to viral hepatitis. Can also present as alcoholic cirrhosis, which is more chronic and insidious in nature. Treatment is supportive; focus on abstinence.

Hepatocellular carcinoma
Increasingly common, presents with signs of liver disease and constitutional symptoms. Treatment is supportive.

Obstructive jaundice

- Cholecystitis is the most common cause and typically presents with severe right upper quadrant pain with a positive Murphy's sign (inspiratory arrest with right upper quadrant palpation) on physical examination, nausea, and vomiting. Treatment is usually supportive, with antibiotics. Severe cases may require surgery, if available.
- Pancreatitis, usually resulting from either gallstones or alcohol use, can also result in jaundice. Treatment is also supportive.

Other diagnostic considerations

- Metabolic diseases, including Gilbert syndrome and Crigler–Najjar syndrome, are typically asymptomatic, but may present with jaundice during periods of stress or illness in childhood. The jaundice is usually self-limited and rarely requires treatment.
- Autoimmune hepatitis (rare) may present with jaundice in the later stages of disease. Primary biliary cirrhosis will typically present with fatigue and pruritus before the onset of jaundice. Primary sclerosing cholangitis coexists with inflammatory bowel disease. Treatment is supportive.

Chapter 23

Lymphadenopathy

Anna MacDonald

Background to lymphadenopathy

Humanitarian settings are diverse and thus the approach to lymphadenopathy will depend on local epidemiology and local resources. Patients with lymphadenopathy may not be acutely ill, nor may this be their chief complaint, but this is a common presentation of significant systemic or local disease. In lower-resourced settings, patients tend to present later and with more advanced disease.

The main causes of lymphadenopathy can be classified as:
• infectious (the most common cause)
• reactive, inflammatory, or autoimmune
• malignant.

A thorough history, physical examination, and knowledge of local patterns of infectious diseases can often lead to a diagnosis. Where resources permit, it may be necessary to perform a fine-needle aspiration (FNA) to clarify the diagnosis in the case of persistent peripheral lymphadenopathy. FNA will be useful especially where TB and HIV are prevalent. In humanitarian settings, FNA may not always be possible; however, it can help to rule in or rule out TB lymphadenitis. HIV status changes the differential diagnosis and therefore it is critical to establish HIV status in the workup of lymphadenopathy, particularly in areas of high HIV prevalence.

In this chapter, we will focus primarily on infectious causes of lymphadenopathy. Not only are infectious causes more prevalent in humanitarian settings, but they are also more readily treatable.

Definitions

Lymphadenopathy
Refers to the simple enlargement of lymph nodes. This can include both inflamed and non-inflamed enlarged nodes. See Fig. 23.1.

Lymphadenitis
Generally refers to the enlargement of nodes due to inflammation or infection, but is often used interchangeably with lymphadenopathy.

Lymphangitis
Refers to the inflammation of lymphatic channels and appears as an erythematous streak in the skin originating from an area of cellulitis or wound infection and progressing proximally towards the trunk. This resolves with the treatment of the original cellulitis or wound infection and therefore will not be discussed further in this chapter.

Causes of lymphadenopathy

Infectious
Begin by inquiring about diseases endemic to the area:
• *Viruses*: HIV, EBV, CMV, adenovirus, dengue fever, hepatitis B.
• *Bacterial infections*: *Mycobacteria*, syphilis, tularaemia, brucellosis, plague (*Yersinia pestis*), typhoid fever, Lyme disease.
• *Fungal infections*: histoplasmosis, cryptococcal disease.

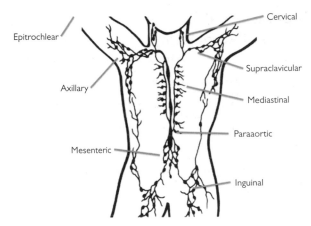

Fig. 23.1 Main lymph node groups. Image released by the National Cancer Institute, an agency part of the National Institutes of Health. This image is in the public domain.

- *Rickettsia*: tick bite fever, scrub typhus, epidemic typhus.
- *Parasitic infections*: toxoplasmosis, visceral leishmaniasis, human African trypanosomiasis, schistosomiasis, lymphatic filariasis, onchocerciasis, loaiasis (inguinal nodes), toxocariasis.

Inflammatory/autoimmune
- Systemic lupus erythematosus.
- Rheumatoid arthritis, juvenile idiopathic arthritis.
- Sarcoidosis.
- Kawasaki disease.
- Dermatomyositis.
- Serum sickness.

Malignancy
- Lymphoma.
- Metastatic disease.

Specific causes common in the humanitarian setting are outlined on
➔ pp. 370–3. The focus here is on conditions whose primary presentation is lymphadenopathy and not those where lymphadenopathy is a minor part of the overall clinical picture (e.g. systemic lupus erythematosus, rickettsial disease, leishmaniasis).

Approach to diagnosis for lymphadenopathy

- Diagnosis begins with a focused history and physical examination first to differentiate between:
  - localized and generalized lymphadenopathy
  - painless versus painful lymphadenitis.
- Consider if there are any associated symptoms, which may point towards an underlying cause.[1]
- Fig. 23.2 outlines a diagnostic approach.

History
Important historical features, and their associations, include:
- Local symptoms: when node(s) first noticed, speed of growth, locations of all enlarged nodes, pain, symptoms in area drained by enlarged nodes, generalized or local lymphadenopathy.
- Systemic symptoms – fever, weight loss, night sweats, anorexia (suggesting TB, malignancy, occult infection).
- Past medical history: HIV status, medications, previous treatments/ assessments for same problem, TB exposure.
- Geography: rural or urban, local or travelled from a different region (helpful regarding risks of infections given diseases endemic to certain areas).
- Bites: tick bites (Lyme disease, tularaemia), flea bites (bubonic plague), animal exposures (cat scratch disease, toxoplasma).

Physical findings
In addition to vital signs, physical examination should include the following:
- Palpation of all common nodal sites (cervical, axillary, inguinal). (See ➌ Fig. 23.1 p. 365.)
- Close examination of site drained by enlarged node(s), looking for evidence of infection or malignancy.
  - E.g. examination of the pharynx and tympanic membrane with cervical adenopathy.
- Systemic signs: hepatosplenomegaly, rash, conjunctivitis, arthritis and mucous membrane lesions (may point towards specific causes, e.g. visceral leishmaniasis, Kawasaki disease, autoimmune).
- Examination of the nodes includes determining size, fluctuance, consistency, fixation, tenderness, and location:
  - firm, fixed, irregular nodes more indicative of malignancy.
  - tender rubbery nodes more likely to be reactive or local infection related.
  - fluctuance associated with bacterial or mycobacterial infection that may require drainage.
- Evaluation of nutritional status (e.g. wasting—suggestive of HIV, TB, or malignancy).
- Evaluation of specific body sites, specifically those which may heighten suspicion of HIV (e.g. oral thrush, oral hairy leucoplakia, or Kaposi's sarcoma).

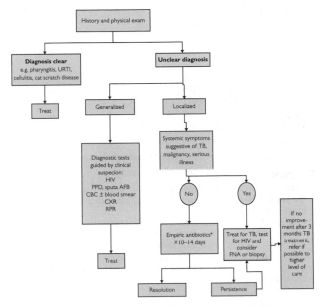

Fig. 23.2 Algorithmic approach to lymphadenopathy. CBC; complete blood count; CXR, chest X-ray (if hilar lymphadenopathy think of TB or Hodgkin's lymphoma); PPD, purified protein derivative (TB skin test); RPR, rapid plasma regain (syphilis test); URTI, upper respiratory tract infection.

* Antibiotics should cover *Staphylococcus aureus* and *Streptococcus pyogenes* (e.g. amoxicillin, cloxacillin, cephalexin) and anaerobes if from a dental abscess (e.g. clindamycin and metronidazole)

Location of affected lymph nodes

The location of the affected lymph nodes can be indicative of the aetiology.[2] The following are the most common conditions associated with specific areas of lymphadenopathy:

Cervical
- Local infections: head and neck.
- Acute bacterial lymphadenitis (*Staphylococcus*, *Streptococcus*).
- Systemic: TB, EBV, CMV, toxoplasmosis.
- Malignancy: head and neck, lymphoma.

Supraclavicular
- Predominantly malignancy:
  - Right sided: mediastinum, lung, oesophagus.
  - Left sided: abdomen.

Axillary
- Local infection: arm, breast, thoracic wall.
- Cat scratch disease.
- Malignancy: breast.

Epitrochlear
Note: this is always pathological.
- Local infection: hand, forearm.
- Systemic: secondary syphilis, tularaemia, sarcoidosis.

Inguinal
- Local infection: e.g. STI.
- Malignancy: genitourinary, leg, rectum.

Other causes of lymphadenopathy tend to present with generalized disease.

Diagnostic techniques
- Often, the cause of lymphadenopathy can be diagnosed and treated on the basis of clinical assessment and limited laboratory tests as indicated in the algorithm in Fig. 23.2.
- In circumstances where lymphadenopathy is localized and subacute or chronic, FNA may aid in diagnosis. This is a relatively simple procedure and the challenge is generally in finding laboratory personnel who can interpret the microscopic slides. In some circumstances, it may be possible to prepare the slides and have them sent out for interpretation in a larger centre.

Fine needle aspiration

- FNA can be used in cases where a cause for the lymphadenopathy is not apparent from history and physical examination.
- It is primarily helpful for the diagnosis of TB or malignancy but can also play a role in other conditions (cryptococcosis, non-TB *Mycobacteria*, sarcoidosis).
- FNA generally is a low-risk procedure and is a less resource-intensive alternative to lymph node biopsy.[3]

Technique

FNA can be done blind or under bedside ultrasound guidance.

- Equipment: a small gauge needle (e.g. 22 G) and a 5–10 mL syringe.
- Larger needles (18 G) may be needed if the node is fluctuant.

Procedure

- Stabilize lymph node with the non-dominant hand.
- Using the dominant hand, place the needle under the skin and apply negative pressure to the syringe.
- Pass the needle in and out of the node a few times to obtain a sample.
- Before exiting the skin, release the negative pressure on the syringe.[4]

Slide preparation

- Only a very small amount of tissue is needed for analysis.
- Apply a drop from the needle onto a slide and use a slide cover to smear.
- Make a few slides for different stains. Allow to air dry.
  - The dried slides can be stained with giemsa (for cytology) or Ziehl–Neelson (ZN) stain (for acid-fast bacilli). One slide can be fixed with a few drops of 95% alcohol and then stained with a Papanicolaou stain for immunofluorescence microscopy if available (for TB).
- ZN or Papanicolaou testing is only useful if the cytology is consistent with TB (granulomas with caseating necrosis).[5]
- If *Cryptococcus* is a concern, an India ink stain can be applied.

Despite the ease of the procedure, the difficulty lies in finding a reliable laboratory technician to read the slide. Additional tests of aspirated material that may prove useful depending on the setting include TB culture and molecular testing for TB.

TB sputa testing

- Xpert® MTB/RIF testing (*Mycobacterium tuberculosis* (MTB) and resistance to rifampin (RIF)) of TB sputa is improving the diagnosis of TB and aspirated lymph node material is showing excellent sensitivity for TB diagnosis when using this method. One study quoted a sensitivity of 97% which is significantly higher than that for ZN stain (~25–45%) or even TB culture (~70%).[5,6]
- If the first attempt is non-diagnostic, repeat aspirations may increase the yield of the test. You might have to familiarize yourself on preparing and reading slides, alongside the local staff.

Specific causes of lymphadenopathy

Acute bacterial lymphadenitis

- Usually involves cervical lymph nodes ± axillary or inguinal.
- May be associated with lymphangitis (painful streaking among lymph channels emanating from wound or infection).
- Most common in children.
- Generally due to staphylococcal or streptococcal infection.

Evaluation

- May have an associated abscess (indicated by a fluctuant area within the inflamed lymph node) that requires incision and drainage for both therapeutic and diagnostic purposes.
- It may be helpful to send the fluid for Gram stain and ZN stain.

Treatment

- When TB lymphadenitis is not strongly suspected on clinical features or available lab testing, empirical treatment with one or two courses of antibiotics is a reasonable first start.
  - Most can be treated with oral antibiotics and first-line choices are cloxacillin, amoxicillin, or cefalexin.[7]
- Admit for IV antibiotics if patient appears toxic, is very young, or shows respiratory compromise. IM antibiotics should be used if patient needs admission but IV is not possible.

> Note: be aware that fluoroquinolones will partially treat TB and possibly delay a TB diagnosis. The same applies to amoxicillin–clavulanate and clarithromycin which are second-line treatment agents for drug-resistant TB. It may be prudent to avoid these antibiotics in areas with high TB endemicity where the diagnosis cannot be confirmed with Gram and ZN stains.

Cat scratch disease (*Bartonella henselae*)

- Usually only single enlarged node.
- Granulomatous changes on FNA (if possible).

Treatment

- Often self-limiting so do not need to treat if only mild symptoms. Otherwise may give azithromycin × 5 days.

TB lymphadenitis

- Lymphadenitis caused by TB is very common in tropical settings, particularly Africa and central Asia.
- Local epidemiological patterns are important as chronic cervical lymphadenopathy can range from 25% to 90% secondary to TB.
  - Seen most commonly in children and those who are HIV+ve.
  - In settings with a high burden of TB, painless and persistent lymph-adenopathy among children (especially with fistulization to the skin) is grounds for empirical TB treatment.
- Usually non-inflammatory, cold, chronic, non-tender lymphadenopathy.

- May be single or multiple, but most commonly bilateral.
- More common in cervical nodes, followed by intra-abdominal (diagnosed by ultrasound), mediastinal, axillary, and inguinal.

Evaluation
- In most settings, the diagnosis is clinical.
- Miliary (or disseminated) TB can also coexist with lymphadenopathy in deeper sites:
  - Chest X-ray may be helpful for mediastinal nodes.
  - Examination and ultrasound may reveal intra-abdominal nodes.
- Purified protein derivative (PPD) is of limited use in the diagnosis of TB lymphadenitis. PPD is positive in most patients, especially where there is high coverage of bacillus Calmette–Guérin (BCG) vaccination and high prevalence of latent TB infection. PPD can also result in a false negative in the context of HIV infections, steroid use, or immunosuppression.
- FNA useful for diagnosis but treat empirically if not available.

Treatment
- Treat according to national TB protocol.
- Successful treatment should result in lymph node resolution in about 3 months.

Non-tuberculous *Mycobacteria*
While the vast majority of mycobacterial infections are due to TB (>95%), non-tuberculosis *Mycobacteria* is an important diagnosis which should not be overlooked.
- Most commonly due to *Mycobacterium avium* complex (MAC).
- More prevalent in immunocompromised patients, can be associated with IRIS (immune reconstitution inflammatory syndrome).
- MAC is seen mostly with advanced HIV (CD4 <50) and is an AIDS-defining illness.

Evaluation
- This has a similar presentation to TB lymphadenitis.
- Diagnosis by FNA culture is probably not possible, thus consider empirical treatment if other empirical treatments fail (e.g. TB treatment and antibiotics).

Treatment
- Treat with antimicrobials (macrolide + ethambutol + rifampicin) for 12 weeks with surgical excision if possible.[8]

Note: BCG lymphadenitis is associated with BCG vaccine, often with local lymphadenopathy in region of vaccine site. More common in immunocompromised patients. If there is no abscess, no treatment is needed.

Malignancy
- Metastatic disease or lymphoma is another significant cause of lymphadenopathy.
- Common presentation with older age, fixed/hard nodes, supraclavicular nodes, and chronic duration.

Evaluation
- Often a diagnosis of exclusion when other empirical treatments fail (e.g. TB treatment and first-line antibiotics), and not explained by persistent generalized lymphadenopathy of HIV.
- FNA, if available, can be helpful.

Treatment
- Most humanitarian settings will be ill equipped to tackle clinical management of malignancy. This does not mean that 'nothing' can be done, and the following should be considered based on the local context and strength of the national health system:
  - Is the national health system equipped to deal with cancer treatment? Some cancers are more easily treatable (e.g. Burkitt lymphoma), and so it should not be automatically assumed that no management options exist.
  - Is the patient in the position to be transferred?
- Further, consider symptomatic management and palliation when/if appropriate (see ➲ Chapter 47).

Burkitt lymphoma

Burkitt lymphoma is a childhood cancer, which is rapid growing, and associated with EBV and HIV infection. This warrants specific mention here as it is common in endemic areas, affects children, has a typical clinical presentation, and has good treatment outcomes. In parts of the world where Burkitt's is endemic, there are often local referral centres that are equipped to treat the condition.

- Commonly presents with facial mass and/or abdominal mass (spleen, ovary, kidney).
- Endemic to parts of equatorial Africa and New Guinea and accounts for 30–50% of all childhood cancers in these regions. Burkitt lymphoma can also be found sporadically outside of these regions as well as in association with immunodeficiency, primarily HIV (regardless of CD4 count).[9]
- In comparison to bacterial infections, Burkitt's will present subacutely (over weeks to months), with no respiratory infection and FNA will not reveal TB.

HIV-positive patients

Many HIV+ve patients will have persistent generalized lymphadenopathy (PGL). PGL is a condition associated with stage 1 HIV and the diagnosis is made if the following criteria are met:
- Greater than two or more separate lymph node regions involved (excluding inguinal).
- In each body region, at least two nodes must be >1 cm in diameter.
- Lymph nodes must be present for >3 months.
- Lymph nodes must not be due to a local infection and are painless.

In addition to the differential diagnosis of lymphadenopathy in immuno-competent patients, some aetiologies are more common in those with HIV:

- TB adenopathy is usually the top diagnosis and should strongly be considered.
- Primary HIV infection.
- *Cytomegalovirus, Toxoplasma,* or *Cryptococcus* (although these tend not to present primarily as lymphadenopathy).
- Other *Mycobacteria* (other than TB).
- Syphilis (when inguinal or epitrochlear nodes are involved).
- Malignancy: Kaposi sarcoma, non-Hodgkin's lymphoma (including Burkitt lymphoma).

References

1. Ferrer R. Lymphadenopathy: differential diagnosis and evaluation. Am Fam Physician 1998;58(6):1313–20.
2. Fletcher RH. Evaluation of peripheral lymphadenopathy in adults. UpToDate. 2018. ℰ https://www.uptodate.com/contents/evaluation-of-peripheral-lymphadenopathy-in-adults
3. Thomas JO, Adeyi D, Amanguno H. Fine-needle aspiration in the management of peripheral lymphadenopathy in a developing country. Diagn Cytopathol 1999;21(3):159–62.
4. Johnson JT. Fine-needle aspiration of neck masses. Medscape. ℰ http://emedicine.medscape.com/article/1819862-overview#a7
5. Ligthelm LJ, Nicol MP, Hoek KGP, Jacob-son R, van Helden PD, Marais BJ, et al. Xpert MTB/RIF for rapid diagnosis of tuberculous lymphadenitis from fine-needle-aspiration biopsy specimens. J Clin Microbiol 2011;49(11):3967–70.
6. Fanny M-L, Beyam N, Gody JC, Zandanga G, Yango F, Manirakiza A, et al. Fine-needle aspiration for diagnosis of tuberculous lymphadenitis in children in Bangui, Central African Republic. BMC Pediatrics 2012;12(1):191.
7. McClain KL, Fletcher RH. Approach to the child with peripheral lymphadenopathy. Causes of peripheral lymphadenopathy in children. UpToDate. 2012. ℰ https://www.uptodate.com
8. Griffith DE, Aksamit T, Brown-Elliott BA, Catanzaro A, Daley C, Gordin F, et al. An official ATS/IDSA statement: diagnosis, treatment, and prevention of nontuberculous mycobacterial diseases. Am J Respir Crit Care Med 2007;175:367–416.
9. Freedman AS, Aster JC. Epidemiology, clinical manifestations, pathologic features, and diagnosis of Burkitt lymphoma. UpToDate. 2018. ℰ https://www.uptodate.com/contents/epidemiology-clinical-manifestations-pathologic-features-and-diagnosis-of-burkitt-lymphoma

Cough and breathlessness

Joseph O'Neill

Cough

Diagnostic clues

The length of time a cough has been present can be helpful in determining its aetiology.

Less than 3 weeks

Although an acute cough could be the first presentation of what turns out to be a subacute or chronic cough, symptoms that are <3 weeks' duration are most often caused by an upper respiratory tract infection, acute sinusitis, pertussis, a chronic obstructive pulmonary disease (COPD) exacerbation, or an allergic or environmentally caused rhinitis.

Immune suppression secondary to HIV increases the chances of *Pneumocystis* pneumonia or other opportunistic pulmonary infections being involved and TB should always be considered regardless of the length of time a cough has been present, especially in a setting of humanitarian crises where people may be living at close quarters under chaotic conditions.

3–8 weeks

Coughs lasting >3 weeks but that eventually resolve in 8 weeks are most likely post-infectious in nature but should increase suspicion for *Bordetella pertussis*.

Longer than 8 weeks

Chronic coughs (> 8 weeks) should prompt consideration of rhinitis (upper airway cough syndrome), asthma or non-asthmatic eosinophilic bronchitis, gastro-oesophageal reflux disease, occupational environmental exposures, or malignancy.

Treatment

Upper respiratory tract infection

- Uncomplicated viral upper respiratory tract infections are self-limiting.
- A 2014 Cochrane review of over-the-counter medications commonly used for acute cough[1] failed to find any evidence for or against their use.
- Although opiates play an important role in the management of chronic cough and breathlessness (see ⊃ Chapter 21), codeine has been found to be no better than placebo in reducing cough associated with acute upper respiratory infections.[2]
- If, however, an acute cough fails to resolve with supportive measures or if there are reasons to suspect a bacterial sinusitis (maxillary toothache, purulent nasal secretions, or abnormalities on transillumination of the sinus) or pneumonia, a course of antibiotics should be considered.

Caution: pertussis, in early stages, can be difficult to distinguish from a viral upper respiratory tract infection. In later stages, however, it can engender the classic symptoms of paroxysms of staccato coughs followed by a 'whoop', vomiting, and exhaustion. It is important to recognize and treat pertussis patients and contacts aggressively.

Other considerations
- Treatment of potential non-infectious causes should be considered. For example, cough caused by:
  - rhinitis due to allergies or by environmental toxins may respond to first-generation antihistamines
  - congestive heart failure (CHF) may improve with diuretics, inotropes, or other targeted therapies
  - bronchospasm should respond to bronchodilators
  - gastro-oesophageal reflux disease can be treated with antibiotics if *Helicobacter pylori* is diagnosed, antacids, histamine blockers, coating agents, proton pump inhibitors, diet modification, and/or head elevation while sleeping
- Inquire about home or work exposures, and stress importance of removal of environmental or occupational irritants.
- There is scant evidence to guide treatment of post-infectious cough. Neurogenic elements are increasingly understood to be involved and some success has been reported with gabapentin.

Non-pharmacological interventions
- Non-pharmacological management of cough should focus on keeping the patient away from smoke and fires, avoiding cigarettes and other forms of tobacco and postural drainage of secretions/sputum.
- Drinks with honey have been found to be helpful in some instances.

Breathlessness

- Dyspnoea can have a broad differential and can arise from both reversible and non-reversible conditions and can present in either chronic or episodic forms.
- Many patients have difficulty in distinguishing between shortness of breath and fatigue, and so a complaint of shortness of breath can trigger as wide a diagnostic search as can be had in medicine.
- A careful history and physical are therefore required to narrow the differential and discover potentially reversible aetiologies.

Diagnostic clues

- If dealing with intermittent air hunger, time spent uncovering what factors may trigger it (environmental, psychological, etc.) is well spent.
- Dyspnoea can arise from wide range of treatable conditions, including bronchospasm, myocardial ischaemia, heart failure, COPD, pulmonary embolus, interstitial lung disease, pulmonary/pleural tumours (primary or metastatic), pleural effusions, and pneumonia.
- Psychological states (anxiety, depression, panic attacks, and others) can also be important contributors.
- Breathlessness can take chronic or episodic forms. While the causes of episodic dyspnoea can vary, consider that the majority of patients with chronic dyspnoea have one of five diagnoses:
  - Asthma
  - COPD
  - Interstitial lung disease
  - Myocardial dysfunction
  - Obesity/deconditioning.

A multidisciplinary approach to dyspnoea management involving physiotherapy, occupational therapy, palliative care, and respiratory medicine has demonstrated survival benefit for patients with COPD and interstitial lung disease.[3] Although it is unlikely that a similar package of complete services will be available in the humanitarian setting, elements of such an approach (e.g. spiritual support, exercises that encourage diaphragmatic breathing, meditation, music, etc.) may be mobilized to good effect.

Treatment

- Treatment for dyspnoea is first directed to any identified underlying disease with the intent of reducing ventilatory demand (e.g. anaemia), improving ventilatory capacity, improving respiratory mechanics, and/or impacting the subjective (affective) experience of dyspnoea.
- In the humanitarian setting, access to these approaches may be limited so an approach that addresses both underlying disease as well as the immediate symptom of dyspnoea are appropriate.
- For management of breathlessness, all reversible underlying conditions need to be ruled out or optimally treated—and then the patient and practitioner should work towards a therapeutic goal of providing comfort and relief from the symptom of breathlessness.

- Regardless of aetiology, the subjective experience of shortness of breath can be mitigated by causing clean cool air to circulate (via a breeze, electric fan, or simply fanning with a magazine) around the patient's face, especially in the area of the distribution of the trigeminal nerve.
- Training the patient in pursed-lip breathing and various relaxation techniques can also help.
- An empiric trial of bronchodilators is often worthwhile if there are no contraindications as can supplementary oxygen if it is available.
- Opiates remain the most important pharmacotherapy for refractory dyspnoea as they have been demonstrated to be effective in curbing the subjective experience of air hunger. Concerns about the rare side effect opiates have of respiratory depression should not outweigh the benefit of improving dyspnoea. See ➔ Chapter 21 for dosing (similar in this setting as in pain management).

References

1. Smith SM, Schroeder K, Fahey T. Over-the-counter (OTC) medications for acute cough in children and adults in community settings. Cochrane Database Syst Rev 2014;11:CD001831.
2. Freestone C, Eccles R. Assessment of the antitussive efficacy of codeine in cough associated with common cold. J Pharm Pharmacol 1997;49(10):1045–9.
3. Higginson IJ, Bausewein C, Reilly CC, Gao W, Gysels M, Dzingina M, et al. An integrated palliative and respiratory care service for patients with advanced disease and refractory breathlessness: a randomised controlled trial. Lancet Respir Med 2014;2(12):979–87.

Chapter 25

Oedema

Anne Aspler

Introduction to oedema

Children and adults will frequently present in humanitarian settings with generalized body swelling, or localized swelling of the abdomen or lower extremities. There can be a broad differential for these presentations, complicated by limited investigations, and a lack of familiarity with common conditions in a low resource or humanitarian setting, which may be infrequently seen in the provider's home country. For example, while non-communicable chronic diseases such as heart failure or malnutrition may be causative agents for generalized oedema, infectious diseases such as TB are also frequently implicated. Further, while patients with oedematous states are generally stable, it is possible to have presentations in extremis for both children and adults.

Pathophysiology

Oedema is palpable swelling, created by an increased interstitial fluid volume that can be local or generalized ('anasarca'). The following pathophysiology may be responsible:

- Decreased plasma oncotic pressure (malabsorption, malnutrition, liver failure, nephrotic syndrome).
- Increased capillary hydrostatic pressure (CHF, cirrhosis, renal failure, pregnancy, venous obstruction, ascites, due to peritoneal TB, should be strongly considered, particularly in regions with HIV).
- Increased capillary permeability (burns, angio-oedema).
- Increased lymphatic pressure (deep vein thrombosis (DVT), neoplasm, lymphadenopathy).

Differential diagnosis of oedema

Especially in low-resource environments, the location and distribution of oedema can offer important guidance as to the aetiology of the underlying condition and can help focus the differential diagnosis.

Generalized oedema causing symmetrical swelling

- Anaphylaxis: presents primarily symmetrical facial and oral oedema.
- Cardiac: presents with pulmonary oedema with symmetrical lower extremity oedema. Causes can include systolic or diastolic dysfunction, constrictive pericarditis, or pulmonary hypertension.
- Hepatic (cirrhosis).
- Renal: causes include nephrotic syndrome, acute nephritis, acute kidney injury (AKI) or chronic renal failure of any aetiology.
- Obstetric: pre-eclampsia.
- Nutritional deficiency (see ➲ Chapter 28).
- Protein-losing enteropathy: this includes conditions in gastrointestinal tract leading to net loss of protein or malabsorption syndromes (e.g. bacterial overgrowth, following intestinal viral infection).

Non-cardiogenic pulmonary oedema causing focal lung oedema

- Acute respiratory distress syndrome (ARDS) (sequel to sepsis, severe malaria, trauma, pancreatitis).
- Intracranial catastrophes (e.g. subarachnoid bleeding can cause increased pulmonary interstitial pressures via CNS damage).
- IV fluid overload.
- Hypoalbuminaemia: such as with liver failure and nephrotic syndrome.
- Drugs/poisons/chemical inhalations.
- Near drowning incidents.

Peripheral oedema causing focal oedema to one extremity

- Venous disease:
  - Due to obstruction: DVT, lymphadenopathy (TB, HIV), pelvic mass. Note: superior vena cava obstruction may result in isolated face and neck oedema.
  - Insufficiency.
- Lymphatic obstruction: i.e. from neoplasm, lymphadenopathy (TB, HIV), filariasis.
- Posterior knee synovial bursa rupture (Baker's cyst).

Localized oedema

- Angio-oedema.
- Burns.
- Trauma (post-traumatic swelling to damaged tissues).
- Cellulitis (note: it is key to differentiate this from underlying osteomyelitis or septic arthritis).

Chronic conditions (chronic heart failure, malnutrition, cirrhosis, chronic renal failure) are more likely to present with profound generalized pitting oedema than acute conditions such as acute heart failure and acute kidney injury.

Clinical evaluation of oedema

The physical examination should be focused on the pattern of oedema (generalized versus focal) and locations of excess fluid (pulmonary, abdominal, and peripheral involvement). (See Table 25.1.)

Clues to aetiology

General appearance
- Pattern of oedema (generalized versus focal).
- Respiratory distress (pulmonary oedema, ascites restricting pulmonary expansion).
- Focal trauma or burns.

Vital signs
- Hypoxia and tachypnoea (pulmonary oedema).
- Hypotension (cardiogenic shock, anaphylaxis, trauma).
- Hypertension (acute heart failure).

Clinical examination
- *Neurological:* mental status changes (hepatic encephalopathy, uraemic encephalopathy, hypertensive encephalopathy in acute nephritis, respiratory failure).
- *Head and neck:*
  - Periorbital oedema (i.e. symmetrical protrusion of lower and/or upper lids) (nephrotic syndrome, malnutrition).
  - Scleral icterus (cirrhosis).
  - Thyromegaly or thyroid nodules (myxoedema).
- *Cardiovascular:*
  - Elevated jugular venous pressure (JVP) (CHF, renal disease).
  - Third heart sound (CHF).
  - Hepatojugular reflex (CHF).
- *Respiratory:*
  - Bibasilar crackles (pulmonary oedema).
  - Decreased air entry (pulmonary effusion).
- *Abdominal:*
  - Ascites (cirrhosis, TB, malignancy, renal failure).
  - Tender hepatomegaly (CHF).
  - Splenomegaly (cirrhosis).

Table 25.1 Physical findings to differentiate oedematous states

Disorder	Pulmonary oedema	Jugular venous pressure	Ascites and/or pedal oedema
Left-sided heart failure	+	Increased	+/–
Right-sided heart failure	–	Increased	+
Cirrhosis	–	Decreased-normal	+
Renal	Variable	Increased	+
Nephrotic syndrome	–	Variable	+
Venous insufficiency	–	Normal	Symmetric pedal oedema

- *Gynaecological*: pelvic mass (ovarian cancer)
- *Musculoskeletal*:
  - Bilateral leg oedema (CHF).
  - Unilateral calf swelling/tenderness (DVT).
  - Pretibial oedema (myxoedema).
  - Unilateral leg swelling (filarial disease).
  - Pitting oedema is due to fluid which has transudated from the venous system (e.g. heart failure or malnutrition with hypoalbuminemia).

Note: non-pitting lymphoedema is due to lymphatic obstruction with causes such as filarial disease or compression of the venous blood supply
- *Dermatological:*
  - Jaundice, spider nevi (cirrhosis).
  - Redness/warmth (cellulitis).
  - Urticaria (angio-oedema).

Investigations
Selective use of the following tests should be based on the suspected underlying pathology:
- Oxygen saturation (*hypoxia may signify pulmonary oedema*).
- Blood pressure (BP) (*hypertension may be seen in acute heart failure or chronic renal failure*).
- Complete blood count and differential (*high WBC may indicate active infection, anaemia is seen in end-stage renal failure*).
- Urinalysis (*proteinuria is associated with nephrotic syndrome*).
- Urine for ova and parasites (*chronic urinary schistosomiasis*).
- Renal function (*renal failure*).
- Liver function (*liver failure*).
- Albumin level (*hypoalbuminemia may indicate heart failure, malnutrition, or cirrhosis*).
- Chest radiography (*for identification of pulmonary oedema, cardiomegaly, and may be suggestive of TB*).
- Point-of-care ultrasound.
  - Inferior vena cava status.
  - Intra-abdominal lymph nodes (FASH exam—focused assessment with sonography for HIV-associated TB) for TB.
  - Echocardiogram: check left ventricular function, rule out pericardial effusion.
  - Pulmonary: pleural effusion, 'B' lines suggesting heart failure.
  - Abdominal:
    —Intraperitoneal fluid (*ascites*).
    —Liver: cirrhosis.
    —Renal: hydronephrosis → obstructive renal failure.
    —Renal: small fibrosed kidney → chronic renal failure.
  - Extremity: DVT.
- HIV testing and CD4 count (*for associated complications and/or opportunistic infections which may be underlying cause of oedema*).
- Acid-fast bacilli (AFB) smear and culture for TB (*ascites*).
- Rapid test or peripheral smear for malaria.
- Locally available filariasis testing.

Oedema: management of cardiopulmonary causes

Treatment of oedema consists of reversal of the underlying disorder. Children with generalized oedema should first be considered for malnutrition, nephrotic syndrome, and heart failure.

Heart failure

Heart failure is a clinical syndrome and not a diagnosis. The patient may have symptoms of exercise intolerance consistent with heart failure, but always search for an underlying aetiology. Causes of heart failure in the humanitarian setting include acute rheumatic heart disease de-compensation; beriberi from thiamine deficiency (in SE Asia in particular); uncontrolled hypertension; ischaemic heart disease, valvular disease (post-rheumatic or due to infectious endocarditis), pericardial disease (i.e. TB); thyrotoxicosis; pregnancy; anaemia.

Diagnosis suggested by:
Exertional dyspnoea, orthopnoea, elevated JVP, bilateral leg oedema, tender hepatomegaly.

Confirmed by:
CXR or echocardiography (if available).

Chronic management of heart failure
- Identify and treat underlying case if possible.
- Treat reversible exacerbating factors.
- Restrict salt and alcohol intake.
- Avoid NSAIDs which can cause fluid retention.
- Thiazide or loop diuretic.
- Monitor diuresis in the long term by measuring the patient's weight.
- See ➋ Chapter 36 for detailed management.

Malaria-associated ARDS

In endemic settings can be a common cause of non-cardiogenic pulmonary oedema. It carries a 50% mortality rate and may occur when the patient is otherwise improving. Excessive fluid replacement exacerbates this complication and is suggested by tachypnoea and hypoxia. Predisposing factors include hyperparasitaemia, renal failure, and pregnancy (may occur suddenly after delivery).[1] Definitive management requires malaria treatment and supportive care.

Acute management of undifferentiated pulmonary oedema
- Sit patient upright to improve ventilation, lower legs to decrease pre-load.
- Provide supplemental oxygen.
- Furosemide 40 mg IV or 80 mg PO (may require higher amounts in patient already taking oral furosemide).
- Nitrates (if available and systolic BP >90 mmHg).
- If patient distressed or has chest pain, consider small amount of IV opioid with antiemetic. Do not give opioids to patients that are drowsy, confused, or not protecting airway.
- Consider inserting urinary catheter and recording urine output to monitor diuresis.

Oedema: management of hepatic causes

Cirrhosis

Chronic liver disease may be a sequel of hepatitis caused by viruses, parasites, bacteria, and toxins (including alcohol). Persistent/recurrent liver injury causes cirrhosis (irreversible destruction of liver cellular architecture by fibrosis with nodular regeneration of hepatocytes).

Clinical features

- Symptoms include malaise, pruritus, and reversal of normal sleep patterns (if encephalopathic). There may be hepatomegaly in early cirrhosis, although fibrotic contraction causes the liver to shrink as the disease progresses.
- Face and skin: jaundice (including scleral icterus), hepatic fetor, excoriations.
- Hands: clubbing, palmar erythema, bruising, asterixis.
- Chest gynaecomastia, loss of body hair, spider nevi, bruising.
- Abdomen: splenomegaly, ascites, testicular atrophy.
- Legs: bilateral oedema (due to hypoalbuminemia), muscle wasting.

Diagnosis suggested by:

Stigmata of chronic liver disease, ascites, ± splenomegaly; elevated (or low) liver enzymes, paracentesis ± ascitic fluid analysis (+TB AFB stain and culture) to exclude other causes, liver ultrasound scan.

Management

Cirrhosis is an irreversible condition, so the aim is to limit further damage, treat complications, and support the patient.

- Avoid alcohol and hepatotoxic drugs (e.g. avoid paracetamol in high doses—low doses are OK).
- Treat dehydration and concurrent infections if present.
- Ensure adequate nutrition/protein intake.
- Treat ascites; therapeutic paracentesis + loop diuretic (furosemide).
- Management and prevention of portal hypertension and oesophageal varices with beta blocker; consider spontaneous bacterial peritonitis prevention with weekly ciprofloxacin or co-trimoxazole.

Oedema: management of renal causes

Oedema[1] is often the presenting feature of nephrotic syndrome, acute nephritis, or renal failure from any underlying cause.

Nephrotic syndrome

Nephrotic syndrome[1] is characterized by proteinuria, hypoalbuminemia, oedema, and hypercholesterolaemia. Most cases of nephrotic syndrome are idiopathic. In field settings, some are secondary to:
- infections, including HIV, hepatitis B virus, and hepatitis C virus
- diabetic nephropathy
- autoimmune disease
- neoplasia
- amyloid (leprosy, TB) and sickle cell disease.

Diagnosis suggested by:
Frothy urine, periorbital oedema + peripheral oedema ± ascites ± pleural effusion.

Confirmed by:
Proteinuria (>3 g/24 hours).

Management
- Ensure an adequate diet with protein.
- Restrict salt use.
- Monitor BP, intake and output, weigh regularly.
- Monitor urinalysis and creatinine.
- Furosemide IV:
  - Higher doses may be required than in patients with normal renal function.
  - Use cautiously since volume depletion may be present.
- Treat the cause in cases of suspected secondary glomerulonephritis (GN):
  - Membranous GN: diagnosis of exclusion when biopsy/pathology not available. Up to 60% may respond to 6 months of treatment with steroids.
  - *HIV-related nephropathy:* generic treatment for GN + initiate highly active antiretroviral therapy (HAART).
  - *HBV-associated GN:* occurs mainly in children who are carriers for HBV. Paediatric management is conservative as most children go into spontaneous remission.

Complications
- Venous thromboembolism: suspect renal vein thrombosis if sudden loss of renal function with haematuria, especially with back pain.
- Infection: consider prophylaxis with phenoxymethylpenicillin during oedematous state (risk of pneumococcal peritonitis).
- Hypovolaemia and AKI: check postural BP, monitor urine output.

Acute nephritis

Most often due to post-streptococcal GN in the tropics occurring 2–3 weeks after streptococcal throat, ear, or skin infection (impetigo, infected scabies, or infected eczema).[1]

Clinical features
Haematuria, oliguria, mild oedema, elevated JVP, hypertension, variable uraemia.

Diagnosis
Haematuria ± red cell casts, proteinuria, elevated blood creatinine and urea.

Management
- Restrict fluid intake, if oliguric, to 500 mL/day + replacement for losses in urine output over past 24 hours.
- Restrict salt and potassium in diet.
- Give diuretics (furosemide) and antihypertensive treatment (non-beta blockers which may precipitate pulmonary oedema).
- Eradicate residual streptococcal infection: oral phenoxymethylpenicillin 500 mg PO four times a day for 10 days; or single-dose benzathine benzyl penicillin 900 mg IM; or if allergic to penicillin, erythromycin 250–500 mg PO four times a day.
- Test for HIV and if positive, treat for stage 4 or advanced HIV with HAART, along with antimicrobial treatment as previously mentioned.

Complications
Hypertensive encephalopathy, pulmonary oedema, rarely rapidly progressive GN, chronic renal failure.

Acute kidney injury
Oedema occurs in both AKI and chronic renal failure due to volume overload: sodium and water intake exceeds the kidney's capacity to excrete them due to loss of glomerular filtration. Causes of AKI are roughly 60% medical, 25% surgical, and 15% obstetric. If AKI is part of multiorgan dysfunction, prognosis is poor. Isolated AKI has a better prognosis and may be completely reversible.

Differential diagnosis of AKI
- Pre-renal: secondary to intravascular volume depletion (dehydration, shock, blood loss, hypotension, or septicaemia). Urine will be concentrated. Requires fluid resuscitation.
- Intrinsic renal: e.g. leptospirosis, falciparum malaria, massive intravascular haemolysis from G6PD deficiency, and drugs/infections, snake bite, post-streptococcal GN, rhabdomyolysis, nephrotoxic drugs.
  - In disaster settings, where there are many blunt trauma or crush victims, rhabdomyolysis may be particularly common.
- Post-renal AKI (obstructive): pelvic mass or large prostate may be causative. Possibly presents with distended bladder, palpable kidneys (hydronephrosis), and ultrasound use is helpful.

Management of AKI
- Examine the patient and assess volume status (JVP, skin turgor, peripheral perfusion, mucous membranes, pulmonary crepitations, peripheral oedema, heart rate, postural BP).
- Optimize fluid balance. Give fluids if dry; if overloaded, try diuretics.
- Catheterize to exclude lower tract obstruction and monitor urine output.

Chronic renal failure

Chronic kidney disease results from progressive and irreversible loss of renal function. In tropical countries, GN, hypertension, diabetic nephropathy, and obstructive uropathy are major causes of CKD.

Clinical features

There are few symptoms of chronic renal failure until the GFR is reduced to <20% when fatigue due to anaemia develops. Uraemia may cause anorexia, vomiting, hiccups, peripheral neuropathy, confusion, and drowsiness.

Management

Treat the underlying cause and reversible contributing factors:
• Relieve obstruction by inserting a catheter.
• Avoid nephrotoxic drugs (e.g. NSAIDs).
• Treat infections.
• Low salt diet if oedematous/hypertensive.
• Low potassium diet if hyperkalaemic.

Prognosis for patients with chronic renal failure may be poor in settings where the definitive management of haemodialysis is not available. See ➋ Chapter 46 for more information.

References

1. Stern SDC, Cifu AS, Atkorn D. Symptom to Diagnosis: An Evidenced Based Guide. 3rd ed. New York: Lange Medical Books; 2006.
2. Sterns RH. Clinical Manifestations and Diagnosis of Edema in Adults. UpToDate®. Last updated 29 August 2016. ⅗ https://www.uptodate.com/contents/clinical-manifestations-and-diagnosis-of-edema-in-adults
3. Wyatt JP, Illingworth RN, Graham CA, Hogg K. Oxford Handbook of Emergency Medicine. 4th ed. Oxford: Oxford University Press; 2012.
4. Llewelyn H, Ang HA, Lewis K, Al-Abdullah A. Oxford Handbook of Clinical Diagnosis. 3rd ed. Oxford: Oxford University Press; 2014.
5. Brent A, Davidson R, Seale A. Oxford Handbook of Tropical Medicine. 4th ed. Oxford: Oxford University Press; 2014.
6. Singer M, Webb AR. Oxford Handbook of Critical Care. 3rd ed. Oxford: Oxford University Press; 2009.
7. Ramrakha PA, Moore KP, Sam A. Oxford Handbook of Acute Medicine. 3rd ed. Oxford: Oxford University Press; 2010.

Chapter 26

Patient with unintentional weight loss

James Maskalyk

Introduction to patient with unintentional weight loss

It is a familiar scenario in any health structure in humanitarian settings, the adult patient who presents with a subacute, indolent history of weight loss (or 'wasting'), in the presence of adequate food availability. These patients, most often, are suffering from chronic diseases, and without treatment, have increased mortality compared to cohorts who have maintained their weight.

In the presence of relatively stable food stores, most people maintain a remarkably consistent weight, fluctuating by only a few kilograms per year. With age, it is common for individuals to experience a slow change in body composition, including a loss of muscle and bone mass. An earlier or greater loss of body weight (>5 kg or >5% of body weight in 6–12 months) should alert the clinician to an unaddressed organic or psychosocial problem.

Broadly, weight loss occurs because of four reasons:
1. Decreased caloric intake (lack of availability, anorexia).
2. Diminished absorption (intestinal loss, pancreatic insufficiency).
3. Impaired cellular metabolism (diabetes).
4. Increased energy requirements (exercise, elevated resting energy requirements from disease states).

Whether unintentional weight loss has been confirmed by history or serial weights, the approach is the same: a detailed medical, dietary, and psychosocial history; a complete physical exam, including swallowing assessment; and if available, focused laboratory, radiological, and microbiological testing.

Differential diagnosis of patient with unintentional weight loss

The variety of diseases and conditions that cause non-intentional weight loss is very broad and can involve nearly every system. With little access to primary care, it is common that disease, infectious and otherwise, might remain undiagnosed until late stages of the illness. The list in Box 26.1, while not exhaustive, is an attempt to capture likely causes found in low-resource settings.

> **Box 26.1 Causes of weight loss**
>
> **Weight loss with anorexia**
> - AIDS
> - TB
> - Malignancy
> - Renal failure
> - Visceral leishmaniasis
> - Amoebiasis/amoebic liver abscess
> - Giardiasis
> - Gut helminths
> - Schistosomiasis
> - Infective endocarditis
> - Brucellosis
> - Hydatid disease
> - Anxiety/depression
> - Drugs.
>
> **Weight loss with preserved or increased appetite**
> - Starvation
> - Gut helminths (variable)
> - Diabetes mellitus
> - Thyrotoxicosis/hyperthyroidism
> - Connective tissue disease (rheumatoid arthritis, vasculitides)
> - Phaeochromocytoma
> - Malabsorption
> - Drugs.
>
> Information from Cook, G.C., P. Manson, and A. Zumla. Manson's tropical diseases. Saunders Ltd, 2009. Print. pp 93–105.

Infectious disease

Although the differential for weight loss is broad, infectious diseases cause the majority of treatable causes of involuntary weight loss in most humanitarian and tropical settings. With a clear geographical influence, chronic infectious disease infection allows for three main mechanisms to occur, generally with some overlap:
1. Chronic inflammation leading to greater energy expenditure.
2. Decreased appetite because of general weakness.
3. Increased caloric requirements due to organism needs.

Viral
- Acquired immune deficiency (e.g. HIV/AIDS).

Bacterial
- TB (pulmonary and extra-pulmonary).
- Infective bacterial endocarditis.
- Chronic infection (including abscess).

Fungal
Fungal infections, in an immunocompetent host, are almost always acquired environmentally and focused on the skin or lungs. In an immunocompromised host, non-endemic, opportunistic fungal infections can invade a patient more deeply and spread in a haematogenous manner. Diagnosis is difficult, often requiring histopathology and so treatment is presumptive. Consider:
- Histoplasmosis.
- Blastomycosis.
- Coccidiomycosis.
- Aspergillosis.

Parasitic
Parasites can cause weight loss by interfering with normal absorption by creating chronic intestinal inflammation and increasing systemic caloric requirements. While gastrointestinal parasites can often be detected through stool samples, systemic parasites vary greatly with exposure and geography and often need more refined diagnostic tests.

Gut
- Helminths: nematodes (roundworms), cestodes (tapeworms), trematodes (flukes).
- Protozoa.
- Giardiasis.
- Amoebiasis.
- Cryptosporidiosis.

Systemic
- Schistosomiasis.
- Echinococcosis.
- Filariasis.
- Leishmaniasis (visceral).
- Trypanosomiasis (African, American).

Approach to patient with unintentional weight loss

History
- Confirm diagnosis of significant weight loss in the presence of adequate food availability.
- In the absence of serial weights, gather information about changes in clothes/belt size, collateral information from family members.
- Assess risk factors for HIV, TB exposure.
- Qualify possible associated constitutive symptoms (fevers, night sweats, rigours).
- Screen for psychiatric comorbidities (depression, anorexia nervosa, etc.).
- Assess social risks (addiction, smoking).
- Determine new medications or changes in doses.
- Determine quantity of food intake, and change over time.

Physical findings
- Vital signs:
  - Fever (infection, malignancy).
  - Tachycardia (anaemia, hyperthyroidism, phaeochromocytoma, sympathomimetic drugs).
  - Respiratory rate (COPD, TB, lung cancer, acidosis).
- Appearance: loss of lean muscle mass, jaundice, uraemic frost (renal failure), hyperpigmentation (adrenal insufficiency).
- Head + neck: jaundice, gum/tooth disease, enlarged thyroid, lymphadenopathy (malignancy), oral candidiasis, swallowing assessment.
- Respiratory: focal sounds, decreased air entry suggesting consolidation or effusion (TB, fungal infection, malignancy).
- Cardiovascular: systolic murmurs (suggestive of endocarditis, or rheumatic disease), elevated JVP, third heart sound (CHF).
- Gastrointestinal: organomegaly, mass (malignancy, liver abscess, hydatid disease, splenomegaly from visceral leishmaniasis), fistula, melena.
- Genitourinary and gynaecological: enlarged prostate, palpable uterus or ovaries, cervical mass, vaginal bleeding.
- Musculoskeletal: focal atrophy or weakness, chronic changes of rheumatoid arthritis.
- Neurological: focal sensory or functional deficit.
- Integumentary: Roth spots, splinter haemorrhages, Janeway lesions (endocarditis), Kaposi's, superficial fungal infections (HIV), clubbing (chronic disease), signs of abuse or neglect (unexplained bruising, burns, etc.).

Investigations

If available, the following tests would help narrow the differential:

Laboratory
- Complete blood count and differential.
- Renal, liver, and thyroid function tests.
- Electrolytes, blood sugar.
- Urine (ketones (starvation, diabetes, alcoholic ketoacidosis), glucose (diabetes), casts (glomerulonephritides).
- HIV test.
- Leishmaniasis rapid test (if endemic).

Microscopic
- Urinalysis (schistosomes, casts).
- Stool examination (parasites, blood, fat globules).
- Sputum (for AFB, hyphae, if productive cough).

Radiological
- Chest radiograph.
- Abdominal ultrasound (organomegaly, liver abscess, hydatid cysts).

Management

- Treatment is best directed towards the causative pathology, and can be accompanied by supplementation with what nutrient-dense food the environment can afford, such that the affected individual can begin to repair their body (target is 40 kcal/kg/day, ± multivitamin).
- Malignancies and chronic non-communicable diseases are often poorly addressed in the low-resource setting, and so clinicians should focus on identifying reversible pathologies, leaving more progressive conditions as diagnoses of exclusion.
- If the physical examination and available investigations fail to provide a diagnosis, empiric treatment of common pathologies should be considered, mostly notably intestinal parasites, and protozoa. This approach is summarized in Fig. 26.1, and might be changed based on local patterns of disease.
- Given how challenging this presentation can be, if the field medical resources cannot yield a causative pathology and empirical treatment does not help, then the patient and family can be considered for referral to a higher level of care, although context and prognosis will determine the feasibility and practicality of this.

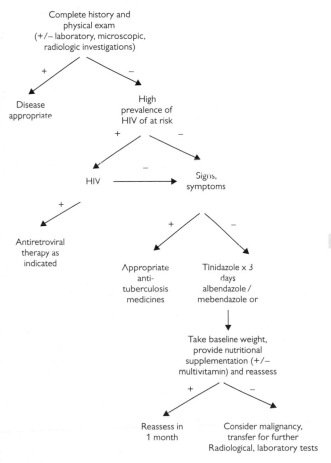

Fig. 26.1 Approach to management of non-intentional weight loss in low-resource settings.

Diarrhoea and vomiting

**Peter Moons, Vincent Buard and
Raghu Venugopal**

Context of diarrhoea and vomiting

Diarrhoea and vomiting are common pathologies in humanitarian contexts, with young children typically most adversely impacted. Globally, diarrhoea is the third leading cause of death among children <5 years of age, primarily due to dehydration and malnutrition. Typically with an infectious aetiology (rotavirus, enterotoxigenic *Escherichia coli* and *Vibrio cholerae* are leading causes), diarrhoea and vomiting are both preventable and treatable.

The 1994 exodus of 500,000–800,000 Rwandan refugees to eastern Congo resulted in a crude mortality rate of 20–35 deaths/10,000 persons/day (50,000 deaths in about 1 month). These rates, which resulted from serial epidemics of cholera and shigellosis, were two- to threefold greater than the highest rates previously reported among refugees or internally displaced populations. More lives could have been saved with more aggressive rehydration, prioritization of basic sanitation and hygiene, provision of sufficient clean water and health outreach.[1]

Evaluation of diarrhoea and vomiting

History

A careful history is essential with the goal being to distinguish acute and chronic cases and within acute cases, between bloody, non-bloody, and watery diarrhoea. To determine this, your history should include the following:

- Frequency of vomiting and stools:
  - Diarrhoea is defined as three or more loose stools per day.
  - Remember: loose, pasty stools by breast-fed babies are normal.
- Duration of complaints:
  - Persistent diarrhoea is defined as diarrhoea with a duration of 14 days or longer.
- Appearance:
  - Vomitus with coffee ground appearance is suggestive of upper gastrointestinal bleeding.
  - Stool with the appearance of rice-water is suggestive of cholera.
  - Stool with frank blood suggests *Shigella*, other bacteria or parasites (e.g. amoebiasis or schistosomiasis).
- History of fever with diarrhoea:
  - Can be due to certain non-enteric infections such as pneumonia, bacteraemia, urinary tract infections, ear infections and malaria.
  - Fever is seen with amoebiasis, schistosomiasis and bacterial and viral enteric infections.
  - *Salmonella typhi* is noteworthy, presenting with sudden-onset, high-grade, prolonged fever and characteristic bowel habits of constipation in week 1 and diarrhoea in week 3.
- Review of relevant symptoms such as convulsions, which are more common in shigellosis.
- Ability to feed, appetite and history of recent food ingested.

Physical examination

Look for:

- signs of dehydration: decreased level of consciousness, irritability, sunken eyes, dry mucous membranes, reduced turgor on skin pinch, fast pulse rate and decreased pulse strength
- localized or general abdominal distension, masses and/or pain.

Be aware that specific microbiological causes of diarrhoea can cause pain in specific locations (see Fig. 27.1):

- Amoebiasis when at the stage of causing diarrhoea will cause pain in the left iliac area upon palpation.
- HIV-related protozoan disease will cause periumbilical pain as well as left iliac pain (due to amoebiasis—a common entity among those who are HIV+ve).
- Typhoid is often found without diarrhoea but rather with fever in peaks and other constitutional symptoms. Pain occurs mostly in the right iliac area, in epigastric area or is diffuse. Often also associated with splenomegaly and hepatomegaly.

- Shigella causes diffuse pain, along with high fever, hypotension, and weakness.
- Schistosomiasis causes diffuse abdominal pain, sometimes localized in the left iliac area.

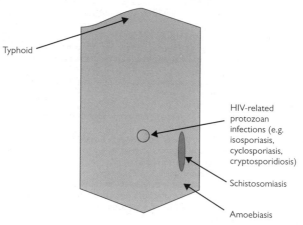

Fig. 27.1 Characteristic sites of pain with particular causes of diarrhoea.

Diagnosis of diarrhoea and vomiting

Acute diarrhoea

The Differential diagnosis for acute diarrhoea depends on the presence or absence of blood in the stools.

Non-bloody acute watery diarrhoea

- Viruses are common causes.
- Gastrointestinal infections: viral or bacterial (e.g. non-typhi *Salmonella*, *Escherichia coli*, *Vibrio cholerae*, *Yersinia*) or parasitic (e.g. giardiasis, cryptosporidiosis).
- Extra-intestinal infections (e.g. malaria and respiratory tract infections).
- Food poisoning

Acute bloody diarrhoea

- Gastrointestinal infections (mainly bacterial infections: *Shigella*, *Campylobacter*, *Yersinia*, *Salmonella*, enteroinvasive or enterohaemorrhagic *E. coli*).
  - *Shigella* accounts for about half of cases of bloody diarrhoea[2] though there are characteristic features.
- Pseudomembranous colitis.
- Inflammatory bowel disease.
- Amoebic infections.
- Intussusception.
- Bilharzia.

> Know the prevalence of particular diseases in your region, such as typhoid, schistosomiasis, cholera, shigellosis, etc. Be alert for local reports of similar complaints which could suggest an outbreak.

Persistent diarrhoea

In persistent diarrhoea (>14 days), the differential diagnosis needs to include the above-mentioned aetiologies plus the following:

- Lactose intolerance.
- *Clostridium difficile*.
- Infectious diseases that are particularly prevalent among HIV+ve and paediatric patients (isosporiasis, cyclosporiasis, cryptosporidiosis, microsporidiosis).

Investigations

- At many sites, diagnosis will be largely clinical.
- Stool examination may reveal parasitic causes such as amoebiasis, giardiasis, or schistosomiasis (*Schistosomiasis mansoni* in particular).
- Cholera rapid tests are useful to establish the presence of initial cases, but once an outbreak is declared, cases can easily be diagnosed on clinical grounds, and rapid tests are generally not routinely used.
- Portable ultrasound can play a very helpful role in assessing hydration by studying the inferior vena cava—particularly among those who are malnourished.

Vomiting

Due to its prevalence in humanitarian settings, this chapter focuses predominantly on diarrhoea, with or without vomiting. Be aware, however, that vomiting has a broad differential diagnosis, and one should not automatically ascribe it to 'gastroenteritis' without careful history and examination. Vomiting, especially in the absence of diarrhoea, should prompt consideration of the broader differential which would include the following:

- Intra-abdominal causes: cholera, gastroenteritis, food poisoning, bowel obstruction, hepatitis, appendicitis, cholecystitis, cholangitis, pancreatitis, peptic ulcer, peritonitis.
- Bilious vomiting in a child should prompt consideration of malrotation with midgut volvulus and intussusception.
- CNS causes: increased intracranial pressure, head injury, meningitis, tumour, migraines.
- Metabolic causes: uraemia, diabetic ketoacidosis, hyponatraemia, alcohol.
- Mental health: stress, anxiety, conversion disorder, depression.
- Other: severe pain, myocardial infarction, sepsis, pregnancy, poisonings.
- Iatrogenic: medication side effects or toxin related (e.g. traditional therapies).
- Non-specific: any general infection (in children in particular) can cause vomiting, after more serious causes have been considered.

Management of diarrhoea and vomiting

Principles
There are four general principles of the syndromic management of diarrhoea:
1. When there is no sign of dehydration, prevent it.
2. When dehydration is present, treat it.
3. Prevent malnutrition by encouraging feeding during and after diarrhoea.
4. Reduce the severity and duration of diarrhoea as well as future episodes with zinc supplementation.

Assessment
In order to determine the appropriate treatment for these four principles, an assessment of the patient needs to be conducted according to Table 27.1.

Treatment guidelines
Treatment will vary for well-nourished[3] versus malnourished children and for adults.

For well nourished-children
Treatment Plan A (no signs of dehydration)
- Give as much extra fluid (ideally oral rehydration solution (ORS)) orally as the child will accept.
  - If the child is 0–2 years: give 50–100 mL after each loose stool.
  - If the child is 2 years old or older give 100 200 mL after each loose stool.
  - A syringe is a good way to help parents administer ORS correctly.
- If a child is still breastfeeding, continue with increased frequency and duration than usual.
  - Educate mothers to increase their own fluid intake to ensure adequate milk output.
  - If exclusively breastfeeding, add ORS or clean water; frequently, in small amounts, as much as the child will accept.
  - Add liquid foods if not exclusively breastfed (i.e. soup or rice water).
- ORS use is key, especially if a patient has already been treated with Plan B or C or if they live far away from medical care.
- Caregivers need to be taught explicitly how to prepare ORS and need two packages for treatment at home.

Treatment Plan B (some dehydration)
- Give ORS 75 mL/kg over 4 hours and if the child wants more, then give more.
- Give extra ORS for each loose stool (as in Treatment Plan A).
- If breastfeeding, continue for as much as the child will take.
- Reassess after 4 hours and reclassify the state of hydration.

Treatment Plan C (severe dehydration)
- If the child can drink, give ORS even during IV therapy.
- If you can start an IV:
  - Give 100 mL/kg of Ringer's lactate or normal saline as follows:
    —<12 months old—first 30 mL/kg in 1 hour followed by give 70 mL/kg in 5 hours.
    —12 months to 5 years old—first 30 mL/kg in 30 minutes followed by 70 mL/kg in 2.5 hours.

- Reassess each 1–2 hours—if not improving, increase the IV rate.
- Give ORS 5 mL/kg/hour when the child can drink.
- Reassess after 6 hours (aged <12 months) and after 3 hours (aged >12 months) and select the appropriate plan (A, B or C).
- Be wary of underlying malnutrition—it is prudent to assume some degree of subclinical malnutrition depending on the environment and some myocardial limit to tolerate a fluid challenge. Careful re-evaluation is prudent.
- In a scenario in which you cannot start an IV within 30 minutes but you can safely insert an NG tube in a child who is awake and with a patent airway:
  - Rehydrate by mouth or by NG tube with 20 mL/kg/hour for 6 hours—note that the rate of success for IV insertion may improve with some oral or NG tube hydration.
  - Reassess each hour—if there is no improvement by 3 hours, pursue a transfer to a higher level of care.
  - Administer fluids at a slower rate if there is repeated vomiting.
  - Some children will improve and will not need to be transferred to a higher level of care. Observe these non-transferred children for another 6 hours to ensure hydration can be maintained.
  - Reassess hydration status at 6 hours.
- If you cannot start an IV within 30 minutes and rehydration by NG tube is not successful:
  - Consider intraosseous needle insertion.
  - Try to refer the child to a higher level of care.

Table 27.1 Assessment of diarrhoea patients for dehydration

LOOK AT: CONDITION[a]	Well, alert	Restless, irritable	Lethargic or unconscious
EYES[b]	Normal	Sunken	Sunken
THIRST	Drinks normally, not thirsty	Thirsty, drinks eagerly	Drinks poorly, or not able to drink
FEEL: SKIN PINCH[c]	Goes back quickly	Goes back slowly	Goes back very slowly
DECIDE	The patient has **NO SIGNS OF DEHYDRATION**	If the patient has two or more signs, there is **SOME DEHYDRATION**	If the patients has two or more signs, there is **SEVERE DEHYDRATION**
TREAT	Use Treatment Plan A	Weigh the patient, if possible, and use Treatment Plan B	Weigh the patient and use Treatment Plan C URGENTLY

[a] Being lethargic and sleepy are *not* the same. A lethargic child is not simply asleep: the child's mental state is dull and the child cannot be fully awakened; the child may appear to be drifting into unconsciousness.

[b] In some infants and children, the eyes normally appear somewhat sunken. It is helpful to ask the mother if the child's eyes are normal or more sunken than usual.

[c] The skin pinch is less useful in infants or children with marasmus or kwashiorkor, or obese children.

Reproduced from The Treatment of Diarrhoea – A manual for physicians and other senior health workers, WHO, 2005, Page 8, with permission.

Practical tips
- ORS can be made at home; 1 litre of clean water with 1/2 teaspoon of salt and 6 teaspoons of sugar.
- Remind caregivers to give ORS in small sips as if it were hot fluid. As a general rule, 1–2 sips every 5 minutes; double after 30 minutes, and double again after 30 minutes.
- If the child vomits, then wait 10 minutes and restart more slowly than before.
- Feed as soon as possible, but start slowly.

For malnourished children
- Most children who die from diarrhoea are malnourished.
- Dehydration tends to be over-diagnosed among children with marasmus and under-diagnosed with kwashiorkor (see ⊃ Chapter 28).
- Signs of dehydration in malnourished children are difficult to assess. Weight changes are a more reliable way of establishing hydration status. Repeated weight measurements are needed and observations such as eagerness to drink, lethargy, extremity coolness, radial pulse and urine output need to be monitored.
- In severely malnourished children, ReSoMal (lower sodium content, higher potassium) is used instead of ORS.
- For prevention of dehydration, the approach is similar to Plan A in well-nourished children with ReSoMal being used instead of ORS. As a general guideline, 50–100 mL ReSoMal is given after each loose stool.
- The use of IV fluids in malnourished children and the possible risk of fluid overload is a field of debate. It is for this reason that many recommendations discourage the use of IV fluids in the malnourished (recommending that IV fluids be reserved for shock).
- In severe dehydration, ReSoMal, by mouth or by NG tube is used:
  - 5 mL/kg every 30 minutes for the first 2 hours, followed by 5–10 mL/kg/hours for 4–10 hours (depending on ongoing losses).
  - Monitor for fluid overload.

For adults
- Most adults initially respond well to 1–2 litres of IV fluid.
- IV fluid boluses should continue until a radial pulse is detected.
- For severe dehydration, such as cholera, aggressive hydration may be required (15–20 litres of fluid may be needed) via two or more large-bore catheters.
- When large volumes of fluid are given, as with cholera, Ringer's lactate is the preferred option.
- Start ORS as soon as possible alongside the infusion.

Supplementation

Zinc supplementation
- In children, zinc supplementation reduces the duration and severity of diarrhoea and has been shown to prevent future episodes.

- Supplementation is recommended for both children <6 months (10 mg) and >6 months (20 mg/day) × 14 days. For small children, zinc can be dissolved into fluid. If a child is receiving ready-to-use therapeutic feeds (which contains zinc), additional supplementation is not needed.

Use of antibiotics and antiemetics

- Avoid antiemetics in children as they often cause sedation and reduced rehydration ability.
- Most episodes of gastroenteritis are viral in origin. Even in acute bacterial gastroenteritis antibiotics are not always indicated.
- Bloody diarrhoea among children is usually caused by *Shigella*, and should be treated with antibiotics. Recommendations for the choice of antibiotics for *Shigella, Giardia, Entamoeba,* and *Schistosoma* species are given in Table 27.2.

> In cholera, hydration is the main treatment, not antibiotics. Antibiotics, however, can reduce the volume and duration of diarrhoea, and reduce the carrier state duration. Give antibiotics for moderately to severely dehydrated patients, those passing large volumes of stools, and those who are hospitalized. ⟩ See Chapter 35 for more information.

Follow-up

- Advise to return immediately if the patient develops any danger signs (lethargy, unconsciousness, convulsions, inability to eat or drink).
- Otherwise, follow-up should be in 5 days if there is no improvement in diarrhoea.

Table 27.2 Antimicrobial treatment

Causative agent	Antimicrobial treatment
Shigella species	Ciprofloxacin, oral, adult dose: 500 mg twice daily, child (>1 month) dose 15 mg/kg/dose twice daily × 3 days
	Note: local susceptibility patterns (e.g. in central Africa) may require other choices such as azithromycin or ceftriaxone[4]
Giardia lamblia	Metronidazole, oral, adult dose 2 g daily; child dose 30 mg/kg daily × 3 days
Entamoeba histolytica	Metronidazole, oral, adult dose 500–800 mg every 8 hours; child dose 45 mg/kg/dose every 8 hours × 5 days
Schistosoma mansoni	Praziquantel, oral, 40 mg/kg, single dose

Prevention of diarrhoea and vomiting

- Breastfeeding reduces the incidence of diarrhoea and should be exclusive until 6 months of age.
- It is critical to emphasize to families *not* to reduce fluid intake, particularly for children. This mistake is often a hidden cause of deaths at home.
- Encourage hand washing among family members before food preparation, after changing clothing soiled with stool or urine, after bathing children and before feeding children or oneself.
- Measures to improve water and sanitation are essential. Liaise with other actors (government organizations or NGOs) involved in Water Sanitation and Hygiene (WASH) to improve the quantity and quality of water available to the population.
- Ensure suitable resources for toileting, bathing and cooking.

References

1. Salama P, Spiegel P, Talley L, Waldman R. Lessons learned from complex emergencies over past decade. Lancet 2004;364:1801–13.
2. Médecins Sans Frontières. Clinical Guidelines: Diagnosis and Treatment Manual. 2017. ℘ https://medicalguidelines.msf.org/viewport/CG/english/clinical-guidelines-16686604.html
3. World Health Organization. Pocket Book of Hospital Care For Children: Guidelines for the Management of Common Childhood Illnesses. 2nd ed. Geneva: WHO; 2013. ℘ http://www.who.int/maternal_child_adolescent/documents/child_hospital_care/en/
4. World Health Organization. Guidelines for the Control of Shigellosis, Including Epidemics Due to Shigella Dysenteriae Type 1. Geneva: WHO; 2005. ℘ http://whqlibdoc.who.int/publications/2005/9241592330.pdf

Malnutrition

Kevin Chan and Jennifer Turnbull

Context of malnutrition

Malnutrition is a spectrum of disorders that can be grossly divided into *macronutrient* and *micronutrient deficiencies*, and into *acute* and *chronic*. There are innumerable terms used in the malnutrition literature: *stunting, wasting, severe acute malnutrition, underweight, marasmus*, and *kwashiorkor*, which can be confusing. During complex humanitarian emergencies, acute malnutrition serves as an important indicator of the severity of the crisis. Recognition and treatment of severe forms of acute micro- and macronutrient deficiency will be a priority in emergency situations, particularly among children.

- The assessment of global acute malnutrition (GAM), which includes moderate acute malnutrition (MAM) and severe acute malnutrition (SAM), is based on the rate of children aged 6–59 months who are below 2 standard deviations (SD) of the norms for weight-to-height.
- This has been shown to act as an indicator of overall population nutritional status. The WHO recognizes GAM levels of 10–14% of the under-five population as serious, and levels ≥15% as critical.[1]

Epidemiology

- Malnutrition is most often encountered in the under-five population and in specific vulnerable subsets of adults, such as those with HIV/AIDS and pregnant women.
- Greater than 90 million children under 5 years of age are underweight globally.
- Of these, 20 million children suffer from SAM, mostly in the WHO African and South-East Asia Region.
- SAM mortality contributes to 35% of under-five mortality globally, and children suffering from SAM have a ninefold risk of dying over normal-weight children with a case fatality rate of 30–50%.[2]

Causes

- Malnutrition occurs when the diet does not provide the calories, protein, and micronutrients required for growth and maintenance of health, or the individual is unable to utilize the nutrients available due to illness.
- The causes of malnutrition are complex, and while food insecurity plays an important role, the populations most affected by humanitarian crises are often chronically undernourished.
- Fig. 28.1 illustrates the interplay of causes at the societal, family, and individual level.[3]

Relationship between infectious disease and malnutrition

- There is a vicious cycle of illness and malnutrition.
- Infections can cause decreased food intake, due to decreased appetite or poor mobility to access food. During acute illness, a precarious nutritional status can deteriorate to SAM and its complications.
- Similarly, malnutrition itself can cause anorexia, through a complex interplay of gut dysfunction, altered microbiome, and intestinal bacterial and fungal overgrowth. As malnutrition worsens, susceptibility to infections rises.
- The leading causes of mortality in malnutrition are infectious.

Conceptual framework of the causes of undernutrition

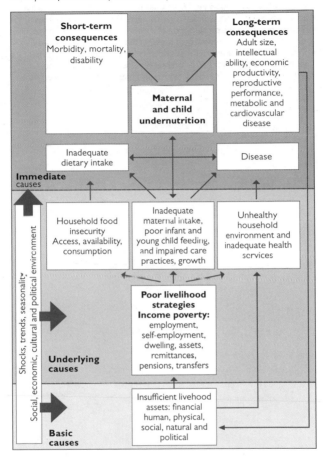

Fig. 28.1 Factors affecting malnutrition. Reproduced with permission from The Sphere Handbook: Humanitarian Charter and Minimum Standards in Humanitarian Response (© The Sphere Project 2011) p146.

Management keys

There are several management/therapeutic keys that reduce mortality:

- Early intervention is essential, prior to malnutrition-related anorexia.
- There should be the presumption of existing infection, whether occult or obvious, and early treatment is essential to decreasing mortality.
- Treatment has evolved to focus primarily on outpatient management with only a small subset of critical cases requiring hospitalization.
- Adherence to protocols on diagnosis and management has been shown to reduce mortality.

Clinical assessment of malnutrition

Early recognition

- All children presenting for medical care should be triaged using the WHO ETAT protocol. See ➲ Chapter 16 for more information.
- Dangers signs signifying severe medical pathology need to be identified and treated as soon as possible (see ➲ Box 28.1).[5]
- Children who present no danger signs can then be assessed for priority signs, including signs of wasting or oedema suggestive of malnutrition.
- The priority in the field will be to quickly identify the child with SAM and to determine if they will require inpatient or outpatient care. All children should be assessed for malnutrition as part of triage and three criteria can be used to diagnose SAM:
  - Mid-upper arm circumference (MUAC): a good screening tool that allows rapid identification of children aged 6–59 months with SAM who have the highest risk of mortality. MUAC can be used as a sole indicator in humanitarian emergencies.
  - Weight-for-height: another measure of malnutrition (a diagnosis of SAM can be made if either MUAC or weight-for-height meet criteria).
  - Bilateral pitting oedema: its presence in the setting of other findings suggestive of malnutrition is sufficient for the diagnosis of SAM, regardless of MUAC or weight-for-height.

History and examination

- Key features of a focused history and physical examination are listed in Table 28.1, p. 416.[5-7]
- Some basic investigations that should be performed are haemoglobin, malaria rapid test if endemic, and blood glucose if suspected hypoglycaemia.
- Other laboratory tests such as electrolytes are of little value in SAM, and can in fact be misleading, despite the fact that electrolytes are commonly unbalanced.[4]
- Other tests can be performed as needed such as chest X-ray and urinalysis (if available, and urinalysis only if there is a question of cause of oedema or possible UTI).

Box 28.1 Danger signs of severe disease in children

- High fever
- Hypothermia
- Increased respiratory rate
- Respiratory distress
- Persistent vomiting
- Persistent diarrhoea or dysentery
- Convulsion, lethargy, apathy, or hypoglycaemia
- Severe pallor
- Severe dehydration
- Inability to feed or breastfed.

Recognition of malnutrition

For simplicity, this section separates macronutrient and micronutrient deficiency. The clinical reality is far more complex and all forms of malnutrition likely represent a spectrum of overlapping deficiencies.

Macronutrient deficiency

There are two distinct clinical spectrums within SAM. These are *marasmus* and *kwashiorkor*. These two syndromes can overlap resulting in findings of both conditions (see Fig. 28.2, p. 417). Table 28.2 compares the clinical features of both syndromes.[8]

Table 28.1 History and physical examination in malnutrition

History	Physical
• Recent weight loss and appetite	• Triage and search for danger signs
• History related to intercurrent illness (fever, cough, vomiting, diarrhoea, signs of upper respiratory infection)	• MUAC, weight-for-height, oedema
	• Temperature, heart and respiratory rate
• Dietary and breastfeeding history	• Head and neck: signs of infection, eye disease, hair changes
• Vaccination and vitamin A supplementation	• Chest: signs of lower respiratory infection
• Family history of TB, HIV, other illness	• Heart: murmur
• Social history: number of children, birth order, living conditions	• Abdomen: hepatosplenomegaly, mass, distention
	• Skin and lymphatic: swollen or draining lymph nodes, desquamation, hyperpigmentation, skin infection
	• Neurological: reflexes, tone, power

Table 28.2 Comparison of marasmus and kwashiorkor

Marasmus	Kwashiorkor
Weight-for-height <3 SD below the norm	Weight-for-height may be preserved
Total caloric malnutrition (simplification as pathophysiology more complex)	Protein malnutrition, sometimes in presence of fair to good caloric intake (simplification as pathophysiology more complex)
Obvious emaciation, loss of subcutaneous fat	Pitting oedema: feet > shins > forehead
Sunken eyes	Skin changes: hyperpigmentation > general desquamation
Lethargic	Irritable
Bradycardia, hypothermia	
Decreased skin turgor, dry mucous membranes, sunken eyes even in absence of dehydration	

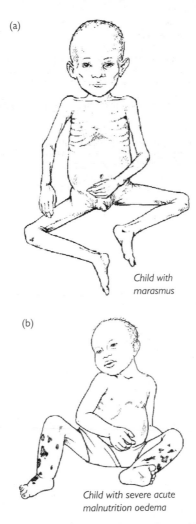

(a)

Child with marasmus

(b)

Child with severe acute malnutrition oedema

Fig. 28.2 Clinical spectrum of macronutrient deficiency. Reprinted from WHO pocketbook for hospital care of children, Second edition, WHO, Chapter: Severe Acute Malnutrition, pages 198–199, Copyright 2013. (www.who.int/maternal_child_adolescent/documents/child_hospital_care/en/).

Micronutrient deficiency

The most common endemic micronutrient deficiencies are iodine, iron, vitamin A, and zinc, affecting at least one-third of the world's population. These deficiencies can increase mortality and susceptibility to infection, and can lead to morbidity such as blindness, decreased cognitive capacity, adverse birth outcomes, lower respiratory tract infections, and diarrhoea in children.

See Table 28.3 for common micronutrient deficiencies and associated clinical signs.

Table 28.3 Clinical signs of micronutrient deficiency

Micronutrient	Clinical signs
Iodine	Goitre, cretinism (growth stunting and developmental delay related to hypothyroidism)
Iron	Tiredness, pallor
Niacin	The '3 Ds': dermatitis, diarrhoea, dementia
Thiamine	Progressive severe weakness and wasting of muscles, heart failure presenting as tachypnoea and cyanosis, paralysis, loss of consciousness, ataxia, long-term consequences such as cognitive impairment
Vitamin A	Night blindness, conjunctival xerosis
Vitamin C	Bleeding, purple, swollen gums; pseudoparalysis, dry skin
Zinc	Lower respiratory tract infections and diarrhoea in children, dermatitis
Essential fatty acids	Dry skin, desquamation, dull hair, brittle nails

Adapted with permission from UNHCR 2011, Guidelines for Selective Feeding: The Management of Malnutrition in Emergencies.

Diagnosis of malnutrition

Children 6–59 months

- SAM in children aged 6–59 months is defined as MUAC <115 mm or/
and weight-for-height <3 SD or/and bilateral pitting oedema.
- It has been shown that children below these cut-offs have a highly
elevated risk of death, and have higher weight gain and faster recovery
when receiving a therapeutic diet.
- Fig. 28.3 shows weight-for-height SD.
- Children with SAM can be further classified into those requiring
inpatient management (complicated SAM), and those who can
be managed in an ambulatory setting (uncomplicated SAM). See
Table 28.4.[7]

(a)   **Weight-for-length reference card (below 87 cm)**

	Boys' weight (kg)				Length	Girls' weight (kg)				
–4 SD	–3 SD	–2 SD	–1 SD	Median	(cm)	Median	–1 SD	–2 SD	–3 SD	–4 SD
1.7	1.9	2.0	2.2	2.4	45	2.5	2.3	2.1	1.9	1.7
1.8	2.0	2.2	2.4	2.6	46	2.6	2.4	2.2	2.0	1.9
2.0	2.1	2.3	2.5	2.8	47	2.8	2.6	2.4	2.2	2.0
2.1	2.3	2.5	2.7	2.9	48	3.0	2.7	2.5	2.3	2.1
2.2	2.4	2.6	2.9	3.1	49	3.2	2.9	2.6	2.4	2.2
2.4	2.6	2.8	3.0	3.3	50	3.4	3.1	2.8	2.6	2.4
2.5	2.7	3.0	3.2	3.5	51	3.6	3.3	3.0	2.8	2.5
2.7	2.9	3.2	3.5	3.8	52	3.8	3.5	3.2	2.9	2.7
2.9	3.1	3.4	3.7	4.0	53	4.0	3.7	3.4	3.1	2.8
3.1	3.3	3.6	3.9	4.3	54	4.3	3.9	3.6	3.3	3.0
3.3	3.6	3.8	4.2	4.5	55	4.5	4.2	3.8	3.5	3.2
3.5	3.8	4.1	4.4	4.8	56	4.8	4.4	4.0	3.7	3.4
3.7	4.0	4.3	4.7	5.1	57	5.1	4.6	4.3	3.9	3.6
3.9	4.3	4.6	5.0	5.4	58	5.4	4.9	4.5	4.1	3.8
4.1	4.5	4.8	5.3	5.7	59	5.6	5.1	4.7	4.3	3.9
4.3	4.7	5.1	5.5	6.0	60	5.9	5.4	4.9	4.5	4.1
4.5	4.9	5.3	5.8	6.3	61	6.1	5.6	5.1	4.7	4.3
4.7	5.1	5.6	6.0	6.5	62	6.4	5.8	5.3	4.9	4.5
4.9	5.3	5.8	6.2	6.8	63	6.6	6.0	5.5	5.1	4.7
5.1	5.5	6.0	6.5	7.0	64	6.9	6.3	5.7	5.3	4.8
5.3	5.7	6.2	6.7	7.3	65	7.1	6.5	5.9	5.5	5.0
5.5	5.9	6.4	6.9	7.5	66	7.3	6.7	6.1	5.6	5.1
5.6	6.1	6.6	7.1	7.7	67	7.5	6.9	6.3	5.8	5.3
5.8	6.3	6.8	7.3	8.0	68	7.7	7.1	6.5	6.0	5.5
6.0	6.5	7.0	7.6	8.2	69	8.0	7.3	6.7	6.1	5.6
6.1	6.6	7.2	7.8	8.4	70	8.2	7.5	6.9	6.3	5.8
6.3	6.8	7.4	8.0	8.6	71	8.4	7.7	7.0	6.5	5.9
6.4	7.0	7.6	8.2	8.9	72	8.6	7.8	7.2	6.6	6.0
6.6	7.2	7.7	8.4	9.1	73	8.8	8.0	7.4	6.8	6.2
6.7	7.3	7.9	8.6	9.3	74	9.0	8.2	7.5	6.9	6.3
6.9	7.5	8.1	8.8	9.5	75	9.1	8.4	7.7	7.1	6.5
7.0	7.6	8.3	8.9	9.7	76	9.3	8.5	7.8	7.2	6.6
7.2	7.8	8.4	9.1	9.9	77	9.5	8.7	8.0	7.4	6.7
7.3	7.9	8.6	9.3	10.1	78	9.7	8.9	8.2	7.5	6.9
7.4	8.1	8.7	9.5	10.3	79	9.9	9.1	8.3	7.7	7.0
7.6	8.2	8.9	9.6	10.4	80	10.1	9.2	8.5	7.8	7.1
7.7	8.4	9.1	9.8	10.6	81	10.3	9.4	8.7	8.0	7.3
7.9	8.5	9.2	10.0	10.8	82	10.5	9.6	8.8	8.1	7.5
8.0	8.7	9.4	10.2	11.0	83	10.7	9.8	9.0	8.3	7.6
8.2	8.9	9.6	10.4	11.3	84	11.0	10.1	9.2	8.5	7.8
8.4	9.1	9.8	10.6	11.5	85	11.2	10.3	9.4	8.7	8.0
8.6	9.3	10.0	10.8	11.7	86	11.5	10.5	9.7	8.9	8.1

(b) **Weight-for-height reference card (87 cm and above)**

Boys' weight (kg)					Height	Girls' weight (kg)				
−4 SD	−3 SD	−2 SD	−1 SD	Median	(cm)	Median	−1 SD	−2 SD	−3 SD	−4 SD
8.9	9.6	10.4	11.2	12.2	87	11.9	10.9	10.0	9.2	8.4
9.1	9.8	10.6	11.5	12.4	88	12.1	11.1	10.2	9.4	8.6
9.3	10.0	10.8	11.7	12.6	89	12.4	11.4	10.4	9.6	8.8
9.4	10.2	11.0	11.9	12.9	90	12.6	11.6	10.6	9.8	9.0
9.6	10.4	11.2	12.1	13.1	91	12.9	11.8	10.9	10.0	9.1
9.8	10.6	11.4	12.3	13.4	92	13.1	12.0	11.1	10.2	9.3
9.9	10.8	11.6	12.6	13.6	93	13.4	12.3	11.3	10.4	9.5
10.1	11.0	11.8	12.8	13.8	94	13.6	12.5	11.5	10.6	9.7
10.3	11.1	12.0	13.0	14.1	95	13.9	12.7	11.7	10.8	9.8
10.4	11.3	12.2	13.2	14.3	96	14.1	12.9	11.9	10.9	10.0
10.6	11.5	12.4	13.4	14.6	97	14.4	13.2	12.1	11.1	10.2
10.8	11.7	12.6	13.7	14.8	98	14.7	13.4	12.3	11.3	10.4
11.0	11.9	12.9	13.9	15.1	99	14.9	13.7	12.5	11.5	10.5
11.2	12.1	13.1	14.2	15.4	100	15.2	13.9	12.8	11.7	10.7
11.3	12.3	13.3	14.4	15.6	101	15.5	14.2	13.0	12.0	10.9
11.5	12.5	13.6	14.7	15.9	102	15.8	14.5	13.3	12.2	11.1
11.7	12.8	13.8	14.9	16.2	103	16.1	14.7	13.5	12.4	11.3
11.9	13.0	14.0	15.2	16.5	104	16.4	15.0	13.8	12.6	11.5
12.1	13.2	14.3	15.5	16.8	105	16.8	15.3	14.0	12.9	11.8
12.3	13.4	14.5	15.8	17.2	106	17.1	15.6	14.3	13.1	12.0
12.5	13.7	14.8	16.1	17.5	107	17.5	15.9	14.6	13.4	12.2
12.7	13.9	15.1	16.4	17.8	108	17.8	16.3	14.9	13.7	12.4
12.9	14.1	15.3	16.7	18.2	109	18.2	16.6	15.2	13.9	12.7
13.2	14.4	15.6	17.0	18.5	110	18.6	17.0	15.5	14.2	12.9
13.4	14.6	15.9	17.3	18.9	111	19.0	17.3	15.8	14.5	13.2
13.6	14.9	16.2	17.6	19.2	112	19.4	17.7	16.2	14.8	13.5
13.8	15.2	16.5	18.0	19.6	113	19.8	18.0	16.5	15.1	13.7
14.1	15.4	16.8	18.3	20.0	114	20.2	18.4	16.8	15.4	14.0
14.3	15.7	17.1	18.6	20.4	115	20.7	18.8	17.2	15.7	14.3
14.6	16.2	17.4	19.0	20.8	116	21.1	19.2	17.5	16.0	14.5
14.8	16.2	17.7	19.3	21.2	117	21.5	19.6	17.8	16.3	14.8
15.0	16.5	18.0	19.7	21.6	118	22.0	19.9	18.2	16.6	15.1
15.3	16.8	18.3	20.0	22.0	119	22.4	20.3	18.5	16.9	15.4
15.5	17.1	18.6	20.4	22.4	120	22.8	20.7	18.9	17.3	15.6

Fig. 28.3 WHO weight-for-length tables. Reproduced from WHO Child Growth Standards and the Identification of Severe Acute Malnutrition in Infants and Children, Geneva: World Health Organization; 2009. English. Available from: www.ncbi.nlm.nih.gov/books/NBK200776/.

Table 28.4 Admission criteria for ambulatory and inpatient care

Ambulatory therapeutic feeding centre (ATFC)	Inpatient therapeutic feeding centre (ITFC)
Weight-for height <3 SD *or*	Weight-for-height <3 SD *or*
MUAC <115 mm *or*	MUAC <115 mm *or*
1+ oedema	2+ or 3+ oedema
No severe medical pathology	Severe medical pathology (see danger signs listed in Box 28.1)
No anorexia	Anorexia (child will not eat ready-to-use therapeutic food (RUTF), such as Plumpy'Nut®)

Grading of bilateral nutritional oedema:
1+: feet or ankles.
2+: feet and pre-tibial lower extremities.
3+: above plus forehead.

Infants aged 1–6 months

- Diagnostic criteria for this age group are similar to those children aged 6–59 months, however MUAC is not used.
- All infants with weight-for-height <-3 SD (or <-2 SD + danger signs) and/or bilateral pitting oedema are considered to have SAM, and should be treated in the inpatient setting regardless of the grade of oedema or absence of severe medical pathology.
- For infants <45 cm in height, SAM is defined as >10% weight loss.

Adults

SAM in adults can be diagnosed based on body mass index (BMI) or MUAC. See Table 28.5.[9]

Table 28.5 Malnutrition in adults

	BMI	MUAC (mm)
Men	<16	<224
Women	<16	<214
Pregnant women (cut-off should be chosen based on number of women falling under each category and the resources available)	N/A	<210 (in emergency settings) <230 (fetus at risk of growth retardation)

Treatment of malnutrition

- Standardized nutritional protocols, adhering to WHO guidelines, are the key to successful treatment of malnutrition.
- In addition to WHO protocols, there are also organizational protocols of NGOs involved in the management of SAM (e.g. MSF, Action Contre la Faim); most countries with high rates of malnutrition have well-established national guidelines.
- The management of SAM involves systematic and nutritional treatment, and the identification and management of life-threatening emergencies.

Systematic treatment

- Systematic treatments are given to all severely malnourished children to address common pathologies seen almost universally, such as infection and micronutrient deficiency (see Table 28.6, p. 423).
- In addition to the systematic treatment, sensory stimulation and emotional support should be provided as most malnourished children have delayed mental and behavioural development. In the inpatient setting, this should include 15–30 minutes per day of structured therapeutic and physical activity once well enough. Maternal involvement and sensitization can include health promotion around hygiene, nutrition, and health planning.

Nutritional treatment

- Re-nutrition is more complex than simply providing calories, protein, and fat as almost all malnourished children have electrolyte imbalances and intestinal dysfunction.
- These imbalances are not properly reflected in serum electrolyte testing, and this testing should therefore be avoided, as it can be misleading. Nutritional treatment aims to correct these electrolyte imbalances, and to allow catch-up growth.
- Regardless of treatment setting, breastfeeding should be encouraged

See → Table 28.4 p. 420 to identify children who can be treated in the ATFC versus ITFC.

Ambulatory

- RUTF is the mainstay of ambulatory nutritional treatment. RUTF should be considered a medication and prescribed based on protocols (see Table 28.7, p. 424).[7]
- RUTF, such as Plumpy'Nut®, adhere to the WHO standards of macronutrient and micronutrient treatment, are easy to transport, and do not require refrigeration.

Inpatient

- Inpatient nutritional treatment is more complex and combines the use of therapeutic milk and RUTF (Table 28.7, p. 424).[7] It is divided into three phases:
  - Stabilization
  - Transition
  - Rehabilitation.
- Each phase has strict criteria (Table 28.8, p. 424) and children in each phase should be physically separated to ensure appropriate protocols.

Table 28.6 Systematic treatment in the management of SAM

Treatment	Dose	Day							
		1	2	3	4	5	6	7	8
Amoxicillin	80 mg/kg/day ÷ twice a day	+	+	+	+	+			
Vitamin A	High dose is only administered if evidence of eye disease related to vitamin A deficiency or measles infection	+	+						+ (Day 15)
Albendazole (praziquantel 40 mg/kg if high schistosomiasis prevalence)	<8 kg: 200 mg ≥8 kg: 400 mg								+
Measles vaccination (review all vaccines)	Defer if intensive care unit or HIV with CD4 ≤25%	+							
Malaria rapid test		+							
Tuberculosis screening[a]	On admission and then every 2 weeks	+							
HIV counselling and testing[b]	Ideally done within a few days of admission	+							

[a] TB screening includes TB+ close contact, respiratory disease not responding to antibiotics, signs of extra-pulmonary TB, unexplained fever >2 weeks, no response to nutritional treatment after 2 weeks, absence of appetite after 2 weeks, chronic diarrhoea, >2 episodes unexplained severe anaemia, HIV+ve.

[b] HIV testing should be performed in contexts where prevalence is >1% and treatment is available.

Adapted with permission from MSF Geneva, MSF OCG and OCBA Feb 2015. Protocols for Management of Nutritional Support in Children with Severe Acute Malnutrition, Table 6.2, p40.

Considerations for phase 1 and 2 patients

ITFC inpatients tend to be sicker and more vulnerable to complications (see ➲ 'Malnutrition emergencies' pp. 426–31). Patients in phase 1 are at particular risk of fluid and electrolyte shifts and require a diet that is low in sodium, fat, and protein. Table 28.9 shows the composition of the therapeutic milks used in the stabilization phase (F-75) and the rehabilitation inpatient phase (F-100).

Table 28.7 Nutritional treatment

Ambulatory therapeutic feeding centre (ATFC)	Inpatient therapeutic feeding centre (ITFC)		
	Phase 1: stabilization (≤7 days)	Transition phase (1–3 days)	Phase 2: rehabilitation
RUTF: 500 kcal/sachet			
<8 kg ≥8 kg	Therapeutic milk: F-75	RUTF or therapeutic milk: F-100	RUTF (or therapeutic milk: F-100)
2/day 3/day (14/week) (21/week)	100 kcal/kg/day (130 mL/kg/day)	130 kcal/kg/day (130 mL/kg/day)	200 kcal/kg/day
	8 meals/day	6 meals/day	6 meals/day
Encourage breastfeeding Offer other nutritionally appropriate foods if still hungry after RUTF	Encourage breastfeeding: offer 30 min *before* therapeutic meals Always offer orally before NG, even in a patient has NG in place Never force a child to eat		

Table 28.8 Criteria for each inpatient nutritional treatment phase

Phase 1: stabilization	Transition phase	Phase 2: rehabilitation
• Anorexia • Severe medical pathology including severe anaemia • Oedema 2+ and 3+ • Children in other phases with re-apparition of oedema or signs of fluid overload (see ➲ 'Malnutrition emergencies' pp. 426–31), or suspected refeeding syndrome	• Oedema 3+ on admission that has not improved during 7 days in phase 1 • Diarrhoea in a child in phase 2 • Children in intensive care beyond 7 days in phase 1	• Ambulatory patients not gaining weight • No severe medical pathology • Good appetite and ability to eat RUTF

Adapted with permission from MSF Geneva, MSF OCG and OCBA Feb 2015. Protocols for Management of Nutritional Support in Children with Severe Acute Malnutrition, Table 6.3.1, p44.

Table 28.9 Composition of therapeutic milks

Constituent	Amount per 100 mL	
	F-75	F-100
Energy	75 kcal	100 kcal
Protein	0.9 g	2.9 g
Lactose	1.3 g	4.2 g
Potassium	3.6 mmol	5.9 mmol
Sodium	0.6 mmol	1.9 mmol
Magnesium	0.43 mmol	0.73 mmol
Zinc	2.0 mg	2.3 mg
Copper	0.25 mg	0.25 mg
Percentage energy from:	5%	12%
Protein	32%	53%
Fat		
Osmolarity	333 mOsmol/L	419 mOsmol/L

Reprinted from Management of Severe Malnutrition: A Manual for Physicians and Other Senior Health Workers, WHO, page 14, Copyright 1999.

Malnutrition emergencies

- Malnourished children have increased susceptibility to a host of conditions compared to well-nourished children.
- Prevention of many emergencies can be achieved through careful monitoring and adhering to protocols.
- Despite efforts, emergency situations can arise during treatment, which should be quickly identified and managed.

Hypothermia

- Malnourished children are at risk due to a lack of adipose tissue and low metabolic rates. Even in some hot climates, night-time temperatures can dip significantly, putting these patients at risk of hypothermia.
- Hypothermia can also signify severe infection and/or hypoglycaemia, and both should be suspected and treated.

Definition
Any temperature <36.5°C in a malnourished child is hypothermia that needs assessment. A temperature <35.5°C is an emergency.

Treatment
- Suspect sepsis/meningitis and treat.
- Suspect hypoglycaemia and treat.
- Prevention is key, particularly at night (hats can be very useful).
- Avoid over-correction (no hot baths or hot water bottles).
- Encourage skin-to-skin contact with the mother (kangaroo method).
- Re-evaluate every 2 hours until core temperature >36°C.

Hypoglycaemia

- Severely malnourished children have less energy reserves and are less able to maintain normoglycaemia in the face of stressors, i.e. infection.
- Hypoglycaemia and hypothermia often occur together and both should be suspected and treated if one is discovered.
- Hypoglycaemia is of particular concern in the convulsing and/or unconscious patient. If unable to test blood glucose, hypoglycaemia should be suspected in all cases of sudden clinical deterioration, lethargy, hypothermia, coma, and convulsion.

Definition
Blood glucose <3 mmol/L (54 mg/dL) in malnourished children.

Treatment
- Prevention is key.
- Treat: give IV glucose 10% solution 5 mL/kg over 2–3 minutes. See
  ➋ Malnutrition: appendix' p. 436 to make glucose 10% when only glucose 50% is available.
- Recheck glucose 30 minutes after first glucose and re-evaluate until clinically stable and glucose normal.
- If repeated boluses necessary, consider switching to IV maintenance.
- In an unconscious patient, avoid treating via the oral or NG route where possible. This can lead to aspiration.

- Alternatively, if awake, feed. Split into four equal amounts and give in half-hourly intervals.
- *Use small, frequent feeds even overnight—every 2 hours.*
- Suspect sepsis/meningitis and treat.
- Suspect malaria and treat (if endemic).

Hypovolaemia

Classic signs of dehydration are not reliable in malnourished patients:
- Marasmus patients have decreased skin turgor, sunken eyes, and dry mucous membranes even in the absence of dehydration.
- Kwashiorkor patients are total body fluid overloaded but can be intravascularly depleted and dehydrated even with oedema.

Treatment
- Prevention is key, monitor fluid losses such as vomiting and diarrhoea and replace losses with rehydration solution for malnourished children (ReSoMal), encourage breastfeeding, and continue therapeutic feeds.
- Except in hypovolaemic shock or in altered mental status, dehydration should be treated *orally*:

ReSoMal
- Except in cases of cholera, ReSoMal should be used in malnourished patients instead of oral rehydration salts (ORS) due to lower osmolarity
- ReSoMal is prepared with 2 litres of water and is composed of less sodium and more potassium, magnesium, zinc, and copper.
- See ➲ Malnutrition: appendix' p. 436 for a ReSoMal recipe if only standard ORS is available.
- Oral rehydration consists of 5 mL/kg every 30 minutes orally of ReSoMal over the first 2 hours, followed by 10 mL/kg each hour orally until dehydration is corrected.
- Each loose stool should be replaced with 5 mL/kg of ReSoMal if the child is only mildly dehydrated.
- ReSoMal can be administered in the *conscious* vomiting patient by NG drop-by-drop using an IV drip set-up.
- In the setting of severe dehydration and inability to tolerate oral or NG rehydration, IV rehydration with glucose 5%/Ringer's lactate at twice maintenance can be used.
- *ReSoMal is only for oral use, never IV use.*
- Even with oral rehydration, patients should be monitored for sudden fluid overload (increased heart and respiratory rate, newly palpable liver edge during treatment).
- Breastfeeding and therapeutic feeding should continue.
- *Hypovolaemic shock*: see Box 28.2, p. 428 for diagnosis of shock and Table 28.10, p. 430 for management.

Infection and septic shock

- Malnourished children suffer from intestinal bacterial overgrowth and have decreased immune function. All malnourished children should be presumed to have some form of infection and antibiotics should be given systematically (see ➲ Table 28.6 p. 423 for systematic treatment).

Box 28.2 Diagnosis of shock (hypovolaemic or septic)
All three criteria:
- Weak pulse, or increased heart rate or bradycardia (for age).
- Cold hands/feet.
- Capillary refill time $\geq$3 seconds.

Other signs commonly seen in shock
- Lethargy or unconsciousness.
- Decreased urine output.
- Increased respiratory rate (due to acidosis).

- Focal signs of infection should be sought and treated but typical signs such as fever may *not* be present.
- Hypoglycaemia, altered mentation, and hypothermia are hallmarks of severe infection.

Treatment
- Give broad-spectrum antibiotics. See country and organizational protocols for treatment and antibiotic choice for different infections.
- *Infection without complications*: oral antibiotics are indicated (e.g. amoxicillin. See ➔ Box 28.1 p. 415).
- *Infection with danger signs, with or without shock*: IV or IM antibiotics are recommended for children:
  - Ceftriaxone 100 mg/kg/day divided in 1 or 2 doses.
  - Consider adding cloxacillin if no response to treatment after 2 days and evidence of skin breakdown.
  - Consider adding metronidazole if gastrointestinal source.
  - Second choice: ampicillin 50 mg/kg IM/IV every 6 hours *and* genta-micin: 7.5 mg/kg IM/IV once daily.
  - Consider TB treatment if not responding to standard antibiotic therapy after 10 days.
  - Consider resistant organisms and systemic fungaemia in non-responders to first- and second-line broad-spectrum antibiotics.
- *Septic shock*: see Box 28.2 for diagnosis of shock; management as follows:

Management of septic shock
Evidence for the type, amount, and infusion rate of IV fluids for shock in children, particularly with malnutrition, is limited or evolving. In the absence of consensus, an attempt should be made to implement protocols that use internationally accepted guidelines, while accounting for resource limitation in humanitarian contexts. See ➔ Chapter 17 'Approach to paediatric care' and Chapter 18 'Shock' for more information. With this in mind, the following protocols are proposed.

Systematic treatment for all malnourished children in shock (septic or hypovolaemic)
- Blood glucose, treat hypoglycaemia.
- Check haemoglobin.
- Rapid testing for malaria.

- Give oxygen if available until recovery. Patients in shock are hypoxic at the vital organ level even in the presence of a normal saturation.
- Keep warm.
- Monitor vital signs: watch for signs of fluid overload during and after IV fluids and re-evaluate regularly for improvement of shock (see Box 28.2, p. 428 for signs of shock).
- If available: blood culture, urinalysis, urine culture, lumber puncture.

Antibiotics: should be given regardless of type of shock

- Ceftriaxone IV/IM 100 mg/kg/day divided in 1 or 2 doses.
- Consider adding another antibiotic if source identified or suspected
- Second choice: ampicillin 50 mg/kg IM/IV every 6 hours *and* gentamicin: 7.5 mg/kg IM/IV once daily
- Treat with antimalarials if malaria +ve.

Hypoxia

Children with respiratory distress due to respiratory infections may be hypoxic. Early detection of respiratory infection saves lives.

Definition

Oxygen saturation <90%. If oximetry is unavailable, assume hypoxia in the presence of central cyanosis, or severe chest indrawing, and grunting and altered level of consciousness.

Treatment

- Lower respiratory tract infections may present with subtle or *no* signs/symptoms in malnourished children (*no* tachypnoea, dyspnoea, desaturation, or crackles). Early treatment of malnourished children for infection prior to the development of these signs is important see (➔ 'Infection and septic shock' pp. 427–8)
- *Streptococcus pneumoniae* and *Haemophilus influenzae* species are the most common bacterial pathogens in lower respiratory tract infections (as in well-nourished children).
- *Staphylococcus* and Gram-negative organisms should also be considered in malnourished children with sepsis due to skin breakdown and intestinal bacteria overgrowth.
- Titrate O_2 therapy to a saturation between 90% and 96%.
- In the absence of oximetry, apply O_2 to all patients presenting with respiratory distress and/or altered level of consciousness.
- Severe respiratory infections require IV or IM antibiotics (see ➔ p. 428).
- Tachypnoea may be caused by lower respiratory tract infections but can also be due to acidosis in the setting of malaria or severe infection. If other signs of shock (see Box 28.2, p. 428), treat for septic shock (Table 28.10, p. 430).

Convulsions

- These can be very obvious or subtle (just eyes or face).
- Malaria is particularly known for producing subtle convulsions.

Treatment

- Manage airway, breathing, and circulation first.

Table 28.10 Management of shock

- Weight.
- O₂.
- Elevate legs (unless suspected cardiogenic shock) and assess liver edge.
- IV or intraosseous.
- Check haemoglobin (Hb), glucose, rapid malaria test, and treat:
  - •Repeat Hb after transfusion, bolus, and at 120 min.
  - •Repeat glucose at 30, 60, 120, 180 min.
- Give IV ceftriaxone.

Shock with severe dehydration		Shock without severe dehydration		
Hb <6 g/dL	Hb ≥6 g/dL	Hb <6 g/dL	Hb 6–10 g/dL	Hb ≥10 g/dL
• Transfuse PRBC 15 mL/kg (or whole blood 20 mL/kg) over 3 hours • Maintenance fluid at 200% with D5/RL while waiting for blood, then reduce to 100% during transfusion (requires 2 IVs) • Reassess and treat according to Hb • Start ReSoMal once all signs of shock have resolved • Start F-75 at feeding times when all signs of shock have resolved	• 15 mL/kg of RL over 1 hour (maximum 2 boluses) • If shock resolved, or maximum boluses given: D5/RL 150–200% maintenance depending on ongoing losses × 2 hours • Reassess every 2 hours • Start ReSoMal once all signs of shock have resolved	• Transfuse PRBC 15 mL/kg (or whole blood 20 mL/kg) over 3 hours • Maintenance fluid at 100% with D5/RL while waiting for blood (requires 2 IVs)	• Maintenance fluid at 100% with D5/RL	• Bolus 10 mL/kg over 30 min • Reassess and repeat bolus if shock persists (maximum 3 boluses)
		• Maintenance fluids and start F-75 at feeding times when all signs of shock have resolved		

- Consider 100 mg IV thiamine slow infusion over 30–60 min via a separate IV:
  - <13 years old: 100 mg every 12 hours × 48 hours
  - ≥13 years old: 200 mg every 12 hours × 48 hours
- •Maintenance (beyond 48 hours): 50 mg/day orally or NG × 1 month (once oral/NG possible)

D5, 5% dextrose; PRBC, packed red blood cells; RL, Ringer's lactate.

- Turn the child on their side into the recovery position and make sure airway is clear of secretions (never deep suction, i.e. beyond hard palate, as this can lead to vomiting or vagal-induced bradycardia).
- Apply O_2 during the convulsion, if available.
- Ensure the surroundings are free from objects that could cause trauma.
- Test and treat for hypoglycaemia.
- If the convulsion continues despite presumptive treatment of hypoglycaemia, give diazepam 0.5 mg/kg rectally (watch for respiratory depression). Can be repeated × 1.
- If convulsions continue despite diazepam × 2 and correction of hypoglycaemia, proceed to IV phenytoin 20 mg/kg over 20 minutes.
- Always consider infection (bacterial, malaria) and treat.
- Consider other causes of prolonged convulsion such as fluid overload and electrolyte disturbances, by carefully reviewing the chart, clinical exam, and vital signs documentation prior to convulsions.
- Benign febrile seizures are a diagnosis of exclusion in humanitarian settings.

Pitfalls in inpatient management

Management of the malnourished child is very nuanced, and careful attention to standardized nutritional protocols greatly reduces the risk of errors and decreases mortality. See Box 28.3 for common errors of inpatient management.

> **Box 28.3 Pitfalls in inpatient management**
>
> *Diagnosis*
> - Failure to prevent, identify, and treat hypothermia.
> - Failure to prevent, identify, and treat hypoglycaemia.
> - Failure to consider and treat infection.
> - Failure to test haemoglobin prior to decisions of shock management.
> - Failure to identify anaemia and treat hookworm infection.
> - Failure to consider HIV or TB in children not responding to treatment after 2 weeks.
> - Overestimation of dehydration (i.e. weight not used to track fluid loss and recovery after oral rehydration).
> - Underestimation of dehydration in kwashiorkor patients (see ➲ 'Hypovolaemia' p. 427).
> - Failure to exclude medical causes of oedema (renal failure, cardiac failure, nephrotic syndrome, etc.).
> - Missing re-feeding syndrome when children may demonstrate congestive heart failure/fluid overload. It can also mimic sepsis and pneumonia, and can involve an altered level of consciousness. In this case, slow down the re-feeding rate by half, and consider adding thiamine.
> - Reliance on blood-work for clinical decisions and treatment (apart from Hb and glucose).
>
> *Medical treatment*
> - Lack of daily clinical assessments of children in phase 1.
> - Failure to separate critically ill patients from others in phase 1.
> - IV fluids administered to patients not in hypovolaemic or septic shock.
> - Poor supervision of required IV fluid administration and missing signs of fluid overload.
> - Treating nutritional oedema with diuretics, despite the exclusion of the medical causes as listed above. This can cause further volume depletion and electrolyte abnormalities in an already sick patient.
>
> *Nutritional treatment*
> - Administration of inappropriate food in the initial phase of re-nutrition (see ➲ 'Treatment of malnutrition' pp. 422–3).
> - Patients left >7 days in the initial phase of re-nutrition.

- No physical organization of the ward to distinguish between phase 1 and phase 2 patients (see Table 28.8 p. 424). Physically dividing up patients into the different phases of treatment avoids the risk of inappropriate therapeutic food being given and allows for increased supervision of patients in phase 1.
- Poor supervision and recording of meals and consumption.
- Absence of meals overnight or long intervals between meals.
- Overuse of NG tubes for re-nutrition and rehydration (NG tubes can be essential but should be removed as soon as the patient is taking oral food).
- Not breastfeeding as soon as the patient is able to do so, in young children and infants.

Monitoring of malnutrition

Patient monitoring

- Due to the vulnerability and potential for high mortality rates in this patient population, strict monitoring is essential.
- Table 28.11 describes the monitoring of children in both the ambulatory and inpatient settings.
- Patients should gain at least 10 g/kg/day during the inpatient rehabilitation phase. Weight gain <5 g/kg/day should prompt an in-depth assessment of the patient, looking for medical pathology (i.e. TB, HIV, diarrhoea.).
- In the ATFC, poor weight gain is a criterion for readmission to the ITFC.

Transition from ITFC to ATFC

- Patients should be assessed for transition between inpatient and ambulatory care (and vice versa), as well as discharge from the malnutrition programme completely. The following criteria are required for transition to ambulatory care:
  - Oedema has started to resolve.
  - Good appetite, eats RUTF (no therapeutic milk in ATFC).
  - No severe medical pathology or danger signs.
  - No injectable treatment.
- The transition is *not* based on percentage weight gain, MUAC, or weight-for-height.

Table 28.11 Patient monitoring guidelines

	ITFC		ATFC
	Phase 1 and transition	Phase 2	Weekly assessment
Weight	Daily	Every 2 days	• Physical exam and history looking for danger signs
MUAC	Once a week	Once a week	
Height	On admission	Once a month	
Oedema	Daily	Every 2 days	• Temperature, heart and respiratory rate
Temperature, heart and respiratory rate	Morning and evening (more if needed due to medical pathology)	Morning and evening for temperature, morning for heart and respiratory rates (more if needed due to medical pathology)	• Weight
• Oedema
• Appetite test
Medical assessment	Daily	Every 2 days	• Height and MUAC every 2 weeks
Observation of meals	Each meal	Each meal	
Inquiry about vomiting and/ or diarrhoea	Each event	Each event	

Adapted with permission from MSF Geneva, MSF OCG and OCBA Feb 2015. Protocols for Management of Nutritional Support in Children with Severe Acute Malnutrition, p39 & 56.

Discharge from malnutrition programme

With good-quality malnutrition treatment, and adherence to standardized protocols, patients will eventually recover enough to be completely discharged from the programme. Criteria for discharge are:

• Absence of oedema for 2 weeks
• Weight-for-height ≥ −2 SD
• MUAC ≥125 mm.

Programme monitoring

• Programme evaluation and data collection are important parts of maintaining the quality of a malnutrition programme.
• Trends in data can indicate the severity of and changes in the humanitarian emergency.

The following are important indicators that should be collected, along with their definitions. Table 28.12 shows target values as well as possible interpretations of the data.

Admissions: number of new patients in a given period

Discharges: total number of patients discharged from the programme

Average length of stay: total length of stay of all discharges (in days) divided by the total number of discharges

Table 28.12 Target values for programme monitoring

Indicator	Interpretation	ITFC	ATFC
• Admissions: • New cases • Discharges • Cured • Deaths • Defaults[a] • Non-recovered[b]	• Evolution of nutritional situation • Food security trends • Programme work load		
Readmissions		<5%	<5%
% cured	• Quality of programme • Quality of medical care • Accessibility	>80%	>80%
% defaults		<10%	<15%
% mortality		<10%	<2%
Length of stay	Quality of care	Stabilized <12 days Discharge <30 days	< 40 days
Average weight gain	Quality of care	>10 g/kg/day	5 g/kg/day

[a] Defaults: classified after third, absence from ATFC, and attempts made to trace patient.
[b] Non-recovered: do not meet programme discharge criteria after 4 months of treatment despite all treatment options being explored.

Adapted with permission from MSF Geneva, MSF OCG and OCBA Feb 2015. Protocols for Management of Nutritional Support in Children with Severe Acute Malnutrition, p71.

Malnutrition: appendix

Recipes for glucose 10% from glucose 50%

- Dilute 1 (50 mL) vial of glucose (D) 50% in 450 mL bag of G5% (i.e. 500 mL bag with 50 mL removed).
- Dilute 1 part G50% in 4 parts sterile water:
  - 10 mL syringe: 2 mL G50% + 8 mL sterile water.
  - 20 mL syringe: 4 mL G50% + 16 mL sterile water.
  - 50 mL syringe: 10 mL G50% + 40 mL sterile water.

Recipe for ReSoMal if only ORS available

- Mix 1 WHO-formulation ORS 1-litre packages in 2 litres of clean water.
- Add 50 g of sugar (10 teaspoons; 1 teaspoon is 5 g).
- Add 40 mL of electrolyte/mineral solution if available (see ETAT resource for composition[10]). It is not recommended to give diluted ORS without this additional solution.

References

1. World Health Organization. The Management of Nutrition In Major Emergencies. 2000. ℘ http://www.who.int/nutrition/publications/emergencies/9241545208/en/
2. World Health Organization. Child Growth Standards and the Identification of Severe Acute Malnutrition in Infants and Children. 2009. ℘ http://www.who.int/nutrition/publications/severemalnutrition/9789241598163/en/
3. The Sphere Project. The Sphere Handbook: Humanitarian Charter and Minimum Standards, 2011. Minimum Standards in Food Security and Nutrition. 2011. ℘ http://www.spherehandbook.org/en/introduction-3/
4. World Health Organization. Guidelines for the Inpatient Treatment of Severely Malnourished Children. 2003. ℘ http://whqlibdoc.who.int/publications/2003/9241546093.pdf?ua=1&ua=1
5. World Health Organization. Pocket Book Of Hospital Care For Children: Guidelines for the management of common childhood illnesses. 2nd ed. Geneva: WHO; 2013. ℘ http://www.who.int/maternal_child_adolescent/documents/child_hospital_care/en/
6. World Health Organization. Management of Severe Malnutrition: A Manual for Physicians and Other Senior Health Workers. 1999. ℘ http://apps.who.int/iris/bitstream/10665/41999/1/a57361.pdf
7. Médecins Sans Frontières, OCG and OCBA. Protocols for Management of Nutritional Support in Children with Severe Acute Malnutrition. February 2015.
8. Marcdante K, Kliegman RM. Nelson Essentials of Pediatrics. Philadelphia, PA: Elsevier Health Sciences; 2014.
9. UNHCR. Guidelines for Selective Feeding: The Management of Malnutrition in Emergencies. 2011. ℘ http://www.unhcr.org/4b7421fd20.pdf
10. World Health Organization. Emergency Triage Assessment and Treatment (ETAT). WHO; 2005. ℘ http://www.who.int/maternal_child_adolescent/documents/9241546875/en/

Further reading

Maitland K, Kiguli S, Opoka RO, Engoru C, Olupot-Olupot P, Akech SO, et al. Mortality after fluid bolus in African children with severe infection. N Engl J Med 2011;364(26):2483–95.
Médecins Sans Frontières. Paediatric Guidelines. February 2017, MSF OCP-OCG and MSF OCBA.
World Health Organization. Handbook IMCI: Integrated Management of Childhood Illness. 2005. ℘ http://apps.who.int/iris/bitstream/10665/42939/1/9241546441.pdf

Part IV

Infectious diseases

Malaria

Elizabeth Ashley

Context

An estimated 3.4 billion people are at risk of malaria worldwide. The WHO estimates that approximately 212 million cases of malaria occur each year with around 429,000 deaths, mainly in African children.[1] Malaria tends to target the most vulnerable groups in communities, such as young children and pregnant women.

It has been estimated that >80% of humanitarian emergencies take place in areas endemic for malaria. In this chapter, we discuss all aspects of malaria control in a humanitarian emergency setting including diagnosis, treatment, prevention, and epidemic preparedness and management.

Malaria biology

Malaria is a parasitic disease caused by the protozoan *Plasmodium* spp. and transmitted by the bite of the female *Anopheles* mosquito. Five species of *Plasmodium* are known to infect humans: *P. falciparum* (PF), *vivax* (PV), *ovale* (PO), *malariae*, and *knowlesi*, the latter being a fairly recent addition to the list. PF and PV malaria are responsible for the main disease burden. PF malaria is most likely to cause severe malaria and death.

Malaria lifecycle

- The female anopheline mosquito injects sporozoites from her salivary glands into the human host.
- Sporozoites travel to the liver, where they develop into intracellular hepatic schizonts. After approximately 8–10 days, these release numerous merozoites into the circulation which invade red blood cells (RBCs). During this period before RBC invasion the infected person is asymptomatic.
- Once inside the RBCs the merozoites develop as ring trophozoites, which mature into schizonts. The schizonts rupture, releasing more merozoites into the circulation which invade RBCs and cause the infection to expand. This is the asexual cycle of the parasite.
- Some of the blood-stage parasites develop into sexual forms or gametocytes. These are responsible for the onward transmission of malaria. A male and female gametocyte, taken up by a female anopheline during a blood meal, will develop and then fuse to form a zygote. The zygote further develops to form a mobile ookinete which penetrates the wall of the mosquito midgut, forming an oocyst. The oocyst releases sporozoites, thus completing the life cycle.
- Variations in life cycles between species include the following:
  - o PV and PO have a dormant liver stage (hypnozoite) in their life cycle, capable of causing subsequent disease relapse.
  - o The intra-erythrocytic asexual developmental stage takes 48 hours in PF, PV, and PO; 72 hours in *P. malariae*; and 24 hours in *P. knowlesi*.
  - o PV prefers younger red cells and invades a smaller sub-population of red blood cells compared to PF. As a result, parasitaemias tend to be lower and severe disease is less frequent.

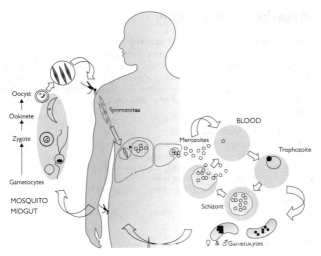

Fig. 29.1 Life cycle of *Plasmodium falciparum*.

Malaria epidemiology

Geographical distribution of species

Malaria is found in tropical and sub-tropical regions although transmission intensity varies depending on factors such as climate, altitude and prevailing vectors. *P. knowlesi* malaria is primarily a zoonotic disease; hence transmission requires the presence of one of the two macaque hosts (long-tailed or pig-tailed). The distribution of the different species is summarized in Table 29.1.

Transmission intensity

- As a general rule, PF transmission is higher in Africa than in Asia.
- In Africa, due to intense exposure and acquired immunity developing in early life, malaria is predominantly a disease of those <5 years old.
- In SE Asia where transmission is lower, there is less opportunity for immunity to develop and all age groups present with symptomatic disease.
- Information on transmission by country is available from the WHO World Malaria Report.[1]

Malaria vectors

There are approximately 40 species of *Anopheles* that commonly transmit malaria. Some species are more efficient vectors than others. The parasite development in the mosquito from gametocytes to sporozoites takes at least 8 days, so the adult female needs to survive for longer than this for malaria to be transmitted. The usual lifespan of the adult female is 1–2 weeks. Adult mosquitoes lay their eggs in water. The eggs will hatch into larvae which may be found in different environments depending on the species.

Table 29.1 Geographical distribution of malaria species

Species	Geographical distribution
P. falciparum	Africa
	Asia
	Latin America (see Fig. 29.2)
P. vivax	Asia (South and Southeast)
	Latin America
	Middle East
	Uncommon in Africa (except Horn and Madagascar)
P. ovale	Sub-Saharan Africa (occasional cases in Asia)
P. malariae	As for PF but much lower incidence
P. knowlesi	Southeast Asia (in particular Malaysia and Borneo)

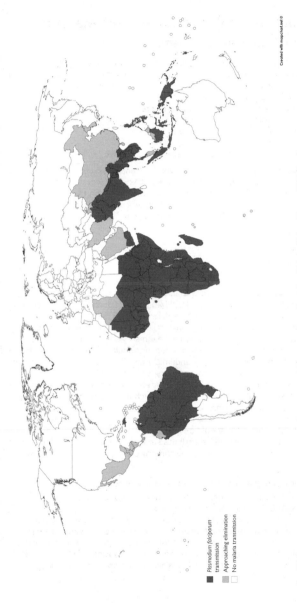

Fig. 29.2 Map of geographical distribution of *Plasmodium falciparum* malaria (based on World Malaria Report 2016 data[1]).

Plasmodium falciparum transmission

Approaching elimination

No malaria transmission

Created with mapchart.net ©

Planning health services and malaria control interventions

Knowledge of the epidemiology of malaria in the region where you are working will help with the initial planning of malaria control activities. You need to know:

• Which species are prevalent?
• Is it an area of high or low transmission?
• Is transmission seasonal or perennial?
• Is there a history of malaria epidemics?
• What are the local malaria vectors?
• Are there any control measures in place already?

Having the answers to these questions will enable you to tailor prevention and control measures appropriately; e.g. if you are working with a population with many young children in an area where malaria transmission is high and seasonal, you may plan a round of malaria chemoprevention before the next malaria season (see ➔ 'Prevention and vector control' pp. 460–1).

Assessment phase

An initial assessment to gather this information and to determine the importance of malaria as a health problem should take <1 week. This could be done as part of an overall situational analysis of the main causes of morbidity and mortality in the setting. Sources of information are likely to include local health authorities, community stakeholders, UN agencies, healthcare personnel, representatives of the MOH/National Malaria Control Program as well as WHO reports, e.g. World Malaria Report and published literature.

The risk of malaria following a natural disaster or in a complex emergency may be increased by breakdown in health services, environmental degradation encouraging mosquitoes to breed, or population movement displacing non-immune persons into an endemic area. The site of a new settlement should be away from vector breeding sites if possible. Different vectors will have different preferred breeding sites but as a general rule they will be areas where water collects, e.g. sites which flood during the rainy season, and slow moving streams.

A mortality survey may have been performed giving an estimate of malaria deaths but results should be interpreted with caution since most deaths associated with fever will be attributed to malaria. If there is very little useful information available, consider performing a rapid clinic-based fever survey yourself.

Conducting a rapid clinic-based fever survey

• A busy clinic should be selected with the aim of collecting data on at least 100–200 patients reporting fever.
• Using rapid diagnostic tests (RDTs) to conduct the survey (and make immediate decisions on treatment) followed by confirmatory expert microscopy of all slides after the survey is over is recommended as the 'gold standard' approach. If expert microscopy is not available, e.g. during an acute emergency, RDTs alone will provide a good enough estimate.

- If slides are taken, aim to read them all within 1 week of the survey to identify and treat missed cases.
- Analyse and interpret the survey results (see Box 29.1).
- The survey can be repeated to monitor trends, or routine surveillance data collection can be set up in all clinics.

Box 29.1 Analyse and interpret the survey results

Typically, in a stable population in a low-transmission setting, you can expect <10% of fever cases to be confirmed as malaria, while in a high-transmission area, >50% of children <10 years old would be parasitaemic and <50% of adults. Interpreting the results in a newly arrived (i.e. refugee) population is more complicated as prior immune status needs to be considered. If a high proportion of all age groups are infected, this could signal low immunity with consequently more symptomatic and severe infections, and an increased risk of outbreaks.

Planning services

The main objectives when planning services should be as follows:

- Ensuring access of the population to early diagnosis and treatment. In a non-epidemic situation, confirmed laboratory diagnosis of all cases is preferable to using clinical case definitions.
- Provision of adequate facilities for case management. This requires safe blood transfusion to be available in referral sites. This does not mean a blood bank but can be laboratory capability to provide rapid screening of stand-by blood donors (for hepatitis B, HIV, and malaria). Patients with severe malaria are managed as inpatients so referral pathways may be needed.
- Personnel already skilled in malaria case management, laboratory diagnosis, or control should be identified. Staff should be trained in triage of malaria patients, recognition of danger signs (described in ⊃ 'Disease presentation' p. 446), diagnosis, and treatment. An integrated community case management approach may be adopted, where community health workers assess children for malaria, pneumonia, or diarrhoea and are equipped to manage all three diagnoses.[2]
- Implementation of standard protocols and procedures.
- Ensuring supply of good-quality antimalarial drugs and RDTs without stock-outs.
- Setting up a basic surveillance system early.
- Implementation of preventive measures, such as provision of insecticide-treated bed nets, targeted intermittent preventive treatment strategies, and spraying with insecticides.

Disease presentation

The time between an infectious bite to the appearance of symptoms is usually around 7–14 days. Clinical malaria is classified as uncomplicated or severe and management of these presentations differs.

Uncomplicated malaria

The standard case definition of uncomplicated malaria is very non-specific, i.e. fever or history of fever associated with symptoms such as nausea, vomiting and diarrhoea, headache, back pain, chills, and myalgia, where other infectious diseases have been excluded.

- Children may present with fever and respiratory symptoms only.
- Examination findings can often be non-specific, e.g. conjunctival pallor, tachypnoea, or hepatosplenomegaly.
- In high-transmission areas, a high percentage of the population may be harbouring parasites at any time without symptoms, due to acquired immunity with repeated exposure. An alternative diagnosis may need to be pursued even if parasites are present.
- Uncomplicated malaria with parasitaemia >10% should be treated as severe malaria because of the risk of a rapid deterioration in the patient's condition.

Severe malaria

Clinical manifestations of severe infection are typically cerebral malaria at any age (PF) or severe anaemia in children. Massive haemoglobinuria ('blackwater fever') and renal or respiratory failure may also occur. Hypoglycaemia is common and acidosis may show as fast deep breathing.

The WHO has defined a list of criteria for the diagnosis of severe malaria; however, in practice, only a few of these can be assessed under field conditions. There is a useful shorter checklist of malaria *danger signs* for staff to use to identify patients with severe disease:

Malaria danger signs
- Drowsiness.
- Repeated vomiting.
- Severe dehydration.
- Inability to sit.
- Inability to feed.

Without prior experience of managing patients with cerebral malaria it may be hard to believe at first that they have a hope of recovering from such a profoundly deep coma which may include teeth-grinding (bruxism) or even extensor posturing. With good care, many patients will recover with no neurological sequelae. However, the more pronounced the neurological signs, the worse the prognosis will be.

Diagnosis

In the acute emergency situation, parasitological diagnosis may not be available and presumptive treatment will have to be given to fever cases. However, biological diagnosis should be implemented as soon as possible. Clinical diagnosis has been practised widely for decades but it is extremely unreliable except when malaria incidence is very high, e.g. an epidemic. Keep in mind that the presence of parasites on a blood film does not always explain the symptoms a patient is presenting with, particularly in high-transmission areas where asymptomatic parasitaemia is common.

See → Chapter 53 for technical diagnostic guidelines. General principles are outlined as follows.

Malaria blood smear

Making a good malaria slide requires skill. A poor slide with too much or too little blood, not dried completely before staining, stained for an inadequate length of time with the wrong concentration of stain that is not fresh, or has not been filtered, and examined down a microscope that has seen better days all threaten the chance of ending up with an accurate diagnosis. Added to this, microscopists may be overworked with too many slides to read or be in need of refresher training. A reasonable average daily workload is 30–50 slides depending on their other duties.

Malaria rapid diagnostic tests

Many programmes now rely on RDTs rather than microscopy for diagnosis, especially if the caseload is high, if community-based case management is being implemented, or if providing microscopy of a good enough standard is not achievable. Staff may be trained in their use relatively quickly (<1 day).

RDTs work by detecting various parasite antigens. The most widely used tests detect either histidine-rich protein 2 (HRP2) a protein produced by PF only, or parasite lactate dehydrogenase (pLDH) which is produced by all malaria species, or a combination of the two. There are different pLDH antigens: one 'Pan' antigen which is common to all malaria species and hence cannot distinguish between them and also species-specific varieties of pLDH which enable differentiation.

There are many different RDTs on the market. Performance between tests varies. The WHO has published selection criteria for procurement of RDTs which have gone through their product testing programme.[3]

Most tests are relatively straightforward to perform, but, as with any diagnostic test, RDTs are not foolproof. Assuming you are working with a good quality test (which you should always question) there are other factors affecting performance and interpretation of the results to be aware of:

- Many tests lose sensitivity at lower parasitaemias.
- Heat stability. Tests may degrade and give unreliable results if stored for prolonged periods in ambient tropical temperatures rather than under ideal conditions.
- HRP2 persists in the circulation for days or weeks after a malaria infection has been treated successfully, during which time the test remains positive. This can present management difficulties if a patient returns symptomatic within days of receiving treatment—is it treatment failure or is there another diagnosis and the test has simply not yet reverted to negative?

- pLDH tests tend to revert to negative within 1 week of treatment; however, gametocytes also produce pLDH, and hence may prolong a positive result in a treated patient.
- In general, performance seems to be poorer for non-falciparum species.
- False-negative results occur occasionally in patients with very high parasite densities.
- Geographical variation in the HRP2 antigen may mean test performance is different in different places.

Many of the uncertainties listed here can be resolved if there is some capacity for slide microscopy. A useful golden rule is: 'If in doubt, treat as falciparum malaria'. This way you will not go very wrong (although there is a risk of later relapse of PV or PO malaria if these species are missed).

Management of uncomplicated malaria

- Most patients with uncomplicated malaria are treated as outpatients.
- Patients with uncomplicated malaria may be febrile, vomiting, and dehydrated. Treating the fever first with sponging and antipyretics is advisable before administering the antimalarials, especially in children.
- There are some paediatric formulations of antimalarials but they are not always available so it may be necessary to crush tablets and make a suspension. Several drugs have a bitter taste which may need to be disguised as children may spit out the tablet immediately.
- If the antimalarial drug is vomited within half an hour of administration, the dose should be repeated. If between 30 minutes and 1 hour, half of the dose should be given. An antiemetic may be prescribed. If a dose is vomited twice, parenteral treatment should be given.
- Failure to adhere to a complete course of antimalarials increases the chance of a population of parasites below the microscopic level of detection recrudescing at a later date. Advise on the importance of completing the course even if symptoms resolve quickly.

Medications

Treatment of uncomplicated falciparum malaria
(See Table 29.2.)
- As a general rule, the choice of drugs will follow the recommendations of the National Malaria Control Program.
- Uncomplicated falciparum malaria, or mixed infections, are treated with one of the recommended artemisinin-based combination therapies (ACTs). ACTs include artemether + lumefantrine, artesunate + mefloquine, artesunate + amodiaquine, artesunate + sulfadoxine–pyrimethamine (SP), dihydroartemisinin + piperaquine, and artesunate + pyronaridine. Artemisinin resistance has emerged in Southeast Asia. ACTs are still being used currently but this may change.[4]
- If an ACT is contraindicated, then alternative treatments are quinine combined with either doxycycline or clindamycin, or atovaquone–proguanil.

Drugs for uncomplicated non-falciparum malaria
(See Table 29.3.)
- Chloroquine is still the drug of first choice for the treatment of uncomplicated PV, PO, or *P. malariae* in most areas except Indonesia where resistance is widespread. Up-to-date recommendations should be consulted.
- *P. knowlesi* should be treated as falciparum malaria (with an ACT) because of the increased risk of developing severe disease.
- Drugs used to treat falciparum malaria will treat non-falciparum infections (with the exception of SP for PV).
- To avoid relapse after an episode of PV or PO malaria, caused by reactivation of the latent hypnozoites in the liver, a course of the 8-aminoquinoline primaquine should be given. This drug causes haemolysis in patients with G6PD deficiency which should be excluded before prescribing primaquine for radical cure. In practice, tests which detect G6PD deficiency are usually not available, hence primaquine is usually not prescribed.

> *Practical point*: Absorption of artemether + lumefantrine is improved by
> coadministration with fat. Treatment failures have been associated with
> low drug concentrations. Mothers should be encouraged to breastfeed
> their infants with each dose, and older children and adults should be ad-
> vised to take the dose with milk or food containing fat if available.

Adverse effects of antimalarials
Common adverse effects of antimalarials:
- Gastrointestinal disturbance with all drugs.
- Skin reactions, e.g. pruritus or rash with chloroquine or quinine (typically
  photosensitive). The artemisinin derivatives occasionally cause rash and
  type 1 hypersensitivity reactions. Patients should not be re-challenged
  should this occur. SP may cause Stevens–Johnson syndrome.
- Cinchonism (dizziness, tinnitus, blurred vision) with quinine.
- Vomiting, dizziness, and sleep disturbance, and rarely neuropsychiatric
  reactions with mefloquine.

Table 29.2 Treatment of uncomplicated falciparum malaria

	Dose
Artemisinin-based combination therapy Artemether + lumefantrine. Fixed dose co-formulation of tablets containing 20 mg artemether (AM) and 120 mg lumefantrine (LF)	Given as 6 doses over 3 days (hour 0, 8, 24, 36, 48, 60). Target dose is 5–24 mg/kg body weight (bw) artemether and 29–144 mg/kg bw lumefantrine Weight-based dosing: 5–14 kg: 20 mg AM + 120 mg LF/dose 15–24 kg: 40 mg AM + 240 mg LF/dose 25–34 kg: 60 mg AM + 360 mg LF/dose ≥35 kg: 80 mg AM + 480 mg LF/dose
Dihydroartemisinin +piperaquine Fixed dose co-formulation of tablets containing 40 mg dihydroartemisinin (DHA) and 320 mg piperaquine (Pip) or 20 mg dihydroartemisinin (DHA) and 160 mg piperaquine (Pip)	Given once daily over 3 days. Target dose is 4 mg/kg DHA+2 mg/kg Pip if bw <25 kg and 4 mg/kg DHA + 18 mg/kg Pip if bw ≥25kg Weight-based dosing: 5–7 kg: 20 mg DHA + 160 mg Pip/dose 8–10 kg: 30 mg DHA + 240 mg Pip/dose 11–16 kg: 40 mg DHA + 320 mg Pip/dose 17–24 kg: 60 mg DHA + 480 mg Pip/dose 25–35 kg: 80 mg DHA + 640 mg Pip/dose 36–59 kg: 120 mg DHA + 960 mg Pip/dose 60–79 kg: 160 mg DHA + 1280 mg Pip/dose ≥80 kg: 200 mg DHA + 1600 mg Pip/dose
Artesunate + amodiaquine Fixed dose co-formulated tablets of artesunate (AS)/amodiaquine (AQ) tablets available in three strengths: 25/67.5 mg; 50/ 135 mg; 100/270 mg	Given once daily over 3 days. Target dose is 4 mg/kg bw/day of AS + 10 mg/kg bw/day AQ Weight-based dosing: 4.5–8 kg: 25 mg AS + 67.5 mg AQ/dose 9–17 kg: 50 mg AS + 135 mg AQ/dose 18–35 kg: 100 mg AS + 270 mg AQ/dose ≥36 kg: 200 mg AS + 540 mg AQ/dose

Table 29.2 (*Contd.*)

	Dose
Artesunate + sulfadoxine–pyrimethamine (SP) Loose tablets: Artesunate 50 mg tablets SP tablets contain 25 mg pyrimethamine + 500 mg sulfadoxine	Artesunate given once daily over 3 days. Only *one* dose of SP is given. Target dose is AS 4 mg/kg bw/day with a single dose of SP (based on 1.25 mg/kg bw pyrimethamine) Weight-based dosing: 5–9 kg: 25 mg AS × 3 days + 250/12.5 mg S/P × 1 10–24 kg: 50 mg AS × 3 days + 500/25 mg S/P × 1 25–49 kg: 100 mg AS × 3 days + 1000/50 mg S/P × 1 ≥50 kg: 200 mg AS × 3 days + 1500/75 mg S/P × 1
Artesunate + mefloquine Fixed dose co-formulation of paediatric tablets containing 25 mg artesunate and 55 mg mefloquine (MQ) HCl (adult tablets contain 100 mg and 220 mg respectively)	Given once daily over 3 days. Target dose is AS 4 mg/kg bw/day and MQ 8.3 mg/kg bw day Weight-based dosing: 5–8 kg: 25 mg AS + 55 mg MQ/dose 9–17 kg: 50 mg AS + 110 mg MQ/dose 18–29 kg: 100 mg AS + 220 mg MQ/dose ≥30 kg: 200 mg AS + 440 mg MQ/dose
Artesunate + doxycycline	Weight-based dosing: Artesunate 2 mg/kg bw/day for 7 days + doxycycline 4 mg/kg bw/day for 7 days
Non-artemisinin-based combination therapy Quinine + doxycycline Loose tablets. Different formulations available	Weight-based dosing: Quinine 10 mg bw/kg three times a day for 7 days with doxycycline 4 mg/kg bw/day for 7 days
Quinine + clindamycin Loose tablets. Different formulations available	Quinine as above + clindamycin 5 mg/kg bw three times per day for 7 days
Atovaquone + proguanil Fixed dose co-formulated tablets available in two strengths: 250 mg atovaquone (ATV) + 100 mg proguanil (PG) (adult) or 62.5 mg ATV+ 25 mg PG (child)	Target dose ATV 20 mg/kg bw/day + PG 8 mg/kg bw/day Weight-based dosing: 5–8 kg: 125 mg ATV + 50 mg PG/dose 9–10 kg: 187.5 mg ATV + 75 mg PG/dose 11–20 kg: 250 mg ATV + 100 mg PG/dose 21–30 kg: 500 mg ATV + 200 mg PG/dose 31–40 kg: 750 mg ATV + 300 mg PG/dose ≥41 kg: 1000 mg ATV + 400 mg PG/dose

Note
- Mefloquine is contraindicated in people with neuropsychiatric disorders. It should not be given again within 2 months of a previous treatment.
- Doxycycline is contraindicated in children <9 years of age and pregnant women.
- Quinine + clindamycin is recommended as first-line treatment in the first trimester of pregnancy.

Table 29.3 Treatment of uncomplicated non-falciparum malaria

	Dose
Chloroquine Chloroquine phosphate (1 tablet contains 250 mg salt, equivalent to 155.3 mg base). Followed by: (in vivax or ovale malaria) *Primaquine*	Dose is 10 mg/kg bw base once a day for 2 days followed by 5 mg/kg bw base on the third day. Primaquine 0.25–0.5 mg base/kg bw daily for 14 days (if G6PD normal)

Note
- Always consult national guidelines as resistance may be emerging in some regions.
- *P. knowlesi* should be treated as for falciparum malaria with an ACT.
- Primaquine is contraindicated in G6PD deficiency, in pregnancy, breastfeeding women, and infants <6 months of age.

Management of severe malaria

Severe malaria is a medical emergency with a high associated mortality. It is diagnosed by the detection of *danger signs* (drowsiness, repeated vomiting, severe dehydration, inability to sit, and inability to feed). Appropriate facilities for managing patients with severe malaria should be able to provide frequent vital sign, fluid balance, glycaemia, parasitaemia, and haematocrit monitoring and administer IV drug and fluid therapy. Referral pathways should be agreed in advance.

Immediate management steps

- Give IV artesunate (or alternative, see Table 29.4). Rectal artesunate (10 mg/kg) should be given to children <7 years of age before transfer if parenteral drugs are not available on site.
- Exclude hypoglycaemia. Hypoglycaemia (glucose <2.2 mmol/L) is a particular risk in quinine-treated patients and pregnant women. Treat with an IV bolus of 20% glucose, 2 mg/kg over 10 minutes, or if unavailable give 50% glucose, 1 mL/kg over 10 min, preferably concurrently with an IV infusion of replacement fluids to protect the veins. Blood glucose levels should be checked at least hourly as rebound hypoglycaemia is common.
- Maintenance with 10% glucose may be necessary in refractory or recurrent hypoglycaemia. This can be prepared by dilution of 50% glucose (usually 50 mL) in 450–500 mL of 5% glucose.

Drugs for treating severe malaria
(See Table 29.4.)
- Parenteral artesunate is preferred and reduces mortality substantially compared to quinine. It may be given IV or IM. If not available, IM artemether *or* IV/ IM quinine may be substituted.
- If quinine is administered IM, it should be given as two divided doses into both anterior thighs to minimize the risk of sciatic nerve injury.
- Parenteral drugs may be discontinued once the patient improves and oral treatment should be started—either a full course of an ACT *or* oral artesunate plus either doxycycline or clindamycin *or* oral quinine plus either doxycycline or clindamycin (see Table 29.2).
- Mefloquine should be avoided as follow-on treatment for severe malaria because of the risk of post-malaria neurological syndrome.

> *Practical point*: artesunate is an unstable compound and the IV preparation comes as a vial containing powder which has to be reconstituted with sodium bicarbonate contained in a separate ampoule. This is then diluted further using 5 mL of normal saline or 5% glucose for IV administration or 2 mL if the drug will be given IM. The correct volume is administered according to the patient's weight. Once prepared, it should be used immediately and any excess drug discarded if not used within 1 hour

Fluid resuscitation
- Blood transfusion. Children with fast deep (acidotic) breathing are frequently hypovolaemic and anaemic. Consider immediate transfusion if haemoglobin <5 g/dL in high-transmission settings or 7 g/dL in low-transmission settings.

Table 29.4 Treatment of severe malaria

Drug	Dose
Artesunate IV (or IM) or	<20 kg body weight: 3 mg/kg on admission, then at 12 hours and 24 hours and then once a day until oral therapy tolerated. Patients weighing 20 kg and above should receive 2.4 mg/kg/dose
Artemether IM or	3.2 mg/kg on admission, then 1.6 mg/kg daily until oral therapy tolerated
Quinine IV (or IM)	20 mg salt/kg *loading dose* on admission (IV infusion or divided IM injections) followed by 10 mg/kg every 8 hours until 48 hours, and then every 12 hours until oral therapy tolerated

- Hypovolaemic patients without severe anaemia should be given crystalloid (*not* colloid). Patients with severe malaria are at risk of both fluid overload with pulmonary oedema (particularly adults) and renal failure so careful fluid management is required.

Current fluid recommendations are:
- Children:
  - Initial fluid resuscitation over 3–4 hours with 0.9% saline at a rate of 3–5 mL/kg/hour and then switch to maintenance 5% glucose (2–3 mL/kg/hour).[5]
  - If solutions containing 0.45% saline/5% glucose are available then these are preferred. Use a burette to give fluids safely to young children if possible.
- Adults:
  - Give 0.9% (normal) saline 3–5 mL/kg/hour during the first 6 hours of admission with frequent vital sign assessment.
  - Then reassess and aim to switch to alternate 500 mL bags/bottles of 5% glucose and 0.9% saline for maintenance fluid replacement (2–3 mL/kg/hour).
  - Monitor urine output, inserting a catheter if necessary.

Practical point: In low-resource settings, if IV glucose is not available, consider the sublingual route. In a study in West Africa, children with hypoglycaemia and severe malaria were given a teaspoon of sublingual sugar every 20 minutes as a replacement for parenteral glucose. Initial recovery from hypoglycaemia was comparable but there was a higher relapse rate in the sublingual group and the authors suggested increasing the frequency of administration. This should be considered as a holding measure only until parenteral therapy is available.[6]

Antiseizure medications
- Treat seizures with IV diazepam 0.3 mg/kg (maximum dose 10 mg) over 2 minutes; or 0.5 mg/kg per rectum, after excluding hypoglycaemia as the cause.
- Prophylactic anticonvulsants are not recommended.[7]

Antimicrobials

Serious bacterial infections may coexist with severe malaria. Give broad-spectrum antibiotics initially to all children presenting with severe malaria in moderate- to high-transmission areas and review the need to continue at 24-48 hours.

Management of the unconscious patient

- Patients with cerebral malaria may be deeply unconscious and need airway management, good nursing care, and turning to avoid pressure sores developing.
- If coma is prolonged, NG feeding should be instituted; however, there is a significant risk of aspiration pneumonia in a non-intubated patient. Delaying until at least 60 hours in adults or 36 hours in children has been advocated by some experts.

Blantyre Coma Scale

Developed to enable monitoring of coma in children with severe malaria. Monitor 6-hourly with vital signs.

- Eye movement:
  - 1: watches or follows.
  - 0: unable to watch or follow.
- Best motor response:
  - 2: localizes painful stimulus.
  - 1: withdraws limb from painful stimulus.
  - 0: no response or inappropriate response.
- Best verbal response:
  - 2: cries appropriately with pain, (or speaks).
  - 1: moan or abnormal cry.
  - 0: none.

Treatment failures

A second episode of malaria up to 9 weeks after treatment may be due to a true treatment failure (recrudescence), a new infection, or, in the cases of PV or PO, a relapse caused by reactivation of previously dormant parasite forms in the liver. These are indistinguishable clinically. A true failure of treatment will be particularly hard to identify in a high-transmission area where patients are re-infected regularly. In practice, most recurrences of malaria occurring within 2 weeks of a course of treatment are likely to be recrudescent infections.

Factors which may predispose to treatment failure are drug resistance, inadequate drug levels, non-adherence to therapy, falsified or sub-standard drugs, and high parasitaemias. Patients re-presenting with malaria within 1 month of an earlier episode should be treated with an alternative regimen if available (see Table 29.2).

If it comes to your notice that many patients seem to be returning with a second symptomatic infection very soon after their first, consider the possibility that resistance has developed to your first-line treatment.

Malaria in at-risk groups

Pregnant women, children, and individuals who are malnourished or co-infected with HIV are all at higher risk from malaria and should be given special consideration.

Malaria in pregnancy

Women become more susceptible to malaria during pregnancy, in particular their first pregnancy. Pregnant women are more likely to develop severe disease than their non-pregnant counterparts and the mortality risk associated with severe malaria in pregnancy is much higher, rising to 50% in cerebral malaria.

- In general, malaria in pregnancy is associated with an increased risk of miscarriage, low-birth-weight infants, and increased anaemia.
- If malaria is suspected in a woman who is pregnant it should be investigated and treated very promptly.
- HIV co-infection in pregnancy puts women at even greater risk from malaria, being associated with higher parasitaemias and higher rates of anaemia, maternal death, and placental malaria.

Prevention of malaria in pregnancy

- Intermittent preventive treatment with SP is recommended by WHO to be given to all pregnant women in high-transmission areas at each antenatal visit, except during the first trimester.[8]
- Daily co-trimoxazole is recommended (*without* SP intermittent preventive treatment) for HIV infected pregnant women (reduces malaria incidence as well as other opportunistic infections).
- Changing drug susceptibility means the most up-to-date recommendations should always be sought.

Treatment of malaria in pregnancy

- ACTs are currently not recommended to treat malaria in the first trimester of pregnancy because of fears of embryotoxicity which has been observed in animals; however, this may change as evidence of safety accrues.
- First trimester: a 7-day course of quinine and clindamycin is recommended (see Table 29.2). Adherence is difficult due to three-times-a-day dosing and side effects are very common, making treatment supervision advisable.
- Second and third trimesters or severe malaria: treatment recommendations are the same as for non-pregnant individuals. In severe malaria, hypoglycaemia is more common, particularly if quinine is given. Regular fetal monitoring should be performed while a pregnant woman is being treated.
- Non-falciparum malaria is treated with chloroquine (or quinine + clindamycin in an area of chloroquine resistance) but primaquine is contraindicated in pregnancy.

Malaria in infants and children: congenital malaria

- Congenital malaria is uncommon but easy to miss. It is most likely to occur when the mother has malaria at or around the time of delivery which may be asymptomatic. If malaria is detected in the mother, infants should be screened regardless of their clinical condition.

- Treatment options are limited since many antimalarials are not recommended for use in babies below a certain weight, e.g. artesunate + amodiaquine is only recommended for those ≥4.5 kg.
- Parenteral artesunate or quinine should be given for PF. They will also treat PV (although chloroquine may be given).
- Primaquine is not recommended below 6 months of age.

Intermittent preventive treatment for infants
- The WHO recommends that infants living in moderate- to high-transmission areas should receive three doses of intermittent preventive treatment with SP at approximately 10 weeks, 14 weeks, and 9 months of age, corresponding to the routine vaccination schedule of the WHO Expanded Programme on Immunization.
- This should not be given in areas where parasite resistance to SP is high (defined as prevalence of PF dihydropteroate synthase mutation ≥50%).
- Children with HIV infection receiving co-trimoxazole prophylaxis should not receive SP.

Seasonal malaria chemoprevention

Children residing in areas of highly seasonal transmission in the Sahel sub-region are a high-risk group and seasonal malaria chemoprevention (SMC) (the administration of full treatment courses of antimalarials during the malaria season to prevent malaria) is recommended by WHO for children aged 3–59 months. A complete treatment course of SP plus amodiaquine should be given at monthly intervals, beginning at the start of the transmission season, up to a maximum of four doses during the malaria transmission season. Intermittent preventive treatment should not be used in SMC areas. Careful planning is needed to ensure an adequate drug supply, staff trained in SMC delivery, and community support. SMC should be monitored for safety, efficacy, and coverage, with involvement of district or regional health authorities. The WHO field guide to SMC outlines different approaches to implementation depending on the context and includes several sample forms.[9]

Malaria and HIV infection

Malaria infection is associated with a temporary increase in HIV viral load, although no differences in survival in HIV-infected patients living in malaria-endemic areas have been described. Conversely, patients infected with HIV are more susceptible to malaria. In general, treatment recommendations are the same as for uninfected patients except that patients taking co-trimoxazole prophylaxis should not receive any kind of intermittent preventive treatment for malaria with an antifolate drug (SP). Also, patients receiving zidovudine or efavirenz should avoid amodiaquine if there is an alternative due to an increased risk of neutropenia and hepatotoxicity respectively.[10]

Surveillance and monitoring

Malaria surveillance is frequently neglected. Linking with local authorities to support the early implementation of a simple surveillance system is highly recommended to allow trends in incidence to be observed, facilitating earlier detection of outbreaks. It can be used to monitor the effectiveness of control measures.

Key indicators for malaria surveillance

- Proportion of fever cases caused by malaria. A fever case is anyone with a history of fever as well as documented fever in the clinic.
- Slide or RDT positivity rate, identified by parasite species. If the RDT used for malaria diagnosis only detects PF or cannot discriminate between species then it will not be possible to get accurate data on incidence of non-falciparum species routinely.
- Number of severe malaria cases.
- Case-fatality rate of severe cases.
- Overall case-fatality rate.
- Malaria incidence rate (note: denominator is the *population at risk*, not just clinic attendees).
- Malaria mortality as a proportion of all-cause mortality. It should be possible to stratify the results into broad age categories (e.g. <5 years, 5 years and over) and pregnant women should be identifiable separately.

Outbreak preparedness and response

Being prepared for an outbreak means having a surveillance system in place to recognize it when it happens, and being able to mobilize sufficient staff, drugs, and laboratory supplies to manage it if it occurs.

There is no specific epidemiological threshold for a malaria outbreak.

Malaria epidemics may be of varying orders of magnitude, from a few hundred cases to very many more such as the disastrous epidemic that occurred in Burundi in 2000–2001 which affected 9 out of 16 provinces and resulted in 3.5 million cases. One of the hardest tasks may be recognizing an epidemic in its early stages, especially as malaria may already be a common disease and an outbreak may easily be mistaken for a seasonal peak.

Assessing the likelihood of an epidemic

Consider the following:

- Is the slide-positivity rate going up compared to previous weeks or the same season in previous years?
- Are there more hospitalized or severe malaria cases?
- Have the numbers of deaths from malaria increased?
- Are there obvious pre-disposing factors, e.g. recent population movements or changes in the environment?
- Is it a place where epidemics are known to occur periodically?
- Are drug or insecticide resistance suspected?

If the answer to any of these questions is yes, this increases the likelihood that there is an epidemic. If there is uncertainty, consider performing a rapid prevalence survey to confirm the epidemic.

Epidemic response

In an epidemic situation you need to be able to manage large numbers of cases efficiently and quickly. Elements of an effective epidemic response which should be prioritized are:

1. *Increase access to treatment.* Interventions to de-centralize care and promote early diagnosis and treatment by improving access should be implemented urgently. Staffing requirements for a basic health post for this purpose would include one person to register patients, record vital signs, and triage; a nurse or medic to assess patients and decide on management; ± a dispenser to give medicine and advice, depending on the caseload. There should be ready access to transportation for severely unwell patients. Artesunate may be given via the IM route (or rectal route in children <7 years), both of which are practical options for pre-referral therapy of severe cases.

2. *Abandon systematic parasitological diagnosis.* If the caseload is high, have a low threshold for treating and restrict testing to doubtful cases only. It is wise to continue to test a proportion of all cases presenting to identify when the epidemic is ending. Routine parasitological confirmation should be reintroduced when the case positivity rate falls <50%.

3. *Pay attention to patient triage.* Training to identify high-risk patients needs to be reinforced with priority for assessment given to patients showing signs of disease severity (danger signs), pregnant women, and young children.

4. *Communicate with the community.* Education to encourage people to seek diagnosis and treatment early is vital as this will save lives.

5. *Anticipate increased capacity needs.* Facilities to manage severe cases and capacity to provide safe blood transfusion may need to be expanded and supported.

Epidemic monitoring and reporting

The number of cases treated needs to be recorded by geographical location and age. Plot an epidemic curve of malaria cases against time using retrospective data and those collected during the epidemic. This should be updated weekly and communicated to all interested parties. Communication channels should include other agencies working with the same population as well as regional and national health authorities.

Other control measures

Early on in the epidemic there may be a role for implementing vector control activities such as indoor residual spraying and ensuring bed net usage is high. Mass drug administration is not usually advisable, particularly in a large-scale epidemic. Seek expert advice if you are considering this.

Prevention and vector control

Bed nets

- Long-lasting insecticide-treated nets (LLINs) have been shown to be protective against malaria and should be deployed.
- LLINs may bring other additional benefits such as a reduction in scabies infestations, common in cramped conditions typical of temporary settlements.
- When procuring LLINs, select one approved by the WHO Pesticide Evaluation Scheme (WHOPES).
- Universal coverage is the goal, which in practice means at least one bed net per two individuals.
- Distribution may be achieved in various ways, e.g. combined with immunization or antenatal care delivery, inclusion in non-food item kits, or mass distribution campaigns. Mass distributions should be followed by intermittent targeted distributions to high-risk groups (pregnant women, young children) to ensure coverage rates do not fall.
- Mass distribution campaigns require careful planning. One method is to set up distribution centres and give each household a coupon which they can use to claim the appropriate number of nets from their local centre.
- Education in bed net use is vital. Mobilizing a team of community health workers to distribute the nets, provide education on the benefits of net usage, and advise individual households on how to hang the nets correctly and take care of them should result in better coverage, improved usage, and improved effectiveness. The national malaria control programme of the country may already have education materials to promote net usage. Some people appreciate bed nets for their effect of reducing nuisance biting by mosquitoes but acceptance is not universal, with bed nets perceived by some to be too hot or uncomfortable to sleep under, and others disliking the smell of insecticide and being reluctant to place their infants under the net.
- Post-distribution surveys to evaluate net use and population coverage are recommended.
- In a refugee camp setting where the population is sleeping in tents, hanging the LLINs may be difficult and insecticide-impregnated tents are preferred. If these are not available, education on correct net usage is crucial to success.

Indoor residual spraying and vector control

Indoor residual spraying (IRS) refers to spraying the inside of houses with a dilute solution of insecticide to kill mosquitoes resting indoors.

The duration of the effect is usually between 4 and 10 months. Other vector control measures employed have been 'mosquito proofing' of shelters with insecticide-treated netting and even application of insecticide to livestock. The WHO has published an operational manual for IRS for malaria transmission control and elimination.[11]

The beneficial effects of LLINs will depend on the local vectors. In many parts of Africa, *Anopheles gambiae* predominate, which typically rest indoors and bite at night; hence bed nets may have a significant impact on malaria transmission. Insecticide (pyrethroid) resistance in *Anopheles gambiae* has emerged in some areas and threatens to reduce the beneficial impact of LLINs to reduce transmission, with the potential to increase malaria morbidity. In Asia, the behaviour of many of the common anopheline vectors is different, e.g. a tendency to bite earlier before dusk, and being less likely to rest indoors, thus the benefit of implementing bed nets will not be so great.

Intermittent preventive treatment strategies

These target at-risk groups such as pregnant women and young children. See ➲ 'Malaria in at-risk groups' pp. 456–7 for details.

Other environmental control measures

Improved drainage of areas prone to flooding and good wastewater management will reduce malaria transmission by reducing the number of mosquito breeding grounds. In emergency situations, common approaches to wastewater management include soakpits, diversion to natural drainage, and infiltration trenches.

Vaccination

The RTS,S/AS01 vaccine is a recombinant vaccine against falciparum malaria which targets the early stage of the parasite life cycle when the sporozoites invade and develop in the host's liver. Results of trials in young children have shown partial protection of the vaccine against clinical malaria and a reduction in severe malaria in children aged 5–17 months who received four doses of the vaccine. WHO has recommended further large-scale pilot evaluations of effectiveness in this age group before firm recommendations are made on deployment.

Malaria and the humanitarian worker

The risks of not taking prophylaxis in a high-transmission setting should not be underestimated, especially if you have no background immunity. The agency you work for may have a policy on taking antimalarial prophylaxis. The choice of suitable drugs is limited and none guarantee 100% protection. In high-transmission areas, mefloquine or atovaquone–proguanil are common options. Mefloquine is not well tolerated by everyone. It can cause nightmares and, rarely, neuropsychiatric side effects. Consider a trial at home for a couple of weeks before departure. Atovaquone–proguanil is usually well tolerated but expensive. Doxycycline is an alternative agent which is often recommended. It is a less potent antimalarial and is a more appropriate choice for low-transmission areas. Photosensitivity and heartburn are well-described side effects. Expert advice should be sought for personnel working in endemic areas for prolonged periods (>1–2 years).

References

1. World Health Organization. World Malaria Report 2016. ℳ http://www.who.int/malaria/publications/world-malaria-report-2016/report/en/
2. World Health Organization. Integrated Community Case Management of Malaria. Last update: 12 July 2016. ℳ http://www.who.int/malaria/areas/community_case_management/overview/en/
3. World Health Organization. Information Note on Recommended Selection Criteria for Procurement of Malaria Rapid Diagnostic Tests (RDTs). March 2016. ℳ http://www.who.int/malaria/publications/atoz/rdt_selection_criteria/en/
4. World Health Organization. Guidelines for the Treatment of Malaria. 3rd ed. 2015. ℳ http://www.who.int/malaria/publications/atoz/9789241549127/en/
5. A World Health Organization. Severe malaria. Trop Med Int Health 2014;19(Suppl 1):7–131.
6. Graz B, Dicko M, Willcox ML, Lambert B, Falquet J, Forster M, et al. Sublingual sugar for hypoglycaemia in children with severe malaria: a pilot clinical study. Malar J 2008;23(7):242.
7. Crawley J, Waruiru C, Mithwani S, Mwangi I, Watkins W, Ouma D, et al. Effect of phenobarbital on seizure frequency and mortality in childhood cerebral malaria: a randomized controlled intervention study. Lancet 2000;355(9205):701–6.
8. World Health Organization Global Malaria Programme. Updated WHO Policy Recommendation (October 2012). Intermittent Preventive Treatment of malaria in pregnancy using Sulfadoxine-Pyrimethamine (IPTp-SP). ℳ http://www.who.int/malaria/iptp_sp_updated_policy_recommendation_en_102012.pdf
9. World Health Organization. Seasonal Malaria Chemoprevention with sulfadoxine-Pyrimethamine Plus Amodiaquine in Children: A Field Guide August 2013. ℳ http://www.who.int/malaria/publications/atoz/9789241504737/en/
10. World Health Organization. Malaria in HIV/AIDS patients. Last update: 27 April 2017 ℳ http://www.who.int/malaria/areas/high_risk_groups/hiv_aids_patients/en/
11. World Health Organization. Indoor Residual Spraying: An Operational Manual for IRS for Malaria Transmission, Control and Elimination. 2nd ed. June 2015. ℳ http://www.who.int/malaria/publications/atoz/9789241508940/en/

Chapter 30

Neglected tropical diseases

Jan Hajek

Introduction

Neglected tropical diseases (NTDs) wreak havoc among the poorest and most disenfranchised people in the world. Despite the availability of safe and inexpensive interventions that can drastically reduce their burden, these diseases continue to kill an estimated 500,000 people every year and millions of people are disfigured, disabled, blinded, and stigmatized.

The disproportionate burden of NTDs perpetuates poverty, ill health, and fosters conflict and political instability. Addressing and prioritizing their elimination is fundamentally a humanitarian endeavour, driven by principles of human rights, social justice, and health equity.

The diagnosis and management of NTDs can be a challenge for health workers who may have little experience with their recognition and may be working in places with very limited diagnostic testing. This chapter cannot comprehensively cover all aspects of the management of these infections, but aims to provide an overview of their main features and management issues.

It is critical that health workers in humanitarian settings can recognize key features of NTDs and understand the basic principles of their diagnosis, treatment, and prevention. Advocacy and awareness of these diseases will improve case management in the field, and foster the implementation of effective public health interventions.

Overview of NTDS

The concept of NTDs emerged in the early 2000s to increase recognition for these poverty-related diseases that lacked funding and political support, and were inadequately targeted by the Millennium Development Goals.

The new *Sustainable Development Goals* explicitly target the NTDs; emphasizing the need for universal health coverage and resolving to end the epidemics of communicable and NTDs by the year 2030.

The NTDs represent a diverse group of diseases; most are vector-borne, zoonotic, or associated with contaminated water. The definitions have evolved over time and vary between agencies, but key features remain:

- They affect almost exclusively poor and marginalized populations, and they have a disproportionately low profile among public health priorities and funding.
- All are endemic in the tropics, but many also occur among marginalized and impoverished communities in temperate and wealthy countries.
- Although rural poverty is the most important determinant of NTDs, conflicts, forced migration, natural disasters, and other humanitarian emergencies can dramatically impact the transmission and severity of NTDs.

17 infectious diseases have been prioritized by the WHO and designated as official NTDs (see Table 30.1). However, there are many other diseases such as hepatitis E, cryptosporidiosis, and snakebite that share similar characteristics. These diseases have been neglected by our international community and require advocacy by humanitarian workers to address their burden among the populations we seek to help.

Table 30.1 The 17 WHO designated NTDs (those marked with an asterisk have also been classified as emerging infectious diseases)

Virus	Bacteria	Parasite	
		Protozoa (unicellular)	Helminths (multicellular)
1. Dengue* 2. Rabies*	3. Leprosy 4. Buruli ulcer 5. Trachoma 6. Yaws	7. Chagas disease (American trypanosomiasis)* 8. Human African trypanosomiasis (sleeping sickness) 9. Leishmaniasis	10. Soil-transmitted helminths 11. Cysticercosis* 12. Dracunculiasis (guinea-worm disease) 13. Echinococcosis 14. Schistosomiasis 15. Food-borne trematodes 16. Lymphatic filariasis (elephantiasis) 17. Onchocerciasis (river blindness)

Elimination and eradication of NTDs

Rather than control, WHO and partner agencies are increasingly calling for the elimination and eradication of NTDs.

Control

Reduction of disease burden to a locally acceptable level as a result of deliberate efforts. Continued measures are required to maintain the reduction.

Elimination

Zero cases in a geographic limited area; control measures needed to prevent re-establishment of transmission. Polio was eliminated from the Americas in 1994. The term 'elimination' is often used imprecisely in reference to elimination of a disease 'as a public health problem'. Epidemiological criteria for such elimination vary depending on the disease (e.g. TB elimination calls for <1 case per million per year and leprosy elimination calls for <1 case per 10,000 people per year).

Eradication

Worldwide interruption of transmission; zero cases globally and control measures no longer needed. Smallpox was eradicated in 1977. Guinea worm was targeted for eradication by 2015.

WHO-endorsed strategic interventions to address NTDs

- Preventative chemotherapy and mass drug administration (MDA).
- Intensified case management.
- Vector control.
- Veterinary public services.
- Improved access to clean water, sanitation, and hygiene services.

NTDs are particular clinical challenges, both in actual recognition of the diseases which may be unfamiliar to the provider as well as due to the contextual difficulties with prevention and management. As such, throughout the chapter, key features and challenges of each NTD will be highlighted for the reader.

Buruli ulcer

Key features

- Painless skin ulcer with characteristic undermining of the edges; can begin as a plaque or nodular lesion.
- Caused by a slow-growing environmental bacteria; *Mycobacterium ulcerans*.
- Treated with a combination of two antibiotics for 8 weeks.

Challenges

- One of the most under-diagnosed diseases.
- Need for a new field-based diagnostic test (microscopy for AFB positive in only about 50%).
- Late diagnosis leads to scarring, contractures, and disability.
- Treatment can be complicated by 'paradoxical reactions'.

Transmission

- Infection likely occurs following minor trauma and direct inoculation of *M. ulcerans* from water and soil.
- >90% of cases occur in Western and Central Africa. Sporadic cases occur in other rural tropical areas around the world.

Clinical features

- Classically presents a single painless skin ulcer on legs or arm with undermined edges.
- Nodular lesions, plaques, or localized oedema may precede ulceration.
- Fever, systemic illness, or lymphadenopathy are *not* typically seen.

See Figs 30.1–30.3.

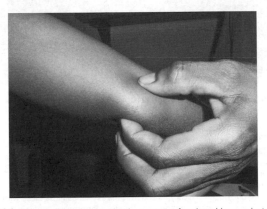

Fig. 30.1 Buruli nodule. Reproduced with permission from http://www.who.int/buruli/photos/nonulcerative/en/.

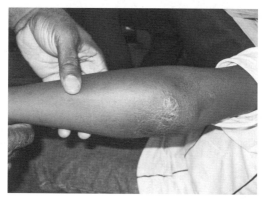

Fig. 30.2 Buruli oedema. Reproduced with permission from http://www.who.int/buruli/photos/nonulcerative/en/.

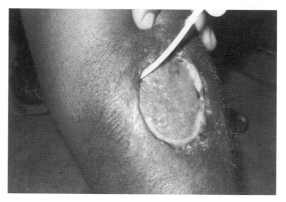

Fig. 30.3 Buruli ulcer. Reproduced with permission from http://www.who.int/buruli/photos/nonulcerative/en/.

Diagnosis
(See Table 30.2.)
- Often unrecognized and misdiagnosed, especially in early and non-ulcerative stages. Progression can lead to ulceration, scarring, and contractures.
- Can be diagnosed clinically in endemic areas as a painless ulcer with characteristic undermined edges. However, laboratory confirmation should be sought.

- Swabs of ulcer edges or needle aspirates of skin lesions should be sent for polymerase chain reaction (PCR) (microscopy for AFB is <60% sensitive).
- A referral network of laboratories capable of doing PCR has been established by the WHO.

Treatment

- Effectively treated with a combination of rifampin 600 mg PO plus one other antibiotic given daily for 8 weeks:
  - *Either* streptomycin (15 mg/kg IV/IM, maximum 1 g daily), *or* clarithromycin 500 mg PO twice daily *or* moxifloxacin 400 mg PO once daily.
- There may be transient, immune-mediated, paradoxical deterioration during or even shortly after completing therapy.
- Wound care is important; ulcers should be cleaned gently without caustic agents and covered with a white soft paraffin gauze to prevent overlying dry gauze bandages from sticking. Surgery may be needed in addition to antibiotics for extensive lesions.

Resources and further reading

- Additional information is available on the WHO Buruli ulcer website (ℜ http://www.who.int/buruli/information/publications/en/index. html) or by email (buruli@who.int).

Table 30.2 Differential diagnosis of ulcers and non-healing wounds seen in areas of humanitarian disaster. Secondary bacterial infections of traumatic wounds may be most common.

Disease	Cause	Features	Diagnosis (field)
Buruli ulcer	*Mycobacterium ulcerans*	Undermined edges, painless, typically no adenitis or fever.	Swab of margins and needle aspirate for AFB and PCR
Pyoderma (ecthyma)	*Staph aureus* or *Strep pyogenes*	Painful, acute, ± local lymphadenopathy	Clinical, response to antibiotics (e.g. cefalexin)
Tropical ulcer	Fusiform anaerobes and mixed bacteria	Painful, usually a single large ulcer on lower leg	Clinical, response to antibiotics (e.g. co-amoxiclav)
Anthrax	*Bacillus anthracis*	Painless, acute onset, central eschar, lots of oedema, ± fevers. History of exposure to animals	Gram stain (Gram-positive bacilli). Clinical response (e.g. ciprofloxacin *not* cefalexin)
Yaws	*Treponema pallidum pertenue*	Painless, typically a raised ulcerative lesion with a red, moist base (usually children)	Syphilis serology
Cutaneous leishmaniasis	*Leishmania* protozoa transmitted by sandflies	Painless ulcer, margins often raised and indurated	Scrapings of ulcer base and needle aspirate for microscopy and PCR
Fungal or mycobacterial	e.g. *Sporothrix shenkii* (fungal) *Mycobacterium marinum*	Typically a single or localized group of nodules or plaques	Biopsy, microscopy, culture, and histopathology
Venous stasis and sickle cell-related ulcerations	Vascular insufficiency, minor trauma, secondary bacterial infections	Usually medial malleolus, may be bilateral, often with lower limb oedema	Clinical, and exclusion of other causes
Pyoderma gangrenosum	Non-infectious. Often associated with systemic illness, e.g. inflammatory bowel disease	Painful, tender, violaceous ulcers; scalloping of ulcer margins	Diagnosis of exclusion; biopsy to rule out other causes

Chagas disease

Key features
- Chagas is a 'silent killer' and a leading cause of heart disease and premature death in Latin America.
- Primarily transmitted by triatomine insects (reduviid bugs) that live in poorly constructed houses.
- >7 million people, 1% of the population of Latin America, are chronically infected, of whom 30% have or will develop heart disease and arrhythmias.
- Available treatment is effective in early stages, but not once cardiac dysfunction has developed.

Challenges
- Most patients with early stages of infection are not aware of the diagnosis or their risk for heart disease.
- Vertical transmission can occur from mother to child.
- Lack of accurate diagnostic tests and therapy for chronic stages.

Transmission
- Caused by the protozoan parasite *Trypanosome cruzii*.
- Transmitted by triatomine (reduviid) bugs that live in cracks in walls of rural houses, and bite people while they are sleeping, shedding *T. cruzii* in their faeces after biting. When the person rubs or scratches at the bite site, the *T. cruzii* is introduced via breaks in the skin, conjunctiva, or mucous membranes. House improvements and insecticide residual spraying can dramatically reduce transmission (see Fig. 30.4).
- Transmission can also occur by blood transfusion or vertical transmission (mother to child), and the latter now accounts for about 25% of all new infections worldwide.

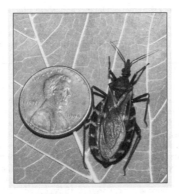

Fig. 30.4 The triatomine or reduviid bug. Reproduced with permission from https://www.cdc.gov/parasites/cme/chagas/course.html with permission from Sonia Kjos.

Clinical features
See Fig. 30.5.

Acute phase
Occurs 1–2 weeks after infection, accompanied by parasitaemia. Most people are asymptomatic or have self-limited fever and non-specific systemic manifestations. Unilateral conjunctivitis or a localized rash at the inoculation site is sometimes seen.

Chronic phase
Parasites become sequestered in the tissues of heart, oesophagus, and colon. Most patients remain asymptomatic, but when present, symptoms fall into three categories:
1. Conduction block or arrhythmias (e.g. palpitations, pre-syncope).
2. Heart failure (e.g. dyspnoea, decreased exercise tolerance).
3. Gastrointestinal involvement (e.g. dysphagia, odynophagia, constipation).

> ECG can reveal early signs of disease; especially right bundle branch block and various degrees of atrioventricular block.

Presentation in people living with HIV/AIDS
Acute reactivation with high levels of parasitaemia can occur in patients with immunosuppression. In patients with HIV/AIDS, Chagas disease can presents as meningoencephalitis mimicking toxoplasmosis.

Diagnosis
- *Microscopy*: blood smears using the same techniques as for malaria, can identify trypomastigotes only in the acute phase and in 50% of infants with congenital infection. Parasitaemia is undetectable by microscopy in the chronic phase.
- *PCR*: has excellent sensitivity in infants and acute infections, but only 30–70% sensitivity in chronic infection.
- *Antibody detection*: usually needed for the diagnosis of chronic Chagas. However, no available test is sufficiently sensitive and specific on its own. Results of multiple tests must be interpreted in combination making an accurate serological diagnosis difficult.

Treatment
There are only two drugs available against Chagas disease: benznidazole has less side effects and is first line; nifurtimox is an alternative. They are both given daily PO for 60 days. Although they are effective in acute infection (>80% cure), treatment of patients with chronic disease has not been shown to significantly reduce deterioration of cardiac function.
  The indications for use of antiparasitic drugs can be controversial:
- *Always recommended* for (1) acute, (2) early congenital, and (3) reactivated infection in setting of immunosuppression.
- *Generally recommended* for children (≤18 years) who tolerate the drugs better than older adults.

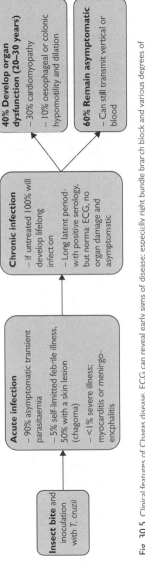

Insect bite and inoculation with *T. cruzii*

Acute infection
– 90% asymptomatic transient parasitaemia
– 5% self-limitted febrile illness, 50% with a skin lesion (chagoma)
– <1% severe illness; myocarditis or meningo-encphalitis

Chronic infection
– If untreated 100% will develop lifelong infection
– Long latent period with positive serology, but norma ECG, no organ damage and asymptomatic

40% Develop organ dysfunction (20-30 years)
– 30% cardiomyopathy
– 10% oesophageal or colonic hypomotility and dilation

60% Remain asymptomatic
– Can still transmit vertical or blood

Fig. 30.5 Clinical features of Chagas disease. ECG can reveal early signs of disease; especially right bundle branch block and various degrees of atrioventricular block.

- *Generally not recommended* for adults (>50 years) and those with already advanced heart disease.
- *Considered* for younger adults without established heart disease.

New, effective treatment for chronic Chagas disease is urgently needed.

Congenital Chagas disease

Congenital transmission occurs in 1–10% of infants born to mothers with chronic infection. Most infections are asymptomatic or non-specific (fever, anaemia, hepatosplenomegaly). Benznidazole is *not* safe in pregnancy, but treatment of infants with congenital infection is effective and prevents future chronic complications.

Screening for congenital infection includes:
- prenatal serology for all pregnant women from endemic areas
- microscopy and PCR of cord blood in seropositive mothers
- serology of baby at 9 months if negative microscopy/PCR at birth.

Dengue

Key features

- Dengue is the most rapidly spreading mosquito-borne viral disease in the world with 50–100 million infections per year.
- Most cases are mild, but there are at least 500,000 severe cases and 25,000 deaths per year
- Supportive care and IV fluids can reduce mortality of severe dengue from >20% to <1%

Challenges

- Lack of vaccine and sustained global mosquito-control efforts.
- Presentation is non-specific and can mimic malaria, bacterial, and other viral infections.
- Massive outbreaks can quickly overwhelm healthcare systems.

- Dengue is an outlier among the 17 NTDs. It affects both rich and poor communities and has drawn increased public health attention, and recent funding for vaccine development has increased exponentially.
- But, in common with NTDs, major implementation gaps still exist in surveillance and vector control. There is a massive unmet need for global access to high-quality supportive clinical care for those with severe illness; similar to sepsis.

Transmission

- Dengue is spread by *Aedes* mosquitoes—day biting, peri-domestic, and breed in rainwater in small discarded containers or old tyres.
- Highest rates occur in urban/semi-urban Asia and Latin America.

Clinical features

Dengue can be clinically indistinguishable from malaria and bacterial and other acute viral infections. Classically it presents with acute-onset fever, headache, retro-orbital pain, and myalgia. Rash occurs in 50%.

There are three phases of illness (see Fig. 30.6):

- *Febrile* phase, accompanied by high viraemia, lasts for 3–7 days.
- *Critical* phase coincides with resolution of fever and drop in viral load. Although most patients improve, there is a transient increase in capillary permeability that can lead to plasma leakage and progression to severe illness in 5–10% of people. This is where intervention with IV fluids may be life-saving.
- *Recovery* phase is marked by a rise in the platelet count and resolution of plasma leakage.

Severe dengue versus dengue haemorrhagic fever

The new WHO classification system emphasizes the recognition of plasma leakage rather than haemorrhage as the most important feature for clinical management of patients with dengue (Fig. 30.7).

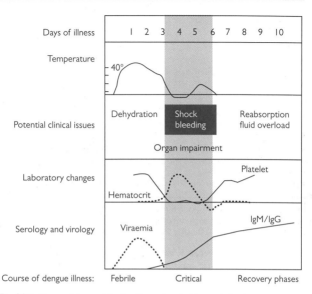

Fig. 30.6 Phases of dengue infection. Reproduced with permission from
Dengue: Guidelines for diagnosis, treatment, prevention, and control, new edition
2009, World Health Organization (WHO) and the Special Programme for Research
and Training in Tropical Diseases (TDR), page 25.

Diagnosis

Clinical diagnosis and the tourniquet test are unreliable outside of outbreak settings—laboratory testing is needed. Rapid point-of-care tests are
commercially available and should be used for diagnosis and surveillance.
Test selection depends on timing and tests may be used in combination to
maximize yield.

- *NS1 antigen* correlates with viremia, is positive early (day 1 of illness)
  but disappears by day 5–7 of illness.
- *Immunoglobulin (Ig)-M antibodies* appear later (beginning around day 5
  of illness). IgM response is lower and may be negative in secondary
  infections in which an early IgG response predominates.

All dengue cases should be reported to health authorities, to document
burden, identify outbreaks, and guide community interventions.

Treatment

- Patients with dengue and warning signs (see Fig. 30.7): should be
  admitted to hospital for close monitoring and supportive care.
- Monitor vital signs closely for signs of compensated shock:
  - Narrowing of pulse pressure.
  - Persistent tachycardia as fever drops.

- Follow Hct every 12–24 hours: a *rise* in Hct with *fall* in platelets indicates plasma leakage, and need for IV fluids.
- Careful IV fluid therapy is critical to management of dengue shock. The WHO handbook helps guide IV fluids and clinical care (⅋ http://www.who.int/csr/resources/publications/dengue_9789241547871/en/).

- Providing care to critically ill patients in low-resource settings is challenging, but supportive care and IV fluids can reduce mortality of severe dengue from >20% to <1%.
- A strong critical care programme can also support patients with influenza, or other causes of sepsis, and should be part of epidemic preparedness planning.

Secondary infection and severe disease

There are four dengue serotypes (DEN-1, -2, -3, and -4). Following infection, patients have life-long immunity to only one serotype. Secondary infections with a different serotype can occur, and are associated with an increased risk for severe dengue—but the overall risk remains low.

Personal precautions and vector control

- Personal protective measures: mosquito repellent (DEET) during the day, protective clothing during the day, and screens on houses are useful. Insecticide-treated bed nets and sheeting can be used in emergency shelters.
- Vector control: peri-domestic insecticide spraying and removal of old tyres or empty containers to reduce mosquito breeding sites.
- Dengue is not spread by contact or droplets in hospital, but because other communicable diseases present similarly, additional precautions may need to be in place before diagnosis.

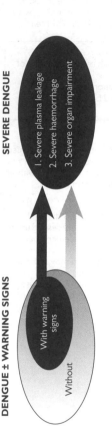

DENGUE ± WARNING SIGNS

SEVERE DENGUE

With warning signs

Without

1. Severe plasma leakage
2. Severe haemorrhage
3. Severe organ impairment

CRITERIA FOR DENGUE ± WARNING SIGNS

Probable dengue

Live in/travel to dengue endemic area.
Fever and 2 of the following criteria:

• Nausea, vomiting
• Rash
• Aches and pains
• Tourniquet test positive
• Leukopenia
• Any warning sign

Laboratory-confirmed dengue
(Important when no sign of plasma leakage)

Warning signs*

• Abdominal pain or tenderness
• Persistent vomiting
• Clinical fluid accumulation
• Mucosal bleed
• Lethargy, restlessness
• Liver enlargment >2 cm
• Laboratory: increase in HCT concurrent with rapid decrease in platelet count

*(Requiring strict observation and medical intervention)

CRITERIA FOR SEVERE DENGUE

Severe plasma leakage

leading to:

• Shock (DSS)
• Fluid accumulation with respiratory distress

Severe bleeding

as evaluated by clinician

Severe organ involvement

• Liver: AST or ALT >= 1000
• CNS: Impaired consciousness
• Heart and other organs

Fig. 30.7 Clinical classification of dengue infection. Reproduced with permission from Dengue: Guidelines for diagnosis, treatment, prevention, and control, new edition 2009, World Health Organization (WHO) and the Special Programme for Research and Training in Tropical Diseases (TDR), page 11.

Human African trypanosomiasis

Key features

- Also known as African sleeping sickness, human African trypanosomiasis (HAT) is caused by a single-cellular protozoan parasite transmitted by tsetse flies
- There are two forms of HAT and both are fatal if not treated
  - In Western and Central Africa—*Trypanosoma brucei gambiense* (G-HAT):
    —*Chronic form*, can mimic mental illness, 98% of all HAT cases.
  - In East and Southern Africa—*Trypanosoma brucei rhodesiense* (R-HAT):
    —*Acute form*, can mimic malaria, occurs sporadically.

Challenges

- It is often misdiagnosed, under-reported, and inadequately treated.
- Poverty and remoteness of affected areas limits access to care.
- Current medications available for CNS stage of R-HAT are toxic.

Transmission

The tsetse fly has a painful bite and patchy distribution throughout sub-Saharan Africa. 90% of all HAT cases occur in the DRC.

Clinical features

There are two clinical stages common to all forms of HAT:

- *First haemolymphatic stage*: characterized by fevers, headaches, and myalgias—without cerebrospinal fluid (CSF) involvement.
- *Second meningoencephalitic (CNS) stage*: characterized by parasite penetration into the CSF causing encephalopathy and behaviour changes that may progresses to coma and death.

The two subspecies of *Trypanosome brucei* that cause HAT are morphologically identical but occur in geographically separate areas and have different disease presentations.

G-HAT accounts for 98% of all HAT cases globally, most of which occur in the DRC. It is indolent and chronic.

- The first stage can be protracted for months with non-specific symptoms such as low-grade fevers and malaise. Posterior cervical adenopathy (*Winterbottom's sign*) may be present.
- The onset of the second stage is often marked by psychiatric or behavioural changes, followed by impairment of speech, cerebellar function, and motor function over months to years leading to coma and death.

R-HAT is a zoonotic infection, the reservoir is mainly wild antelope. It occurs sporadically in people.

- The first stage is much more acute with more prominent fever and systemic illness than G-HAT. Patients may even die of myocarditis or multiorgan failure before reaching the CNS stage. A skin lesion (chancre) develops in 20–50% at the site of the tsetse fly bite. CNS manifestations are similar to G-HAT but the time-course is much faster.

Diagnosis

- R-HAT is diagnosed by *microscopy* of blood films (like malaria).

- G-HAT has much lower levels of parasitaemia but is easier to diagnosis thanks to the availability of serologic tests such as the card agglutination test (CATT) and point-of-care rapid tests (RDTs).
- Because treatment varies depending on the stage, lumbar puncture is required for all patients even in absence of CNS symptoms. CSF should be examined for trypanosomes and number of WBCs.
- Second CNS stage = >5–20 WBC/mL or any parasites seen in the CSF.

Treatment

- Treatment depends on disease type and stage (see Table 30.3.) All drugs are provided free of charge through the WHO and administered according to national guidelines.
- Treatment of G-HAT has been revolutionized by eflornithine.
- Treatment for R-HAT remains challenging. Eflornithine lacks efficacy against R-HAT and melarsoprol causes potentially fatal encephalopathy in about 5% of treated individuals

Table 30.3 Differentiation of G-HAT and R-HAT

Parasite/disease	Gambiense (G-HAT)	Rhodesiense (R-HAT)
Distribution	Central and Western Africa	Eastern and Southeastern Africa
Incidence	~98% of all HAT cases reported ~20,000 cases/year	~2% of all HAT cases reported
Presentation	Indolent: low-grade fever, headache Often misdiagnosed as mental illness	Acute: fever, headache ± myocarditis Often misdiagnosed as malaria
Incubation period	Months–years	1–3 weeks
Posterior cervical lymphadenopathy	Characteristic	Absent
Skin chancre	Absent	Characteristic
Parasitaemia	Uncommon/low	Common/high
Serology testing	Yes	No
Vector	Riverine tsetse flies	Savanna tsetse flies
Primary reservoir	Humans	Antelope (zoonotic disease)
Occurrence in travellers	Very rare among travellers, occasionally seen in immigrants	Occasionally among travellers to safari parks
Treatment		
First stage	Pentamidine	Pentamidine or Suramin
Second (CNS) stage	Nifurtimox + eflornithine combination therapy (NECT)	Melarsoprol Prednisone may decrease risk of CNS toxicity

Leishmaniasis

Key features
- Caused by a protozoan parasite transmitted by sandflies,
- Three clinical syndromes (visceral VL, cutaneous CL, and mucosal ML)
  - *Skin lesions* (CL), the most common form, can be stigmatizing.
  - *Systemic febrile illness* (VL), the most severe form, is fatal without treatment.
- Epidemics occur in areas of conflict and humanitarian disaster.

Challenges
- Lack of simple field-based diagnostic tests and lack of uniformly reliable treatments for CL.
- Social stigma and community misconceptions about CL can lead to devastating isolation and marginalization of those with facial lesions.

Transmission
- Sandflies (one-third the size of mosquito) in either urban or rural settings.
- Depending on the region, the reservoir host can be predominantly animals (dogs and rodents) or people.

Clinical features
Clinical manifestations depend on the species, geographic location, and host response. There are three distinct clinical syndromes (Table 30.4).

Viscera leishmaniasis (kala-azar)
In endemic areas, VL is a disease of childhood, often occurring below 5 years of age. In outbreaks all ages may be equally affected.

Clinical features
- Fever ($\geq$2 weeks).
- Splenomegaly (can be massive).
- Weight loss.
- Pancytopenia.

Diagnosis
- *Serology* is the primary means for diagnosis. The rk39 point-of-care antibody test and additional serological testing, such as the direct agglutination test (DAT) should be available in endemic areas.
- A positive serological test in a patient with compatible presentation is enough to establish the diagnosis and start treatment. Splenic or bone marrow aspirates can be reserved for cases of relapse.

Treatment of VL
There are three principal medications used for treatment of VL. The recommended regimens vary by region and national guidelines.
- *Liposomal amphotericin B (L-amB)* is the most effective anti-leish medication; just one 10 mg/kg dose is curative in India, longer courses (e.g. 3–5 mg/kg daily × 10 days) are recommended in East Africa and Latin America.
- *Miltefosine* is the only oral medication with proven efficacy against VL. A 30 day course is safe and generally well tolerated.

Table 30.4 Clinical syndromes of leishmaniasis

	Visceral leishmaniasis (VL) 'Kala-azar'	Cutaneous leishmaniasis (CL)	Mucosal leishmaniasis (MCL)
Cases/year globally	200,000–400,000 cases/year	0.7–1.3 million cases/year	<10,000 cases/year
Species	*Leishmania donovani, L. infantum*	Old world: *L. tropica, L. major* New world: *L. braziliensis, L. mexicana*	New world: *L. braziliensis*
Regions affected	≥90% of cases occur in either: 1. India (Bihar), Bangladesh, and Nepal 2. Sudan 3. Brazil	≥90% of cases occur in: 1. Iran, Saudi Arabia, and Syria 2. Afghanistan 3. Brazil and Peru	Only in Latin America (New World) ≥90% of cases occur in: Bolivia, Peru, or Brazil
Clinical features	Systemic febrile illness Anaemia, weight loss, and splenomegaly Fatal if untreated	Skin lesions Typically ulcers on exposed skin Most self-cure Can cause permanent scars and stigma	Destructive lesions of naso- and oropharynx Typically 1–5 years *after* CL skin lesions Occurs in 2–5% of patients with *L. braziliensis*

- *Pentavalent antimony (Sb^{5+})* is the historical gold standard for VL. However, as a heavy metal compound, Sb^{5+} has severe toxicities (e.g. arrhythmias and pancreatitis), particularly in patients with HIV. There is increasing resistance to Sb^{5+} especially in India.

Combination treatment can improve efficacy and prevent resistance. Combination therapy with L-amB plus miltefosine is becoming the treatment of choice for VL in patients with HIV.

> *HIV and leishmaniasis:* VL is an opportunistic infection. Patients with HIV have a much higher risk of developing VL, an increased risk of treatment failure, and very high rates of relapse. L-amB 3 mg/kg every 3 weeks is often used for secondary prophylaxis, but standard regimens have not yet been established.

Cutaneous leishmaniasis

Clinical features
- Typically starts as a small papule, which ulcerates and enlarges to form a single painless ulcer with a raised indurated border. (See Fig. 30.8.)
- CL can be atypical; lesions may be multiple or plaque-like. Almost any skin lesion in an endemic area could be CL.

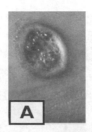

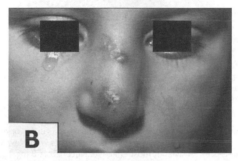

Fig. 30.8 Cutaneous leishmaniasis develops at the site of a sandfly bite, typically begins as a small area of erythema or papule, and can have variable manifestations; a high index of suspicion is required for diagnosis.

A) Shows a classic wet ulcerative lesion with a characteristic raised border on the forearm. Reproduced from Ahmad Fawad Jebran et al, Rapid Healing of Cutaneous Leishmaniasis by High-Frequency Electrocauterization and Hydrogel Wound Care with or without DAC N-055: A Randomized Controlled Phase IIa Trial in Kabul, PLOS Neglected Tropical Diseases: 13/02/2014 (http://journals.plos.org/plosntds/article?id=10.1371%2Fjournal.pntd.0002694). Copyright: Creative Commons Attribution (CC BY 4.0).

B) Shows a dry crusting plaque-like lesion on the face. Reproduced with permission from Elie Alam et al, Cutaneous Leishmaniasis: An Overlooked Etiology of Midfacial Destructive Lesions, PLOS Neglected Tropical Diseases: 10/02/2016 (http://journals.plos.org/plosntds/article?id=10.1371/journal.pntd.0004426#pntd-0004426-g001). Copyright: Creative Commons Attribution (CC BY 4.0).

Diagnosis
- In endemic areas, CL is typically diagnosed clinically but laboratory confirmation should be sought if possible.
- Ulcer scrapings, needle aspirates, or punch biopsy can be examined for parasites by microscopy (60% sensitive) or sent to reference laboratories for PCR (>95% sensitive). (See Fig. 30.9.)

Treatment
- Most cases of CL resolve on their own without medical treatment. Minor skin lesions need only wound care.
- Response to treatment is variable and region specific—there is no 'one-size-fits-all' treatment for CL.
- Local therapies include topical paromomycin ointment, cryotherapy, or intralesional injections of Sb^{5+}.

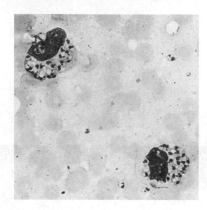

Fig. 30.9 Leishmania parasites can be recognized by microscope as small, round intracellular structures within macrophages with two distinct pieces of chromatin; a larger nucleus and a smaller kinetoplast, a mitochondria-like structure. Reproduced from https://www.cdc.gov/dpdx/leishmaniasis/ with permission from CDC DPDx.

- Systemic therapy (similar to VL) is used in facial, disfiguring, or extensive disease and may prevent mucosal disease in patients with New World CL. L-amB is expensive but most effective. Fluconazole 8 mg/kg/day × 6 weeks PO has recently been shown to be a promising alternative for both Old and New World CL.

Mucosal leishmaniasis

Clinical features
- Mucosal lesions are painless, slowly progressive, and destructive.
- The nasal septum, palate, and nasopharynx are typically affected. Lips are only rarely involved.
- MCL typically begins as nasal itchiness or epistaxis. Patients with New World CL should be counselled and actively examined for mucosal involvement.

Diagnosis
Similar to CL, MCL can be diagnosed by tissue scrapings sent for microscopy and PCR.

Treatment
- Systemic therapy is necessary and effective.
- Treatment options are similar to VL, with L-amB and miltefosine being most effective. A prolonged course of therapy is generally required, expert advice should be sought.

Resources and further reading
The WHO has published region-specific and practical guidelines on diagnosis and management of leishmaniasis (⌘ http://www.who.int/leishmaniasis/resources/en/). National guidelines should also be consulted.

Yaws

Key features
- Painless skin lesions including plaques and ulcers.
- Caused by bacteria very similar to those that cause syphilis *Treponema pallidum*.
- Transmitted by direct contact, in conditions of poverty, overcrowding, and poor hygiene.
- Most cases occur in children (ages 5–10 years).

Challenges
- Yaws occurs in remote settings *'where the road ends, yaws begins'*.
- If untreated, yaws can affect nasal cartilage and long bones; leading to deformity and disability
- Effective treatment with single-dose azithromycin offers promise of eradication by 2020.

Transmission
Transmitted by direct skin to skin contact in warm, tropical environments with crowding, and poor hygiene.

Clinical features
Like syphilis, there are characteristic stages of yaws:

Early (infectious)
- Primary yaws begins as a papule and can evolve into a round 2–5 cm raised lesion—often a painless ulcer with a red, moist base.
- Secondary yaws occurs weeks later and is characterized by additional primary-yaws-type skin lesions and patches of thickened/cracked skin on palms and soles. There can be painful inflammation of tibial bones (periostitis) and fingers (dactylitis).

See Fig. 30.10.

Late (non-infectious)
Late or tertiary yaws is now very rarely seen. But, if untreated, in about 10% of cases yaws can lead to deformities of the nose and long bones.

Diagnosis
Clinical diagnosis is confirmed with serology; using the same tests used for syphilis, including VDRL and new point-of-care rapid tests. Serology cannot distinguish between yaws and syphilis.

Treatment
- Azithromycin 30 mg/kg (maximum 2000 mg) single dose.
- Benzathine benzylpenicillin 1.2 million units IM single dose.

Eradication
Treatment with single-dose azithromycin is effective and community-wide treatment interventions offer promise of eradication by 2020.

(a)

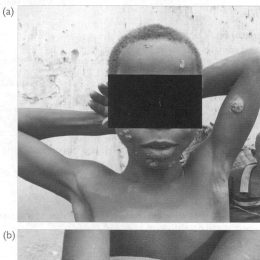

(b)

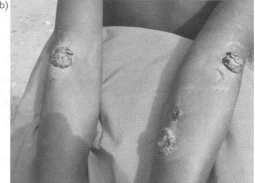

Fig. 30.10 Photograph of typical painless 'framboise' yaws lesions in children from Côte d'Ivoire. Reproduced with permission from http://www.who.int/yaws/photos/en/index2.html.

Leprosy

Key points

- Leprosy is a stigmatizing, disfiguring, and disabling disease of the skin and peripheral nerves caused by *Mycobacterium leprae*.
- Despite public perception, leprosy is not very contagious and is entirely treatable.
- Early diagnosis and prompt treatment of *neuritis* is necessary to prevent nerve damage.

Challenges

- The stigma of leprosy is severe and can be worse than the disease (using the term *Hansen's disease* may reduce the sense of stigma).
- Treatment with clofazimine can cause (reversible) darkening of the skin and increase stigma.
- Patient (and family) education and opportunity for discussion is essential.

Leprosy is an ancient disease. It has been eliminated from most countries, but in 2014 there were still >200,000 new cases reported.

Transmission

The exact mechanism is unknown, but leprosy is probably transmitted via respiratory droplets. 95% of people are naturally immune to the disease. Once on effective treatment patients are no longer infectious. Because of the very low risk of transmission, patient isolation or additional contact or droplet precautions are not recommended.

Clinical features

Manifestations of leprosy occur along a spectrum between two forms, tuberculoid and lepromatous, depending on the host immune response:

Tuberculoid leprosy: paucibacillary

- Strong cell-mediated immune response—AFB rarely seen in tissue.
- Only a few skin lesions.
- Skin lesions are characteristically *hypoaesthetic* (i.e. numb).
- Peripheral nerve involvement is limited to one or two superficial nerves that may be palpably enlarged.

Lepromatous leprosy: multibacillary

- Weak cell-mediated immune response—many AFB are seen in tissue.
- Diffuse skin involvement.
- Skin lesions are *not* hypoaesthetic and there may be thickening of earlobes and loss of eyebrows.
- Peripheral nerves show glove and stocking sensory loss.

Borderline leprosy

- Lies somewhere between tuberculoid and lepromatous.
- Multiple, asymmetric lesions with variable sensory impairment and nerve involvement.
- Immunologically unstable and reversal reactions are very common

See Figs 30.11–30.14.

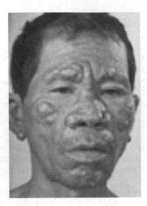

Fig. 30.11 Characteristic *leonine* faces of lepromatous leprosy (symmetrical, widespread skin infiltration, thickened ears, and loss of eyebrows). Skin slit smears or biopsy would show multiple AFB and confirm the diagnosis of MB leprosy. Reproduced with permission from Guinto, Ricardo S., Abalos, Rodolfo M., Cellona, Roland V., and Fajardo, Tranquilino T., An Atlas of Leprosy; 1983, Tokyo, Sasakawa Memorial Health Foundation.

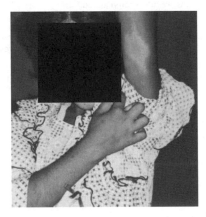

Fig. 30.12 Skin patches with definite loss of sensation are diagnostic of leprosy. This young girl with a single hypoaestheic patch should be carefully examined for any peripheral nerve involvement and started on treatment for leprosy. Reproduced with permission from McDougall, A. Colin, and Yuasa, Yo, A New Atlas of Leprosy, 2002, Tokyo, Sasakawa Memorial Health Foundation.

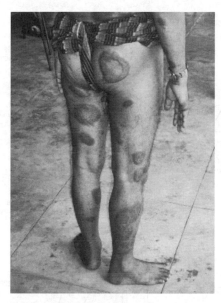

Fig. 30.13 Numerous irregular rings with 'punched out' centres characteristic of borderline leprosy. Many lesions showed loss of sensation and there were three enlarged peripheral nerves confirming the diagnosis of leprosy. Reproduced with permission from McDougall, A. Colin, and Yuasa, Yo, A New Atlas of Leprosy, Sasakawa Memorial Health Foundation, Tokyo, 2002.

Diagnosis

There are three cardinal signs, any *one* of which is diagnostic of leprosy:

1. Skin lesion with definite loss of sensation.
2. Enlarged peripheral nerves.
3. AFB seen on microscopy of skin slit smear.

Physical exam

- A complete skin and a careful neurological examination are essential.
- Sensory loss may be occult and not noticed by the patient. Palpate peripheral superficial nerves for swelling and check sensation and strength in the hands and feet.

Skin slit smears

Laboratory testing is not needed for diagnosis if there is a distinct hypoaesthetic skin patch. However, skin slit smears are useful for the diagnosis of lepromatous leprosy. Procedure: on one earlobe and an area of affected skin, make a small slit (1–2 mm deep), then with the edge of the scalpel held perpendicular gently scrape the exposed dermis, smear the material on a slide, stain for AFB, and examine by microscopy.

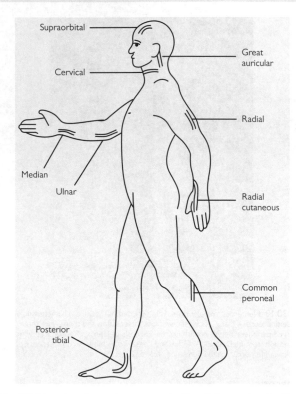

Fig. 30.14 Locations of nerves most commonly affected in leprosy; they should be palpated for swelling and tenderness. Other affected nerves include the facial, posterior auricular, median, and radial nerves. Reproduced with permission from Hastings RC and Opromolla DVA (eds). Leprosy, 2nd edn. Churchill Livingstone, 1994.

Treatment

The WHO has simplified the diagnosis and treatment of leprosy. Standardized, programmatic, multidrug drug therapy (MDT) is offered according to two categories:
- *1–5 skin lesions* = paucibacillary: treated with two drugs for 6 months (rifampin and dapsone).
- *>5 skin lesions* = multibacillary: treated with three drugs for 1 year (rifampin, dapsone, and clofazimine).

Treatment pearls
- Patients should be cautioned that clofazimine can cause (reversible) skin darkening.
- Once-monthly treatment with rifampicin, ofloxacin, and minocycline (ROM) may be just as effective as the WHO daily MDT.
- Patients should be advised about the possibility of neuritis and instructed to present to medical attention if they notice any nerve impairment.
- Neuritis and leprosy reactions are treated with prednisone. Early recognition and steroid treatment is needed to prevent nerve damage.

Reactions

Leprosy reactions are immune-mediated inflammatory complications that occur in 30–50% of patients. They can occur before or during MDT treatment and are a leading cause of nerve damage.

Type 1 reactions are caused by an upgrading of the cell-mediated immune response. Existing skin lesions become inflamed and affected nerves may become swollen and tender—weakness or sensory loss may develop. *Prednisone*, starting at 40–60 mg per day and tapering slowly over 6 months can reduce the inflammation and is about 50% effective in preventing permanent damage.

Type 2 reactions (erythema nodosum leprosum (ENL)) are systemic reactions to immune complex deposition in patients with lepromatous disease—similar to serum sickness. New subcutaneous nodules may develop, accompanied by fever, lymphadenitis, arthritis, and/or iritis

---

Corticosteroids increase the risk for three key infections

1. TB: screen for latent TB infection with skin testing and consider providing treatment for latent TB infection.
2. Hepatitis B: screen with serology and monitor carefully for liver inflammation if positive.
3. Strongyloidiasis: empiric treatment is recommended if using steroids in settings with high prevalence of strongyloidiasis (e.g. ivermectin 200 mcg/kg on 2 consecutive days or 2 weeks apart).

Prophylaxis and treatment of contacts
Although chemoprophylaxis is not universally provided, treatment of contacts with a single-dose of rifampicin has been shown to reduce the risk of leprosy.

Patient education
It is essential to have an open discussion with patients and family members about misconceptions, stigma, and transmission. Using the term Hansen's disease may reduce sense of stigma.

Patients need to be carefully counselled about the risks of impaired sensation to prevent secondary damage to neuropathic areas.

Filariasis

Filaria are thread-like, tissue dwelling roundworms transmitted by fly or mosquito vectors.

The three principal filarial infections are lymphatic filariasis, onchocerciasis, and loiasis (see Table 30.5). Each has two developmental stages: macrofilaria (adult worms) and microfilaria (larval offspring). The presence of endosymbiotic *Wolbachia* bacteria makes lymphatic filariasis and onchocerciasis susceptible to doxycycline.

Lymphatic filariasis

A leading cause of permanent disability. >1 billion people live in areas at risk and 120 million people are chronically infected. The most common manifestations are chronic lymphoedema and hydrocele.

Clinical features

Asymptomatic microfilaraemia:

The majority of infected people are asymptomatic. Many have eosinophilia, low-level, intermittent microfilaraemia and are reservoirs for disease transmission.

Acute adenolymphangitis (ADL):

Recurrent episodes of ADL are due to bacterial superinfection and impaired lymphatic drainage. Fevers may be the predominant symptom. ADL typically resolves on its own within 5 days, but contributes to disease progression and lymphoedema.

Chronic disease:

Over years, lymphatic obstruction and recurrent episodes of ADL lead to overt lymphoedema or hydrocele (men) which can be unilateral or bilateral. In women, axillary node involvement can lead to breast oedema.

Table 30.5 Key filarial infections

Filarial infection	Vector	Region most affected	Location of macrofilariae	Location of micro-filariae	Clinical features	Wolbachia present
Lymphatic filariasis (elephantiasis)	Mosquito	SE Asia, India, Africa, Pacific	Lymph vessels	Blood	Foot swelling Lymphoedema Hydrocele	Yes
Onchocerciasis (river blindness)	Black fly	West and Central Africa	Subcutaneous nodules	Skin and eye	Itchiness Dermatitis Blindness	Yes
Loiasis (*Loa loa*) (African eyeworm)	Deer fly	West and Central Africa	Migratory (subcutaneous tissues)	Blood	Painless migration across conjunctiva	No

Diagnosis of lymphatic filariasis
- Often diagnosed clinically in endemic areas as painless, chronic asymmetric leg swelling or hydrocele.
- Microfilaria seen on thick blood films can provide definitive diagnosis; but it is intermittent, usually nocturnal and, often very low level. Passing blood through a filter may help increase the yield.
- Rapid tests for circulating filarial antigen are more sensitive than microscopy, but may also be negative in late stages.
- In men, ultrasound can often detect adult worms in dilated scrotal lymphatics—the 'filarial dance sign'.

Treatment of individual patients
- *Doxycycline* (200 mg daily × ≥6 weeks) by targeting the *Wolbachia* bacteria can kill the adult worms and improve lymphoedema
- Careful skin care, washing the leg daily with soap and water, and use of antibiotics for superinfections can prevent progression.
- Large hydroceles can be treated surgically.

Elimination of lymphatic filariasis
- The WHO recommends MDA with single-doses of albendazole plus either ivermectin or diethylcarbamazine (DEC) to kill microfilaria and interrupt transmission.
- Unlike doxycycline, MDA with albendazole does not kill the adult worms and must be repeated annually for several years.

Onchocerciasis (river blindness)
Onchocerciasis is a leading cause of preventable blindness in Africa; >30 million people are chronically infected and >1 million are blind or severely visually impaired. It also causes dermatitis which can be intensely itchy and is often misdiagnosed as scabies or eczema.

Life cycle
Threadlike adult worms live in subcutaneous nodules (0.5–3 cm in size) typically over the iliac crest or chest wall. They release tiny microfilaria into the skin that cause inflammation in the skin and eyes.

Clinical features
- *Dermatitis*: characteristically itchy, can mimic eczema, presents as a papular rash or just itchy skin.
- *Eye disease*: begins with corneal opacities that progress to scarring and blindness. Chorioretinitis contributes to visual impairment.

Diagnosis
- In endemic low-resource areas, onchocerciasis is often diagnosed clinically and treated empirically (see ➔ p. 494).
- Corneal opacities can be seen at late stages; slit-lamp and fundoscopy is needed to detect early punctate keratitis and chorioretinitis.
- Skin snip biopsy, if available, can confirm the diagnosis (see Fig. 30.15.

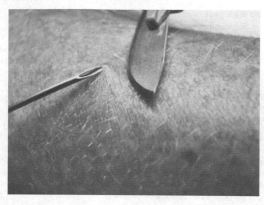

Fig. 30.15 Skin snip can be done by carefully slicing off a tiny piece of superficial dermis, about 1 mm deep. Several non-bloody skin snips can be placed in saline on a slide and examined ≥3 hours later with microscopy for microfilaria which emerge from the skin. Reproduced with permission from https://www.cdc.gov/parasites/onchocerciasis/health_professionals/.

Treatment
- Ivermectin—a single dose clears microfilaria and reduces the itch. But it does not kill the adult filarial worms so treatment must be repeated every 3–6 months for up to 10 years until adults die.
- Doxycycline 200 mg daily × 6 weeks can kill the adult worms and should be used for management of individual patients instead of repeated doses of ivermectin.
- DEC should not be used in people who may have onchocerciasis because it can trigger inflammation and ocular damage.

Elimination of onchocerciasis
The WHO recommends MDA with single-doses of albendazole plus ivermectin to kill microfilaria and interrupt transmission.

Loiasis
Loiasis, African eyeworm, is endemic in ten countries in Western and Central Africa; an estimated 13 million people are infected.

Clinical manifestations
Threadlike adult macrofilaria migrate through subcutaneous and connective tissues and release tiny microfilariae into the bloodstream.

Surprisingly, most patients are completely asymptomatic. Migration of the adult worm across the conjunctiva of the eye is dramatic but not harmful. Transient episodes of localized angio-oedema can occur characteristically at the wrist (Calabar swellings).

Diagnosis
Diagnosis can be made by patient self-report of a migrating 'eyeworm' or by detecting *Loa loa* microfilariae on a blood film.

Treatment
- Treatment is complicated by adverse reactions to antiparasitic treatment. Rapid killing of circulating *Loa loa* microfilaria in the blood by DEC, and less commonly ivermectin, can trigger an inflammatory reaction and encephalopathy.
- Albendazole is safe and can gradually bring down the microfilaremia—over months. Doxycycline is not effective because *Loa loa* do not depend on *Wolbachia* bacteria.

Neurocysticercosis

Key points
- Caused by the cyst stages of pork tapeworm (*Taenia solium*).
- Leading cause of adult-acquired seizure disorder worldwide.
- It is found globally, most commonly in areas of poor sanitation where pigs (and humans) are in contact with human faeces.

Challenges
- Requires neuroimaging (computed tomography (CT) or magnetic resonance imaging (MRI)) for diagnosis.
- Antiparasitic treatment and killing the cysts can trigger inflammation and seizures. It should be given with steroids.

Life cycle
- Only humans carry intestinal pork tapeworms acquired by eating infected pork meat. These people are asymptomatic, but shed eggs in stool and play an essential role in disease transmission.
- When people (or pigs) ingest eggs excreted by intestinal tapeworm carriers, the larvae form small cysts in muscles and body tissues.
- When cysts form in the brain, the condition is called neurocysticercosis (NCC).

Clinical features
- Most people with NCC are asymptomatic. After a variable number of years, the cysts begin to degenerate and can elicit an inflammatory response.
- Cysts in brain parenchyma present with seizures. People are generally well and asymptomatic in between seizure episodes.
- Extraparenchymal cysts (in ventricles or subarachnoid space) are less common and typically associated with hydrocephalus.

Diagnosis
- Serology has excellent (≥98%) sensitivity for ≥2 cysts, but only approximately 60% sensitive for single or calcified cysts.
- CT or MRI is needed for diagnosis of NCC. A single 1 cm cyst is most common, but the number and appearance of cysts are variable. Other infections including TB always need to be considered. Identification of a scolex—a small nodule within the cyst—is the only pathognomonic radiological finding.

Treatment
- Antiparasitic therapy with albendazole or praziquantel can kill the cysts and reduce the future risk of seizures. Although individual practice varies, a combination of albendazole 800 mg/day + praziquantel 50 mg/kg/day in two divided doses × 10 days is often used. Longer courses are required for extraparenchymal cysts.
- Corticosteroids should be given with antiparasitic therapy to manage the transient inflammation as cysts die. Prednisone 1 mg/kg/day for 10 days, followed by a gradual 8–12 week taper.
- Household contacts of patients with NCC should be screened by stool microscopy. Those with pork tapeworm eggs can be treated with a single 600 mg dose of praziquantel.

Rabies

Key points
- Rabies should be considered in all patients who present with acute encephalitis.
- Rabies is 100% preventable, but once symptomatic it is almost 100% fatal.
- All animal bites and scratches should be carefully assessed for rabies risk.
- Rabies elimination is possible through mass vaccination of dogs.

Challenges
- Access to effective rabies post-exposure prophylaxis (PEP) is limited in areas of rural poverty.
- Rabies still causes >50,000 deaths annually.

Transmission
- Rabies is transmitted by saliva of an infected animal; primarily by bites, but also scratches with contaminated claws, or licking mucosa and broken skin.
- Worldwide >99% of rabies deaths are from dog bites. Dramatic reductions are possible through mass vaccination of dogs and careful management of dog-bite victims.

Clinical presentation
- Symptoms usually begin about 1 month after exposure but can range between 7 days to >2 years. Classic symptoms include:
  - pain or paraesthesia at the site of the bite wound
  - hydrophobia, dysphagia, and hypersalivation
  - alternating periods of lucidity, agitation, and confusion.
- The 'furious' form (80% of human cases) is dominated by hyper-reactivity, agitation, and spasms. The 'paralytic' form is characterized by paralysis that often starts at the bite site and can mimic Guillain–Barré syndrome.

Diagnosis
Clinical diagnosis can be challenging; a history of animal bite may not be provided and wounds may have healed. A high index of clinical suspicion is necessary. Public health or MOH programmes should be contacted for confirmatory testing at a reference laboratory.

Treatment
Rabies can be very dramatic, and spasms and agitation can be extremely distressing. Management should be palliative with IV diazepam and morphine. Death usually occurs within 2 weeks.

Prevention
Local wound care
As a first step, immediately flush and wash the area with soap and water × 15 minutes to inactivate the virus.

Post-exposure prophylaxis

As a rule of thumb, the default practice should be to administer PEP unless there is reliable information indicating that is not required. All dog bites in rabies-endemic countries are high risk, especially if the bite was unprovoked, or if the animal was behaving abnormally. (See Table 30.6.)

PEP should be given as soon as possible, carefully following WHO-approved schedules and dosing protocols. Providers seeing patients in low-resource settings need to advocate and support patients to ensure they can receive the full PEP schedule, particularly those who live far from health facilities.

Rabies vaccine

There are several WHO-approved PEP regimens requiring three to five clinic visits. See WHO website (⌘ http://apps.who.int/iris/handle/10665/85346).

Rabies immunoglobulin (RIG)

If RIG is indicated and not immediately available, vaccination should not be delayed. RIG can be given later—but not >7 days after the first dose of vaccine because an active antibody response will have already started.

10-day observation period

In countries where canine rabies is rare or eliminated, if a dog appears healthy and can be observed for 10 days, PEP can be deferred. However, in countries where canine rabies is prevalent, PEP should be started immediately. If the animal remains healthy for the 10-day observation period, PEP can then be discontinued.

Table 30.6 Rabies post-exposure prophylaxis for categories of contact

Categories of contact with suspect rabid animal	PEP
Category I—touching, licks or secretions on intact skin	None
Category II—minor scratches or bites of uncovered skin without obvious bleeding	Vaccine alone Local treatment of the wound
Category III—bites or scratches that penetrate the skin, licks or saliva on broken skin or mucous membranes	Vaccine *plus* Immunoglobulin* Local treatment of the wound

* Rabies immunoglobulin can be omitted in patients who have been previously vaccinated using a 3-dose pre-exposure regimen.

Schistosomiasis

Key points
- Caused by a short flatworm known as a trematode or fluke.
- Acquired by direct contact with contaminated fresh water.
- At least 200 million people are affected and 90% of cases occur in sub-Saharan Africa.
- Schistosomiasis affects the liver (portal hypertension), urogenital tract, and intestinal system.

Challenges
- Chronic stages cause liver fibrosis and portal hypertension with oesophageal varices and risk of massive gastrointestinal bleeding.
- Female genital ulceration is common and increases the risk of HIV acquisition.

There are three main species of *Schistosoma*: *S. mansoni, haematobium, and japonicum*. All cause liver fibrosis and portal hypertension.

S. haematobium also affects the bladder and genitourinary system.

Transmission
Schistosomiasis is acquired by direct skin contact with freshwater in lakes or rivers that have been contaminated by stool or urine of patients with schistosomiasis. Snails act as intermediate hosts.

Clinical features
Acute schistosomiasis syndrome
- Acute schistosomiasis, *Katayama fever*, is a hypersensitivity reaction that presents as a non-specific febrile illness typically with urticaria and eosinophilia about 2–8 weeks after initial exposure.
- Typically seen in travellers and previously un-exposed individuals.

Chronic schistosomiasis
- Chronic schistosomiasis occurs as a result of chronic inflammation and fibrosis in response to the eggs deposited in various tissues. It does not present as a febrile illness.
- *Hepatosplenic schistosomiasis*: presents as portal hypertension with splenomegaly, ascites, and variceal bleeding. Unlike cirrhosis from viral hepatitis or alcohol, jaundice is rare and hepatocellular function is relatively preserved.
- *Intestinal schistosomiasis*: chronic intestinal inflammation can cause intermittent abdominal pain, anorexia, diarrhoea, and iron deficiency.
- *Urinary schistosomiasis*: can lead to haematuria, strictures, obstructive renal failure, and an increased risk for bladder cancer.
- *Female genital schistosomiasis:* underappreciated, friable lesions of cervix/vulva can increase risk of HIV acquisition by two- to threefold.
- *Neuroschistosomiasis*: ectopic migration to the spinal cord triggers inflammation. It can present as transverse myelitis and accounts for >5% of cases of non-traumatic paraplegia in endemic settings. Corticosteroids manage inflammation.

Diagnosis

- Diagnosis of acute schistosomiasis is challenging. Stool and urine microscopy are still negative. Eosinophilia is common and serology may be positive. Exposure history is important.
- For chronic schistosomiasis, stool and urine microscopy can detect eggs, but has low sensitivity and multiple samples or concentration techniques are recommended. Serology is positive (although not widely available in low-resource settings).
- New rapid point-of-care urine tests that have excellent sensitivity and specificity are now commercially available.

Treatment

- A single dose of *praziquantel* 40 mg/kg is usually effective for *S. haematobium* and *S. mansoni*. For *S. japonicum*, the dose is repeated in 6–12 hours.
- *A repeat dose 2 weeks later may increase the cure rates, especially for heavy infections.*
- Praziquantel only works against adult worms and chronic stages of schistosomiasis. It does not work against immature forms or as PEP immediately following exposure to freshwater.
- Treatment of acute schistosomiasis, a hypersensitivity reaction, is typically prednisone 30 mg/day × 5 days. Praziquantel is generally administered 6 weeks later to eliminate adult worms.

Control and elimination

- In some areas of sub-Saharan Africa the prevalence of infection can be very high; >50% of school-aged children can be affected.
- Annual community-wide MDA with single doses of praziquantel is used in endemic areas to reduce the burden of disease. Unfortunately, MDA reaches <50% of the >200 million people who need to be treated.
- Access to sanitation that adequately separates human excreta from open water and human contact is an essential intervention to interrupt transmission and eliminate schistosomiasis.

Soil-transmitted helminths

Key points
- Soil-transmitted helminths are a group of intestinal worms whose transmission depends on a period of development in warm soil. Diagnosis is by stool microscopy.
- Transmission occurs through inadvertent ingestion of eggs or direct skin penetration by larvae when walking on contaminated soil.
- To reduce disease burden in endemic areas, annual MDA with single-dose albendazole is recommended.

Challenges
- >1 billion people are infected.
- Most are asymptomatic but morbidity can be devastating from growth retardation and iron deficiency, especially in children.

Roundworm (*Ascaris lumbricoides*)
- Ascaris is non-invasive and generally benign. Intestinal obstruction can occur in children with chronic exposures and many worms.
- Treatment: albendazole 400 mg single dose—additional doses are recommended if heavy burden of disease.

Hookworm (*Ancylostoma duodenale* and *Necator americanus*)
- Hookworm is a major cause of iron deficiency worldwide among children and pregnant women. Each 1 cm-long worm can suck up to 0.25 mL of blood per day. Eosinophilia is common.
- Treatment: albendazole 400 mg single dose—similar to *Ascaris* additional doses are needed for cure if heavy burden of disease.

Whipworm (*Trichuris trichuria*)
- Heavy infections in children can lead to iron deficiency, growth retardation, colitis, proctitis, and rectal prolapse.
- Treatment: albendazole 400 mg/day for 5–7 days.

Strongyloidiasis (*Strongyloides stercoralis*)
- Unlike most helminths *Strongyloides* worms can complete their life cycle and multiply in the human host.
- In people with a normal immune response, the numbers of worms are kept low and the infection is usually asymptomatic.
- *Hyperinfection* can occur following immunosuppression especially with steroids—even after a short course of prednisone. Hyperinfection syndrome is associated with Gram-negative sepsis and often fatal. Patients who receive steroids in areas of high strongyloidiasis prevalence should be empirically treated.
- Stool microscopy has very low sensitivity, except in hyperinfection.
- Serology has excellent sensitivity, but is not often available.
- Treatment: for asymptomatic *Strongyloides* infection, ivermectin 0.2 mg/kg/day × 2 days is preferred; albendazole 400 mg/day × 7 days is an alternative. For hyperinfection, ivermectin (≥2 weeks) may be given subcutaneously, in combination with albendazole.

Trachoma

Key points

- Eye infection, conjunctivitis, caused by *Chlamydia trachomatis* and a leading cause of preventable blindness.
- Recurrent minor infections causes inverted eyelashes that scratch the corneal surface.
- Single-dose azithromycin clears the infection, but a simple surgical procedure is needed to correct the inverted eyelashes.

Challenges

- Occurs in areas of poverty and may be missed by health workers.
- >200 million people are at risk; an estimated 1.8 million are visually impaired, and 0.5 million are blind.

Transmission

Trachoma is spread by contact from person to person, especially among children and their caregivers in areas of poverty, crowding, and water shortages, particularly in Africa and the Middle East.

Clinical features

Recurrent episodes of conjunctivitis lead to scarring and inversion of the upper eyelid. It is the painful scraping of the inverted upper eyelashes against the cornea that leads to keratitis and visual impairment.

Diagnosis

Trachoma is a clinical diagnosis:

- In early stages, trachomatous conjunctivitis is diagnosed by everting the upper eyelid and identifying an inflamed conjunctiva with multiple pale 0.5–2 mm follicles.
- Late stages of trachoma are easy to recognize based on inversion of the upper eyelid and eyelashes and associated corneal opacities.

See Fig. 30.16.

Treatment

- *Antibiotics*: a single dose of azithromycin PO, or a 1-week course of topical tetracycline ointment, clears the infection, but infection usually reoccurs. In endemic areas, MDA of azithromycin for everyone every 6 months is recommended.
- *Surgery*: a simple surgical procedure is needed to correct inverted eyelashes. About 7 million people are waiting for this operation to prevent visual loss.

Most control efforts follow the *SAFE strategy*:
- Surgery to correct inverted upper eyelids.
- Azithromycin MDA.
- Facial cleanliness to reduce transmission.
- Environmental improvement, access to water and sanitation.

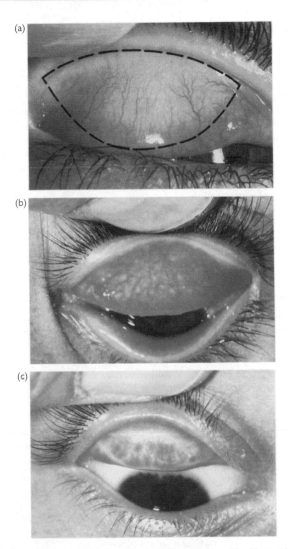

Fig. 30.16 Trachoma images. Reproduced with permission from http://www.who.int/blindness/causes/trachoma_documents/en/. (a) Normal tarsal conjunctiva (×2 magnification). The dotted line shows the area to be examined. (b) Trachomatous inflammation - follicular (TF). (c) Trachomatous scarring (TS).

Food-borne trematode infections

Key points
- Food-borne trematode infections are a group of neglected parasitic infections caused by short flatworms (flukes) acquired through ingestion of contaminated food—typically freshwater plants, fish, or crabs.
- 10% of the world's population is at risk and >50 million people are chronically infected. The highest burden of disease is in Southeast Asia and South America.

Transmission
Transmission occurs by eating raw fish, crustaceans, or aquatic plants that have been raised in freshwater that has been contaminated by faeces of people or animals harbouring chronic infection.

Clinical presentation
- Chronic infection can cause severe liver and lung disease.
- Specific clinical features are listed in Table 30.7.

Diagnosis
- Eosinophilia with liver or lung lesions on imaging are clinical clues.
- Stool microscopy is diagnostic but has low sensitivity.
- Serology is very useful, but not available in most endemic countries.

Treatment
- Praziquantel (25 mg/kg three times daily for 3 days) is used for *Clonorchis*, *Opisthorchis*, and *Paragonimus* spp.
- Triclabendazole (10–20 mg/kg single dose) is required for treatment of *Fasciola* spp. It can be ordered free of charge through WHO.

Prevention and control
Prevention requires changes in dietary and cultural practices to avoid eating uncooked foods. MDA with single-dose triclabendazole or praziquantel is recommended by WHO to reduce the burden in highly endemic communities.

Table 30.7 Characteristics of the common food-borne trematodes

Food-borne trematode	Acquired by eating	Epidemiology	Clinical features
Oriental liver flukes: e.g. *Clonorchis* *Opisthorchis*	Freshwater fish: Raw or undercooked	China Southeast Asia	Intermittent biliary obstruction, cholangitis Bile duct cancer
Common liver flukes: e.g. *Fasciola*	Aquatic plants: Watercress Water chestnuts	Global: Sheep/cattle rearing areas	Intermittent biliary obstruction, cholangitis
Lung fluke: *Paragonimus*	Raw crustaceans: 'Drunken crab'	Far East West Africa South America	Can mimic TB with chronic cough and haemoptysis

Echinococcosis

Key points

- Also called hydatid disease, cystic echinococcosis is a zoonotic parasitic disease caused by the dog tapeworm *Echinococcus granulosus*.
- It primarily affects the liver, causing a slow growing cyst that can grow >10 cm and cause a mass effect.
- Cystic echinococcosis affects >1 million people and is often diagnosed incidentally by abdominal ultrasound.
- Alveolar echinococcosis, caused by *E. multilocularis* is much less common and causes a slow-growing tumour-like mass

Challenges

- Treatment is challenging and needs to be individualized.
- Surgery or interventional radiological procedures are often required in conjunction with antiparasitic medications.

Transmission

- Cystic echinococcosis has a global distribution. The burden of disease is highest in South America, East Africa, Central Asia, and China.
- Dogs are asymptomatic carriers of the small intestinal tapeworms and pass eggs in their faeces. If people accidentally ingest the eggs they develop into larvae and form cysts in the liver, lungs, or other organs.
- Sheep and cattle are the usual targets of disease—humans are also susceptible through contaminated food and water.

Clinical features

- Cystic echinococcosis results in slowly expanding cystic lesions in the liver (80%) and lung (20%).
- Patients are usually asymptomatic until the cysts grow large enough to cause complications through a mass effect.
- Fever of systemic illness is not typically seen.

Diagnosis

- The cysts often have a characteristic appearance and diagnosis is usually made by evaluation of ultrasound or CT scan.
- Serology, if available, can be used to help confirm the diagnosis.
- Cyst contents can be carefully obtained by needle aspirate and examined under the microscope for tapeworm scolices (hooklets).

Treatment

- Drainage is required for large cysts. There is a small risk of spillage with the procedure that can result in a hypersensitivity reaction and intra-abdominal dissemination. Therefore, albendazole should be given peri-procedure and continued for at least 8 weeks.
- Instillation of scolicidal agents (e.g. 10% saline) can be done after aspiration to prevent recurrence but requires technical expertise,
- Prolonged courses of daily albendazole (≥1 year) are used for smaller or multiple cysts not amenable to drainage.

Chapter 31

Tuberculosis and HIV in humanitarian contexts

Peter Saranchuk

Introduction

In this chapter, you will find management of human immunodeficiency virus (HIV) and tuberculosis (TB) presented together. Although it may initially seem surprising to have two diseases covered in the same clinical section, this unconventional approach is done purposefully for several reasons:

- There is often a high burden of both TB and HIV in humanitarian contexts, where these two diseases can be viewed as 'two sides of the same coin': TB is the leading cause of morbidity and mortality among people living with HIV (PLHIV) and a significant percentage of TB patients are co-infected with HIV. In fact, in many sub-Saharan settings, the majority of TB patients are co-infected with HIV (see Fig. 31.1).

- Antiretroviral therapy (ART, the treatment for HIV) reduces the risk that PLHIV will develop active TB by approximately two-thirds, plus it lowers the risk of mortality by about half in those who do develop TB.

- Clinical and programmatic experience has shown that there are significant advantages to addressing HIV and TB in a coordinated manner. In *high-burden* settings, TB and HIV services are increasingly being integrated, including at the primary care level, thereby allowing co-infected patients to be managed on the same day, by the same provider, in the same health facility. Not only is this more patient friendly, but it can improve treatment outcomes and make service delivery more efficient.

- Even in *low-burden* settings, it is useful to include TB and HIV management within primary healthcare services. All TB patients need to be tested for HIV and all HIV-infected patients need to be screened for active TB disease at every consultation, both of which can be performed by trained primary healthcare staff.

This chapter aims to guide the health provider through the assessment and management of HIV and TB patients. As national policies can vary, always check the national guidelines in the country in which you are working for context-specific guidance.

Estimated HIV prevalence in new and relapse TB cases, 2014

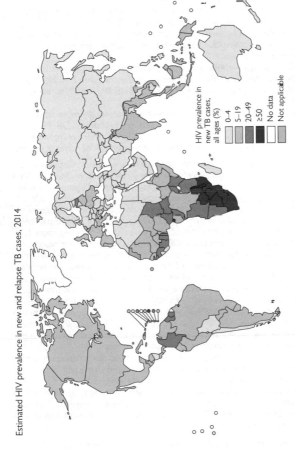

Fig. 31.1 Estimated HIV prevalence in new and relapse TB cases. Reproduced with permission from Global Tuberculosis Report 2015, World Health Organization: Figure 2.5 (http://apps.whc.int/iris/bitstream/10665/191102/1/9789241565059_eng.pdf).

Context

Although the global TB burden has been slowly declining each year, its prevalence can be significantly higher in humanitarian contexts for a number of reasons:

• TB transmission is increased in settings where people are forced to live in overcrowded conditions.

• The malnutrition that often accompanies such situations increases the risk that TB infection will progress to active TB disease.

• The TB situation in many countries has become more complicated over the past few decades due to both the HIV epidemic and the rise of drug-resistant strains.

  • Due to their weakened immune systems, PLHIV are much more likely to develop active TB disease, so countries with high HIV burdens have experienced steep rises in TB incidence and TB-related mortality.

  • Drug-resistant TB (DR-TB) has become increasingly more common in both low- and high-HIV-burden settings. Not only is DR-TB more difficult to diagnose, but its treatment is longer, more complex, exceedingly expensive, and carries an increased risk of adverse events.

Regarding HIV, there has been tremendous progress over the past decade, namely through increased knowledge among healthcare workers (HCWs) and access to ART, including in many resource-limited settings. First-line ART regimens are much less expensive now and newer antiretroviral medications (ARVs) have fewer drug-related side effects, so less treatment monitoring is required than previously. As a result, some HIV-related medical activities have been 'task-shifted' to trained and supervised lower-level HCWs in settings where there are limited human resources for health.

We now know that starting a person on ART earlier has a number of benefits including reduced risk of progression to acquired immunodeficiency syndrome (AIDS) and reduced mortality, including from non-AIDS-related causes. Because of this, the WHO now recommends that lifelong ART be given to all those living with HIV, regardless of a person's immune status.[1] These simplified WHO recommendations will hopefully stimulate improved access to ART in those settings where HIV care and treatment remain woefully inadequate, despite a high prevalence in the general population and/or specific groups (e.g. injection drug users).

Evidence has also shown that HIV treatment can prevent transmission: the landmark HPTN Study 052 demonstrated that early initiation of ART in a person living with HIV could reduce the risk of HIV transmission to HIV-uninfected partners by ~96%, compared with delayed ART.[2] When viewed in a public health context, a broad 'treatment as prevention' strategy that increases access to ART among all PLHIV can be expected to reduce transmission at the community level.

Epidemiology of HIV/TB in humanitarian contexts

TB epidemiology

Mycobacterium tuberculosis (TB) is a slow-growing bacillus that is transmitted by inhalation of tiny infectious droplets produced by a person with active *pulmonary* disease, mainly through coughing. It is estimated that one-third of the world's population have inhaled TB bacilli at some point in their lifetime and thus become infected with TB. Such infection rarely progresses to active TB disease in healthy people (<10% lifetime risk). However, development of active TB is common in those with weakened immune systems, including young children, the elderly, the malnourished, and especially those living with HIV (in whom the risk can be ~10% annually in high-TB-burden settings).

Despite declining mortality and incidence rates in most countries, the global burden of TB remains high. WHO estimates that 9.6 million people developed active TB disease in 2014, including 1 million children, and that 1.5 million died that year, including ~400,000 who were HIV-positive.[3]

DR-TB is a growing threat with 3.3% of new cases of active TB and 20% of previously treated cases estimated to be multidrug resistant (MDR-TB) to both isoniazid and rifampicin, the two most important first-line anti-TB drugs.[3] Almost half a million new cases of MDR-TB emerge each year and despite improvements in its detection, the majority of MDR-TB cases go undiagnosed and untreated.

HIV epidemiology

There are two major HIV subtypes, HIV-1 and HIV-2. The former is largely responsible for the worldwide epidemic that was first documented in the 1980s, while the latter continues to be found mostly in West Africa. HIV is present in blood and body fluids of infected people and transmitted most commonly during unprotected sexual activity. Mother-to-child transmission of HIV can occur *in utero*, during labour and delivery, or during the breastfeeding period. Other common modes of transmission include uncontrolled blood transfusions (common in resource-limited settings) and unsafe use of needles and syringes.

Although there were ~2 million new HIV infections globally in 2014, bringing the total number of people living with HIV worldwide to ~37 million people, the annual number has fallen greatly since the peak of the epidemic.[4] There has been good progress on prevention of mother-to-child transmission, as shown by a 58% decrease in new childhood HIV infections since 2000.[5] AIDS-related deaths are at their lowest since the peak in 2004, having declined by 42%,[5] in large part because of increased access to ART in many parts of the world. TB remains the number one cause of morbidity and mortality in PLHIV.

Unique challenges in humanitarian contexts

Managing TB and HIV can be challenging in resource-limited humanitarian settings. Confirmation of TB and other HIV-related conditions will often not be possible, either because a diagnostic test is not accessible or its sensitivity is not sufficient. Clinicians must instead rely on a thorough history and physical examination, together with clinical judgement, and in many cases initiate patients on treatment empirically.

Diagnosis of TB in children is particularly challenging for several reasons: good diagnostic tools for pulmonary disease in children are lacking, extrapulmonary disease is common, obtaining specimens for testing can be difficult, children tend to have less bacilli in their specimens, and chest X-ray interpretation can be difficult.

Once diagnosis is made and treatment started, 'retention in care' in TB and HIV programmes can be a challenge and long-term adherence can require innovative solutions. Adherence support measures could include the use of treatment education by 'peer supporters' and 'adherence counsellors' that visit patients in the communities where they live.

Stigma and discrimination can create real barriers that prevent patients from utilizing available HIV and TB care and treatment services. Patients may fear that their attendance at health facilities will raise suspicion among family and their community, thereby leading to indirect disclosure of their HIV and/or TB status. Providers need to be aware of and address these contextual factors to ensure uptake of services.

If essential *diagnostic* tests and/or treatments are lacking in your setting, consider advocating for their introduction:

- For example, if HIV testing is not available, how will you know which pregnant women should be offered straightforward treatments that are known to successfully prevent mother-to-child transmission of HIV?
- Programme managers may have been reluctant in the past to introduce rapid HIV testing due to lack of an adequate medical infrastructure and/or concerns around sustainability related to treatment (ART). However, even if lifelong ART cannot be guaranteed in a setting, patients found to be HIV-positive can still be educated in behaviour change that can prevent transmission, as well as given prophylactic medications (e.g. co-trimoxazole (CTX)) to prevent certain opportunistic infections (OIs).
- Point-of-care HIV- and TB-related diagnostics now exist that are especially useful in contexts where specimen (and patient) transport to distant health facilities is often not possible.
- Discuss the introduction of any missing but essential diagnostic tests with the relevant health authorities, including potential benefits, assurance of quality control, and how the test's implementation might be able to reduce healthcare costs (e.g. by reducing the need for other more costly investigations).

Key programmatic strategies

- Implementation of new HIV and TB services should be done in partnership with relevant local health authorities.
- There is likely to be a shortage of skilled HCWs in most humanitarian contexts. The workload can be alleviated by *shifting certain tasks* to properly trained and supervised lower levels of HCWs, e.g. distribution of ARVs.
- *Case-finding* for both TB and HIV should be intensive in high-burden settings.
  - TB symptom screening should be performed routinely on each patient presenting to a health facility in a high-TB-burden setting.
  - HIV testing and counselling (HTC) should be offered routinely by HCWs in high-HIV-burden settings, with patients being given the opportunity to 'opt-out' if they prefer.

- An active *screening* process should be in place to allow for early detection and management of the most common OIs that cause morbidity and mortality in PLHIV. Note that these OIs can vary by region (e.g. Penicilliosis is common in Southeast Asia, but not elsewhere).
- TB and HIV services should be *decentralized* as much as possible, ideally being incorporated into primary healthcare services, close to where affected people live. Decentralization of HIV treatment and care can increase access to and improve retention in care.[1]
- *Collaboration* of TB and HIV services (and *integration* in high-burden settings) can not only improve diagnosis and treatment outcomes (for both TB and HIV), but also offers the opportunity to make healthcare delivery more efficient.
- Avoid the temptation to start too big. Introduce new TB and HIV activities in a manageable number and size; then scale-up those activities that are working well.
- Investment in diagnosis and management of TB and HIV in humanitarian contexts, including conflict settings, will *prevent* many new cases in the future. Treatment is prevention!

Disease assessment

TB: disease presentation

Cases of TB can be classified as follows:

- *Bacteriologically confirmed* by smear microscopy, culture, or a WHO-approved rapid diagnostic test such as the molecular test Xpert® MTB/RIF (also known as GeneXpert®).
- *Clinically diagnosed* TB case, i.e. not bacteriologically confirmed but diagnosed by a clinician (including on the basis of an X-ray finding) who has decided to give the patient a full course of TB treatment.

Classification can also be based on the anatomical site of TB disease:

- Pulmonary tuberculosis (PTB) involves the lung parenchyma or the tracheobronchial tree.
- Extrapulmonary tuberculosis (EPTB) involves organs other than the lungs: lymph nodes, abdomen, meninges, pleura, etc. EPTB is often difficult to diagnose in resource-limited settings, so is often under-diagnosed.

Children, especially those <5 years of age, are more likely to have EPTB (especially lymphadenopathy, meningitis, and miliary forms) or clinically diagnosed PTB (i.e. not bacteriologically confirmed). This is also true for *PLHIV*, especially those with advanced immunodeficiency. Active TB disease in PLHIV tends to involve more rapid clinical deterioration, leaving a relatively short 'window of opportunity' for diagnosis before mortality. If a young child or PLHIV presents with symptoms or signs suggestive of TB but there is not yet bacteriological confirmation, clinical diagnosis and a full course of TB treatment is reasonable to reduce the risk of early mortality.

TB: symptoms and signs

- Active TB disease most commonly involves the lungs. *PTB* usually presents with a cough lasting >2 weeks, sputum (sometimes blood-stained), and pleuritic chest pain. Chest symptoms are often associated with systemic ones such as fever, night sweats, and loss of appetite and weight.
- In the presence of a compromised immune system (due to HIV, malnutrition, etc.), pulmonary symptoms tend to be less obvious, while fever and weight loss become more pronounced. In such patients, extrapulmonary forms of TB are also more common.
- Active TB disease can involve essentially any part of the body and mimic other diseases. Symptoms and signs of *EPTB* will depend on exactly which part of the body is involved. See Box 31.1.
- *Miliary TB* refers to widespread dissemination of TB bacilli throughout the body. The diagnosis can be confirmed by visualization of a miliary pattern on chest X-ray and sometimes choroidal tubercles on funduscopic examination. See Fig. 31.2.
- The symptoms and signs of *DR-TB* are the same as those of drug-sensitive strains.

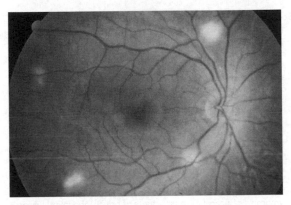

Fig. 31.2 Four choroidal tubercles can be seen on this retinal image.

Not all those with a chronic cough have TB! The differential diagnosis to consider in a coughing HIV-positive patient will vary by setting, but typically includes:
- bacterial bronchitis/pneumonia (including atypical causes)
- bronchiectasis with bacterial superinfection
- lung abscess or empyema
- *Pneumocystis jirovecii* pneumonia (PCP)
- disseminated fungal infections
- nocardia
- non-tuberculous mycobacteria (NTM)
- Kaposi sarcoma of the lung
- other cancers, including bronchial carcinoma and lymphoma
- congestive heart failure

HIV: disease presentation

Natural evolution
- In the first few weeks after infection with HIV, many people will develop fever and other non-specific symptoms related to *primary infection*, as the virus rapidly replicates within CD4 cells.[*]
- Following recovery, most people feel well for an extended period of time (often years), apart from infrequent, minor infections. During this period of time, many will be unaware of their HIV status.
- As HIV replicates and destroys CD4 cells over time, there is a progressive decline in strength of the immune system. If the CD4 count drops to <200 cells/μL, that person is at risk of a number of serious (and often life-threatening) OIs and other HIV-related conditions. See Table 31.1. This natural evolution can be interrupted (and reversed) at any time by the initiation of ART.

[*] Also known as 'helper' T lymphocytes, these white blood cells express cluster determinant 4 (CD4) and help to activate an immune response.

Box 31.1 Extrapulmonary TB manifestations

- TB-related pleural effusion (often unilateral) is commonly seen in high-TB/HIV-burden settings and presents with pleuritic chest pain and/or shortness of breath.
- A person with TB lymphadenopathy presents with one or more enlarged, painless nodes in the cervical (most commonly), axillary, or inguinal regions. Enlarged nodes are often bilateral and eventually become fluctuant and develop fistulas that drain caseous material.
  - Intra-abdominal and mediastinal TB-related lymphadenopathy are common sites of involvement but require ultrasound or chest X-ray for identification.
- The symptoms of abdominal TB are usually non-specific (pain, alteration in bowel habit, etc.). If there is seeding of the peritoneum, ascites will be present. Another (somewhat subjective) sign of abdominal TB is the presence of a 'doughy' abdomen on palpation.
- Those having TB-related pericarditis may present with chest pain and symptoms of heart failure (shortness of breath, abdominal fullness, and swelling of the lower limbs). Signs include a rapid heart rate, distended neck veins, and pericardial friction rub.
  - TB pericarditis can cause acute cardiac tamponade, for which Beck's triad of signs is pathognomonic: low arterial BP, distended neck veins, and distant/muffled heart sounds.
- TB meningitis presents with headache, confusion, and fever. If not diagnosed and treated early, it will progress to include neck stiffness, vomiting, and represent a medical emergency.
  - TB meningitis is common in children with active TB disease. Beware that symptoms of meningitis in young children tend to be much more non-specific (e.g. drowsiness, irritability, and poor feeding).
- Joint involvement usually presents as a relatively painless, chronic monoarthritis involving a hip, knee, or elbow. If this goes undiagnosed and untreated, destruction of the joint will result.
- Pott's disease of the spine occurs when active TB disease affects the vertebrae and intervertebral discs. Destruction and deformation of the spine is preceded by localized pain. If the disease process goes untreated, neurological complications may result.

HIV-related clinical staging and laboratory testing

Note: unlike for HIV-1, viral load assays that reliably measure HIV-2 are not currently available on a commercial basis.

Physical exam

It is important to spend some extra time assessing those with advanced immunodeficiency, including a thorough physical examination. Areas not to overlook include the following:

- *All four vital signs*: these help to identify clinically unstable patients, who in turn require referral to a hospital for admission. According to the World Health Organization (WHO), clinical danger signs include one or more of the following: unable to walk unaided, respiratory rate >30 per minute, fever >39°C, and pulse rate >120 per minute.

- *Dyspnoea* (could indicate PCP, miliary TB, and/or dehydration):
  - Look for nasal flaring in children.
  - An O_2 saturation <90% requires admission to hospital and should increase clinical suspicion of PCP.
- Signs of *dehydration* (increased respiratory rate, tachycardia, low BP, decreased skin turgor).
- *Weight* at every visit.
- *Height* at the first visit and calculation of body mass index (BMI).
- *Oral cavity* for evidence of oral candidiasis (thrush) and/or lesions of Kaposi sarcoma.
- *Enlarged lymph nodes* in the cervical, axillary, and inguinal areas (often related to TB, but could also represent Kaposi sarcoma or lymphoma).
- Chest (for signs of respiratory distress, and/or pleural effusion).
- Abdomen (for hepatomegaly, epigastric tenderness).
- Genital exam (for signs of STIs and enlarged inguinal nodes).
- Skin (for Kaposi sarcoma lesions and disseminated OIs such as cryptococcosis).
- CNS (especially for meningeal irritation and/or focal neurological signs).
- *Funduscopic* exam is useful since a number of HIV-related conditions can have retinal manifestations, including disseminated TB, toxoplasmosis, CMV retinitis and cryptococcal meningitis (CCM) (the latter as papilloedema). See Fig. 31.2 on page 575 and ➔ Fig. 31.8 on page 601.

Table 31.1 Risk of HIV-related conditions by CD4 cell count

CD4 count level	Condition
Any CD4 count	TB (pulmonary and extrapulmonary)
	Herpes zoster (shingles)
	Bacterial pneumonia
	Cervical intraepithelial neoplasia (CIN)
	HIV-related thrombocytopenia
	Lymphocytic interstitial pneumonitis (LIP)
	Parotid gland enlargement
<200 cells/μL (= opportunistic infections)	Oral candidiasis (also known as thrush)
	Oesophageal candidiasis
	Pneumocystis jirovecii pneumonia (PCP)
	Cryptosporidiosis
	Lymphoma (non-CNS)
	Kaposi sarcoma
	HIV-associated dementia
<100 cells/μL	Toxoplasmosis
	Cryptococcal meningitis (CCM)
	Cytomegalovirus (CMV) retinitis
<50 cells/μL	Disseminated non-tuberculous infection (e.g. *Mycobacterium avium* complex)
	Lymphoma (CNS)
	Progressive multifocal leucoencephalopathy (PML)
	Cytomegalovirus infection (brain or disseminated)

Adapted from the MSF HIV/TB Clinical Guide, 2015 [7]

Approach to diagnosis

TB diagnosis

Screening for TB

TB screening should be performed *routinely in* humanitarian settings having a high TB burden, especially in those known (or suspected) to be infected with HIV. TB symptom screening is straightforward and can be performed quickly by (adequately trained) lower-level HCWs.

Adults and adolescents just need to be asked about the presence of four symptoms: current cough, fever, weight loss, and night sweats. *Children* (and/or their caregivers) should be asked about current cough, fever, poor weight gain, and contact history with a TB case.

Those infected with HIV not reporting one or more of the above-mentioned symptoms are unlikely to have active TB disease.[8] An important exception is those with advanced immunodeficiency: 'subclinical TB' is common in this group in high-burden settings, so *routine* TB investigations should be considered, even in the absence of TB symptoms.

Evaluation for TB

Those reporting one or more TB symptoms need *evaluation* for TB, which involves a thorough physical examination and appropriate diagnostic tests. Thus, evaluation is much more complex than the *screening* process mentioned previously.

Clinical findings that warrant immediate TB treatment

The presence of one of the following clinical findings in those with TB symptoms in a high-TB-prevalence area is enough to warrant *immediate initiation* of TB treatment:

- Non-painful lymphadenopathy in children, with fistulization to the skin surface.
- Angle deformity of the spine in children (i.e. Pott's disease).
- Choroidal tubercles on funduscopic examination (see ➜ Fig. 31.2 , p. 515).
- Unilateral pleural effusion (that is 'straw-coloured' on aspiration) in PLHIV.

Diagnostic modalities

- Sputum smear microscopy has been the traditional method to diagnose TB in most humanitarian contexts, but its low sensitivity in children and PLHIV means that it will miss many cases of PTB. Neither can it identify drug-resistant strains.
  - Important: a 'negative' smear result does not rule out active TB disease, especially in children and people living with HIV!
- Xpert® MTB/RIF (also known as GeneXpert®) is a molecular test that can detect TB, including rifampicin-resistant strains, in pulmonary and extrapulmonary specimens. *N.B. WHO recommends GeneXpert® as the initial diagnostic in adults and children suspected of having HIV-associated TB or MDR-TB.*
- TB culture is a sensitive diagnostic that can also be combined with drug susceptibility testing (DST) to detect drug-resistant strains.

- N.B. WHO recommends that DST be performed at the start of TB therapy in all those previously treated for TB and all those co-infected with HIV.
- Determine® TB LAM (lipoarabinomannan) is a lateral flow assay (i.e. 'dipstick') that can detect disseminated, TB-specific antigen in urine. However, this test should be reserved for those with low CD4 counts (e.g. <100 cells/μL) since it is much less sensitive at higher CD4 counts.
- Chest X-ray is helpful in diagnosing active PTB and some cases of EPTB disease:
  - In HIV-negative adults, X-ray findings of PTB typically include upper lobe infiltrates, often with cavitation.
  - With advanced immunodeficiency, chest X-ray findings in PLHIV with active PTB can be atypical and even normal. See Box 31.2.

Even in resource-limited settings, the following investigations can and should be used by trained clinicians to aid in diagnosis of EPTB:
- Needle aspiration of fluctuant lymph nodes to look for AFB.
- Thoracentesis of a pleural effusion (if large enough).
- Lumbar puncture for testing of cerebrospinal fluid (CSF).
- Ultrasound to look for signs of EPTB: pericardial effusion, intra-abdominal nodes, splenic hypodensities, and/or ascites.

Box 31.2 Chest X-ray presentations of TB in PLHIV

Chest X-ray presentations of active TB in PLHIV are now well character-ized and should no longer be considered atypical for TB in HIV-prevalent settings.[9] These include:
- miliary or diffuse shadowing (Fig. 31.3)
- large heart (especially if symmetrical and rounded) (Fig. 31.4)
- pleural effusion (Fig. 31.5)
- enlarged lymph nodes inside the chest (Fig. 31.6).

TB diagnostic algorithms

TB diagnostic algorithms can assist clinicians in making a timely diagnosis of active TB, especially in PLHIV, in whom smear microscopy is often reported as 'negative' despite the presence of active TB disease. Check the national guidelines where you are working for setting-specific algorithms. WHO also has some standard TB diagnostic algorithms that may be helpful.[9]

TB treatment considerations
- Since active TB is often difficult to confirm in PLHIV and children, don't delay treatment in someone who is clinically unwell. If TB is strongly suspected on clinical grounds, then initiate empiric TB treatment while continuing to try to confirm the diagnosis.
- If it has been necessary to start someone on empiric TB therapy, close follow-up is necessary to document the response to therapy and exclude other diagnoses.
- If a person is not improving on TB treatment, the differential diagnosis should include DR-TB. Immune reconstitution inflammatory syndrome (IRIS) is another possibility in PLHIV having recently been initiated on ART (see ➲ 'Immune reconstitution inflammatory syndrome' pp. 525–6).

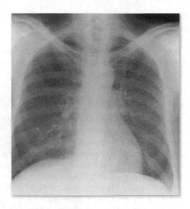

Fig. 31.3 Chest X-ray showing fine miliary pattern. Reproduced with permission from Edward C. Rosenow, III, Mayo Clinic Challenging Images for Pulmonary Board Review, OUP: 2010.

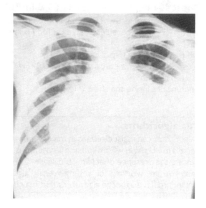

Fig. 31.4 Posteroanterior chest X-ray of a patient with a large pericardial effusion. The heart shadow is greatly enlarged and globular in shape. Those parts of the lung fields that can be seen are normal. Reproduced with permission from Warrell, David, et al. Oxford Textbook of Medicine, OUP: 2014, Fig 16.8.1.

HIV diagnosis

In many settings, the majority of HIV-infected people are *unaware* of their status. This needs correcting, since the earlier that people know they are infected and access care, the less likely they are to suffer HIV-related morbidity and mortality and transmit the virus to others.

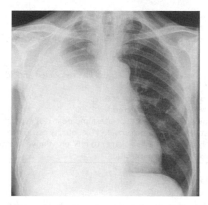

Fig. 31.5 Posteroanterior chest X-ray showing a large pleural effusion filling much of the right chest. Reproduced with permission from Darby, M J., et al, Oxford Handbook of Medical Imaging, OUP: 2011, Fig 4.32.

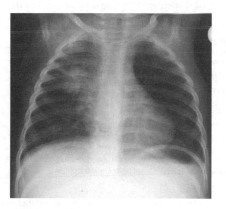

Fig. 31.6 Enlarged lymph nodes (in a child). Reproduced with permission from Starke, Jeffrey R. and Donald, Peter R. Handbook of Child and Adolescent Tuberculosis, OUP: 2015, Fig 8.9.

Testing and counselling

HIV testing and counselling (HTC) should be offered in humanitarian contexts through a variety of *active* approaches.

• WHO recommends that routine, provider-initiated testing and counselling (PITC) be considered in clinics where TB, malnutrition, sexually transmitted infection (STI), and antenatal services are offered, as well as health services for key populations.[1]

- Community-based testing approaches should include sites where high-risk groups tend to congregate.
- All children of a parent living with HIV should be routinely offered HIV testing.

According to the WHO, the 5 Cs should be respected and adhered to by all models of HTC services:
- *Consent* must be given prior to testing.
- *Confidentiality* must be respected.
- Accompanied by appropriate pre-test and post-test *counselling*.
- *Correct* test results must be provided (i.e. quality assurance).
- With timely *connection* (i.e. linkage) to HIV preventive, treatment and care, following a positive result.

Diagnostic modalities

Rapid HIV tests

- Rapid HIV testing is used in adults and older children to detect HIV antibodies in capillary blood taken by 'finger prick'. These typically give point-of-care (POC) results within 20 minutes.
- There is evidence to show that trained and supervised lay providers can perform safe and effective HIV testing using such rapid tests.
- Point-of-care screening tests tend to be very *sensitive*, so 'false-positive' results are possible. Thus, all positive results must be confirmed through testing of a separate specimen by a second operator.
- In settings where the population being tested has a <5% HIV prevalence, WHO now recommends the use of three sequential reactive tests before making an HIV-positive diagnosis.[1]

Virological testing

- Virological assays that detect the virus or its components are recommended to diagnose HIV infection in infants and children <18 months of age. Rapid HIV antibody tests are inappropriate in such cases because they can give 'false-positive' results due to circulating maternal antibodies in this age group.
- Specimens for virological testing can be collected from infants using the dried blood spot (DBS) sampling technique.

Additional notes

- *Infants exposed to HIV*, i.e. born to an HIV-infected mother, should have virological testing done at 4–6 weeks of age. If negative, HIV testing should be repeated until the child is no longer at risk (e.g. following discontinuation of breastfeeding). *Check the national HTC guidelines in the country in which you are working and/or latest WHO recommendations for more information.*
- With data showing that effective HIV treatment dramatically reduces the likelihood that someone living with HIV will transmit the virus to his/her uninfected sexual partner,[2] voluntary HTC should be increasingly offered to *couples/partners*, together with support for mutual disclosure.

- A number of baseline laboratory tests are usually offered at enrolment into an HIV care and treatment programme (e.g. CD4 testing, pregnancy tests in women), although these will differ by availability and setting. Baseline CD4 count testing (especially if done at point of care) is useful for identifying patients requiring urgent linkage to care and treatment, as well as alerting clinicians to the risk of certain HIV-related conditions (see ➜ Table 31.1 p. 517).

Treatment options

Treatment of TB

If a child or adult with active TB disease is able to adhere to an appropriate treatment regimen for the prescribed number of months, then there is a good chance of achieving a *cure*.

Drug-sensitive TB can be cured with a standard regimen of four first-line anti-TB drugs (isoniazid, rifampicin, pyrazinamide, and ethambutol) taken as part of a 6-month regimen.

MDR and even extensively drug-resistant (XDR)* strains of TB can also be cured, but these treatment regimens have conventionally been difficult, exceedingly expensive, and required 20 months or more of a combination of second-line anti-TB drugs, which carry a high risk of adverse events.

- A shorter regimen of 9–12 months is now recommended in selected cases of MDR-TB or rifampicin resistance.[13]
- Patients with MDR-TB should be treated using mainly *ambulatory* care rather than models of care based principally on hospitalization, as there is no evidence that the latter leads to more favourable treatment outcomes.
- It is important that mono-resistant and polydrug-resistant (PDR) strains† are treated adequately, in order to prevent amplification of drug resistance and development of MDR-TB.
- *All* TB patients co-infected with HIV should be initiated on ART (see p. 526 for optimal timing of ART).
- Treatment strategies must include adequate support for patients to help overcome barriers to adherence: psychological support, education about the disease, early diagnosis and management of side effects, and the provision of 'enablers' (e.g. food, transport) in some cases.
- *Check the National TB Program (NTP) guidelines in the country in which you are working and/or latest WHO recommendations for more information on standard treatment regimens for drug-sensitive and DR-TB.*

TB treatment delivery

As part of an overall TB strategy, WHO recommends that TB treatment be directly observed in all patients by an independent and trained third party. In addition to ensuring that patients adhere to treatment and increase the chance of cure, directly observed treatment has been championed as a way to reduce the risk of development of DR-TB.

However, in settings where human resources for health are limited, directly observed treatment is not always being implemented effectively, and TB patients sometimes have to self-administer therapy while being followed by a healthcare worker. As in all settings, it is important that the delivery of TB therapy in humanitarian contexts be done in such a way as to protect the health of the community (i.e. by maximizing cure rates and minimizing default rates) while remaining patient centred (using ambulatory and community-based approaches, offering patient education, etc.).

---

* XDR-TB is a strain of TB that is resistant to rifampicin and isoniazid, plus one or more of the injectable drugs (capreomycin, kanamycin, amikacin) and any fluoroquinolone (e.g. ofloxacin).

† Mono-resistance refers to resistance against one first-line anti-TB drug only, while *poly-resistance* refers to more than one first-line anti-TB drug, other than both isoniazid and rifampicin.

Treatment of HIV

HIV cannot be cured, but the disease can be well controlled if a combination of ARVs, commonly referred to as 'triple therapy' or antiretroviral therapy (ART), is taken indefinitely. By reducing HIV replication, ART dramatically increases the life expectancy of PLHIV. There are a number of classes of ARVs, based on where they act in the lifecycle of HIV (see Table 31.2).

Initiating treatment

Before initiating ART in HIV-infected children or adults, all serious OIs and other HIV-related conditions should be diagnosed and treatment started in order to reduce the risk of IRIS (see ➔ 'Immune reconstitution inflammatory syndrome' pp. 525–6). This implies that clinicians need to have an understanding of the most common serious OIs where they are working, and screen for each of them prior to initiating ART in PLHIV.

ART in resource-limited settings has traditionally been 'rationed' by a CD4 count eligibility threshold, e.g. given only to those having a CD4 count <200 cells/µL. Based on good evidence showing better outcomes, WHO now recommends that ART be initiated in everyone living with HIV *at any clinical stage and at any CD4 count.*[1] This includes all those with active TB co-infected with HIV.

- If implemented, this expansion in ART eligibility criteria will result in better prevention of HIV transmission from mother to child and those in serodiscordant relationships.
- Check the national ART guidelines in the country in which you are working for their current eligibility criteria.

Immune reconstitution inflammatory syndrome

Following ART initiation, replication of the virus slows and levels of circulating HIV decline; as a person's immune system strengthens, new OIs become less likely to occur. In the short term, however, the recovering immune system can produce inflammatory reactions against any existing active infections. Thus, new symptoms and signs that develop (or worsen) within the first few months of a person starting ART may be the result of IRIS.

Table 31.2 Classes of ARV medication

Nucleoside/tide reverse transcriptase inhibitors (NRTIs)	Lamivudine (3TC)
	Emtricitabine (FTC)
	Zidovudine (AZT)
	Abacavir (ABC)
	Stavudine (d4T)
	Didanosine (ddI)
	Tenofovir (TDF)
Non-nucleoside reverse transcriptase inhibitors (NNRTIs)	Efavirenz (EFV)
	Nevirapine (NVP)
Protease inhibitors (PIs)	Lopinavir (LPV)
	Atazanavir (ATV)
	Ritonavir (/r) is often used to 'boost' the effect of other PIs.
Integrase inhibitors	Dolutegravir (DTG)
	Raltegravir (RAL)

IRIS presentation and management
- TB is a common cause of IRIS. Those already on TB treatment can develop 'paradoxical worsening' of TB symptoms several weeks or months after starting ART. IRIS can also unmask subclinical/undiagnosed TB in those not yet on TB treatment.
- IRIS against CCM can be life-threatening so ART should be deferred in those with a recent diagnosis of CCM and other types of meningitis (see *following timing section*).
- Clinicians must view IRIS as a diagnosis of exclusion, i.e. rule out other causes prior to concluding that any new symptoms are due to IRIS.
- Management of patients with IRIS is directed at the underlying infection, plus supportive therapy and sometimes corticosteroids; the latter should be used with caution however.

Timing of ART
The following groups of PLHIV should be '*fast-tracked*' to start ART within 2 weeks, if possible:
- Patients with low CD4 counts (especially if <50 cells/μL).
- All those in clinical stage 4, unless meningitis is present (as this requires a delay in ART initiation).
- Pregnant women.
- Young children.

In those with *newly diagnosed TB disease* who are co-infected with HIV, TB treatment should be initiated first:
- TB patients with very low CD4 counts (e.g. <50 cells/μL) should begin ART within ~2 weeks of starting TB treatment.
- To avoid intracranial IRIS in those with TB meningitis, ART should be delayed for 4–8 weeks after initiation with anti-TB drugs and steroids.
- ART can be delayed in those with higher CD4 counts being started on drug-sensitive TB treatment (unless other serious HIV-related conditions are present) in order to reduce the risks of additive drug side effects, pill burden, and IRIS. A lengthy delay should be avoided, however, with ART generally being initiated within the first 8 weeks.

Immediate ART initiation is also not recommended in patients with Cryptococcal meningitis (CCM) due to the risk of life-threatening intracranial IRIS. In those with a recent diagnosis of CCM, ART initiation should be deferred until there is evidence of a sustained clinical response to antifungal therapy; this interval will be shorter if amphotericin B is included in the regimen.

Treatment regimens
ART regimens in resource-limited settings tend to be standardized. If available, fixed-dose combinations (FDCs) help to reduce the 'pill burden' and improve adherence (see Table 31.3).[1]

Table 31.3 Preferred first-line ART regimens

Adolescents and adults (including pregnant and breastfeeding women)	TDF + 3TC (or FTC) + EFV	Advantages include once-daily dosing, fewer side effects, and availability as a fixed-dose combination. An integrase inhibitor (e.g. dolutegravir) can be used in place of EFV to initiate ART. Stavudine (d4T) is no longer recommended due to the high risk of toxicity.
Children aged 3 to <10 years	ABC + 3TC + EFV	AZT or TDF can be used in place of ABC.
Children aged <3 years	ABC or AZT + 3TC + LPV/r	This combination is recommended regardless of any prior ARV exposure (e.g. if NVP was given to mother and/or infant as part of a prevention of mother-to-child transmission intervention). In those <3 years on simultaneous TB treatment, a triple NRTI regimen (e.g. ABC + 3TC + AZT) is recommended because of the interaction between rifampicin and PIs.

Important: since recommendations are regularly updated as new evidence becomes available, please consult the latest WHO and/or national guidelines in the country in which you are working.

HIV drug resistance

It is possible for an HIV strain to mutate and become *resistant* to one or more ARV drugs. If viral replication is suspected in the presence of a first-line ART regimen, it is necessary to review adherence and offer enhanced support. If there is ongoing viral replication on ART despite good adherence, this is termed *treatment failure*. It requires a switch to a second-line regimen containing new ARVs in order to halt replication and regain control of the disease process. The composition of the second-line ART regimen will depend on which ARVs were used in the prior one. If HIV viral load testing is not available in your setting, it is possible to make a diagnosis of ART failure based on clinical or immunological criteria (see ➔ 'Treatment monitoring' pp. 529–30).

Check the national ART guidelines in the country in which you are working and/or the latest WHO recommendations and/or experienced HIV clinicians for guidance on diagnosing treatment failure and which drugs should be considered in a second-line ART regimen.

Adherence

Adherence to TB and HIV treatments is vital for several reasons: poor adherence can lead to treatment failure (with resulting disease progression), the development of resistant strains, and ultimately, increased transmission in the community. Interventions known to promote adherence to ART (and likely to TB treatment as well) include peer counselling, cognitive behavioural therapy, use of reminder devices, mobile phone text messaging, behavioural skills and medication adherence training, plus fixed-dose combinations and once-daily regimens.[1]

Community-based 'treatment supporters' have been used to support adherence to DR-TB treatment. Specific populations (e.g. nomadic groups, migrants) may require additional, tailored adherence support.

Malnutrition is a common problem in PLHIV and those with active TB disease due to decreased appetite and additional energy needs. Those with weight loss should be followed closely, since weight loss is a strong predictor of morbidity and mortality in PLHIV.

In many humanitarian contexts, provision of ART will have to be complemented by a food supply programme. Nutritional supplementation should be considered at the very least for those having dangerously low BMIs (e.g. $\leq$16 kg/m^2).

Clinical signs of *micronutrient* deficiencies include:
- a goitre (iodine deficiency)
- Bitot's spots or corneal xerosis/ulceration (vitamin A deficiency)
- hair loss, skin lesions, diarrhoea, and poor growth in children (*zinc* deficiency)
- pallor (*iron* deficiency anaemia)

Treatment monitoring

Patients on TB medication and ART require monitoring for three reasons:
1. To determine response to therapy.
2. Allow for early recognition of adverse events, including drug-related side effects.
3. Earlier detection of drug resistance.

TB therapy response monitoring

- The foundation for monitoring response to TB therapy is a good clinical examination, especially in resource-limited settings.
- Those improving on treatment for PTB will have less coughing, improved appetite and weight gain, plus an increasing ability to perform activities of daily living.
- If the person is on empiric TB treatment and not clinically improving, additional testing is necessary to detect other conditions (including disease due to a DR-TB strain).
- Follow-up smear microscopy is also important. If these patients do not 'convert' from positive to negative and the person is not improving clinically, additional specimens must be sent for DST to check for *TB drug resistance*.
- There may be a lag or delay in improvement of chest X-ray findings in those on TB treatment, but radiological *deterioration* together with clinical deterioration is concerning.

TB adverse events monitoring

- Monitoring for adverse events in someone on drug-sensitive TB treatment is mainly clinical; use of routine blood tests should be considered in those at high risk for specific adverse events (e.g. routine ALT testing if active viral hepatitis coexists).
- If a skin rash appears during TB treatment, it will often be necessary to stop all of the TB drugs temporarily, especially if there are symptoms and signs of a generalized hypersensitivity reaction. Determining the offending drug can be difficult, since any of the first-line TB drugs can cause a hypersensitivity reaction (although streptomycin, ethambutol, and pyrazinamide are the most likely culprits, in that order).
- Hepatitis can be caused by any of the first-line anti TB drugs, but results most commonly from isoniazid and pyrazinamide. If one does not already exist, consider creating a *setting-specific protocol*, including the order of drug re-challenge, to guide management of hepatitis during TB treatment.
- Monitoring for adverse events during DR-TB therapy relies more heavily on laboratory and other monitoring tests.

Check the national TB/DR-TB and HIV/ART guidelines in the country in which you are working for a list of recommended monitoring interventions (clinical and laboratory) in those on treatment.

ART response monitoring

- Monitoring the response to ART can be done clinically, immunologically (with CD4 count tests), and virologically (with viral load tests).

- HIV viral load testing is preferred over CD4 count testing for monitoring, since the former allows for much earlier detection of adherence issues and treatment failure.
- Dried blood spot sampling from venous or capillary whole blood allows for easier transport of specimens and therefore increased access to viral load testing in resource-limited settings.[10]

ART adverse events monitoring

Monitoring for adverse events during ART often relies on laboratory testing in addition to clinical examination. In addition to allergic reactions, watch for the following possible side effects (also see Table 31.4 for associated symptoms and initial management):

- TDF: renal dysfunction, bone mineralization defects.
- EFV: psychological.
- AZT: anaemia, neutropenia.
- NVP: hepatitis, rash (including Stevens–Johnson reaction).
- ABC: hypersensitivity reaction.
- PIs (LPV/r and ATV/r): gastrointestinal, hepatitis.
- ddI: pancreatitis, lactic acidosis.
- d4T: lactic acidosis, peripheral neuropathy, lipodystrophy.
- 3TC: well tolerated.
- DTG: headache, liver problems, but generally well tolerated.
  Co-trimoxazole (CTX): hepatitis, rash, renal dysfunction (N.B. CTX is not an ARV but is included here since it is often given simultaneously and can have overlapping side effects).

N.B. If you suspect that someone has had a hypersensitivity reaction to NVP or ABC, then never re-challenge as that could be life-threatening!

Side effects

Serious side effects occur less commonly with the newer ARVs being used. However even mild side effects should be taken seriously for two reasons: they could represent early grades of potentially life-threatening ones and if the symptoms are significant, patient adherence may be compromised. See Table 31.4 for initial management.

Prevention of life-threatening lactic acidosis

A number of different ARVs can cause high lactate levels, for which clinicians need to maintain a high index of suspicion. Symptoms of hyperlactatemia are non-specific and include nausea and vomiting, abdominal pain, dyspnoea, fatigue, and weight loss. If the offending ARV is not discontinued, life-threatening lactic acidosis can develop. Since the treatment for lactic acidosis is mainly supportive, its *prevention* should be the goal through early identification of hyperlactatemia.

Drug interactions

Drug–drug interactions are common, especially in people taking both TB drugs and HIV-related drugs simultaneously. A resource to recognize/avoid drug–drug interactions can be found at ℜ http://www.hiv-druginteractions.org/.

Table 31.4 Symptoms and management of ART-related side effects

Symptom	Think of ...	Important actions
Severe nausea ± vomiting	Hepatitis Pancreatitis, if associated with abdominal pain High lactate, if >4 months on d4T or ddl	Correct any dehydration Antiemetic as needed (PRN) Blood work prn (ALT, lipase, lactate, etc.) Stop d4T (or ddl) if lactate level high
Abdominal pain	Pancreatitis Hepatitis	Blood work (lipase, ALT, etc.) and treat accordingly
Rash	Drug related cause (NVP, CTX, TB drugs)	Grade the rash and treat accordingly Don't ignore what might be an early case of Stevens–Johnson syndrome
Weight loss	Not a side effect, but could represent an undiagnosed OI Ask about chronic diarrhoea Screen for TB symptoms High lactate, if >4 months on d4T or ddl	If one or more TB symptoms, evaluate for active TB disease If diarrhoea, treat for most likely causes Stop d4T (or ddl) if lactate level high
Confusion	Need to rule out infectious causes (meningitis, etc.) prior to blaming this on a drug (EFV, second-line TB drugs).	Lumbar puncture Consider substituting EFV with another ARV
Weakness	Anaemia if on AZT Renal failure if on TDF High lactate, if >4 months on d4T or ddl	Blood work (haemoglobin, lactate, etc.) Check creatinine and calculate CrCl; if <50 mL/min and on TDF, substitute with another ARV Stop d4T (or ddl) if lactate level high
Fever, rash, and constitutional symptoms (malaise, aches, etc.)	Hypersensitivity reaction (HSR) to ABC Infectious cause	Investigate infectious cause If on ABC and HSR suspected, stop ABC immediately and do not re-challenge. Substitute ABC with another ARV

ALT, alanine aminotransferase; CrCl, creatinine clearance; PRN, as needed.

Key opportunistic infections

People with advanced immunodeficiency are at increased risk of OIs and other HIV-related conditions. The weaker a person's immune system (i.e. the lower the CD4 count), the greater the number of conditions to be considered (see Table 31.1).

Prevention of OIs

The best way to prevent OIs in PLHIV is to prevent immune systems from becoming severely compromised in the first place, i.e. through early initiation of ART. In addition, certain medications can be used to prevent OIs as follows.

Co-trimoxazole preventive therapy (CPT) helps to prevent PCP and toxoplasmosis, plus certain bacterial infections and malaria:

- CPT should be given to *all* infants, children, and adolescents living with HIV. Eligible adults include all those with active TB, advanced clinical disease (stages 3 or 4) and/or having a CD4 count <350 cells/μL. CPT is also recommended for *all* adults living in settings where malaria and/or severe bacterial infections are highly prevalent.
- The usual dosage for adults is 960 mg daily, whereas dosing for children is weight based.[11]
- CPT can be discontinued in adults who are clinically stable on ART and have evidence of immune recovery and viral suppression, except in settings where malaria and/or severe bacterial infections are highly prevalent, where it should be continued.

See the national HIV/ART guidelines in your setting and/or latest WHO guidelines for up-to-date recommendations on the use of OI preventive medication, including eligibility criteria, paediatric dosing tables, and when to discontinue.

Isoniazid preventive therapy (IPT) prevents development of active TB. WHO recommends at least 6 months of IPT for HIV-infected adults and adolescents, as long as they are unlikely to have active TB. This recommendation is irrespective of the CD4 count, and includes those already on ART, those previously receiving TB treatment, and pregnant women.[8] TB skin testing is not a pre-condition for IPT. *See ➔ 'TB prevention' pp. 540–1 for more information on IPT, including its use in children and HIV-negative individuals.*

Common opportunistic infections

Diagnosis of OIs is often made clinically in low-resource settings due to a lack of access to sensitive diagnostic tests; the use of empiric treatments implies the need for good follow-up to assess the response to therapy. Note that two or more infections may coexist in one patient at any one time. It is important to get to know the disease profile in your setting, since the rate of certain conditions can vary significantly by region.

TB is almost always the most common cause of morbidity and mortality in PLHIV in humanitarian settings.

Cryptococcal disease

- Cryptococcal disease is the second most common OI in many settings, typically presenting as meningitis (CCM).
- Presentation: symptoms of CCM are similar to other types of meningitis but tend to be less acute in onset. Headache is usually the main symptom, often together with a change in mental status.

- Diagnosis: HIV-infected adults, adolescents, and children with suspected first episode of CCM should have this confirmed, whenever possible and as long as there is no contraindication,* through lumbar puncture and testing of CSF with India ink staining and/or a rapid cryptococcal antigen (CrAg) assay. If lumbar puncture is not feasible, or clinically contraindicated, CrAg testing can be performed on serum. Normal opening CSF pressure ranges from 10 to 20 cmH$_2$O in an adult lying supine; if not available, a rudimentary manometer can be created using IV tubing that has been pre-marked (using a tape measure) and attached to an IV pole.
- Treatment: the induction phase of treatment should include IV amphotericin if possible, as its fungicidal activity gives better treatment outcomes. 'Ampho B' must be accompanied by pre-emptive hydration, electrolyte replacement, and toxicity monitoring and management (for hypokalaemia, nephrotoxicity, etc.)[†].
  - IV amphotericin is commonly given together with fluconazole for 2 weeks in the induction phase, followed by a consolidation phase consisting of oral fluconazole alone for 8 weeks.
  - A smaller, maintenance dose of fluconazole is then given daily as secondary prophylaxis until discontinuation criteria are met.[1]
  - High intracranial pressures due to CCM should be aggressively managed with repeated therapeutic lumbar punctures.
  - Initiation of ART should be delayed for ~4–6 weeks and/or until a response to therapy has been observed.
- Screening: in settings where cryptococcal disease is common, all *adults* presenting with advanced immunodeficiency (e.g. with CD4 <100 cells/µL) should be screened prior to initiation of ART, by clinical examination and rapid testing of serum or plasma, preferably with a rapid CrAg lateral flow assay.

Toxoplasmosis
- Presentation: cerebral toxoplasmosis ('toxo') most commonly presents with a headache and focal neurological deficit. It can also be associated with new-onset seizure activity.
- Diagnosis: in resource-limited settings, it is acceptable to start empiric treatment in those clinically suspected to have cerebral toxo, even on an outpatient basis. If there is no response to therapy, other causes must be considered (tuberculoma, lymphoma, etc.).
- Treatment: high doses of CTX tend to be used in resource-limited settings due to its affordability over alternative regimens (such as sulfadiazine and pyrimethamine). Folic acid is also given since CTX can quickly deplete folic acid stores. Start ART within 2 weeks if possible.
- Prevention: CTX daily.

---

* *Contraindications* to lumbar puncture include significant coagulopathy or suspected space-occupying lesion based on focal neurological signs, recurrent seizures, or confirmed on CT scan. Raised intracranial pressure is not a contraindication to lumbar puncture. Contraindication may include major spinal deformity and consistent patient refusal.[12]

† Lipid formulations (e.g. liposomal amphotericin) are better tolerated and have less risk of toxicity compared to conventional amphotericin, but can be significantly more expensive.

Table 31.5 Diagnosis and management of common, serious opportunistic infections in people living with HIV

HIV-related condition	Presentation	Diagnosis	Treatment	Screening and prevention
Pulmonary TB (PTB)	Cough that persists (often blood-stained in HIV-negative vs dry cough in HIV-positive)	Use a setting-specific TB diagnostic algorithm consisting of elements of clinical exam and locally available tests (GeneXpert®, microscopy, chest X-ray, Hb, CRP, etc.)	A new case of TB requires a 6-month regimen involving four first-line drugs	IPT can be given for 6 months or longer to prevent TB infection from becoming active TB disease
	Fever		If a DR-TB strain is suspected, then DST should be performed; DR-TB treatment regimens should include at least four second-line anti-TB drugs likely to be effective	
	Night sweats			
	Loss of appetite and weight			
Extrapulmonary TB (EPTB) Note: the symptoms mentioned here are usually associated with systemic ones such as fever, night sweats, and loss of both appetite and weight EPTB and PTB symptoms can occur together	TB-related pleural effusion can present with pleuritic chest pain and/or shortness of breath	Pleural tap revealing straw-coloured fluid (i.e. not pus) is enough evidence to begin TB treatment in a person with TB symptoms in a high-TB-burden setting	Use of steroids has been shown to reduce mortality in those with TB meningitis	
	TB lymphadenitis presents with one or more enlarged lymph nodes, usually painless	Needle aspiration of a fluctuant node and examination of the aspirate		
	Located in the cervical, axillary, or inguinal areas	Fine needle aspiration biopsy of a non-fluctuant node and investigation of its contents		
	Fistulization to the skin surface often eventually occurs	NB A draining, enlarged lymph node in a child with TB symptoms is sufficient to make a clinical diagnosis and immediately initiate TB treatment		

Abdominal TB presents with non-specific abdominal symptoms (pain, alteration in bowel habit, etc.)

Ascites (if seeding of peritoneum)

A 'doughy' abdomen on clinical exam

Clinical suspicion

Abdominal ultrasound

Paracentesis and examination of ascitic fluid (if present)

TB meningitis presents with sub-acute headache, confusion, and fever

Progresses to neck stiffness

NB Symptoms are much more non-specific in children and include irritability, poor feeding and excessive drowsiness

Lumbar puncture and examination of CSF using GeneXpert® or smear microscopy

TB pericarditis presents with chest pain and symptoms of heart failure

Signs include a rapid heart rate, distended neck veins, and a pericardial friction rub

Large, round heart on chest X-ray

(Continued)

Table 31.5 (Contd.)

HIV-related condition	Presentation	Diagnosis	Treatment	Screening and prevention
	Joint involvement presents as a relatively painless, chronic monoarthritis involving a hip, knee, or elbow	If the joint is draining, send a specimen for smear microscopy X-ray can show joint destruction if the presentation is late		
	Pott's disease presents as a spinal deformity ± distal neurological compromise	*NB A new deformity of the spine in a child with TB symptoms is sufficient to make a clinical diagnosis and immediately initiate TB treatment*		
	Disseminated TB is often diagnosed late, as the symptoms are systemic and non-specific	Choroidal tubercles on funduscopy Miliary pattern on chest X-ray Anaemia and elevated CRP are common Urine LAM testing is recommended only for HIV-positive adults having low CD4 counts and/or are seriously ill		
Oesophageal thrush	Difficult and/or painful swallowing	Usually accompanied by oral thrush	Oral fluconazole	
CCM	Headache Confusion Less acute in onset than other types of meningitis May also present with extensive rash consisting of umbilicated papules	Lumbar puncture and testing of CSF with India ink and/or CrAg assay If lumbar puncture is contraindicated, CrAg testing can be performed on serum or plasma	Induction phase should include IV amphotericin, plus oral fluconazole Followed by a consolidation phase with oral fluconazole	Screen all adults with CD4 <100 prior to ART initiation, by testing *serum or plasma* with CrAg, preferably using the newer LFA

Toxoplasmosis	Focal neurological deficit Headache ± New-onset seizures	Clinical suspicion Response to empiric anti-toxo treatment	High-dose CTX, together with folic acid	CPT
CMV	Most commonly presents as retinitis which is often initially asymptomatic Sometimes presents as gastrointestinal (e.g. esophagitis) or neurological disease	Typical findings on funduscopy	Systemic treatment with daily oral valganciclovir or daily IV ganciclovir Weekly intravitreal ganciclovir (if sight-threatening retinitis) Start ART immediately	Funduscopic screening in all those with CD4 <100 allows for early diagnosis and prevention of vision loss
PCP	Shortness of breath Cough (usually dry)	Diagnosis usually made clinically Supported by low O₂ saturation Chest X-ray findings in some cases	Oxygen as necessary High-dose CTX together with folic acid Steroids	CPT
Kaposi sarcoma	One or more purplish nodules on the skin and/or within the oral cavity Less commonly, there is pulmonary or gastrointestinal involvement	Diagnosis usually made clinically	IV pegylated liposomal doxorubicin or other chemotherapy And/or radiotherapy Start ART	

CCM, cryptococcal meningitis; CPT, co-trimoxazole preventive therapy; CrAg, Cryptococcal antigen; CRP, C-reactive protein; CSF, cerebrospinal fluid; CTX, co-trimoxazole; Hb, haemoglobin; LFA, lateral flow assay; LP, lumbar puncture; PCP, Pneumocystis pneumonia.

Pneumocystis jirovecii pneumonia (PCP)
- Presentation: dyspnoea due to hypoxaemia and non-productive cough.
- PCP commonly affects children.
- Diagnosis: in humanitarian settings, a diagnosis is often made clinically, supported by a low O_2 saturation and chest X-ray result (often non-specific but may show widespread interstitial infiltrate with reticulonodular markings more pronounced in the lower lobes). See Fig. 31.7.
- Treatment: if the patient is severely dyspnoeic/hypoxic, then admit to hospital. Treat with high-dose CTX, together with folic acid. Add high-dose steroids initially, followed by a tapering course. Start ART within 2 weeks.
- Prevention: CTX daily.

Cytomegalovirus
- CMV disease is one of the more common OIs seen in those having advanced HIV disease in Southeast Asia.
- Presentation: usually presents as vision loss due to retinitis, but can also affect the gastrointestinal tract (oesophagitis, colitis) and neurological systems.
- Diagnosis: typical findings of CMV retinitis include dense retinal whitening that follows vessels, with 'satellite lesions' extending from an irregular border, and variable amounts of haemorrhage. See Fig. 31.8.
- Treatment: daily oral valganciclovir is preferred. The addition of weekly intravitreal injections of ganciclovir can help to preserve vision in sight-threatening cases. Start ART immediately.
- Prevention and screening: routine funduscopic screening is advised in all those presenting with advanced HIV disease (e.g. CD4 count <100 cells/µL) in high-burden settings; vision loss is usually irreversible, so early detection and treatment (i.e. before eye symptoms develop) is paramount.

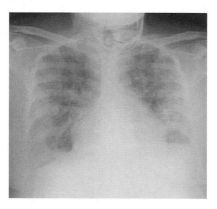

Fig. 31.7 Chest X-ray showing PCP. Reproduced with permission from Caplivski, Daniel and Scheld, W. Michael, Consultations in Infectious Disease: A Case Based Approach to Diagnosis and Management, OUP: 2012, Figure 7d.1.

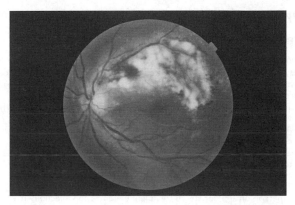

Fig. 31.8 Active CMV retinitis is characterized by dense retinal whitening having an irregular border, 'satellite lesions', and variable haemorrhage. It tends to follow vessels and as it spreads centrifugally, 'central clearing' can be seen. If the retinitis affects the fovea and/or optic disc (as is imminent in this case), significant vision loss will occur. Photo credit: Dr. Gary Holland.

Kaposi sarcoma (KS)

- Kaposi sarcoma is a cancer that originates from the inner lining of blood vessels, caused by human herpes virus, type 8.
- Presentation: it can affect any part of the body (e.g. lung), but lesions will be most often observed on the skin and inside the oral cavity. They begin as dark purple papules that will progressively enlarge/multiply unless treated.
- Diagnosis: clinical.
- Treatment: chemotherapy with IV pegylated liposomal doxorubicin is preferred and/or radiation. Start ART immediately.

Other conditions

Additional conditions that are under-diagnosed in those with advanced immunodeficiency include:

- disseminated fungal infection (e.g. cryptococcosis, histoplasmosis)
- non-tuberculous mycobacteria, especially disseminated *Mycobacterium avium* complex
- common bacterial infections, including UTI and sepsis.

Prevention

TB prevention

Context

TB is an airborne disease, transmitted through inhalation of tiny infectious droplets produced by a person with active pulmonary disease, mainly through coughing.
- These 'droplet nuclei' can remain airborne for several hours in a poorly ventilated room.
- A person with undiagnosed/untreated smear-positive pulmonary disease is estimated to infect between 10 and 20 people per year.
- TB transmission can increase in situations where people are forced to live in overcrowded conditions, such as in refugee camps. The malnutrition that often exists in such contexts increases the risk that infection with TB bacilli will lead to active TB disease.
- A person on appropriate TB treatment becomes non-infectious in a matter of days to weeks.

Preventing airborne transmission

The following infection control measures can reduce TB transmission in health facilities, homes, and community settings:
- Administrative measures aim to limit the amount of infectious TB droplet nuclei in the air. They are typically the least costly but most effective of infection control measures. An example is 'cough etiquette' in which patients are taught to cough into a tissue (or a sleeve).
- Environmental measures reduce the concentration of droplet nuclei in the air. In resource-limited settings, this can simply consist of opening windows in rooms where coughing people spend time. In health facilities, waiting areas are best placed outdoors.
- Personal protective measures complement (but do not replace) the above two types of measures by reducing an individual's risk of inhalation of infectious droplet nuclei. Respirator masks (e.g. N95) should be available and used by all those caring for people with infectious TB.
- Ideally, infection control committees should be formed to develop setting-specific infection control policies, oversee their implementation in health facilities (and elsewhere), and perform regular infection control assessments.
- Don't forget to regularly monitor all health workers in your setting for TB symptoms, so that prompt diagnosis, care, and treatment can be provided.

Intensified TB case finding

- The definitive way to prevent TB transmission is through early diagnosis and treatment of all active TB cases. Intensive case-finding strategies are necessary for this and should include tracing and assessing all close contacts of infectious TB cases.

- Although challenging in humanitarian contexts, 'contact tracing' is especially valuable for young children and PLHIV, since they are at high risk of mortality from active TB disease.
- Contacts found to have one or more TB symptoms should be *evaluated* for active TB disease, while those not having any TB symptoms can be considered for IPT (see next section).

Preventing development of active TB disease

Isoniazid prevention therapy

- IPT is inexpensive, safe, and effective at preventing development of active TB disease.
- WHO recommends at least 6 months of IPT in HIV-infected adolescents and adults having an unknown or positive TB skin test and unlikely to have active TB, as part of a comprehensive package of HIV care.
- Children living with HIV unlikely to have active TB should be offered IPT in specific circumstances, including after successful completion of TB treatment (as a sort of secondary prophylaxis).
- IPT also has a role in preventing active TB in *HIV-negative* contacts of infectious cases, especially newborns and children <5 years.
- If you are working in a high burden setting and IPT is not currently being implemented, a good place to start would be in young children, since they are at such high risk of developing active TB.
- *Consult the national TB guidelines for IPT recommendations in the country where you are working.*

BCG vaccine

Immunization with a single dose of BCG vaccine protects HIV-uninfected children against severe types of TB (e.g. miliary TB and TB meningitis). As a live vaccine, it should be delayed until HIV status is known and avoided in infants and children known to be HIV-infected.

Prevention of HIV

As mentioned earlier, HIV treatment itself can prevent transmission: by dramatically reducing the viral load in bodily fluids, ART greatly reduces the risk that HIV will be transmitted from an infected person (on ART) to an uninfected person. This so-called treatment as prevention can also reduce the risk of transmission from a public health perspective, if there are sufficient strategies in place to expand HIV testing and access to care and treatment.

- Prevention of HIV transmission begins with local capacity to perform HTC.
- Community education campaigns are useful in creating awareness about modes of HIV transmission and risky behaviours, use of condoms and uptake of medical male circumcision.
- More recently, evidence has shown that HIV-*uninfected* individuals can take the ARV tenofovir (TDF) daily to prevent acquisition of the virus. WHO now recommends that such *pre-exposure prophylaxis* (PrEP) be offered as a prevention choice to all those at substantial risk of HIV infection.[1] Adherence is key.

Prevention of mother-to-child transmission

If there are no HIV services in the humanitarian context in which you are working, introduction of activities that prevent mother-to-child transmission (PMTCT) would be a good place to start.

- HTC should be offered to all pregnant women in all high-prevalence settings as a routine part of antenatal care services. If the HIV test result is negative, it should be repeated one or more times, so as not to miss those women who become infected during pregnancy or the breastfeeding period.
- If the HIV test result is positive, pregnant women should be 'fast-tracked' to start ARVs; the HIV viral load needs to be as low as possible during labour and delivery, since this is the most effective way to prevent mother-to-child transmission.
- WHO guidelines now recommend giving *lifelong* ART to all pregnant and breastfeeding women living with HIV, regardless of CD4 count.[1]
- Following delivery, the 'HIV-exposed' infant at high risk (e.g. the mother not yet stable on ART) should be given ARV medication as a sort of 'post-exposure prophylaxis' (PEP) for the first 6 weeks of life (e.g. AZT twice daily and NVP once daily).

Feeding of HIV-exposed infants

Although HIV can be transmitted through breast milk, the use of commercial infant formula is not necessarily the best feeding option in many humanitarian contexts. The risk of HIV transmission needs to be weighed against that of mortality from diarrhoea, pneumonia, and malnutrition in infants who are not exclusively breastfed.

- In most resource-limited settings, *breastfeeding* is recommended for HIV-infected mothers (who should already be on ART).
- Breastfeeding should be done *exclusively* for the first 6 months, i.e. the infant receives only breast milk, no other liquids (including water) or solids. The only exceptions are medications and oral rehydration solution when necessary.
- After 6 months, appropriate complementary foods should be gradually introduced.
- Breastfeeding should continue for the first 12 months of life, and only be stopped once a 'nutritionally adequate and safe diet' can be provided.[1]
- *Guidance on breastfeeding by HIV-infected mothers is setting-specific, so be sure to consult national and/or local guidelines.*

Post-exposure prophylaxis (PEP)

A protocol and supply of ARV medication should be available in all health facilities in humanitarian settings in order to allow for PEP following exposure of an individual to potentially HIV-infected body fluids, whether it is due to sexual violence, occupational in nature, or through other means.

- In all cases of exposure, an initial *risk assessment* should be performed promptly so that a decision can be made as soon as possible as to eligibility for a preventive course of ARVs. If the benefit outweighs the risk, PEP should be offered immediately. The first dose should be taken as early as possible and not any longer than 72 hours after the incident.
- In the case of an occupational needlestick injury, the risk of HIV transmission is already relatively small (~1/300), but can be further reduced through use of first aid measures (e.g. washing but not squeezing any wound).
- If the incident involved a splash into the person's eye, it should be irrigated immediately with isotonic saline solution (NaCl 0.9%), not soap or disinfectant.
- If determined to be necessary following the risk assessment, the same ARV regimen recommendations are used for occupational and non-occupational exposure, including sexual violence.

ARV drugs for PEP

A combination of three drugs is preferred, for a duration of 28 days. Recommended regimens:
- TDF + 3TC + LPV/r (or ATV/r) for adolescents and adults.
- AZT + 3TC + LPV/r for children <10 years of age.

- Nevirapine (NVP) should *not* be used in any PEP regimen (due to the risk of adverse events).
- Since many people will have trouble adhering to the entire 28-day regimen, adherence support measures should be provided.
- It is important to note that ARV drugs are just one element of a support and care package needed for those potentially exposed to HIV.[1] Other essential elements include psychological support (since possible exposure to HIV is likely to result in much anxiety), clinical and lab monitoring, linkage to treatment and prevention services, and careful documentation/reporting.
- HIV testing at baseline and follow-up is important, but voluntary counselling and testing should neither be viewed as mandatory nor delay initiation of PEP.
- Be sure to maintain patient confidentiality at all times.
- Don't forget to protect against hepatitis B virus.
- Prophylaxis against other potential sexually transmitted infections will also be required in cases of sexual violence.

Check for PEP guidance within the national ART guidelines in the country where you are working and/or the latest WHO recommendations for ARV dosages, plus specific considerations for the support and care package required for different categories of exposure.[11]

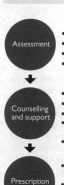

Assessment
- Clinical assessment of exposure
- Eligibility assessment for HIV post-exposure prophylaxis
- HIV testing of exposed people and source if possible
- Provision of first aid in case of broken skin or other wound

Counselling and support
- Risk of HIV
- Risks and benefits of HIV post-exposure prophylaxis
- Side effects
- Enhanced adherence counselling if post-exposure prophylaxis to be prescribed
- Specific support in case of sexual assault

Prescription
- Post-exposure prophylaxis should be initiated as early as possible following exposure
- 28-day prescription of recommended age-appropriate ARV drugs
- Drug information
- Assessment of underlying comorbidities and possible drug-drug interactions

Follow-up
- HIV test at 3 months after exposure
- Link to HIV treatment if possible
- Provision of prevention intervention as appropriate

Fig. 31.9 Care pathways for people exposed to HIV. Reproduced with permission from WHO, Guidelines on PEP for HIV and the use of Co-trimoxazole Prophylaxis for HIV-related infections among adults, adolescents and children: Recommendations for a Public Health Approach, 2014, Figure 4.1 (http://www.who.int/hiv/pub/guidelines/arv2013/december2014supplementARV.pdf).

References

1. World Health Organization. Consolidated Guidelines on the Use of ARV Drugs for Treating and Preventing HIV Infection. 2nd ed. 2016. ℘ http://www.who.int/hiv/pub/arv/arv-2016/en/
2. Cohen MS, Chen YQ, McCauley M, Gamble T, Hosseinipour MC, Kumarasamy N, et al. Prevention of HIV-1 infection with early antiretroviral therapy. N Engl J Med 2011;365:493–505. http://www.nejm.org/doi/full/10.1056/NEJMoa1105243
3. World Health Organization. Global TB Report 2015. ℘ http://apps.who.int/iris/bitstream/10665/191102/1/9789241565059_eng.pdf
4. UNAIDS. The Gap Report. 2014. ℘ http://www.unaids.org/en/resources/documents/2014/20140716_UNAIDS_gap_report
5. UNAIDS. AIDS by the Numbers. 2015. ℘ http://www.unaids.org/sites/default/files/media_asset/AIDS_by_the_numbers_2015_en.pdf
6. Bemelmans M, Baert S, Goemaere E, Wilkinson L, Vandendyck M, van Cutsem G, et al. Community-supported models of care for people on HIV treatment in sub-Saharan Africa. Trop Med Int Health, 2014;19(8):968–77. http://onlinelibrary.wiley.com/wol1/doi/10.1111/tmi.12332/abstract
7. Médecins Sans Frontières. HIV/TB Clinical Guide. 2015 edition. ℘ https://samumsf.org/en/resources/msf-hivtb-clinical-guide-2015
8. World Health Organization. Guidelines for Intensified TB Case-Finding and IPT for People Living with HIV in Resource-Constrained Settings. 2010. ℘ http://whqlibdoc.who.int/publications/2011/9789241500708_eng.pdf
9. World Health Organization. Improving the Diagnosis and Treatment of Smear-Negative Pulmonary And Extrapulmonary TB Among Adults and Adolescents: Recommendations for HIV-Prevalent and Resource-Constrained Settings. 2007. ℘ http://whqlibdoc.who.int/hq/2007/WHO_HTM_TB_2007.379_eng.pdf

10. World Health Organization. Technical and Operational Considerations for Implementing HIV viral Load Testing. Interim Technical Update. July 2014. 𝒮 http://www.who.int/hiv/pub/arv/viral-load-testing-technical-update/en/

11. World Health Organization. Guidelines on PEP for HIV and the Use of Co-trimoxazole Prophylaxis for HIV-Related Infections Among Adults, Adolescents and Children: Recommendations for a Public Health Approach. 2014. 𝒮 http://www.who.int/hiv/pub/guidelines/arv2013/december2014supplementARV.pdf

12. World Health Organization. Rapid Advice on Diagnosis, Prevention, and Management of Cryptococcal Disease in HIV-infected Adults, Adolescents, and Children. 2011. 𝒮 http://whqlibdoc.who.int/publications/2011/9789241502979_eng.pdf

13. World Health Organization. WHO Treatment Guidelines for Drug-Resistant Tuberculosis. 2016 update. 𝒮 http://www.who.int/tb/areas-of-work/drug-resistant-tb/treatment/resources/en/

Clinical suspicion of Ebola

Tim Jagatic and Craig Spencer

Introduction

Note: as this chapter was written as a guideline to assist clinicians dealing with a clinical suspicion of Ebola prior to confirmation, it is not meant to be a comprehensive guide to the management of Ebola virus disease. Ebola virus disease is classified as a biohazard safety level four (BSL-4) pathogen, the highest rating that exists, which is directly related to the lethality of the virus.

As the signs and symptoms of Ebola are similar to other diseases that exist in sub-Saharan Africa, there can be difficulty in identifying the diseases and delays in recognizing and declaring an outbreak. As health providers, particularly those working in remote regions, are often the first to encounter cases, as well as the increase in numbers of outbreaks and cases in recent years, this chapter provides the essential guidance to clinicians when there is suspicion of Ebola virus disease.

This chapter includes an outline of the basic measures that medical staff should follow, including whom to alert if there is a suspected Ebola case. There are also some basic measures the staff can take while waiting for trained personnel to arrive. The medical staff should follow the WHO alert procedures as quickly as possible. The confirmation of an outbreak will be done by WHO and if an outbreak is declared (only one case needs to be confirmed to declare an outbreak), properly trained teams from a variety of organizations will assume responsibilities of outbreak management.

Background

Virology

Ebola is an enveloped, non-segmented, negative-sense RNA virus. Each Ebola virion (complete viral particle) is enveloped in a lipid bilayer coat and heavy glycosylation which is believed to contribute to the virus's ability to avoid an immune response.

Epidemiology

Ebola virus disease was discovered in 1976 when simultaneous outbreaks of the previously unknown virus occurred in Yambuku, Zaire (present Democratic Republic of Congo) and Nzara, Sudan. Since then, five different subspecies—Zaire, Sudan, Taï Forest, Bundibugyo, and Reston—have been discovered in geographically separate areas. Only Reston is not known to cause disease in humans. The deadliest of the five, Zaire, can have a mortality rate as high as 90%.

The disease was classified as a viral haemorrhagic disease but has since been renamed Ebola virus disease due to <20% of cases developing any signs of haemorrhage. Since the first known outbreak there have been sporadic outbreaks throughout sparsely populated areas of central sub-Saharan Africa.

Since 2000, there has been an increase in the number of outbreaks and the number of cases per outbreak. Increasing human contact with potential reservoirs through changes in land use and increases in deforestation and mining are believed to be contributing factors. March of 2014 marked the largest outbreak to date, occurring in West Africa. The number of cases in this outbreak surpassed the total number of cases that have been reported in all outbreaks since 1976 combined. The total number of cases surpassed 28,000.

Vector and reservoir

There is ongoing investigation to verify the reservoir of Ebola virus, and there is evidence that fruit bats of various species host the virus.

Evidence of Zaire Ebola virus in naturally infected fruit bats was documented by the detection of viral RNA and antibodies in three tree-roosting species: *Hypsignathus monstrosus, Epomops franqueti*, and *Myonycteris torquata*. Despite such strong evidence of the reservoir, the virus itself has yet to be identified in an arthropod vector. There has been no evidence in any outbreaks to date that arthropod vectors could be linked to human transmission.

Infection rates

There is currently evidence that suggests Ebola virus has been present in West Africa since the 1990s. Some weaker evidence shows it was present as far back as the 1970s. Overall, infections have most likely been under-reported primarily due to a lack of public health surveillance systems, as well as under-reporting of suspicious cases due to poor understanding of disease or political or social stigma.

Presentation

Signs and symptoms

- The virus is transmitted by direct contact of a bodily fluid containing the virus with an abrasion in the skin, and/or mucosal surface, the use of an infected needle, or ingestion of infected meat/fluid.
- Often, the initial sign of Ebola virus infection is the onset of abrupt fever following an incubation period of 2–21 days (mean 4–10 days).
- Early in the disease process, the fever is often accompanied by malaise, myalgia, and chills. These initial signs and symptoms typically last for the first 2–3 days before evidence of multisystem organ involvement manifests.
- The organ systems affected include:
  - gastrointestinal (anorexia, nausea, vomiting, diarrhoea, abdominal pain)
  - cardiac (palpitations, shortness of breath, sudden cardiac death)
  - respiratory (chest pain, cough, nasal discharge)
  - vascular (conjunctival injection, ecchymoses, postural hypotension, oedema)
  - neurological (headache, confusion, neuropathic pain, coma).
- A maculopapular rash is often observed, typically presenting between days 5 and 7 of the disease process.
- Haemorrhagic signs present in roughly 20% of cases and often manifest as petechiae, ecchymoses, uncontrolled oozing from venepuncture sites, mucosal haemorrhage, and haematochezia or melena.

Laboratory findings

- Early leucopenia is often seen (as low as 1000 cells/μL) followed by thrombocytopenia (50,000–100,000 cells/μL).
- High levels of serum aminotransferases correlate to the virus's affinity for the liver early in the disease.
- Patients with non-fatal outcomes are able to mount specific immunoglobulin M and immunoglobulin G responses against the virus with a strong inflammatory reaction early on.

Treatment

There is currently no approved treatment for Ebola virus although there have been some preliminary and promising results involving monoclonal antibody treatment as well as a vaccine.

Despite the lack of a specific therapeutic agent, a decrease in mortality rates has been observed with the implementation of intensive supportive medical care. A supportive treatment protocol has been established by the WHO that is used to treat symptoms as well as a presumptive treatment for any comorbidities the patient might have. Low-resource settings and critical shortages of trained staff have made the implementation of intensive care extremely difficult.

> Note: treatments given to a patient with a clinical suspicion of Ebola should be done with extreme caution. No invasive procedures should be conducted, including the placement of IV lines, until properly trained personnel arrive.

The following is a treatment protocol using oral/non-invasive drugs from the WHO list of essential medicines necessary to treat Ebola:
- *Fever*: paracetamol (acetaminophen) is given for fever and mild pain. Dose for adults: 1 g PO 6 hours as required, max. 4 g/24 hours. For children: 15 mg/kg (maximum dose 1 g).
- *Vomiting*: ondansetron 8–24mg as loading dose depending on severity of vomiting then 8 mg/12 hours as needed. If there are signs of hepatic impairment, do not exceed 8 mg/day.
- *Anxiety*: anxiety is common. Diazepam (e.g. 5 mg PO three times a day) might be given to manage severe anxiety.
- *Antibiotics*: broad-spectrum antibiotics such as cefixime or azithromycin (for patients allergic to penicillin) can be given for a minimum of 5 days to cover co-infections such as typhoid fever or upper respiratory tract infection that are commonly seen throughout sub-Saharan Africa and may increase mortality in patients co-infected with Ebola virus. The course of antibiotics can be lengthened at the discretion of the physician.
- *Antimalarials*: all patients should receive a full course of antimalarial treatment with artemether–lumefantrine preferred.
  - Antimalarials are strongly encouraged for all patients, as the mortality for patients with a coinfection with malaria can exceed 90%.
  - The use of amodiaquine and SP is discouraged due to the effects on the liver.
- Supplementation: immune boosting and neuroprotective vitamins are provided to patients. These include:
  - vitamin A: 200,000 international units PO
  - vitamin B complex: 1 tablet per day
  - multivitamin: 1 tablet per day.

Management of suspected cases

- Given the similarity of signs and symptoms of Ebola virus disease with many other diseases found throughout sub-Saharan Africa and the sporadic nature of Ebola outbreaks, clinicians should frequently consider Ebola virus disease in their differential diagnosis.
- Clinical suspicion is developed by combining patient histories, clinical observations, and epidemiological data that supports the possibility of an Ebola outbreak.
- Clinically, suspicion arises when multiple patients over a period of time are observed to lack a resolution of symptoms with treatments typically curative for those treatments (this includes witnessing mortality rates higher than those typically associated with the diseases being treated).
- Treatment failure can be used as an initial point of suspicion of Ebola, however, complications of these diseases must be ruled out before investigation into Ebola begins.
- When complications are ruled out, investigation of patient histories for evidence of possible Ebola infection should begin. Because Ebola virus is spread through close contact with body fluids of infected individuals, it is important to investigate if the patient had any contact with a person (or animal) who had similar symptoms.
- Questions to ask the patient and family members include:
  - Has the patient had contact with bats or primates in the 21 days prior to the start of symptoms?
  - Did the patient consume any undercooked bush meat?
  - Did the patient care for someone with similar symptoms?
  - Have other people within the community experienced similar symptoms? If so, when?
  - Have any people within the community sought healthcare at the hospital and were given treatment but the treatment didn't seem to work? If so, did they contact a traditional healer? (Oftentimes, traditional healers bring sick and healthy people together in close quarters, which can propagate an outbreak.)
  - Did the patient attend a funeral of someone who had died within 21 days of the beginning of their symptoms?
- If there is a pattern of closely related individuals seeking care for symptoms similar to diseases typical for the area (malaria, typhoid, etc.), but who are not responding to treatment, a suspicion of Ebola could be warranted.

Alert

The WHO has developed an alert system through the Strategic Health Operations Centre (SHOC) in the case of a suspected Ebola outbreak that can be followed by a medical team experiencing a clinically suspicious case.

Six main criteria are used to determine whether a reported disease event constitutes a cause for international concern:
1. Unknown disease.
2. Potential for spread beyond national borders.
3. Serious health impact or unexpectedly high rates of illness or death.
4. Potential for interference with international travel or trade.
5. Strength of national capacity to contain the outbreak.
6. Suspected accidental or deliberate release.

These are the factors that must be addressed and documented when contacting the WHO SHOC. These factors will allow the Ebola task force to determine the level of suspicion.
- A suspicion of Ebola virus should be dealt with by contacting the national MOH and the WHO. A focal point should be identified among the group to provide all the necessary information to the WHO and MOH when contact has been made.
- The WHO along with the MOH will assess the situation and, if warranted, begin with its emergency preparedness protocol. The protocol states that MSF will be notified and blood samples will be obtained by trained personnel.
- All healthcare workers not working with WHO or the Ebola management team are strongly advised not to engage in invasive procedures once there is a suspicion of Ebola. When clinical suspicion is met, there should be no physical contact between the symptomatic patients by anyone, medical staff included.
- In the absence of training on the use of personal protective equipment (PPE) and the proper decontamination process, staff should not attempt any medical procedures. The highest risk of infection for care providers come during the PPE removal process. The removal of PPE can only be done under the supervision of trained staff.
- Despite the need for strict measures regarding contact with the patient, it is possible to provide a basic level of care provided that basic precautions are used which can include mask, goggles, gloves, and boots. Staff must not come within 1 metre of the suspected case and no physical contact should occur. A neutral area (e.g. bedside table) can be used as a place to leave medication for the patient.
- The use of basic protection does not provide the same level of protection as PPE designated for the treatment of Ebola. Basic protection is not adequate to engage in any form of physical contact with the patient.
- Contact with all body fluids must be avoided until properly trained personnel arrive.

- Oral medications and oral rehydration can be given to a patient that is properly isolated but direct contact must be avoided.
- Strict measures must be maintained to ensured prevention of contact of non-suspected individuals with suspected patients, and any materials that enter the isolation area must remain there until properly trained staff properly dispose of them. However, staff are encouraged to provide basic provisions including medications, food, water, and clothing to the patient according to the protocol provided. By keeping a distance of at least 1 metre between patient and care provider this can be done with a low risk of disease transmission.
- The patient should be equipped with resources that manage bodily fluids which might be excreted (buckets, absorbent pads).
- Any individuals who have had contact with a symptomatic patient should have their contact information recorded, so proper surveillance can be done in the case of a confirmed outbreak.
- It is important to maintain detailed notes about the patient and their history, including date of onset of symptoms, the geographical location of the patient when the symptoms started, and if there are any suspected cases that haven't presented to healthcare.
- If there is any contact with a body fluid, the area should be washed with warm water and soap. Soap will destroy the lipid envelope of the virus. If a 0.05% chlorine solution is prepared, then that can be used to clean skin as well.

Confirmation of disease

In the case of a confirmed Ebola virus disease outbreak, a more comprehensive Ebola management guide should be consulted, such as the WHO guidelines for Ebola management.

Chapter 33

Venomous animal bites and stings and marine poisoning

David A. Warrell

Venomous animals

In most parts of the world, venomous animals pose a risk, mainly to rural inhabitants whose agricultural and hunting activities expose them and their children to these primeval environmental and occupational hazards. Visiting humanitarian workers will have the responsibility of preventing and treating venomous bites and stings both in the local community as well as among their team members. These may be unfamiliar problems giving rise to anxieties about their own personal safety. Risk can be reduced by finding out in advance about the local hazards, behaving cautiously, wearing protective clothing, using a light when walking about at night, and being prepared to respond appropriately if a venomous accident occurs.

If the work location is known to be infested with venomous animals, the decision must be taken in advance whether to rely on local medical resources or to stock the specific antidote(s), antivenom(s) (also known as antivenin, or anti-snakebite serum, ASV), ancillary drugs, and other materials in sufficient quantities to meet patients' requirements, rather than relying on in-country supplies. Antivenoms are usually scarce commodities. The ability to administer antivenom is especially important if the project site is more than a few hours' evacuation time from medical care (the local referral hospital), and is possible only if your team includes someone capable of injecting antivenom intravenously (IV) and dealing with a possible complicating anaphylactic reaction. The team's medical officer should acquire basic knowledge about preventing and treating envenoming (= 'envenomation' in America/Australia).

Snakebite

In parts of West Africa, Southeast Asia, the Indian sub-continent, New Guinea, and the Amazon region, snakebite causes many fatalities and disabilities. In India, there are 46,000 and in Bangladesh 6000 snakebite deaths each year. There is a high burden of chronic physical and mental morbidity in survivors.

Be aware of the important species in the geographic area of work, and the associated clinical features. The medically important families are elapids, vipers and pit vipers, colubrid (back-fanged) snakes, and atractaspid burrowing asps, distributed as follows:

Medically important species

Europe
Vipers only, such as the common adder (*Vipera berus*).

Africa and the Middle East
Elapids—cobras and spitting cobras (*Naja* species), mambas (*Dendroaspis* species); vipers—saw-scaled vipers (*Echis* species), puff adder (*Bitis arietans*), desert horned-vipers (*Cerastes* species); colubrids—boomslang (*Dispholidus typus*), twig snake (*Thelotornis* species); and atractaspids—burrowing asps (*Atractaspis* species).

Asia
Elapids—cobras (*Naja* species) and kraits (*Bungarus* species); vipers—Russell's vipers (*Daboia* species), saw-scaled vipers (*Echis* species); pit vipers—Malayan pit viper (*Calloselasma rhodostoma*), green tree vipers, habus, and mamushis (*Trimeresurus, Protobothrops, Gloydius* species, etc.); Colubrids—keel-backs (*Rhabdophis* species).

Oceania
Elapids only—taipans (*Oxyuranus* species), black snakes (*Pseudechis* species), brown snakes (*Pseudonaja* species), tiger snakes (*Notechis* species), and death adders (*Acanthophis* species).

Americas
Elapids—coral snakes (*Micrurus* species); pit vipers—lance-heads (*Bothrops* species), moccasins (*Agkistrodon* species), bushmasters (*Lachesis* species), and rattlesnakes (*Crotalus* species).

Indian and Pacific Oceans
Elapids—sea-snakes.

Clinical features

Elapids
Most cause local pain and mild/moderate local swelling, with regional lymph node enlargement; African spitting cobras and Asian cobras cause severe local swelling, blistering, and tissue damage (necrosis); descending paralysis progressing from bilateral ptosis and external ophthalmoplegia to life-threatening bulbar and respiratory muscle paralysis; generalized rhabdomyolysis and acute kidney injury. In addition, Australasian elapids also cause incoagulable blood and spontaneous systemic bleeding.

African and Asian spitting cobras and rinkhals
Can squirt venom defensively for a metre or more into the eyes of an aggressor, causing agonizing chemical conjunctivitis with profuse tearing, leucorrhoea, and blepharospasm. Corneal ulceration, infection, and permanent blindness may result.

Vipers and pit vipers
Cause local pain, swelling, bruising, blistering, regional lymph node enlargement, and tissue damage (necrosis); incoagulable blood (as assessed most simply by the 20-minute whole blood clotting test—see p. 559) and spontaneous systemic bleeding from gums, nose, skin, gut, and genitourinary tract; shock (hypotension); with a few species, descending paralysis progressing from ptosis and external ophthalmoplegia to bulbar and respiratory muscle paralysis; generalized skeletal muscle breakdown (rhabdomyolysis) associated with generalized myalgia, muscle tenderness, and myoglobinuria; acute kidney injury.

Colubrids
Cause slight local envenoming but incoagulable blood and spontaneous systemic bleeding (see p. 559) and acute kidney injury.

Atractaspid burrowing asps
Usually cause local pain, swelling, and necrosis and rare cardiovascular fatalities.

Treatment

First aid treatment of snakebite
- Reassure the terrified victim.
- Leave the bite site undisturbed but remove tight bands, bangles, bracelets, etc. from the bitten limb.
- Immobilize the victim, especially their bitten limb, using pressure immobilization by pressure pad or bandage (see pp. 558–9).
- Arrange urgent evacuation to medical care. Victims may vomit and so should be placed in the recovery position.
- Treat pain initially with paracetamol (acetaminophen) not with aspirin or non-steroidal anti-inflammatory agents. Give codeine phosphate, tramadol, or stronger opioids if pain is persistent/severe.
- Do not attempt to catch or kill the snake but if it has been killed, take it safely with the patient to hospital or take several close-up i-phone images.
- Avoid all traditional, herbal, and 'quack' remedies, including incisions, suction, instillation of chemicals or herbs, electric shock, tourniquets, ice, etc.

Pressure immobilization by pressure pad or pressure bandage
These are especially important for elapid bites that can cause rapidly-evolving paralysis. However, since snake identification is usually uncertain, immediate application of pressure immobilization is recommended for all bites unless or until an elapid bite can be excluded. The aim is to compress lymphatics and veins draining the bitten limb (in the case of pressure bandage) or draining the bite site (in the case of pressure pad), to prevent

spread of venom neurotoxins into the systemic circulation using an external pressure that feels tight (as for binding a sprained ankle, approximately 50–70 mmHg). If the bandage is too tight, peripheral pulses will be occluded, fingers/toes will become cyanosed, finger nail capillary refill will be abolished, and the limb will become very painful.

Pressure pad: a pad approximately 8 × 8 × 3 cm thick is applied directly over the bite site, using a broad, non-elastic circumferential bandage around the bitten limb (Fig. 33.1). The whole limb is splinted to prevent movement of any of the joints.

Pressure bandage: the whole bitten limb is bound from fingers or toes to axilla or groin, using elastic bandages (10 cm wide, 4.5 m long), incorporating a splint (Fig. 33.2).

Hospital treatment

After urgent clinical assessment and resuscitation, the crucial decision is whether or not the patient needs antivenom.

Indications for antivenom treatment

- Spontaneous systemic bleeding from gums, nose, or in vomitus, urine, etc.
- Incoagulable blood: failure of the patient's blood to clot solid when placed in a new, clean, dry, glass vessel and left un-disturbed for 20 minutes or persistent bleeding (>30 minutes) from the fang punctures or other wounds, including venepuncture sites.
- Shock: low or falling blood pressure or cardiac arrhythmia.
- Paralysis (starting with bilateral ptosis and external ophthalmoplegia, then progressing to paralysis of other muscles innervated by the cranial nerves and, ultimately, involving bulbar and respiratory muscles).
- Black/dark red-brown urine (indicating rhabdomyolysis or massive haemolysis).
- Local swelling: involving more than half the bitten limb or swelling after bites on the fingers and toes or swelling after bites by snakes whose bites have a high risk of causing necrosis.

Choice of appropriate antivenom

- Most antivenoms are polyvalent, neutralizing venoms of the medically most important venomous species of a specified region.
- Monovalent antivenoms will be appropriate if only one dangerous species occurs in the area (i.e. *Vipera berus* in many European countries), or if the snake has been reliably identified as a rare but dangerous species for which only a monovalent antivenom is available (i.e. boomslang—*Dispholidus typus*—in Africa).
- Ideally, antivenoms should be stored in a +4°C refrigerator or the coolest place which may be under earthenware water pots. Freeze-dried antivenoms are more resistant to high ambient temperatures than liquid ones, but both types retain activity for up to a month in tropical temperatures. Stated expiry dates are unnecessarily early, but no liquid antivenom should be administered if it contains visible particles or has become opaque.

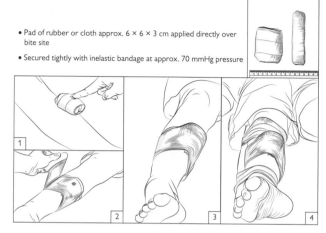

- Pad of rubber or cloth approx. 6 × 6 × 3 cm applied directly over bite site
- Secured tightly with inelastic bandage at approx. 70 mmHg pressure

Fig. 33.1 Pressure-immobilization method A: pressure-pad method.

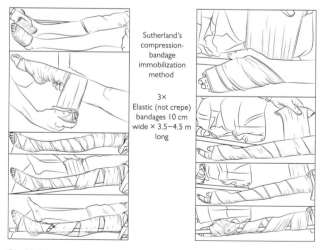

Sutherland's compression-bandage immobilization method

3× Elastic (not crepe) bandages 10 cm wide × 3.5–4.5 m long

Fig. 33.2 Pressure-immobilization method B: pressure-bandage method.

Administration of antivenom
- Give prophylactic adrenaline/epinephrine, adult dose 0.25 mg of 0.1% subcutaneously (SC) before starting antivenom to reduce the risk of a severe reaction.
- Administer antivenom by slow IV injection (2 mL/min) or IV infusion diluted in isotonic fluid over 10–60 minutes.
- Initial dose depends on the type of antivenom, species of snake, and severity of symptoms.
- For at least 2 hours after starting antivenom, watch the patient closely for signs of anaphylaxis, including restlessness, fever, itching, rash, angio-oedema, tachycardia, breathlessness, wheezing, etc.
- Treat anaphylaxis immediately; see Box 33.1

Box 33.1 Treatment of anaphylaxis

- Adrenaline/epinephrine, adult dose 0.5 mL of 0.1% (1 in 1000) solution IM (antero-lateral thigh); this can be repeated every 10 minutes until it is effective. Asthmatic reactions require additional inhaled bronchodilator.
- Histamine anti-H_1 blocker such as chlorphenamine maleate (10 mg for adults; 0.2 mg/kg for children) should be given IV to combat the effects of histamine released during anaphylaxis.
- Once features of anaphylaxis have subsided, cautiously resume and complete IV antivenom dose.

Repeat initial dose of antivenom after 6 hours if the blood remains incoagulable when retested, or after a few hours if life-threatening bleeding, shock, or paralysis are undiminished.

Note: paralysis caused by Asian cobras and Australasian death adders may respond to anticholinesterases such as neostigmine. Atropine 0.6 mg is given IV followed by 0.02 mg/kg neostigmine by IM injection (all adult doses). If there is an improvement in muscle power within the next 20–30 minutes, treatment can be continued with SC neostigmine.

Treatment of complications
- Hypovolaemic shock: results from extravasation of blood and tissue fluid into a swollen limb or systemically. Check for postural drop in blood pressure from lying to sitting up. Treat with crystalloids such as 0.9% saline or Hartmann's solution. See ⊃ Chapter 18 for more details.
- Respiratory failure: results from respiratory muscle paralysis or airway obstruction. Treat by clearing the airway and with assisting ventilation, mouth-to-mouth, or by bag valve mask connected to a tight-fitting face mask, endotracheal tube, laryngeal mask airway, or i-gel®.
- Acute kidney injury: if urine output declines, correct hypovolaemia with IV fluid until the JVP becomes visible at 45°, then restrict fluids to match urine output, check plasma urea/creatinine/K^+, and consider renal replacement therapy.
- Local infection should be treated with co-amoxiclav or chloramphenicol. Tetanus toxoid boosting is appropriate in all cases.

- Surgical complications: necrotic tissue becomes visible and demarcated after a few days and should be debrided and a split skin graft applied. Although the appearance of snake-bitten limbs may suggest compartment syndrome, intra-compartmental pressures are usually normal and fasciotomy is rarely if ever indicated. Surgery must not be undertaken until normal haemostasis has been restored with adequate antivenom treatment.

Spitting cobra-induced eye injuries

African and South-East Asian spitting cobras can spray venom defensively for a metre or more into the eyes of perceived aggressors. Agonizing chemical conjunctivitis results with profuse tearing, leucorrhoea, and blepharospasm with a risk of corneal ulceration, infection, and permanent blindness.

Emergency treatment

Irrigate the eye(s) immediately with generous volumes of any available bland fluid, ideally water under the tap (but milk or even urine is better than nothing). Treat pain with single treatment of 1% tetracaine eye drops but beware of the risk of corneal injury to the anaesthetized eye. If possible, exclude corneal abrasions by fluorescein staining or slit lamp examination if available, or apply prophylactic topical tetracycline or chloramphenicol. Prevent posterior synechiae etc. with topical 2% atropine. Use topical antihistamine for allergic keratoconjunctivitis. Antivenom is contraindicated because it is irritant and unnecessary since all venom will have been removed from the conjunctival sac by irrigation. Topical corticosteroids should be avoided because they promote herpetic keratitis.

Prevention of snakebites

Effective reduction of the risk of a snakebite is based on understanding snake and human behaviour and the circumstances under which most bites occur. In snake-infested areas, refugee camps and residential areas should be cleared of undergrowth, particularly near dwellings. Paths should be kept clear and, if possible, lit at night. Dwellings should not be constructed in a way that allows snakes to live in roof or under-floor spaces. There are no safe and effective snake-deterrent chemicals. Domestic animals, such as poultry, should not be kept close to or inside human dwellings as they encourage rodents, and, in turn, snakes. Staff and community should be educated to observe the following precautions for their personal protection:

- Avoid all snakes, even if they are said to be harmless or appear to be dead and keep clear of snake charmers.
- Open and shake out sleeping bags, clothing, and shoes before use.
- Wear boots, socks, and long trousers (pants) in snake country.
- Use a torch/flash light at night and prod the ground ahead of you with a stick.
- Be cautious and wear gloves when collecting fire wood.
- Remember that banks of rivers, streams, and lakes are common snake haunts.
- Sleep off the ground (hammock or camp bed), or use a sewn-in ground sheet, or a well tucked-in mosquito net.

Arthropod bites and stings

Bee, wasp, hornet, yellow jacket, and ant (Hymenoptera) sting hypersensitivity and anaphylaxis. Bees (Apidae) and wasp-like insects including yellow jackets and hornets (Vespidae), occur worldwide; fire ants (*Solenopsis*) in the Americas and jumper ants (*Myrmecia*) in Australia (especially Tasmania). Stings are a common nuisance but can cause rapidly evolving systemic anaphylaxis in 2–4% of the population who have become hypersensitive to their venoms. In a separate group of people, delayed, massive and persistent local swelling and inflammation may occur without systemic anaphylaxis.

Anaphylaxis

Symptoms can evolve in seconds, including urticaria ('nettle rash' or hives), angio-oedema, shock, unconsciousness, bronchoconstriction (asthma), nausea, vomiting, diarrhoea, incontinence, and uterine colic. See ➲ Box 33.1 p. 561 for a management protocol of anaphylaxis.

Prevention: those at risk must carry self-injectable adrenaline (e.g. Emerade®, EpiPen®, Anapen®) with them at all times. Desensitization is effective for those with evidence of specific venom hypersensitivity.

Mass attacks

Bees, wasps, and hornets may attack en masse if their nest is threatened. Some accidents are preventable by seeking local advice. In the face of an attack, run away very fast, ideally into undergrowth, or immerse yourself under water. Multiple stings can cause haemolysis, rhabdomyolysis, bronchospasm, pneumonitis, and acute kidney injury attributable directly to the large dose of injected venom. In the absence of a specific antivenom, treatment is with histamine anti-H_1 blockers, corticosteroids, and support of respiratory, circulatory, and renal failure.

Blister beetles ('Spanish fly', 'Nairobi eye')

These beetles are distributed worldwide save for New Zealand, Antarctica, and some regions of Oceania. They exude blistering fluid on contact, causing erythema, itching, and formation of large, painless, thin-walled blisters. 'Spanish fly' (*Cantharis vesicatoria*, family Meloidae) is iridescent green. 'Nairobi eye' and similar blistering conditions in Australia and South East Asia are caused by secretions of rove beetles (*Paederus*, family Staphylinidae). Treatment is symptomatic.

Moth and caterpillar sting ('lepidopterism','erucism')

In most parts of the world, contact with a variety of species of brightly coloured, hairy caterpillars, can cause local pain, inflammation, nettle rash, blistering, and arthritis. However, in South America, fatal systemic bleeding, incoagulable blood, and acute kidney injury may follow stings by *Lonomia* caterpillars (Saturniidae). Treatment is symptomatic (antihistamines, corticosteroids, analgesics) but a specific antivenom is available in Brazil for *Lonomia* envenoming.

Scorpion sting

Scorpions abound in dry, dusty, tropical environments including deserts, but some species thrive in South American conurbations. Stings by most species are excruciatingly painful, but the following can produce life-threatening systemic envenoming even in adults:

- North Africa and the Middle East: *Leiurus quinquestriatus, Androctonus* spp., *Hemiscorpius lepturus*, and *Buthus* spp.
- South and North-East Africa: *Parabuthus* spp.
- North America and especially Mexico: *Centruroides* spp. Arizona reports 15,000 *C. exilicauda* stings per year.
- Latin America (including conurbations such as Rio de Janeiro and Sao Paulo) and the Caribbean: *Tityus* spp.
- Indian subcontinent: *Hottentotta tamulus*.

Symptoms

Systemic symptoms include vomiting, abdominal pain, bradycardia, salivation, nasolacrimal secretion, generalized sweating, priapism, piloerection, hypertension, tachycardia, pulmonary oedema, and electrocardiogram (ECG) abnormalities. *Centruroides* envenoming causes erratic eye movements, fasciculations, muscle spasms resembling tonic–clonic seizures, and respiratory distress. *Parabuthus* envenoming causes ptosis and skeletal and respiratory muscle paralysis. *Hemiscorpius lepturus* (Iran, Iraq, Pakistan, Yemen) sting is painless, causing local erythema, bruising, blistering and necrosis, bleeding, myocardial damage, haemolysis, and acute kidney injury with high case fatality.

Treatment

Pain is best treated with local anaesthetic (e.g. 1–2% lidocaine), infiltrated by digital block into stung digits. In the hospital, hypertension, acute left ventricular failure, and pulmonary oedema may respond to vasodilators such as prazosin and hypotension to dobutamine.

Antivenoms are produced for African/Middle Eastern, South African, Indian, Australian, and American species.

Prevention

At night, reveal scorpions in prospective camp sites using ultraviolet light. They hide in cracks, crevices, and under rubbish. They can be eliminated from homes using residual insecticides. Always wear shoes and sleep off the ground under a permethrin-impregnated bed net. Shake out footwear before putting them on.

Spider bite

Bites by black and brown widow spiders (*Latrodectus*) of the Americas, southern Europe, Southern Africa, Australia, New Caledonia; wandering, armed, or banana spiders (*Phoneutria*) of Latin America; and Sydney funnel web spiders (*Atrax, Hadronyche*) of Australia; are neurotoxic, causing severe radiating pain, cramping truncal pains suggesting acute abdomen or myocardial infarction, muscle spasms, weakness, profuse sweating, salivation, gooseflesh, fever, nausea, vomiting, priapism, anxiety, and fluctuating pulse rate and blood pressure. Local pain, sweating, and piloerection ('goose flesh' or 'goose bumps') at the site of a bite are diagnostic. Effective antivenoms are produced in South Africa, Australia, Mexico, and Brazil. Analgesics and muscle relaxants may be needed.

Bites by recluse spiders (*Loxosceles*) of the Americas, southern Africa, and Mediterranean usually happen when the victim brushes against a spider that has crept onto curtains, clothes, or bedding. They cause delayed local pain after a few hours and the classic 'red-white-and-blue sign' evolving into full-thickness necrotic eschar. Rare systemic effects include fever, scarlatiniform rash, haemoglobinuria, coagulopathy, and acute kidney injury. Antivenoms are produced in Mexico and South America but are of uncertain effectiveness. Early surgical debridement of necrotic lesions should be avoided. The role of dapsone and other ancillary drugs is unproven.

Other venomous invertebrates

Centipede stings are painful. Millipedes squirt irritant secretions, causing blistering and staining. No specific treatment is available. Some ticks in North America (e.g. *Dermacentor* spp.), Brazil, and eastern Australia (*Ixodes holocyclus*) have neurotoxic saliva, causing ascending flaccid paralysis. The most urgent treatment is to discover and detach the tick which is often hidden in a body cleft or orifice. Antivenom is no longer available. Paralysed patients may require mechanical ventilation.

Venomous marine animals

Sea-snake bite

Sea-snake bites cause myalgia and muscle tenderness with trismus, myoglobinuria, ptosis, descending paralysis, and acute kidney injury. Treat as for other snakebites.

Fish sting

Dangerous species include stingrays (marine and freshwater), catfish, weevers, scorpion fish, stone fish, sharks, and dogfish. Their venomous spines are in the gills, fins, or tail.

Clinical

Immediate excruciating pain is followed by local swelling and inflammation. Vomiting, diarrhoea, sweating, arrhythmias, fall in blood pressure, spasm or paralysis of muscles, including respiratory muscles, and seizures may occur. Stingrays' barbed spines can cause fatal trauma (pneumothorax, penetration of thoracic or abdominal organs).

Treatment/first aid

The agonizing local pain is dramatically relieved by immersing the stung part in hot but not scalding water not exceeding 45°C. Alternatively, 1% lidocaine (lignocaine) or some other local anaesthetic can be injected, ideally as a digital block. Use antivenom if available and appropriate and monitor closely for development of infection with usual marine pathogens.

Prevention

Adopt a shuffling gait when wading. Avoid handling fish (dead or alive) and keep clear of fish in the water, especially in the vicinity of tropical reefs. Footwear, the thicker the better, protects against most species except stingrays.

Cnidarian (coelenterate) sting: jellyfish, Portuguese man o' war ('blue bottle'), sea nettle, sea wasp, cubomedusoids, sea anemones, stinging corals, etc.

Cnidarian tentacles are studded with millions of stinging capsules (nematocysts) triggered by contact to fire their venomous stinging hairs into the skin at enormous velocity, producing distinctive lines of painful blisters and inflammation. Sensitization from successive stings may lead to recurrent urticarial rashes and life-threatening anaphylaxis. The notorious box jellyfish (*Chironex fleckeri* and *Chiropsalmus* spp.) of Northern Australian and Indo-Pacific waters, have caused >70 deaths since 1883.

Symptoms

- Systemic envenoming can cause cardiorespiratory arrest within minutes of the stings. 'Irukandji' syndrome from *Carukia barnesi* stings comprises musculoskeletal pain, anxiety, trembling, headache, piloerection, sweating, tachycardia, hypertension, and pulmonary oedema starting within 30 minutes of the sting and persisting for hours.
- Portuguese men o' war (*Physalia*) occur worldwide and have caused a few fatalities and local gangrene attributable to arterial spasm.

Stomalophis nomurai of the north-west Pacific, China, and Japan can cause fatal pulmonary oedema.

- The sea nettle (*Chrysaora quinquecirrha*) is widely distributed, but most common in Chesapeake Bay, USA. The mauve stinger (*Pelagia noctileuca*) swarms in enormous numbers causing stinging epidemics in the Adriatic and other parts of the Mediterranean.
- Coral cuts cause painful grazes and cuts. Mechanical injury from the spiky calcified crust combines with envenoming and the risk of a marine bacterial infection.

Treatment
- Rescue the victim from the water to prevent drowning.
- Prevent further discharge of nematocysts on fragments of tentacles stuck to the skin:
  - For *Chironex* spp. and other cubozoans, including Irukandji (Indo-Pacific region and Caribbean), apply commercial vinegar or 3–10% aqueous acetic acid solution. This is not recommended for stings by other jellyfish.
  - For *Chrysaora* spp., apply baking soda and water (50% weight/volume).
  - Tentacles should be washed off, removed by hand or with a shaving razor.
  - Avoid alcoholic solutions (methylated spirits, suntan lotion) that discharge nematocysts.
- Analgesia:
  - *Chironex* spp. and *Physalia*—immersion in hot water.
- For severe envenoming:
  - Cardiopulmonary resuscitation on the beach.
  - Australian antivenom covers box jellyfish (*C. fleckeri*).
- Coral cuts: clean and debride, irrigate, and clean with antiseptic.

Poisonous marine fish and shellfish

Along the shores of many tropical oceans, various species of fish and shell-fish commonly become toxic and cause acute gastroenteritis and, in some cases, fatal paralysis, if ingested. These marine poisons are not destroyed by cooking or boiling. If working in an area where ciguatera, tetrodotoxic, or scombroid fish poisoning or paralytic shellfish poisoning occurs, make sure to review existing protocols to facilitate the prevention, recognition and treatment of such conditions.

Advice on venomous bites and stings

United Kingdom

TOXBASE® Administered by National Poisons Information Service (Edinburgh) website (registered users): ℅ http://www.toxbase.org
24/7 poisons information in the UK: 0344 892 0111

United States

American Association of Poison Control Centers 24/7, help line: 1-800-222-1222 ℅ https://www.webpoisoncontrol.org/
℅ https://www.aza.org/antivenom-index
Miami-Dade Fire Rescue Anti-Venin Bank: Emergency number 1-786-336-6600 ℅ http://www.venomousreptiles.org/pages/antbnk

Snakebite in South and South-East Asia
℅ http://apps.who.int/iris/handle/10665/249547

Snakebite in Africa
℅ http://www.afro.who.int/en/clusters-a-programmes/hss/essential-medicines/highlights/2731-guidelines-for-the-prevention-and-clinical-management-of-snakebite-in-africa.html

Worldwide
℅ http://www.toxinology.com/
℅ http://www.vapaguide.info/

Antivenoms: general
℅ http://globalcrisis.info/latestantivenom.htm
℅ http://www.who.int/bloodproducts/snake_antivenoms/en/
℅ http://www.toxinfo.org/antivenoms/Index_Product.html

Australian antivenoms
℅ http://www.seqirus.com.au/pis

South African antivenoms
℅ http://www.savp.co.za/

Chapter 34

Global impact
of antimicrobial resistance

Catherine Berry

Introduction

The twentieth century witnessed the golden age of antibiotics. Effective, safe, and relatively inexpensive, antibiotics have saved millions of lives. Therapies such as complex surgery and chemotherapy are only possible when backed up by effective agents, but their wide availability has also led to abuse.

Unfortunately, we are seeing exponential increases in resistance to the most effective classes of antibiotics—worryingly, among our most potent antibacterial agents. Annual deaths from drug-resistant infection are projected to increase from 700,000 to 10 million by 2050, at a cumulative cost of US$100 trillion.[1] (See Fig. 34.1.)

Drug development has been slow to respond. Antibiotics such as colistin, previously thought too toxic to ever be used in humans, are being brought into use. The world may face a scenario where the burden from infection is on a scale not seen in over 80 years. Described by the WHO as a major global health security threat, the impact will undoubtedly be greatest in LIC and MIC.

This chapter focuses on antibacterial resistance. Multi-drug resistant tuberculosis, drug-resistant malaria and HIV are often considered separately (see chapters 29 and 31), however a collaborative approach will be key to tackling all forms of AMR.

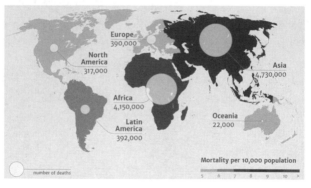

Fig. 34.1 Deaths attributable to antimicrobial resistance every year compared with other major causes of death. Reproduced from Antimicrobial Resistance: Tackling a crisis for the health and wealth of nations, Dec 2014 (https://amr-review.org/Publications.html), under Creative Commons Attribution 4.0 International Public Licence.

Impact in humanitarian settings: current status

Antimicrobial resistance is causing morbidity and mortality in resource-poor settings

The impact of antibacterial resistance has been demonstrated in settings where bacteriology can be accessed. For example, very high rates of resistance have been documented in sub-Saharan Africa and outbreaks of resistant *Klebsiella* spp. have caused problems in adult and neonatal intensive care units worldwide.[2] Overall, there is a significant gap in access to quality surveillance data to guide programme managers in assessing whether antibiotic protocols are appropriate.[3]

Antibiotics are misused

WHO recommends an antibiotic prescribing rate of 30% in out-patient settings; however, in reality rates are much higher. Data from a hospital in Afghanistan showed a prescribing rate of 62% with rates of prescribing for diarrhoeal complaints approaching 100%.[4] Qualitative research has indicated limited knowledge in many communities—at all income levels—around how antibiotics work and the concept of antimicrobial resistance. Expectations from patients to provide antibiotics for common symptoms are drivers of prescribing.[5]

This is coupled with self-treatment, often with poor-quality formulations. Use is widespread in animals. In addition, poor hygiene and sanitation means contaminated water and food can then further circulate resistant organisms in community settings.

Standardized antibiotic protocols cannot be applied to all settings

Existing surveillance data has shown high rates of resistance to first-line antibiotics such as gentamicin and ceftriaxone in many settings.[3] Given the heterogeneity in global resistance, a rational antibiotic protocol that is effective in South Sudan may not be useful in South Asia. This is most prominent in infections such as skin-soft tissue infections, methicillin-resistant *Staphylococcus aureus* (MRSA), urinary tract infections (*Escherichia coli* and *Klebsiella* spp.), typhoid and non-typhoid salmonella, and gonorrhoea.

Last-line antibiotics may be indicated in some settings but are at risk of overuse without careful protocols, diagnostic support, and oversight. Barriers exist in many settings to implement antibiotic stewardship structures—i.e. using a third-party expert to guide and target antibiotic therapies. 'The Review in Antimicrobial Resistance' has called for an expansion in dedicated human resources globally.[6]

Infection control in inpatient departments is often inadequate

Resistant and invasive bacteria have been shown to circulate in intensive therapeutic feeding centres[7] and neonatal intensive care facilities. Recognition of vulnerable or immunocompromised patient populations such as HIV, elderly, diabetic, and/or malnourished children is required and infection control should be prioritized accordingly.

Facilities often struggle with administrative governance to prioritize patient safety activities such as infection control. Adherence to the most cost-effective interventions such as hand washing is poor globally.

Additionally, there is little evidence on how to target infection control interventions in very resource-poor settings, e.g. in temporary hospitals for IDPs or in facilities where beds are shared. Basic water and sanitation must be considered but understanding the role of infrastructure is key in prioritizing investment.

Morbidity from antibacterial resistance: what are the causes?

- Acquiring preventable bacterial infections:
  - Limited access to basic hygiene and safe water.
  - Increasingly complex and vulnerable patients, e.g. neonatal care, war injury, and diabetes.
  - Inadequate infection control in health facilities.
- High rates of resistance in community bacteria:
  - Inadequate governance and regulation.
  - Overuse of antibiotics in humans and animals.
  - Poor community understanding and high rates of self-treatment.
  - Access to poor-quality or ineffective antibiotics.
- Inadequate diagnostics and surveillance data:
  - Limited access to good-quality bacteriology.
  - Slow development of simple rapid diagnostic tests.

Approaches for humanitarian organizations

- *Establish a governance structure to tackle antimicrobial resistance with high-level executive support*. At an administrative level, this would include adequate accountability linked to key clinical and process indicators, typically with associated investment. At a local level, engaging regional health services and hospital directors to clarify needs and support appropriate prevention and control. Additionally, identifying local thought leaders among clinicians and the community is key to any implementation plan. A business case demonstrating cost savings associated with preventative programmes can be useful to convince stakeholders to engage in change management. See Box 34.1 for high-impact and practical interventions to get started.
- *Establish a multidisciplinary approach* to daily patient care, incorporating infectious diseases specialists, microbiologists, infection control professionals, and pharmacists as essential specialties.[6] While this approach might not be feasible at the project level, it is important that support structures have the necessary expertise.
- Use a *targeted approach* to better understand project needs and mechanisms for quality improvement adapted to each setting.
- *Develop standard clinical indicators to detect antimicrobial resistance-related morbidity*. This should be both outcome and process measures. Examples may include rates of nosocomial infections (such as surgical site infections and late-onset neonatal sepsis), hand hygiene audits, and surveys of antibiotic appropriateness.
- *Investigate background resistance rates in country of operation*. This can be accessed via contacting local laboratories, regional reference laboratories, or accessing international data via ℘ http://www.who. int/ or ℘ https://resistancemap.cddep.org/.
- Develop systems of bacteriological surveillance to *create cumulative antibiograms where data does not exist* for relevant geographical or patient groups. Contribute data to international surveillance programmes such as GLASS (Global Antimicrobial Resistance Surveillance System).
- Focus on *infection prevention* through use of vaccines (such as pneumococcal conjugate vaccine), optimizing surgical quality (e.g. caesarean sections), and advocating for adequate water, sanitation, and hygiene.
- *Optimize infection control standards*. Simple interventions such as attention to hand hygiene can have a profound effect on infection rates in both community and hospital settings. The WHO 'Clean Your Hands' campaign has been effective in reducing the emergence and spread of resistant bacteria in hospitals, including in low-income settings. Appropriate accountability and targets can improve the impact of this intervention.[8]

Goals in humanitarian settings
- Ensure good individual patient outcomes.
- Improve overall patient safety.
- Manage costs.
- Reduce contribution to community resistance.

- *Improve antibiotic usage* through awareness and education. Engage the community, civil society, and healthcare providers to take ownership of appropriate antibiotic use. This should be aimed at clinicians, community leaders, and government officials as well as target populations. Clinicians should adhere to national or regional protocols that ensure rational use of antibiotics. Antibiotic stewardship programmes have been shown to be feasible in resource-limited settings[9] and can use models adapted to the available human resources, e.g. with nurse or pharmacist leadership. Good stewardship should be committed to ensuring *access to adequate antibiotic therapies* in areas with high levels of resistance but needs to be done with careful oversight.
- *Invest in innovative diagnostics and advocate for development of new and affordable agents.*

Box 34.1 Practical steps to control antibacterial resistance

Infection control
- A hospital with >50 beds should have an infection control professional (ICP) or focal point supported by an infection control committee.
- Mandate there should be one patient per bed separated by 1 metre.
- Where feasible, hospitals should consider following WHO hand hygiene guidelines including indicators and alcohol-based hand rub.
- The ICP should conduct regular hand hygiene audits every 3–6 months.
- Ensure standards of hospital cleanliness are set and maintained.
- In complex and high-risk settings, such as neonatal intensive care, there should be at least intermittent access to bacteriology for surveillance and consider isolating and/or cohorting patients with multiresistant organisms.

Antibiotic stewardship
- Optimize antibiotic management using locally appropriate clinical guidelines.
- Use adapted antibiotic stewardship models with clinical pharmacist chart review and feedback.
- Hospitals should monitor their antibiotic consumption of third-generation cephalosporins and fluoroquinolones using defined daily doses or days of therapy/100 occupied bed days and track this over time.

References

1. O'Neill J. Antimicrobial resistance: tackling a crisis for the health and wealth of nations. Rev Antimicrob Resist 2014;December:1–16.
2. Leopold SJ, van Leth F, Tarekegn H, Schultsz C. Antimicrobial drug resistance among clinically relevant bacterial isolates in sub-Saharan Africa: a systematic review. J Antimicrob Chemother 2014;69(9):2337–53.
3. World Health Organization. Antimicrobial Resistance: Global Report on Surveillance, 2014. Geneva: World Health Organization; 2014.
4. Bajis S, Bergh R Van Den, Bruycker M De, Mahama G, Overloop C Van, Satyanarayana S, et al. Antibiotic use in a district hospital in Kabul, Afghanistan: are we overprescribing? Public Health Action 2014;4(4):259–64.
5. Burtscher D, Al-Kourdi Y, Mahama G, van Overloop C, Leto C, Bajis S, et al. 'They eat it like sweets' Perceptions of antibiotics and antibiotic-use by patients, prescribers and pharmacists in a district hospital in Kabul, Afghanistan. Presented at Médecins Sans Frontières Scientific Day. 2015. https://f1000research.com/posters/1000006
6. O'Neill J. Tackling Drug-Resistant Infections Globally: Final Report and Recommendations. The Review on Antimicrobial Resistance. London: HM Government and the Wellcome Trust; 2016.
7. Woerther P-L, Angebault C, Jacquier H, Hugede H-C, Janssens A-C, Sayadi S, et al. Massive increase, spread, and exchange of extended spectrum β-lactamase-encoding genes among intestinal Enterobacteriaceae in hospitalized children with severe acute malnutrition in Niger. Clin Infect Dis 2011;53(7):677–85.
8. Luangasanatip N, Hongsuwan M, Limmathurotsakul D, Lubell Y, Lee AS, Harbarth S, et al. Comparative efficacy of interventions to promote hand hygiene in hospital: systematic review and network meta-analysis. BMJ 2015;351. http://www.bmj.com/content/351/bmj.h3728. abstract
9. Wertheim HFL, Chandna A, Vu PD, Pham C Van, Nguyen PDT, Lam YM, et al. Providing impetus, tools, and guidance to strengthen national capacity for antimicrobial stewardship in Viet Nam. PLoS Med 2013;10(5):e1001429.

Response to epidemic disease

AnneMarie Pegg

Introduction

Epidemic diseases in humanitarian settings can be explosive and cata-strophic for the health of the population. Events such as armed conflict or natural disaster can disrupt already weak local infrastructures and can include interruption of routine health services such as vaccination and cause disruptions in water and sanitation, leading to an increased risk of disease outbreak. This is further exacerbated by mass population displacements, which lead to precipitants for outbreaks including overcrowding and lack of access to health services, and possibly poor pre-existing health status. Even within a context of conflict or natural disaster, the impact of infectious disease is capable of quickly overtaking that of injuries and immediate sequelae of the original event/conflict.

There are four main diseases with epidemic potential discussed in this chapter (cholera, dysentery, measles, and meningitis) and the principles of epidemic response have broader application. Ebola, a viral haemor-rhagic fever, is covered separately (see ➲ Chapter 32) due to the funda-mental differences in recommendations, focusing on recognition and not management.

Advance planning for epidemics should include the ability to rapidly mobilize supplies for emergency responses and anticipation of necessary laboratory services and sample transport, surveillance, and notification. Basic hygiene principles should not be overlooked in epidemic settings. The following should be observed in all settings. Specific hygiene guidelines for particular epidemic contexts are included in the sections dedicated to their management.

- Soap and large quantities of water should be provided for hand washing, in easily accessible, highly visible locations.
- Hands should be washed with soap or a dilute solution of chlorine before and after examining each patient.
- Water and other supplies for patients with dysentery should be kept separately from the water and supplies for other patients.
- The collection, transport, and disposal of waste should be organized separately from that for other patients; stools of patients with bloody diarrhoea should be disposed of in a specific, regularly disinfected, latrine.
- Porters and laundry staff should take measures to protect themselves against infection—personal protective equipment such as gloves, goggles, and aprons should be provided, along with access to adequate soap and water, and instructions regarding proper hygiene.
- Movements of people between wards should be kept to a minimum.

See ➲ Chapter 27 for estimation of volume depletion and protocols for rehydration.

Key epidemiological concepts

- Regardless of the aetiology, data related to the number of cases, mortality rates, age, and geographic origin of cases must be collected.
- Weekly statistical collection should occur with calculation and analysis of weekly incidence rates, attack rates, and case fatality rates.
- Examples of simple forms to track morbidity and mortality for various diseases of epidemic or public health significance can be found in Fig. 35.1 and Fig. 35.2.

Weekly incidence rate

- Weekly incidence rate (WIR) is the rate of new cases within a given period of time (usually 1 week). WIR can be expressed per 100 people (percentage) or per 10,000 people. (See Box 35.1.)
- WIR = number of new cases during the week × 100/population exposed during the same week.
- A patient who arrives deceased should be counted both as a case and a death.

Attack rate

- Attack rate (AR) is the cumulative incidence of a disease over a defined period of time, e.g. 1 year, or the whole duration of the epidemic. AR is usually expressed as a percentage. (See Box 35.2.)
- AR = total number of cases during time interval/average population during the same period × 100 (or 10,000, or 100,000).

Case fatality rate

- Case fatality rate (CFR) is the proportion of fatal cases within a specified period of time, expressed as a percentage. (See Box 35.3.)
- CFR = number of deaths caused during time interval/number of new cases diagnosed during the same time interval × 100.

Box 35.1 Example of weekly incidence rate

In the Martissant region of Port-Au-Prince, Haiti (population 250,000), new cholera cases are tallied each day. The following is a chart compiling results from all cholera treatment centres in the area for 1 week in October 2011:

	Mon	Tues	Wed	Thurs	Fri	Sat	Sun
Cases	28	34	42	36	32	27	41

To determine the WIR, per 100,000 population:

Total cases = 28 + 34 + 42 + 36 + 32 + 27 + 41 = 240

$$\frac{240\ cases}{250,000\ population} = \frac{96\ cases}{100,000\ population}$$

Thus, the WIR for this week is 96/100,000.

Box 35.2 Example of attack rate
Between October 2010 and October 2012, there were 604,634 cases (source: WHO) of cholera reported. The population was estimated at 10,400,000 inhabitants. Calculate the attack rate for the epidemic to this point.

$$AR = 604,634/10,400,000$$
$$= 0.058$$
$$= 5.8\%$$

Thus, the attack rate for the epidemic period of October 2010–October 2012 is 5.8%.

Box 35.3 Example of case fatality rate
In the same time period as in Box 35.2, there were 7436 deaths from cholera (source: WHO). Calculate the CFR:

$$CFR = 7,436/604,634$$
$$= 0.012$$
$$= 1.2\%$$

Thus, the CFR during this period was 1.2%.

Province/state: Region/District:

Hospital or health facility/post:

Admission Date (DD/MM)	Name	Patient address (area, town, village, quarter)	Age	Sex	Treatment	Outcome[3]			Previous vaccination?		
						R	D	T	Yes (card)	Yes (by hx)	No

- R = Recovered D =Died T = Transferred

Fig. 35.1 Sample outbreak investigation worksheet. Adapted from MSF, Management of a Measles Epidemic 2013, p149 (http://refbooks.msf.org/msf_docs/en/measles/measles_en.pdf).

These forms can be used to track diseases/conditions with epidemic potential, as well as any condition that may be of relevance to a particular context. (reference: MSF: Refugee health an approach to emergency situations)

CAUSES of MORTALITY- sources should be noted: hospitals, health facilities, home visit investigation, cemetery records, etc

Place: _____   Reported by: _____
Reporting period: from (D/M/Y)_____To (D/M/Y)_____

Disease	<5 years			>5 years			Total deaths			Percent
	Male	Female	Total	Male	Female	Total	Male	Female	Total	
Watery diarrhea										
Bloody diarrhea										
Measles										
Meningitis (suspected)										
Other as relevant										
Other as relevant										

CAUSES of MORBIDITY - summary of all health facilities (OPDs, health posts, hospitals, feeding centres. Take care to avoid double registration)

Place: _____   Reported by: _____
Reporting period: from (D/M/Y)_____To (D/M/Y)_____

Disease	<5 years	>5 years	Total deaths	Incidence
Watery diarrhea				
Bloody diarrhea				
Measles				
Meningitis (suspected)				
Other as relevant				
Other as relevant				

Fig. 35.2 Examples of surveillance forms. Adapted from MSF, Refugee Health: An approach to emergency situations p.365/366 (http://refbooks.msf.org/msf_docs/en/refugee_health/rh.pdf).

Principles of epidemic response

- For certain diseases (e.g. meningitis) endemic to a region, an epidemic threshold exists (set by WHO); that is, a number of cases above which an epidemic is impending or can be declared.
- Response in an outbreak situation requires coordination through an epidemic response committee to ensure coordination between partners, determine priority areas for intervention, avoid duplication of efforts, and participate in public information sharing.
- Individuals to include in this committee should include broad representation including from the MOH, health partners, and municipal officials. Religious leaders, refugee camp coordinators, and others should be included as appropriate.
- In epidemic situations, a simple *case definition* must be agreed upon and used:
    - Determined by WHO, or, in some cases, other relevant health actors, these case definitions are not perfect—they may include patients who are not true cases due to lowered specificity, or miss cases due to lowered sensitivity.
    - Cases identified through the case definition system form the basis for the outbreak monitoring system.
- The response and *capacity* of the local health system must be assessed, and should include:
    - number of beds
    - number of skilled staff (day and night)
    - availability of drugs and other medical supplies
    - reliability of supply lines (can drugs and supplies be restocked in a timely manner?)
    - transport capacity (both to the facilities and to referral centres if necessary)
    - cost associated with care.
- An evaluation of the water and sanitation capacity and quality should be prioritized and include:
    - water sources (boreholes, wells, rivers, etc.)
    - seasonal variability of water quantity or quality
    - type of water treatment, if any
    - quality control related to water treatment/supply
    - maintenance of water supply (including human resource availability and reliability).
- Education efforts need to teach about disease transmission and proper infection control procedures.
- High-risk areas should be identified through evaluation of known risk factors and statistical analysis with targeted interventions for containment, and/or priority intervention. These areas can change over the course of the epidemic.
- Mobile teams are essential for case finding and referral—vulnerable groups are often the least able to access health resources.
- Rapid scale-up of vaccination programmes, particularly for measles and meningitis, should be initiated. Vaccination against pneumococcal disease (particularly for children) could also be considered.

Cholera

- Cholera is extremely contagious. Transmission is by the faecal–oral route, most commonly person to person, or through contaminated water and food.
- The majority (80–90%) of people infected with cholera suffer only a mild-to-moderate illness course, indistinguishable from other diarrhoeal illnesses. These patients are an important potential transmission source, however, as a single millilitre of cholera fluid can contain up to 10^8 bacteria.
- Risk factors linked to more severe cholera infection are similar to those associated with high risk for other disease: poor overall immune status, poor nutritional status, and extremes of age.
- Breastfeeding has consistently been shown to be protective.
- The acute watery diarrhoea and vomiting can cause rapid dehydration, which can be quickly fatal if not properly corrected.
- Infected people, both symptomatic and not, can carry and transmit cholera bacteria for 1–4 weeks; a small number of individuals can remain healthy carriers for several months.
- Corpses of cholera patients are highly infectious through body fluids still present after death.

Precipitating factors/risk factors

- Geography:
  - Cholera is caused by the Gram-negative bacteria *Vibrio cholerae*.
  - Between 1817 and 1921, six pandemics have occurred caused by *V. cholerae* O1, classical biotype. The seventh pandemic caused by *V. cholerae* O1, El Tor biotype, started in Indonesia in 1961 and currently has spread worldwide. A new strain appeared in 1992, *V. cholerae* O139 (Bengal), and has potential to emerge as the eighth pandemic.
- Seasonality:
  - Epidemics frequently start at the end of the dry season or at the beginning of the rainy season, when water sources are limited. This concentrates water-gathering activities at fewer water sources, which increases risks of contamination and transmission.
  - Heavy rains can also provoke the emergence of cholera: flooding of contaminated water from sewage systems, latrines, or septic tanks may contaminate wells or other water sources.
- Age:
  - Those at the extremes of age are particularly vulnerable; however, cholera can attack even healthy, immunocompetent people, and cause rapid dehydration and death within several hours.
  - Be highly suspicious for cholera when hearing reports of previously healthy adults dying of diarrhoeal disease.

Case definition
All organizations working in cholera response are using the *same* case definition. Anyone falling into the definition is considered to have cholera, regardless of the period of time that symptoms have been present.
   The WHO Standard Case Definition is:
• In an area where the disease is *not* known to be present: a patient aged ≥5 years develops severe dehydration or dies from acute watery diarrhoea.
• In an area where there is a cholera epidemic: a patient aged ≥5 years develops acute watery diarrhoea, with or without vomiting.

In areas where cholera is known to be endemic, an outbreak is defined as an unusual increase in new cases:
• If no data exist, this can be a doubling of the number of cases over 3 consecutive weeks.
• If data from previous years are available, a doubling of this non-epidemic average indicates a risk of outbreak.

Clinical features
• Typically, a sudden onset of profuse, painless, watery stools (i.e. 'rice water stools'), often accompanied by vomiting. There is no fever.
• Dehydration appears within 12–24 hours, which can rapidly become severe and lead to cardiovascular collapse.
• Cholera can cause as high as 20–50% mortality if case management is not adequate. Conversely, the death rate can be low (<2%) if proper treatment of associated dehydration is followed.

Diagnosis in epidemic (or possible epidemic) setting
• Bacteriological confirmation is compulsory on the first suspected cases (approximately five to ten cases) for confirmation, identification of the strain, biotype and serotype, and antibiotic sensitivity.
• Rapid tests can give a quick confirmation of a cholera diagnosis, however, they do not provide information on antibiotic sensitivity nor can they be used for biotyping.
• Write down information on name, age, sex, address of patient, clinical symptoms, and date, and send together with the sample.

Complications
• Complications can include electrolyte abnormalities (hyponatraemia, hypokalaemia, hypoglycaemia), acute kidney injury, and pulmonary oedema during treatment (children and the elderly are at risk).
• While testing for electrolyte abnormalities is not always feasible in low-resource contexts, it forms the rationale for the solutions utilized in the treatment of cholera (ORS and IV infusion).
• Pregnant women are at risk for spontaneous abortion (treatment protocol remains the same).

Case management

- Assessment of the patient's level of hydration and fluid management is the backbone of cholera treatment.
- Be aware that fluid deficits can be massive and require significantly higher than usual volumes for resuscitation. The amount of rehydration required for a cholera patient can be impressive: up to 20 litres in certain cases over a 24-hour period.
- Input of fluids and output of stool should be followed closely. Assessment of improving or worsening hydration should be frequent (at least every hour initially).
- The majority of patients are cured by rehydration and do not need antibiotics. Antibiotics are only indicated only for patients with severe dehydration and are given after IV rehydration.
- Before introducing antibiotics, initial samples should be sent to a WHO-approved reference laboratory if at all possible to confirm the strain and antibiotic sensitivity:
  - Doxycycline 300 mg for an adult.
  - Doxycycline 6 mg/kg for a child between 1 and 14 years of age is the first choice antibiotic as it is given as a single dose. Alternative includes children >12 months (azithromycin 20 mg/kg: one dose).
  - Although usually contraindicated in pregnant or breastfeeding women and in children <8 years of age, doxycycline may be used if indicated in the national protocol for treatment. A single dose typically does not have adverse effects. Alternative for pregnant women: azithromycin 1000 mg: one dose.
  - Due to increasing resistance to tetracyclines, other oral antibiotics can be used (check sensitivity): erythromycin, co-trimoxazole, chlor-amphenicol, or furazolidone, but not as a single dose.

Population-level interventions

- Improved water and sanitation are essential for the eradication of cholera, and for limiting its epidemic potential including infrastructure and smaller-scale (home and health facility) efforts. Any management strategy must include a plan for access to clean water and for the appropriate disposal of human waste.
- A stock of chlorine solution should be available for disinfection and spraying in health facilities can limit the spread of infection.
- Systemic chlorination of water points should also be an objective. Home-based chlorination kits can be used until wider safe-water strategies are in place. Depending upon the type of chlorine available, a 1% solution can be prepared in various ways, and then added to filtered drinking water.
- Two WHO-approved vaccines provide short-term (2–3 years) protection. Vaccination alone has not been shown to be helpful in outbreak settings and it is imperative that WASH activities remain the backbone of cholera prevention strategies, but vaccination can be useful in certain settings, particularly the arrival of large numbers of vulnerable people to an endemic area.

Dysentery (including all infectious causes of bloody diarrhoea)

Shigella infection is most commonly associated with epidemic dysentery. However, epidemics have been caused by enterohaemorrhagic *Escherichia coli* (EHEC). Other causes of dysentery one may find in humanitarian settings include *Campylobacter jejuni*, non-typhoidal *Salmonella* spp., *Entamoeba histolytica*, and *Schistosoma mansoni*. (See Table 35.1.)

Case definition
'Diarrhoea with visible blood in the stool.'

Precipitating factors/risk factors

- Geography: epidemic dysentery most often develops in settings with already high rates of endemic dysentery. Refugees and IDPs are at especially high risk.
- Seasonality: peak incidence occurs during rainy season related to an increased contamination of water supplies or seasonal worsening of nutritional status (increasing vulnerability to infection).
- Age: while endemic dysentery is a childhood disease, epidemic dysentery affects all age groups, with the highest incidence among adults. Extremes of age, non-breastfed children, and those recovering from measles are at risk for severe disease.

See Table 35.1 for the mode of spread and clinical presentation.

Diagnosis

- Outbreaks of dysentery should prompt surveillance and testing for the main microbial causes of bloody diarrhoea (i.e. EHEC).
- If culture and antibiotic sensitivity testing are not available, the following stepwise approach can be applied in the event of a suspected outbreak of dysentery:
  - Routine microscopy of fresh stool looking for faecal leucocytes (which suggests bacterial aetiology).
  - Treatment of cases meeting the case definition can begin using standard therapy (see ➡ pp. 598–9).
  - Microscopic evidence of *Entamoeba* trophozoites containing red blood cells provides sufficient evidence to treat for amoebic dysentery caused by *E. histolytica* (bear in mind, however, that chronic infection with this species is common and in the setting of an outbreak may not be the responsible agent, particularly when cysts or trophozoites are found without red blood cells in a blood stool).
  - If cholera is suspected, vibrios can be identified using dark field microscopy.
- A definitive diagnosis of *Shigella* requires the following:
  - Isolating the organism from stool and serotyping the isolate. Culture and antibiogramme is also required to determine antimicrobial sensitivity.
  - As antimicrobial susceptibility of *Shigella* differs by geographic area and time, treatment need be tailored to local isolates.

Table 35.1 Causes of dysentery

Species	Incubation period	Mode of spread	Clinical presentation	Duration
Shigella dysenteriae	1–7 days (average 3)	Contaminated food/water Direct person-to-person contact (unwashed hands) Inadequate sewage disposal associated with larger-scale outbreaks	Abdominal pain and mucoid diarrhoea most common Bloody diarrhoea, fever, vomiting also common Generally 8–10 stools per day without the copious losses seen in other infections Can also be associated with haemolytic–uraemic syndrome (HUS), which carries a higher mortality rate (up to 40%) than EHEC-associated HUS	3–7 days, if untreated, in immunocompetent hosts
EHEC	1–9 days (average 3–4 days)	Contaminated food	Visibly bloody diarrhoea, abdominal tenderness Fever generally absent Can be associated with HUS	–
Campylobacter jejuni	1–7 days (average 3 days)	Contaminated food (notably poultry) Direct contact with infected animal products Outbreaks can be associated with contaminated water	Abdominal pain and cramping In 1/3 of cases, diarrhoea may be preceded by high fever, rigors, and malaise Diarrhoea, with stools becoming bloody after 2–3 days	7–10 days (excretion of Campylobacter in faeces continue for up to 5 weeks)

Salmonella spp. (including *S. typhi*)	5–21 days	Faecally contaminated food or water (animal or human) Faecal–oral following contact with infected humans/animals	Fever, generally preceding abdominal symptoms (classically a 'relative bradycardia' is described, in reality this is a rare finding) Diarrhoea may not be predominant symptom Can be bloody if present 'Rose spots' (faint, pink macules on trunk and abdomen rarely appreciable in darker skin tones)	7–21 days
Entamoeba histolytica	1–3 weeks	Contaminated food or water	Most infections asymptomatic May be associated with fever and/or abdominal pain In rare cases associated with colitis and/or bowel perforation Extraintestinal complications include amoebic liver cysts	Cysts can pass in the stools of infected individuals for long periods of time; symptoms can resolve but transmission continues until treated
Schistosoma mansoni	Once introduced into circulation, the parasite migrates to the liver, maturing over 2–4 weeks Adult worms migrate to mesenteric venules of the colon, where eggs are deposited after 1–3 months Eggs move to the lumen of the intestine and are eliminated in faeces Adult worms generally survive 5–7 years (although can persist for up to 30)	Exposure to freshwater in which the snails acting as intermediate hosts are found	Chronic, intermittent abdominal pain, poor appetite, diarrhoea For non-immune hosts (which could occur in the context of population displacement to and endemic area) acute schistosomiasis syndrome can occur: Fever, urticarial, angio-Oedema, chills myalgias—all due to acute eosinophilia	Without treatment, can be long term, chronic infection in endemic areas is common

Complications
Serious complications may occur, including metabolic abnormalities (hyponatraemia, hypokalaemia, hypoglycaemia), sepsis, convulsions, rectal prolapse (particularly in children), toxic megacolon, intestinal perforation, and HUS.

Case management
- During an outbreak, treatment with antibiotics for shigellosis should be initiated in the context of acute bloody diarrhoea, without waiting for possibly delayed microbiological testing.
- If information about local resistance patterns is unavailable, ciprofloxacin (formerly used as a back-up drug to treat shigellosis) is now the drug of choice for all patients with bloody diarrhoea, irrespective of age (risk outweighs benefits).
  - Ciprofloxacin 500 mg orally, twice a day for 3 days (adults), or 15 mg/kg twice a day for 3 days (children).
- Alternative antibiotics should only be used when local strains of *Shigella* are known to be resistant to ciprofloxacin:
  - Azithromycin is an alternative for adults.
  - Pivmecillinam (amdinocillin pivoxil) and ceftriaxone are the only antimicrobials effective for multiresistant strains of *Shigella* in all age groups.
- When an effective antimicrobial is given, improvement should be noted within 48 hours. This includes fewer stools, less blood in stools, less fever, and improved appetite. Failure to improve should suggest possible resistance.
- Management of dehydration, continued feeding (particularly for breastfed infants), and treatment of fever and pain are integral.
- Supplemental zinc is recommended for children <5 years of age.
- Patients with bloody diarrhoea requiring treatment in a health facility should be kept in a designated, separate diarrhoea ward/area.

Specific infection control measures
- The collection, transport, washing, and disinfection of clothes and bedding should be frequent and exclusive to patients with bloody diarrhoea. Health workers caring for patients with bloody diarrhoea should not prepare/serve food.
- Only one relative should attend each patient.

Population-level interventions
- Vaccination: no vaccine exists against organisms causing dysentery.
  - Measles infection greatly increases the risk of severe dysentery in children, and so active measles vaccination should occur in settings where an outbreak is suspected or populations are at risk.
  - The age group targeted by measles vaccination campaigns may vary according to the risk profile of the population, as well as available resources. Typical campaigns target, at minimum, children aged 6 months to 5 years, as this is the age group most susceptible to serious infection and complications.
  - Vaccination is provided regardless of previous vaccination status.
  - In certain contexts, the target age group may be expanded.

- The following public health strategies can reduce incidence of all diarrhoeal disease:
  - Hand washing with soap.
  - Ensuring the availability of safe drinking water.
  - Safely disposing of human waste.
  - Breastfeeding of infants and young children.
  - Safe handling and processing of food.
  - Control of flies.

Measles

Precipitating factors/risk factors

- Geography: no geographic preponderance exists—although the burden is higher in developing countries, where rates of immunization are lower.
- Seasonality: not apparent.
- Age: primarily a disease of children <5 years old. Unvaccinated children are at the highest risk, although any non-immune person can become infected.
- Nutritional status: low vitamin A is linked to a higher rate of complications (notably corneal blindness) and higher death rates.

Case definition

Any person in whom a clinician suspects measles infection (for those familiar with the diagnosis), *or* any person with fever and maculopapular rash (i.e. non-vesicular) and cough, coryza (i.e. runny nose), or conjunctivitis (i.e. red eyes).

Transmission and carriers

- Highly contagious viral disease, spread by respiratory droplets, capable of surviving on surfaces or air for several hours.
- The incubation period usually lasts 10 days (can range from 7 to 18 days) from exposure to the onset of fever.
- Communicable from slightly before the prodromal period to 4 days after the appearance of the rash. Natural infection produces a lifelong immunity.

Clinical features

- Prodromal fever, conjunctivitis, coryza, cough, and Koplik spots (reddish spots with a white centre) on the buccal mucosa.
- A characteristic red rash appears on the third to seventh day beginning on the face, then becoming generalized, and lasting 4–7 days.

See Figs 35.3–35.5.

Diagnosis

- When an outbreak is suspected, an investigation must be carried out to confirm the diagnosis, assess the extent of the outbreak, and identify the population at risk.
- A sample outbreak investigation worksheet which includes the key information regarding clinical syndrome and immunization status is shown in ➔ Fig. 35.1 p. 581.
- Blood samples must be collected from the initial ten reported cases. Laboratory diagnosis is indicated by either a fourfold increase in antibody titre (at least), isolation of measles virus, or presence of measles-specific IgM antibodies.
- If no laboratory is available, a clinical definition can be used—but samples should still go to a reference lab for confirmation.

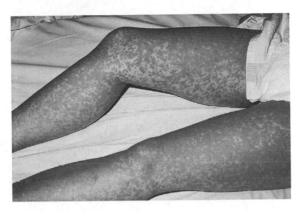

Fig. 35.3 Generalized morbilliform measles rash. Reproduced with permission from D A Warrell, Oxford Textbook of Medicine (5th ed) OUP: May 2017 update. Figure 7.5.6.8a.

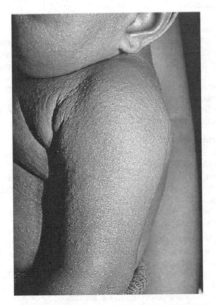

Fig. 35.4 Measles rash in a dark-skinned child. Reproduced with permission from Oxford Textbook of Medicine (5th ed) OUP: May 2017 update. Figure 7.5.6.9.

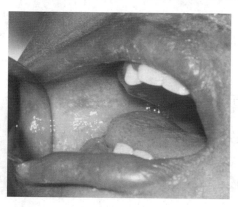

Fig. 35.5 Koplik spots. Courtesy of the late Dr B.E. Juel-Jensen, Reproduced with permission from Oxford Textbook of Medicine (5th ed) OUP: May 2017 update. Figure 7.5.6.7.

Complications

- Measles can lead to life-long disabilities, including blindness, brain damage, and deafness.
- Infection is followed by a period of relative immunosuppression for several weeks and increases susceptibility to other infections. These complications are more frequent in developing countries and can be anticipated in at least 75% of cases in these regions.
- The three major causes contributing to the high case-fatality rate are pneumonia, diarrhoea, and croup.
- The case fatality rates in developing countries are normally estimated to be 3–5%, but may reach 10–30% in some situations.

Case management

Examine the child for specific signs and symptoms to ensure that those with severe complications are properly treated:

- Ask if the child has had any change in the level of consciousness or feeding/drinking, cough, convulsions, diarrhoea, ear pain, discharge from eyes, or loss of vision.
- Look for tachycardia, wasting, sore red mouth, dehydration, respiratory distress, ear infection, and eye disease.

Case management of uncomplicated measles

- Many children will experience uncomplicated measles and will require only supportive measures.
- Give vitamin A (dose depending on child's age, see Table 35.2: WHO guidelines).
- Provide nutritional support: continue breastfeeding or give weaning foods and fluids at frequent intervals and treat mouth ulcers.
- Control fever (tepid sponging or antipyretics).

Table 35.2 Vitamin A dosage depending on child's age

Age	Dose on diagnosis (IU)	Dose on following day (IU)	2–4 weeks later (if eye symptoms noted) (IU)
<6 months old	50,000	50,000	50,000
6–11 months of age	100,000	100,000	100,000
12 months and older	200,000	200,000	200,000

- Instruct to return for further treatment if the child's general condition worsens or any of the danger signs develop: rapid or difficulty breathing, severe cough, worsening dehydration, bloody diarrhoea, seizures, or altered mental status.
- Explain risks of complications to family and advise them to seek medical advice early.
- Immunize close contacts, if identified within 72 hours of exposure.

Case management of complicated measles

- Refer to health facility for further management.
- Ensure that two doses of vitamin A are given.
- Clean eye lesions and treat with 1% tetracycline eye ointment three times a day for 7 days.
- For corneal lesions, cover the eye with a patch. Vitamin A is key minimize the risk of blinding eye lesions so give a third dose of vitamin A 2–4 weeks later using the same dosage.
  - Never use steroid eye drops to treat eye symptoms associated with measles.
- Clean ear discharge and treat with antibiotics.
- Refer suspected encephalitis to hospital.
- Treat concurrent conditions such as dehydration, malnutrition, and pneumonia.

Population-level interventions

- Vaccination:
  - Sadly, in the majority of outbreaks, immunization occurs too late to affect the impact of the outbreak. Supplementary vaccination activities should focus on unaffected areas where the epidemic is more likely to spread.
  - Routine immunization of children should continue.
  - In refugee camps, vaccination of all children <5 years of age is indicated as soon as they arrive at the camp.
- Public health strategies:
  - Health education related to limiting contact between infected children and immunocompromised community members could be included in epidemic response efforts.
  - Specific containment strategies outside of healthcare facilities are not recommended.

Meningitis

- Meningitis is the acute inflammation of the brain and spinal cord membranes, or meninges, which can be rapidly fatal if not recognized and treated effectively.
- Although causes are varied, the primary concern in the humanitarian setting are infectious causes of meningitis, specifically bacterial, which spread rapidly, have an aggressive clinical course, and have been implicated in outbreaks of the disease.
- *Neisseria meningitidis* is a common cause of bacterial meningitis, and can progress from non-specific symptoms to death in hours.
- Untreated, meningococcal meningitis is fatal in 50 to 80% of cases. Case management can reduce the case fatality rate to 8–15%.

Precipitating factors/risk factors

- Geography: bacterial meningitis epidemics are most likely in sub-Saharan Africa, within the 'meningitis belt', an area stretching from the Red Sea to the Atlantic. Major epidemics generally occur every 8–10 years in this region.
- Seasonality: epidemic onset is typically in the middle of the dry season (December to February), often ending spontaneously at the beginning of the rainy season in May/June.
- Age: during epidemics, in the endemic regions, it affects children aged >6 months, adolescents, and young adults. However, in epidemics that have occurred outside the meningitis belt, higher attack rates have been reported among those >30 years of age

Case definition

For children <1 year: a *suspected* case is one presenting with a fever *and* bulging fontanelle *or* petechial rash.

- For adults and children >1 year, *suspect* meningitis in those with a sudden onset of fever and neck stiffness *or* petechial rash.
- A *probable* case includes the above criteria in the context of on ongoing outbreak, and/or cloudy CSF at lumbar puncture.
- A *confirmed* case is a suspected/probable case with a positive rapid test (latex agglutination test), or positive CSF culture.

Transmission and carriers

- Humans are the only reservoir for meningitis-causing bacteria and transmission is via respiratory droplets.
- Healthy carriers can play a major role in the transmission as the carrier state persists for 5–15 weeks (up to 9–16 months in some cases) but mass chemoprophylaxis to prevent or control outbreaks is not recommended due to risks of antibiotic resistance.

Clinical features

- In children >1 year of age and adults: neck stiffness, photophobia, fever, headache, nausea, vomiting, and purpura (localized or generalized). (See Fig. 35.6.) Conjunctival petechiae can also be seen (See Fig. 35.7.)
- For children <1 year of age, symptoms are less specific and diagnosis more difficult. Signs and symptoms include reduced oral intake,

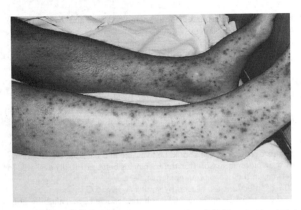

Fig. 35.6 Purpura on the foot of an adult with meningitis. Reproduced with permission from Oxford Textbook of Medicine (5th ed) OUP: May 2017 update. Figure 7.6.5.8.

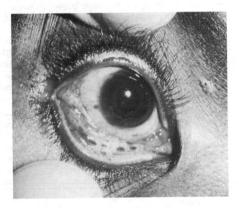

Fig. 35.7 Conjunctival petechiae in an African child with meningococcal group A meningitis. Reproduced with permission from Oxford Textbook of Medicine (5th ed) OUP: May 2017 update. Figure 7.6.5.9.

diarrhoea, vomiting, drowsiness, abnormal cry, seizures, hypo- or hypertonia (neck stiffness often absent in infants), bulging fontanelle when not crying (late sign, poor prognosis), coma, and purpura

- If available, a lumbar puncture will reveal cloudy CSF.
- *A clinical suspicion of meningitis should trigger rapid initiation of treatment.* Treatment should not be withheld while confirmatory testing takes place, nor should it be delayed in order to ensure laboratory or other investigations.

- If an outbreak is suspected, cases should be tallied and treated rapidly, even if the diagnosis is not confirmed.
- Neurological sequelae are a major problem, with up to 20% of the cured patients left with serious sequelae, including deafness, hemiplegia, facial paralysis, mental retardation, and epilepsy.

Diagnosis and confirming outbreaks

- Epidemic bacterial meningitis is caused by *Neisseria meningitides* with confirmation via testing of CSF samples to determine the serogroup(s) involved. Once the serogroup is confirmed, and an outbreak declared, CSF testing should not be done routinely.
- Latex agglutination tests are rapid tests to identify different pathogens and serogroups. These should be available in the field at the beginning of the epidemic season (for the meningitis belt), or rapidly available for delivery in the event of an epidemic alert.
- 90% of infections are caused by strains A, B, and C.
- At the start of an epidemic, CSF culture, followed by an antibiogram, must be carried out to determine the sensitivity of the meningococcus to locally available antibiotics.

If it is not possible to send samples to a reference laboratory, a minimum level of testing which should be available regionally is as follows:
- Collection of a CSF sample and qualitative examination of fluid: turbid, cloudy, or bloody.
- Measurement of the WBC count in the CSF (by microscopy): in meningitis this is generally >1000 cells/mm^3 (and >60% polynuclear cells).
- Gram stain, showing Gram-negative diplococci (for *N. meningitidis*). If Gram stain is not possible, use methylene blue stain.
- If possible, measurement of protein level in CSF: in cases of meningitis this is generally >0.8 g/litre.

> The attack rate during an epidemic can exceed 20/100,000/week (which is the average rate per year, during non-epidemic periods).
> The epidemic threshold confirms an epidemic and can range from 15/100,000 for populations >30,000 people to 5 cases/week or a doubling of cases from 1 week to the next for 3 consecutive weeks for smaller populations.

Case management

The key objectives for during a meningitis outbreak are rapid access to treatment and prioritized, targeted vaccination campaigns.

First-line treatments for epidemic meningitis
- *Children 2–23 months:*
  - Ceftriaxone 100 mg/kg once daily by IM injection for 7 days. In young children, other pathogens (*Haemophilus influenzae*, *Streptococcus pneumoniae*) are common even during a meningococcal meningitis epidemic and ceftriaxone is also effective against these.
  - If ceftriaxone is not available, oily chloramphenicol may be used in children >2 months of age: administer one dose of 0.5 g, then refer in order to provide more adapted treatment.

- *Children <2 months of age:*
  - Ceftriaxone is not effective against *Listeria*, a common causative organism in young children, therefore treat as septicaemia, and give a combination of antibiotics (i.e. ampicillin + gentamicin).
- *Children >2 years and adults:* ceftriaxone (first line) or oily chloramphenicol as a single dose:
  - Ceftriaxone:
    —Single dose 100 mg/kg (maximum 4 g) IM injection—administer half the dose in each buttock.
    —Presumptive treatment with a single IM dose of ceftriaxone should *not* be used in non-epidemic contexts—here, bacterial meningitis (mainly due to *S. pneumoniae* and *H. influenzae*) requires a treatment for 7–10 days. Using single-dose ceftriaxone in non-epidemic contexts poses a risk for the patient, and may have consequences for the sensitivity of the various pathogens to this antibiotic.
    —Treatment of choice in pregnant, breastfeeding women
    —Contraindications, adverse effects, precautions: may cause (rarely) diarrhoea or nausea.
  - Oily chloramphenicol:
    —Oily suspension, 100 mg/kg as a single dose (maximum 3 g) as an *IM injection only*.
    —*Never* give IV or mix drugs in the syringe.
    —The dose should be divided into two different deep IM injections sites (upper, outer quadrants of the buttocks).
    —If there is no clinical improvement or deterioration after 24 hours, review the diagnosis. If no alternative diagnosis, administer ceftriaxone IM for 7 days (100 mg/kg once daily in children and 2 g once daily in adults).
    —Contraindications, adverse effects, precautions: contraindicated during pregnancy and breastfeeding; may rarely cause agranulocytosis.
  - Supportive therapy:
    —Treatment of fever, seizures (note: prophylaxis is not recommended), fluids for those in shock.
    —Maintain clear airway in those with altered mental status/coma.
  - Isolation:
    —Patient isolation is neither justified nor recommended as cases only represent a small proportion of the reservoir and spread occurs by way of healthy carriers.

Chemoprophylaxis of contacts is *not* recommended; however, close contacts of the patient should be considered priority targets for vaccination.

Population-level interventions
- Mass vaccination against meningococcal meningitis of vulnerable groups is key to limiting spread, morbidity, and mortality.
- Within the meningitis belt, bivalent A + C vaccine is currently the most commonly used.

- Antibodies are detected 5–8 days after a single injection. Vaccine effectiveness is 85–90%, decreasing progressively over 3–5 years' time. Studies have shown that after 3 years, only 65% of the vaccinated population is protected. Protection diminishes even more quickly in children.
- Since 2010, countries in high-risk regions of sub-Saharan Africa are introducing a new meningococcal A conjugate vaccine (MenAfriVac®), which is expected to confer both long-lasting individual protection as well as improved population immunity.

Further reading

Médecins Sans Frontières. MSF Cholera Guideline. 2004. ℘ https://www.humanitarianresponse.info/en/operations/iraq/document/msf-cholera-guidelines-2004

World Health Organization. Cholera. ℘ http://www.who.int/topics/cholera/about/en/index.html

World Health Organization. Guidelines for the Control of Shigellosis, Including Epidemics Due to Shigella Dysenteriae Type 1. Geneva: WHO; 2005. ℘ http://whqlibdoc.who.int/publications/2005/9241592330.pdf

World Health Organization. Meningococcal Meningitis. ℘ http://www.who.int/csr/disease/meningococcal/en/

World Health Organization. Treating Measles in Children. 2004. ℘ http://www.who.int/immunization/programmes_systems/interventions/TreatingMeaslesENG300.pdf?ua=1&ua=1

Part V

Clinical guidelines

Cardiac conditions

Saleem Kassam

Cardiology in low-resource settings

The cardiovascular system is affected by the spectrum of health conditions, from infectious to degenerative. Cardiovascular conditions are the cause of significant morbidity and mortality in low-resource contexts. Cardiovascular diseases accounted for 31% of all global deaths in 2012, with the greatest burden and largest increases over time, in LIC to MIC. (See Fig. 36.1.) The majority of population attributable risk for coronary heart disease is from modifiable risk factors, where early detection and management can lead to significant prevention of society disease burden.[1]

In resource-poor settings, one must be prepared to encounter the whole spectrum of diseases. This can include presentations not commonly seen in more developed settings, such as congenital conditions (e.g. patent ductus arteriosus and aortic coarctation). Symptoms may manifest in early adulthood, where conditions such as rheumatic mitral stenosis and dilated cardiomyopathy may present as dyspnoea, syncope, or frank congestive heart failure (CHF) secondary to the haemodynamic stress of childbirth.

Cardiovascular diseases can be challenging to treat in low-income settings: symptoms may be subtle or manifest only in the late stage, such that patients may not self-present when there is an important change in condition, diagnostic tools may be unavailable, and long-term follow-up may be difficult for patients on the move, or far from points of care. Access and affordability of cardiac medications also may be a challenge for patients. This chapter aims to offer providers guidance for the recognition and management of the most common cardiovascular conditions found in humanitarian settings, including those with acute *and* chronic presentations.

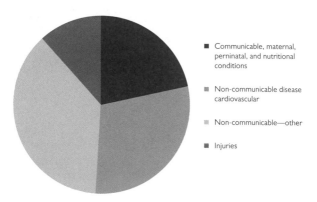

- Communicable, maternal, perinatal, and nutritional conditions
- Non-communicable disease cardiovascular
- Non-communicable—other
- Injuries

Fig. 36.1 Causes of death in low- and middle-income countries, age 5 and older. Data aggregated from Mathers CD, Murray CJL, Lopez AD (2006). The burden of disease and mortality by condition: data, methods and results for the year 2001. In: Lopez AD, et al. (eds) Global burden of disease and risk factors. Oxford University Press.

Approach to cardiac conditions

History taking
In low-resource settings, without access to advanced diagnostic tests, history takes on high importance. Since early disease may be asymptomatic, and treatment at an early stage may be important, one should ask about risk factors as well as specific symptoms.

Cardiovascular risk factors
Major risk factors
- Smoking.
- Hypertension.
- Diabetes.
- Dyslipidaemia.
- Family history (coronary artery disease (CAD) before age 60 in first degree relative). This may also be the only clue to familial dilated cardiomyopathy or malignant arrhythmia (CHF/sudden death).

Minor risk factors
- Obesity.
- Unusual stress (such as displacement, loss of family, or large-scale conflict).
- Lifestyle factors: alcohol abuse.
- Recreational drugs.
- Sedentary lifestyle.

Infectious disease history
Ask about an infectious disease history, which is especially relevant in developing countries and tropical settings. For example, rheumatic fever in childhood can cause valve disease and is estimated to account for 15% of all patients with heart failure in endemic areas; Chagas disease is the most common cause of CHF in South America.

Symptoms
The routine history for cardiovascular disease includes questions about common symptoms, which can suggest a diagnosis:
- Chest pain, dyspnoea, diaphoresis → myocardial ischaemia.
- Dyspnoea, paroxysmal nocturnal dyspnoea, and orthopnoea → increased ventricular filling pressures.
- Dependent oedema, ascites → right-sided overload.
- Syncope and pre-syncope, effort intolerance → low cardiac output.
- Palpitations, sudden pre/syncope → disturbances in rate/rhythm.

Functional status
In compensated conditions, symptoms are often absent at rest, so understanding relationship to effort is important. The New York Heart Association functional classification system is a validated effort tolerance scale which stratifies people as having low-risk and high-risk/unstable cardiac symptoms (See Table 36.2.).

In low-resource settings, patients often present in advanced stages of their illness. Severe cardiac failure may present as circulatory shock, and carries a grave prognosis. Tachycardia, low pulse pressures, oliguria, and cool or mottled extremities are signs of low-output states, for which severe pump failure may be a cause. Differentiating this from sepsis (usually 'warm' shock—hypoperfusion with normal or elevated body temperature) or low effective circulating volume (low JVP/evidence of hypovolaemia), is critical as CHF usually requires diuresis and low effective circulating volume needs fluid replacement.

- Look for the JVP which can direct fluid therapy
- If you cannot see the JVP, lower (towards 0° or supine) and raise the head of the bed (up to 90° or upright), or perform the abdominojugular reflux manoeuvre until it is visible.
- Feeling a displaced or sustained cardiac apex may signify cardiac structural disease.

Consider cultural context

In certain settings, patients may have little knowledge of previous conditions, diagnosed or not, and may never have had previous treatments. Cultural context may be of importance and here clinical acumen plays a particularly important role. Consider how you might be able to gather information. For example:

- Asking if shoes no longer fit, which may be a clue to ankle oedema.
- Problems during childbirth, such as respiratory or circulatory decompensation, may be a clue to otherwise silent myocardial or valvular pathology.
- Syncope may be misinterpreted as 'fits' or seizures.
- Cachexia may be denied for fear of stigmatization due to the association with TB or HIV infection.
- Increasing waist size when wearing trousers may be a sign of chronic cardiac failure.
- Asking about effort required for daily tasks (i.e. walking to market, carrying water, preparing meal) can provide a lot of information about effort tolerance. Can they keep up with peers? Inability to do household chores may a sign of diminished functional ability.

Assessment

General appearance: in many cultures, patients may not volunteer much at all, and may not realize how advanced their condition is. Careful observation can contribute a lot. Are they uncomfortable or in even mild distress? Are their extremities cool? Are they diaphoretic? Are they fully alert or somewhat obtunded?

Specific cardiovascular assessment

- On respiratory examination, assess if patients are tachypnoeic, or if there is evidence of basal crepitations, wheeze, and pleural effusions suggesting pulmonary oedema.
- Assess the apex beat looking for cardiac chamber enlargement: turn the patient in the left decubitus position with expiration if it is difficult to feel while supine. This brings the cardiac apex closer to the chest wall. Make note of its size: >2.5 cm in diameter is considered abnormal.

- Listen for a bi- or triphasic rub indicating pericardial irritation.
- Assess the heart sounds for the presence of murmurs (systolic vs diastolic) suggesting valvular pathology. See Fig. 36.2.
- Palpate the liver edge for enlargement, which may indicate right-sided volume overload, or pulsation, a sign of tricuspid regurgitation.
- Palpate the abdominal aorta for enlargement or aneurysm and assess for bruits to indicate atherosclerosis and possible obstruction.
- Assess peripheral pulses for symmetry, femoral bruits, and evidence of arterial insufficiency.
- Assess for dependent oedema which may suggest right-sided cardiac failure.
- Funduscopy where available can demonstrate atherosclerotic changes in retinal vessels.
- Assess JVP: head of bed at 30–45°, legs flat, and an obliquely positioned light.

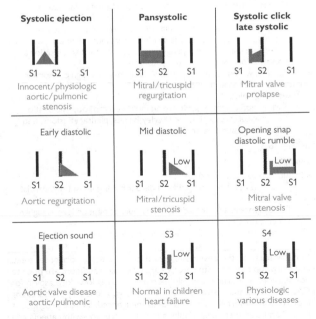

Fig. 36.2 Murmur refresher.

Further testing

12-lead ECG basics

- Assess rate and rhythm for irregularity (seen in atrial fibrillation) and grouped beating (atrioventricular conduction disease).
- A widened QRS (duration >120 ms) signifies conduction disease or left ventricular (LV) dysfunction.
- The presence of Q waves may point to previous myocardial infarction.
- LV hypertrophy on an ECG may indicate LV enlargement or thickening (not specific under age 40). Specific findings may include increased QRS voltages, intraventricular conduction delay, or ST depression representing a so-called strain-pattern.

CXR basics

- Ideally a posteroanterior (PA) film is used to assess heart size.
- Assess for chamber enlargement:
  - LV enlargement in the PA projection is suspected when the cardiac shadow is more than half of the thoracic diameter. In a lateral film, LV enlargement obscures the space between infra-cardiac aorta and the diaphragm. Right ventricular (RV) enlargement is best seen in a lateral film, when the cardiac shadow abuts more than the lower half of the sternum. These findings may support a cardiac cause for a presentation with suspicious symptoms.
- Mediastinal widening (>8 cm on a PA film) may be a sign of thoracic pathology such as an aortic aneurysm.
- Assess lung fields:
  - Radiographic signs of CHF are an increased cardiothoracic ratio >0.5, vascular redistribution/Kerley B lines, pleural effusions, and diffuse air-space disease if advanced.

See Fig. 36.3.

Blood work

- In addition to basic blood tests,
  - Troponin I or T are the gold standard for ruling in/out myocardial infarction.
  - For dyspnoea, an increased brain natriuretic peptide level is highly specific for CHF.
  - Be sure to check local lab reference ranges and cut-off values.

In many parts of the developing world, the facilities to diagnose, treat, and follow up patients with chronic cardiovascular conditions are poor to non-existent. Focusing on simple therapies, such as low-dose aspirin for CAD, or salt/water restriction for CHF, may go a long way in addressing morbidity and mortality, and should not be ignored. Where prognosis is limited and treatment unavailable, a realistic discussion with patients and families is critical.

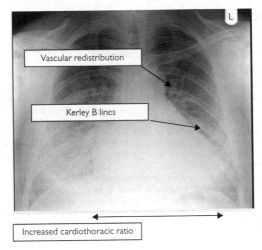

Fig. 36.3 Chest X-ray depicting congestive heart failure. Reproduced with permission from Ali, Usman, et al, Painless aortic dissection presenting as congestive heart failure; BJMP 2011;4(1):a401 (http://bjmp.org/files/2011-4-1/bjmp-2011-4-1-a401.pdf).

Hypertension

Definition
Hypertension is defined as BP >140/90 mmHg.

Context
The magnitude and scope of high BP and its devastating effects in low-resource settings cannot be overstated: hypertension is the most common modifiable risk associated with stroke worldwide, and in particular, in developing contexts. Hypertension is present in more than one-third of adults in Africa and in over half of people screened in Mexico and Latin America. Poorly controlled BP is responsible for approximately half the deaths from stroke and CAD, and is the leading cause of CHF worldwide.

A profound lack of screening, limited healthcare contact, poor patient education, and lack of symptoms, result in long periods of undiagnosed and/or untreated high BPs. The threshold above which antihypertensive treatment is started in long-standing hypertension must be in line with the overall national guidelines, the project goals, and the context and include consideration of resources availability for treatment and follow-up/sustainability.

Presentation
Usually, there are no symptoms. If severe, symptoms may include headache, confusion, neurological symptoms, chest pain, and dyspnoea.

Diagnosis
- The diagnosis of hypertension should not be made until the BP has been measured on at least three visits, spaced over a period of weeks to 3 months.
- Guidelines for measuring BP include, where possible, using a quiet room and taking three readings at least 5 minutes apart, with the patient in a relaxed state. In addition, BP should be measured in both arms at least once to exclude aortic coarctation or peripheral arterial stenosis. In older individuals (>75 years of age) or those with potential orthostatic symptoms, postural measurements should also be taken.

Management
Various guidelines exist, but in its simplest terms, treatment is generally initiated for BP values consistently >140/90 mmHg. Higher values, and greater cardiovascular risk should lower the threshold for initiating treatment (see Table 36.1).[2]

> The WHO has published a risk prediction chart for initiation of treatment in high-, middle-, and low-income countries (M http://www.who.int/cardiovascular_diseases/guidelines/Chart_predictions/en/).

Table 36.1 Guidelines on management depending on cardiovascular risk

Other risk factors, asymptomatic organ damage, or disease	Blood pressure (mmHg)			
	High normal: SBP 130–139 or DBP 85–39	Grade 1 HT: SBP 10–159 or DBP 90–99	Grade 2 HT: SBP 160–179 or DBP 100–109	Grade 3 HT: SBP ≥180 or DBP ≥110
No other RF		Low risk	Moderate risk	High risk
1–2 RF	Low risk	Moderate risk	Moderate to high risk	High risk
≥3 RF	Low to Moderate rsk	Moderate to high risk	High risk	High risk
OD, CKD stage 3 or diabetes	Moderate to high risk	High risk	High risk	High to very high risk
Symptomatic CVD, CKD stage ≥ 4 or diabetes with OD/RFs	Very high risk	Very high risk	Very high risk	Very high risk

BP, blood pressure; CKD, chronic kidney disease; CV, cardiovascular; CVD, cardiovascular disease; DBP, diastolic blood pressure; HT, hypertension; OD, organ damage; RF, risk factor; SBP systolic blood pressure.
Reproduced with permission from Gregory YH Lip and Sunil Nadar, Hypertension 2e: OUP (2015).

Interventions

- Ideally, the goal is to achieve targets with respect to all modifiable cardiovascular risks, and comply with long-term therapy where possible.
- All patients should be counselled to limit salt intake (<3 g/day); an intervention that may translate to a mean reduction of 3–5 mmHg in BP alone.[3]
  - It is important to familiarize yourself with the availability of common antihypertensive drugs at your health structure and regional pharmacies.
  - Choice of drug therapy should be tailored to the patient's co-morbidities or other cardiovascular conditions or risks.
  - A suggested algorithm for outpatient BP management in all settings may be as per Fig. 36.4:

Management notes

- Titrate drug doses every 2 weeks until goal reached or maximum dose/side effect, then add next (second-, followed by third-) line therapy.
- An angiotensin-converting enzyme inhibitor (ACEI) and angiotensin receptor blocker (ARB) are not to be used in combination, and avoided if pregnancy or breastfeeding is a concern. They may be less effective in the black population, where a calcium channel blocker or thiazide-type diuretic, alone or in combination, would be first-line therapy.[4]
- Beta blockers are preferred as second line if there is a history of myocardial infarction/LV dysfunction. Avoid if bronchospasm/elderly (>75 years).

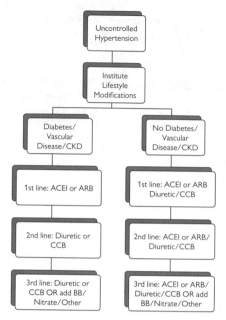

Fig. 36.4 Hypertension treatment algorithm. ACEI, angiotensin-converting enzyme inhibitor; ARB, angiotensin receptor blocker; BB, beta blocker; CCB, calcium channel blocker; CKD, chronic kidney disease.

- Creatinine clearance and potassium level fluctuations are common with ACEI/ARBs and diuretics. If possible, follow serum creatinine/electrolytes when adjusting doses
- Diuretics should be used as second-line if signs of volume overload are present; some formulations, such as hydrochlorothiazide 25–50 mg or furosemide 40 mg orally, are relatively cheap and often effective at lowering BP.[5]

See ♦ p. 629 for standard BP-lowering drugs that may be found in developing country catalogues.

Hypertensive crisis (or emergency)

Definition: severe hypertension (diastolic BP >120, and/or systolic BP ≥180 mmHg) and evidence of end-organ damage (i.e. coronary ischaemia, CHF, aortic dissection, altered mental status, renal failure/oliguria, pre-eclampsia).

Management
- Patients with hypertensive crisis should be admitted when possible.
- Secondary conditions or complications should be looked for and treated: stroke or intracerebral haemorrhage, myocardial infarction, aortic dissection.
- The degree to which BP should be lowered depends on the clinical condition:
  - In the setting of stroke, mild reductions to achieve values of <180/120 mmHg are adequate.
  - In the setting of CHF, aggressive afterload reduction (lowering systemic vascular resistance, or systemic BP) should be instituted.
- In general, previous antihypertensives should be re-started as soon as possible if a gap in therapy is responsible.
- If treatment-naive, single therapy should be started to achieve a BP reduction of 25% over the first few hours.

Congestive heart failure

Definition

CHF is a clinical syndrome characterized by increased ventricular filling pressures with or without impaired systemic perfusion. It is often the final common manifestation of advanced structural cardiac changes and decompensation.

Aetiology

In developed countries, CHF is among the most common causes of hospital admission, and is projected to rise over time. Its prevalence in developing contexts appears to be similar. In a recent African registry, 90% of presentations for decompensated CHF were caused by:

- hypertension
- cardiomyopathy
- rheumatic heart disease.

In all three cases, the 6-month mortality rate was 18%, suggesting a grave prognosis.[6]

Other causes of CHF include the following:

- Ischaemic heart disease: this is a leading cause of CHF, so consider this where the history is suggestive, or where ECG evidence of myocardial damage, such as Q waves, is present.
- HIV infection: its treatment, and AIDS may lead to CHF.
- Other infectious causes are overwhelmingly viral.
- Alcoholism and/or associated thiamine deficiencies.
- Sarcoidosis: this has the highest prevalence among black patients and can manifest in myocardial and cardiac conduction system defects.

Presentation

Diagnostic signs and symptoms include dyspnoea, fatigue, and fluid retention. CHF can often be clinically distinguished from other causes for dyspnoea by:

- an elevated JVP (>5 cm above the sternal angle)
- peripheral oedema
- basilar crepitations or wheeze.

Diagnosis

CHF is a clinical diagnosis, relying on findings of congestion and/or systemic hypoperfusion. In low-resource settings, patients often present in advanced stages of their illness. (See Table 36.2.) Severe cardiac failure may present as circulatory shock, and carries a grave prognosis. Tachycardia, low pulse pressures, oliguria, and cool or mottled extremities are signs of low-output states, for which severe pump failure may be a cause.

- Differentiating CHF from sepsis (usually 'warm' shock—hypoperfusion with normal or elevated body temperature) or low effective circulating volume (low JVP/evidence of hypovolaemia) is critical as fluid management varies greatly between the two. While CHF usually requires diuresis, low effective circulating volume mandates aggressive fluid replacement.

Table 36.2 New York Heart Association (NYHA) classification of heart failure

Class	Patient symptoms
Class I (Mild)	No limitation of physical activity. Ordinary physical activity does not cause undue fatigue, rapid/irregular heartbeat (palpitation) or shortness of breath (dyspnoea)
Class II (Mild)	Slight limitation of physical activity. Comfortable at rest, but ordinary physical activity results in fatigue, rapid/irregular heartbeat (palpitation) or shortness of breath (dyspnoea)
Class III (Moderate)	Marked limitation of physical activity. Comfortable at rest, but less than ordinary activity causes fatigue, rapid/irregular heartbeat (palpitation) or shortness of breath (dyspnoea)
Class IV (Severe)	Unable to carry out any physical activity without discomfort. Symptoms of fatigue, rapid/irregular heartbeat (palpitation) or shortness of breath (dyspnoea) are present at rest. If any physical activity is undertaken, discomfort increases.

Original source: Criteria Committee, New York Heart Association, Inc. Diseases of the Heart and Blood Vessels. Nomenclature and Criteria for diagnosis, 6th edition Boston, Little, Brown and Co. 1964, p 114.

- Look for the JVP: a deliberate, systematic look at the JVP may immediately direct fluid therapy (between volume loading vs careful diuresis) and mastery of this skill is strongly recommended.
- If you cannot see the JVP, lower (towards 0° or supine) and raise the head of the bed (up to 90° or upright), or perform the abdominojugular reflux manoeuvre until it is visible.
- A displaced or sustained cardiac apex signifies the presence of cardiac structural disease and hints to the cause of decompensation.

In some hospital settings, you may have access to an ultrasound probe. Gaining even rudimentary familiarity in its use can greatly simplify diagnosis in situations where gross cardiac pathology is suspected. Learning how to recognize left versus right ventricular chamber enlargement or dysfunction, can immediately help differentiate cardiac versus pulmonary or other causes of haemodynamic compromise. Identifying pericardial effusions can change the treatment pathways significantly.

Management of CHF

Symptoms of CHF are usually related to volume overload. Diuresis and afterload reduction are the cornerstone of therapy. Reducing demand can be acutely managed by reducing anxiety and the work of breathing.

Acute decompensated heart failure management

- Diuresis: in the acute setting, IV therapy achieves faster diuresis, however oral therapy can be very effective when the context permits. IV furosemide 40–80 mg is the most common initial choice. The expected therapeutic response in a person with normally functioning kidneys is to achieve diuresis at 30 minutes, peaking at 1–2 hours (if no diuresis at 30 minutes, increase dose).

- Oxygen, if available, is calming.
- Morphine IV (2–4 mg) can reduce anxiety of breathlessness and provides pre-load reduction (venous dilation), thereby unloading the heart.
- Nitrates, either transdermal (longer acting) or sublingual or aerosolized (short acting) can be helpful to reduce afterload when BP is elevated.
- Digoxin if symptoms of CHF persist after first-line therapies have been instituted.
- Lower BP if ≥180/110 mmHg.

Chronic management

Once symptoms are managed, long-term therapeutic goals include reducing symptoms and re-hospitalization, and prolonging life. Disease-modifying agents are the mainstay for chronic CHF management. See Table 36.3 for recommendations

- All drugs that may contribute to heart failure should be avoided. This includes NSAIDs, antiarrhythmic drugs, calcium channel blockers, and thiazolidinediones.
- Appropriate preventative care includes pneumococcal and annual influenza vaccination if available.
- Salt restriction (<2 g/day) and water restriction (1.5 litres/day) is important to prevent recurrence.
- ACEIs lower BP, and beta blockers cause decreased heart rate and BP—these findings should not prohibit their use unless symptomatic. Generally, symptoms resolve over weeks, and can be minimized by introducing medications one at a time, and up-titrating every 2–4 weeks.
- Diuretics help maintain circulating volume, as outlined below p. 629.

Diuresis

- Oral diuresis is only necessary until normal circulating volume has been achieved; however, in chronic heart failure it may be required indefinitely to avoid symptoms. Commonly available diuretics include furosemide 20–200 mg daily, hydrochlorothiazide 25–50 mg daily, and spironolactone 25–100 mg daily.
- When switching from IV to oral dosing, twice the daily IV dose is considered the oral equivalent.
- Potassium-supplementation should parallel diuretic use. Advise the patient to eat potassium-rich foods (i.e. bananas, oranges).
- In the setting of severe systolic LV dysfunction, mineralocorticoid receptor antagonists should be used in addition to, or instead of, potassium if renal function and potassium can be monitored as an out-patient.

Table 36.3 Recommended CHF drugs/treatment

Evidence-based therapy	Examples in class	Relative mortality risk reduction	Contraindications
Renin–angiotensin system inhibitors	Enalapril, ramipril, perindopril, lisinopril candesartan, valsartan	20%	Hyperkalaemia, advanced renal impairment, history of angio oedema, pregnancy or breastfeeding
Beta blocker	Carvedilol, bisoprolol, metoprolol,	31%	Bradycardia, active bronchospastic disease
Mineralocorticoid receptor antagonist	Spironolactone, eplerenone	25%	Advanced renal disease, hyperkalaemia

Data from Fonarow GC, Yancy CW, Hernandez AF, et al. Potential impact of optimal implementation of evidence-based heart failure therapies on mortality. Am Heart J 2011;161:1024.

Peripartum cardiomyopathy

Definition

There is no universally recognized definition of peripartum cardiomyopathy. It is generally recognized as:
- development of CHF towards the end of pregnancy or in the months following delivery
- absence of another identifiable cause for the CHF
- LV systolic dysfunction typically occurs, and the LV ejection fraction is nearly always <45%.

Context

It is not uncommon to see young women presenting with this condition in certain geographic areas, with an incidence ranging from 1:4000 live births in the United States to 1:1000 in South Africa, 1:300 in Haiti, and 1:100 in Zaria, Nigeria. African descent is an established risk factor.[7]

Signs/symptoms

Symptoms are identical to other forms of CHF. They may be masked by naturally occurring changes during late pregnancy, or be mistaken for pulmonary embolic disease, respiratory infection in a woman at risk, or rheumatic valvular heart disease.

Diagnosis

In the field, the diagnosis can be made on clinical grounds if necessary.

Management

The treatment of peripartum cardiomyopathy parallels that of CHF in the adult with a few exceptions:
- Renin–angiotensin inhibitors (ACEIs, ARBs) and mineralocorticoid receptor antagonists (spironolactone or eplerenone) should be avoided during pregnancy and if breastfeeding, as they are teratogenic.
- Early delivery with caesarean section may be considered depending on the balance between maternal and fetal conditions; this requires a multidisciplinary discussion.
- Contraception should be discussed in a culturally appropriate way: the risk of recurrence with subsequent pregnancies is variable but highest when:
  - there is incomplete recovery of LV systolic function, or
  - the initial presentation is severe when the estimated ejection fraction is <25%.
- Medical treatment should continue for at least 6 months after complete LV systolic functional recovery, and indefinitely otherwise.

Coronary artery disease

Chest pain is the second most common life-threatening complaint in emergency rooms across the developed world and aetiologies can range from the benign to the life-threatening.

Although the differential diagnosis of chest pain is broad, the likelihood of CAD as the cause for chest pain is related to age (usually a direct relationship when >40 years) and the presence of the following three characteristics:

1. Retrosternal chest discomfort.
2. Exertional precipitants or relief with rest
3. Resolution with glyceryl trinitrate.

For coronary ischaemia, the chest discomfort is classically described as a squeezing and is shown with a clenched fist (universal sign). It may also manifest as back, shoulder, neck, or abdominal pain. Accompanying diaphoresis or dyspnoea increases the specificity for CAD as a cause. Bilateral arm and elbow pain with activity is among the most specific symptom of angina or ischaemic chest pain.

Note: in patients with diabetes, which may be underdiagnosed and advanced in low-resource settings, dyspnoea (without chest pain) may be the only symptom of angina.

Myocardial infarction

Acute myocardial infarction (AMI) is caused by complete and sudden occlusion of a major coronary artery. This is overwhelmingly the result of long-standing atherosclerosis, leading to plaque vulnerability, followed by plaque rupture, thrombus formation, and ultimately lumen occlusion. AMI is less common in rural and underdeveloped regions, but the incidence is increasing where patients have established major vascular risk factors. It may be encountered more commonly in contexts where people have migrated to more urbanized areas.

Symptoms

- Sudden, prolonged symptom of chest pain or equivalent (shortness of breath). There may be radiation to the neck, jaw, back, or arms and patients may have the classic description of an 'elephant sitting on my chest'.
- Associated symptoms: diaphoresis, nausea/vomiting, syncope or near-syncope. Often patients feel a sense of impending doom.
- Symptoms are unrelenting and last >15 minutes. There may be limited or no response to three sequential nitro-sprays 5 minutes apart.

Physical examination

- Patients generally present with mild hypertension (pain related) and mild tachycardia, but in extreme cases, there may be haemodynamic instability with hypotension or signs of shock.
- In large infarctions, CHF is seen, but this is usually a late finding (hours after symptom onset).
- Bradycardia is a prominent feature of inferior infarction with dominant vagal symptoms, including nausea and hypotension.

ECG

The diagnosis is acutely confirmed by typical ECG findings making this the gold standard (see Fig. 36.5). The presence of new or presumed new ST-segment elevation is the hallmark finding.

AMI: >1 mm contiguous ST elevation in at least two contiguous limb or precordial leads (>2 mm in V3). Often, there is reciprocal ST depression in un-involved leads:

- Anterior myocardial infarction: ST elevation in precordial lead ± lateral leads (I/AVL).
- Inferior myocardial infarction: ST elevation in II, III, and AVF.
- Posterior myocardial infarction: ST depression V1–V3 and any degree of ST elevation in V7, V8, and V9 (15-lead tracing).

> The most common life-threatening event in the acute setting is ventricular fibrillation. If working in a hospital or similar setting, all patients suspected of having an AMI should be on ECG monitoring (with defibrillation capacity close by) immediately and preferably for a minimum of 48 hours.

a) Anterior myocardial infarction.

b) Inferior myocardial infarction.

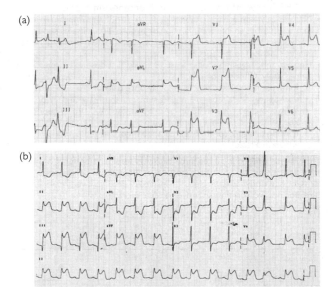

Fig. 36.5 12-lead ECG demonstrating new ST elevation, or new dynamic ST depression (non ST-elevation myocardial infarction). Image A reproduced from Myerson, Saul G., et al, Emergencies in Cardiology 2nd ed, 2009, and image B reproduced from Warrell, David A. Oxford Textbook of Medicine, 2010, both with permission from Oxford University Press.

Treatment

Myocardial necrosis and subsequent mortality are time dependent and need prompt recognition and management. In high-level care centres, establishing reperfusion is done via primary angioplasty or, if not available, by IV fibrinolysis. Streptokinase is the most common fibrinolytic, and is on the WHO essential drug list.

Optimal management

- Place monitor/defibrillator pads on patient.
- Establish IV access.
- Oxygen for comfort.
- Aspirin: 160 mg to be chewed (for mucosal absorption); Even this intervention alone has a relative-risk reduction for mortality of 20–25%.[8]
- Clopidogrel 300 mg PO bolus, then 75 mg PO once daily.
- Pain relief for comfort.

- Beta blocker if haemodynamically acceptable:
  - Metoprolol 25 mg PO twice a day or the equivalent could be used. Such agents should be avoided in the presence of decompensated CHF, bradycardia, hypotension, or bronchospasm.
- Nitrates (glyceryl trinitrate tablets or spray) for BP or symptom relief. In the setting of an inferior infarction or hypotension, nitrates should be avoided and IV fluid boluses would be appropriate (normal saline or Ringer's lactate) to support BP.
- Heparin anticoagulation for at least 48 hours: first dose to be given immediately. Choose one of:
  - fondaparinux 2.5 mg subcutaneously once daily or
  - enoxaparin or dalteparin 1 mg/kg subcutaneously twice daily or
  - unfractionated heparin 70 units/kg bolus, then 1000 units/hour to keep activated partial thromboplastin time as 60–100 seconds
  - fibrinolytic agent (primary percutaneous coronary intervention where available).

If the needs exceed local resource capacity, consider transfer if available. High priority for an acute care hospital includes those unrelenting symptoms, or haemodynamic or electrical instability (incessant ventricular tachycardia or bradycardia unresponsive to usual therapy).

Atrial fibrillation

Definition

Cardiac arrhythmia, characterized by irregular RR intervals (without repetitive pattern), and the absence of distinct P waves on the ECG.

Aetiology

Atrial fibrillation (AF) occurs in states of acute illness, typically cardiothoracic illness (pneumonia, pericarditis), and less commonly for thyrotoxicosis, or other acute systemic conditions. Chronically, it occurs in direct relation to increasing age >65 years, hypertension and chronic lung disease, as well as sleep apnoea.

Presentation

Symptoms may be intermittent in the paroxysmal form, or constant/predominant in the persistent form. These may include palpitations, chest fluttering, chest pain, and dyspnoea, and rarely presyncope or hypotension.

Diagnosis

The diagnosis is made by the ECG, characterized by an irregularly irregular rhythm without organized atrial (p wave) activity.

Management

Where sudden-onset AF is thought to provoke coronary ischaemia, CHF, or haemodynamic instability, direct-current electrical cardioversion is indicated. Whether paroxysmal or permanent, the treatment is essentially the same, with two goals:

- Symptom management:
  - Symptoms are most common in new-onset, or paroxysmal AF.
  - Heart rate control can be established using beta blockers (preferred—in the absence of contraindications), non-vasoselective calcium channel blockers (diltiazem or verapamil), or digoxin.
  - The goal is to relieve symptoms and keep resting heart rates <110 bpm.
  - Antiarrhythmics should generally be avoided.
- Systemic embolic prevention:
  - In the short term, anticoagulation is warranted in most patients in the absence of contraindications.
  - The presence of any of the following features, where bleeding risks are low, would warrant consideration for long-term/chronic anticoagulation:
    —Age >75 years.
    —Previous ischaemic stroke/transient ischaemic attack.
    —CHF.
    —Hypertension.
    —Diabetes.

The decision to anticoagulate must consider prohibitive bleeding risks, access, and affordability of indicated treatments. Of agents likely to be available in low-resource settings, warfarin requires regular blood monitoring and dose adjustment to target a therapeutic international normalized ratio which may not be feasible. Low-dose aspirin (80–100 mg daily) or clopidogrel (75 mg daily) may be considered where anticoagulation is not feasible.

Pericardial disease

Definition

Irritation of the fibroelastic sac surrounding the heart. Diseases may be isolated to the pericardium, or be part of a larger systemic presentation.

Aetiology

With the resurgence of TB in the setting of increased HIV infection, tuberculous pericarditis is the leading cause of pericardial disease in sub-Saharan Africa, and arguably the world.[9] See Box 36.1.

> ### Box 36.1 Tuberculous pericarditis
>
> TB pericarditis has a variable clinical presentation and should be considered in the evaluation of all cases of pericarditis without a rapidly self-limited course. Effusion usually develops insidiously, with systemic symptoms, such as fever, night sweats, fatigue, and weight loss. Chest pain, cough, and shortness of breath/breathlessness are common, while typical pericardial pain is rare. The diagnosis can be made by pericardial fluid with a positive acid-fast stain or the presence of tuberculous bacilli, or by the presence of pericardial fluid with evidence of tuberculous infection elsewhere.

Signs/symptoms

- The principal manifestations of pericardial disease are:
  - pericarditis, as an acute, subacute, or chronic fibrinous process
  - pericardial effusion
  - cardiac tamponade and constrictive pericarditis, generally as long-term complications.
- Typical symptoms include:
  - pleuritic-type chest pain; sharp retrosternal discomfort that is exacerbated by breathing, worse when supine, and better when upright
  - in chronic pericardial disease, these symptoms are replaced by fatigue, cachexia, and increasing peripheral oedema.
- Signs can include:
  - tachycardia and low-grade fever (acutely)
  - a multiphasic pericardial rub may be heard: typically scratchy and intermittent
  - chronic disease may demonstrate an elevated JVP with soft/distant heart sounds
  - peripheral oedema dominates the picture in chronic disease.

Pericardial tamponade occurs when extrinsic pericardial pressure impairs cardiac filling, resulting in the classic triad of an elevated JVP, soft heart sounds, and hypotension. Drainage is indicated, and is typically an indication for referral to a high-level centre.

Diagnosis
- Typical symptoms and an early response to therapy are enough to make the diagnosis.
- Other supportive findings where available, would include leucocytosis on the blood count, elevated acute phase reactant (C-reactive protein, erythrocyte sedimentation rate), and suspicious ECG changes (diffuse ST elevation and PR depression).
- The finding of new pericardial effusion on cardiac sonography is highly specific, although rarely available.

Treatment
- Acute pericarditis is usually viral and/or inflammatory, and treatment generally consists of:
  - high-dose NSAIDs tapered after 1 week for a total of 2–3 weeks and
  - colchicine 0.6 mg PO twice daily for 2 weeks.
- If no improvement after 48 hours, NSAIDs can be switched to prednisone 40–80 mg once daily in divided doses, tapered over 2–4 weeks.
- Treatment of TB pericardial disease is highly sensitive to antituberculous chemotherapy.

Prevention of cardiovascular disease

General recommendations apply to all patients with established vascular disease, regardless of whether they have had an ischaemic event or not. With the realities in low-resource settings, the opportunity for long-term follow-up is often poorly available. General counselling and lifestyle advice, when adhered to, is very potent in preventing recurrent events. Try to have this discussion with patients at the outpatient encounter, and prior to discharge for in-patients. If possible, link them to ongoing follow-up. Needless to say, all lifestyle advice must be culturally sensitive and consider the economic, social, and environmental contexts at hand.

Most guidelines advocate treating all diabetics over the age of 40 years with one additional major cardiovascular risk factor as having established cardiovascular disease, and therefore eligible for secondary prevention treatment, described on p. 628.[10]

Diet
- Low fat: it is recommended that fat be limited to 30% or less of daily caloric intake.
  - Simple advice would include avoiding saturated oils such as peanut oil and animal-based oil. Limit egg yolks to three or fewer per week, and limit red meat (avoid fatty meat) to less than once per week.
- Increased consumption of vegetables and fruits: the 'Mediterranean diet' is the only proven regimen associated with reduction in myocardial infarction or cardiovascular disease death.[11] It typically consists of a 'base' of vegetables, fruits, whole grains, beans, nuts, seeds, and olive oil taken daily, with at least twice-weekly portions of fish, and poultry, and less-frequent portions of red meat and sweets, as well as moderate red wine consumption (1 glass/day).
- Salt: recommend <2–3 g/day; the equivalent of 2 teaspoons; whether used in cooking or added to the food on the plate.
- Water: restrictions (<1.5 litres of water or fluid/day) are only recommended in patients with CHF.

Lifestyle
- Tobacco cessation.
- Avoidance of excessive alcohol (<2 servings/day for females, <3/day for males).
- Cardiovascular physical activity: moderate physical exercise, such as a brisk walk; 30 mins, 5×/week (total 150 minutes/week), or demanding/intense physical exercise, 25 minutes, 3×/week (total 75 minutes/week).
- Appropriate weight maintenance: a BMI (weight in kilograms/square of height in metres) <25. An easier measure is waist circumference <102 cm in men, <88 cm in women.

Drug therapy

In the absence of contraindications, the following generalizations can be made:

- *All* patients with established cardiovascular disease should receive aspirin 80–100 mg and a moderate-to-high-potency statin medication daily, such as atorvastatin 40–80 mg, or rosuvastatin 20–40 mg (Table 36.4).
- The first choice for hypertensive therapy is an ACEI or ARB where contraindication or intolerance does not exist.
- In the setting of previous myocardial infarction, a beta blocker should be added.
- For the first year following a myocardial infarction or coronary arterial intervention/revascularization, clopidogrel 75 mg daily (or ticagrelor 90 mg twice daily) should be added.
- *All* adults with high low-density lipoprotein (>5 mmol/litre) should receive statin therapy for primary prevention (see Table 36.4).
  - Other patients may benefit, depending on their long-term risk for cardiovascular events.
  - For a specific patient scenario, you can consult a WHO risk prediction chart if needed.

See Table 36.5 for standard BP-lowering drugs.

Table 36.4 HMG-CoA reductase inhibitor (statin) equivalency and potency

LDL-C lowering (potency)	Fluvastatin (mg)	Pravastatin (mg)	Rosuvastatin (mg)	Atorvastatin (mg)	Simvastatin (mg)
<30% (low)	20–40	10–20			10
30–50%	80	40	5–10	10–20	10–20
>50% (high)			20–40	40–80	

Table 36.5 Standard blood pressure-lowering drugs that may be found in developing country catalogues

Drugs	Type	Relative cost per unit
Amlodipine 5 mg tab.	Calcium channel blocker	0.41
Atenolol 50 mg tab.	Beta blocker (BB)	0.41
Bisoprolol 1.25 mg tab.	BB	
Bisoprolol 5 mg tab.	BB	
Enalapril 2.5 mg tab.	ACE inhibitor (ACEI)	
Enalapril 5 mg tab.	ACEI	0.02
Furosemide 40 mg tab.	Loop diuretic	0.01
Hydralazine 25 mg tab.	Direct vasodilator	0.03
Hydralazine 50 mg tab.	Direct vasodilator	3.78
Hydrochlorothiazide 12.5 mg tab.	Thiazide-type diuretic	
Hydrochlorothiazide 25 mg tab.	Thiazide-type diuretic	0.06
Hydrochlorothiazide 50 mg tab.	Thiazide-type diuretic	0.01
Hydrochlorothiazide oral liq. 50 mg/5 mL	Thiazide-type diuretic	
Labetalol hydrochloride 200 mg tab.	Combined alpha and BB	0.00
Labetalol 5 mg/mL, 20 mL amp.	Combined alpha and BB	5.97
Methyldopa 250 mg tab.	Central alpha-2 agonist	0.03

Data from Médecins Sans Frontières, MSF Cardiovascular Field Manual 2014.
NB Costs do not necessarily reflect field-realities.

References

1. Yusuf S, Hawken S, Ounpuu S, Dans T, Avezum A, Lanas F, et al. Effect of potentially modifiable risk factors associated with myocardial infarction in 52 countries (the INTERHEART study): case-control study. Lancet 364(9438):937–52.
2. SPRINT Research Group, Wright JT Jr, Williamson JD, Whelton PK, Snyder JK, Sink KM, et al. A randomized trial of intensive versus standard blood-pressure control. N Engl J Med 2015;373(22):2103–16. (See more at M http://www.jwatch.org/na39551/2015/11/09/sprint-trial-intensive-blood-pressure-lowering#sthash.9O110U23.dpuf)
3. He FJ, MacGregor GA. How far should salt intake be reduced? Hypertension 2003;42(6):1093–9.
4. James PA, Oparil S, Carter BL, Cushman WC, Dennison-Himmelfarb C, Handler J, et al. 2014 Evidence-based guideline for the management of high blood pressure in adults: report from the Panel Members Appointed to the Eighth Joint National Committee (JNC 8). JAMA 2014;311(5):507–20.
5. Médecins Sans Frontières. MSF Cardiovascular Field Manual 2014. Paris: MSF.
6. Sliwa K, Mayosi BM. Global burden of cardiovascular disease: recent advances in the epidemiology, pathogenesis and prognosis of acute heart failure and cardiomyopathy in Africa. Heart 2013;99:1317–22.
7. Veille JC. Peripartum cardiomyopathies: a review. Am J Obstet Gynecol 1984;148(6):805–18.
8. ISIS-2 (Second International Study of Infarct Survival) Collaborative Group. Randomised trial of intravenous streptokinase, oral aspirin, both, or neither among 17,187 cases of suspected acute myocardial infarction: ISIS-2. Lancet 1988;2(8607):349–60.

9. Mayosi BM, Burgess LJ, Doubell AF. Tuberculous pericarditis. Circulation 2005;112:3608–16.
10. American Diabetes Association. Standards of medical care in diabetes—2015. Diabetes Care. 2015;38(suppl 1):S1–93.
11. Estruch R, Ros E, Salas-Salvadó J, Covas MI, Corella D, Arós F, et al. Primary prevention of cardiovascular disease with a Mediterranean diet. N Engl J Med 2013;368(14):1279–90.

Further reading

World Health Organization: Global Atlas on Cardiovascular Disease Prevention and Control. Geneva: WHO; 2011. M http://www.who.int/cardiovascular_diseases/publications/atlas_cvd/en/

Respiratory illness

Aditya Nadimpalli and Philippa Boulle

Context of respiratory conditions

Respiratory pathologies are the leading cause of death in LIC and precarious contexts, such as refugee camps. This is especially pronounced in children, where pneumonia accounts for 15% of all deaths of children <5 years old, killing an estimated 922,000 children in 2015. Unfortunately, the nature of the humanitarian context makes diagnosing and treating respiratory pathologies challenging. Consider the difficulties clinicians in developed settings have in trying to distinguish between bacterial versus viral pneumonias or between congestive heart failure and COPD. Then extrapolate these difficulties to low-resource settings where children with pneumonia may also suffer from malnutrition; where there are no X-ray machines; where lack of electricity can limit oxygen concentrators; or where patients cannot access hospitals due to distance or violence.

Understanding burden of disease

Each context will have different disease profiles with which the provider should be familiar. For example, respiratory complaints in a country with high HIV prevalence such as Mozambique will be markedly different than in a Syrian refugee camp. Research the specific context in which you will work, prior to departure. Good sources include:
• MOH website from each country
• WHO country profiles (http://www.who.int/countries/en/)—for respiratory issues, pay special attention to the data about HIV/AIDS, pneumonias, malaria, and TB.

Vaccine coverage

It is also very important to understand vaccine schedules and vaccination coverage rates, which can vary significantly. This information can usually be found via the following sources:
• MOH website from each country.
• UNICEF (http://www.unicef.org/infobycountry/).

From a respiratory viewpoint, check vaccination rates for the following:
• Diphtheria, pertussis, and tetanus (DPT) and *Haemophilus influenzae* type b (Hib): low DPT coverage can cause pertussis outbreaks and Hib is a frequent cause of bacterial pneumonia. Note that sometimes these vaccines are administered together using a pentavalent vaccine (DPT, Hib, hepatitis B vaccine).
• Pneumococcal conjugate vaccine (PCV): can decrease *Streptococcus pneumoniae* infections, but not all countries have started this vaccine due to cost.
• Measles: when vaccination rates fall below 90%, the risk of a measles outbreak markedly increases. In outbreaks, one of the leading causes of death is superimposed respiratory infections.
• BCG: context dependent, but low coverage may promote TB.

Antibiotic resistance

Most likely found through local contacts or reference laboratory, this can help tailor antibiotic protocols to resistance patterns.

Respiratory resources mapping

In order to make appropriate decisions for patients with complex or critical respiratory disorders, it helps to have a resource map done before hand. The best source of information will be the national staff of your hospital—their input will be your most vital resource.

Internal capacity of your hospital/clinic

- Respiratory medical:
  - Oxygen concentrators: these need an electric supply (generator or grid).
  - Oxygen cylinders: these need to be refilled periodically.
  - Oxygen splitters: for both concentrators and cylinders, they can multiply the number of patients treated.
  - Nebulizer machines: you will also need the proper tubing and medications.
  - Ventilators: check if any are available. If not, it is possible to at least make a field-level continuous positive airway pressure (CPAP) ventilator called a 'bubble CPAP' for stabilizing critical infants. (See ➔ 'Further reading' p. 645.)
- Pharmacy: understand current and expiring stock.
- Radiology:
  - X-ray machine: determine if it works properly, if it uses manual or digital developing, and if you can print films for patients once they leave.
  - Ultrasound machines can be helpful for respiratory pathologies, including pneumothoraces, pleural effusions, and even alveolar pathology. If there is an ultrasound machine, determine if it works properly and if there are providers trained to use it.
  - For both, remember that an electric supply is necessary.

External capacity

Transferring patients:

- Additional resources: determine if other hospitals have higher capacity, including artificial ventilation and surgical capability.
- Cost: understand if it will be free for the patient or the cost will be borne by the patient or your hospital.
- Transport: determine if your hospital has an ambulance or if patients will need to find their own transportation. For critically ill patients, oxygen supply may be necessary for transport along with one or two accompanying clinicians. Finally, depending on the context, evaluate the safety of travel, especially at night.

Respiratory epidemiology

Understanding the trends of respiratory disease can alert you to outbreaks or need to re-orient hospital resources. All hospitals have to report monthly data along with 'early-trigger' diseases to the local MOH. If this system works adequately, follow it closely and be alert for specific pathologies in your hospital. If the public health system is not functioning, perhaps due to conflict or rapid population migration, ensure that your own hospital tracks at least the following pathologies related to respiratory issues: lower respiratory tract infections (LRTIs), TB, pertussis, and measles.

Respiratory triaging and stabilization

- Patients with both pulmonary and non-pulmonary pathologies can present with severe respiratory symptoms. The most common severe pulmonary pathology is a primary LRTI, especially bacterial pneumonias and TB. On the other hand, the most common *non*-pulmonary cause of respiratory distress is anaemia due to malaria. Frequently, patients will present with signs and symptoms that could represent multiple diseases. Proper triaging will help identify the sickest patients rapidly.
- There are both outpatient triaging (e.g. ETAT/SATS) and inpatient triaging (e.g. ITAT/PEWS) that can be used by physicians and non-physicians alike. See ➔ Chapter 16 for further information.
- Respiratory stabilization of critically ill patients at triage:
  - If a patient has any abnormal respiratory vital sign or red flag as listed in Box 37.1, transfer to the resuscitation area and start oxygen to keep saturation >90%.
  - Minimum tests generally needed are rapid malaria test, capillary glucose, and Hb.
  - Additional tests as per local resources include X-ray, ultrasound, and other laboratory tests.

Box 37.1 Respiratory age-specific vital signs and respiratory warning signs

Age-specific respiratory tachypnoea
- 0–2 months: >60 breaths/minute.
- 2 months–1 year: >50 breaths/minute.
- 1–5 years: >40 breaths/minute.
- >5 years: >20 breaths/minute.
- Oxygen saturation: <90%.
- Central cyanosis: blueness to lip or oral mucosa.
- Stridor: inspiratory hoarse noise, especially in calm child.
- Grunting: expiratory short repetitive noise produced by partial closure of the vocal cords.
- Chest in-drawing: spaces between, above, or below the ribs indent with each breath.

Associated warning signs
- Inability to feed.
- Variable temperature control (hypo- and hyperthermia).
- Decreased level of activity/consciousness.
- Convulsions.

Note: in addition to having a scoring triage system, a well-trained nurse scanning busy outpatient waiting areas can expedite rapid triaging for sick patients.

Lower respiratory tract infection/pneumonia

Definition
Any form of lung infection caused by bacteria, viruses, or other organisms.

Due to the key differences in aetiology, presentation, and management in LRTIs in younger children as compared to older children as adults, these population groups will be covered separately on → p. 637–8.

Management of LRTI in children <5 years old

Epidemiology
- Most common causes are viruses, *Streptococcus pneumoniae*, and *Haemophilus influenza*.
- Severe pneumonia can have a case fatality rate of 15–25%, with most deaths in the first 3 days. Therefore, early recognition and treatment is critical.

Presentation
Presentation can vary within age group:
- <2 months—variable:
  - Inability to feed.
  - Variable temperature control (hypo- and hyperthermia).
  - Decreased level of activity.
  - Convulsions.
- All children <5 years:
  - Fast breathing.
  - Chest in-drawing.

Respiratory red flag signs in children <5 years old
- Not able to drink.
- Persistent vomiting.
- Convulsions.
- Lethargic or unconscious.
- Stridor in a calm child.
- Severe malnutrition.

Clinical assessment
- Vital signs:
  - Tachypnoea and oxygen saturations are most helpful. Fevers are frequently variable, though hypothermia in children <2 months of age and those suffering from malnutrition can be ominous.
- Pulmonary examination:
  - Observation: stridor and grunting are serious signs, while chest in-drawing is frequently seen.
  - Auscultation: abnormal sounds, especially crackles, are specific but not very sensitive.

Children with no chest in-drawing and no tachypnoea are most likely to have an upper respiratory infection (URI). These are usually viral and/or self-limited, requiring only symptomatic treatment, not antibiotics.

For both paediatric and adult presentations, diagnosis of LRTI is primarily clinical. Chest X-rays are usually unavailable and even when available, they usually show non-specific findings. They should only be used for un-improving or worsening patients. Ultrasound findings, on the other hand, have recently been shown to be useful and in the near future, it might have an expanded role in pneumonia diagnosis.

Diagnosis
In children <5 years of age, the diagnosis of LRTI is based on the presence of fast breathing and/or chest in-drawing. These children are divided into two categories:
- *Pneumonia*: children with isolated fast breathing and/or chest in-drawing.
- *Severe pneumonia*: children with fast breathing and/or chest in-drawing PLUS any red flags.

Treatment
- General therapy:
  - *Pneumonia*: home therapy with oral amoxicillin.
  - *Severe pneumonia*: referral for inpatient care with IV antibiotics (this includes all infants <2 months old).

Specific therapy for different age groups and categories is as follows:

Note: all children <2 months of age are treated as 'severe pneumonia' given the varied presentation and very high mortality risk.

Treatment: age <2 months—hospitalize all children
- <7 days, <2 kg:
  - Ampicillin IV/IM 50 mg/kg two times a day × 10 days.
  - Gentamicin IV/IM 3 mg/kg once a day.
- <7 days, >2 kg:
  - Ampicillin IV/IM 50 mg/kg three times a day × 10 days.
  - Gentamicin IV/IM 5 mg/kg once a day for 7 days.
- 7–59 days <2 kg:
  - Ampicillin IV/IM 50 mg/kg three times a day × 10 days.
  - Gentamicin IV/IM 5 mg/kg once a day for 7 days.
- 7–59 days >2 kg:
  - Ampicillin IV/IM 50 mg/kg four times a day × 10 days.
  - Gentamicin IV/IM 5 mg/kg once a day for 7 days.
- No improvement after 48 hours:
  - <7 days, <2 kg: cloxacillin 25 mg/kg IV two times a day.
  - <7 days, >2 kg: cloxacillin 25 mg/kg IV three times a day.
  - >7 days, <2 kg: cloxacillin 25 mg/kg IV three times a day.
  - >7 days, >2 kg: cloxacillin 25 mg/kg IV four times a day.

Treatment: age 2–59 months with pneumonia (excluding severe pneumonia)

- Amoxicillin orally: 40 mg/kg/dose twice a day × 3 days in low HIV-prevalence settings and 5 days in high HIV-prevalence settings.
- Follow-up in 48–72 hours.
- If unimproved: add azithromycin 10 mg/kg orally once a day.
- If worse: referral to inpatient service for treatment of severe pneumonia.

Treatment: age 2–59 months—severe pneumonia

- Parenteral antibiotics:
  - Ampicillin 50 mg/kg or benzylpenicillin 50,000 U/kg IM/IV every 6 hours for at least 5 days (can extend if not improving) *plus*
  - Gentamicin 7.5 mg/kg IM/IV once a day for 5 days (can extend if not improving).
  - If no improvement or worsening after 48 hours, switch to ceftriaxone 50 mg/kg IV/IM once a day for at least 5 days.
  - If improved after 3 days, switch to amoxicillin oral to complete 7 days of total treatment.

- Empiric co-trimoxazole 50 mg sulfamethoxazole + 20 mg trimethoprim/kg twice a day to treat *Pneumocystis jirovecii* (previously *Pneumocystis carinii*—PCP) should be given to children aged 2 months–1 year who are HIV+ve or HIV-exposed with pneumonia with chest in-drawing or severe pneumonia.
- Once >1 year of age, these patients *do not* need empiric co-trimoxazole.

Management of LRTI in children >5 years old and adults

Epidemiology

Most common aetiologies are viruses, *S. pneumonia, H. influenza* and atypical bacteria (*Mycoplasma pneumonia* and *Chlamydia pneumonia*).

Presentation

- Fever.
- Age-specific tachypnoea.
- Cough and thoracic pain.
- Adventitious sounds are variable and insensitive.

Clinical assessment

High risk patients:

- HIV+ve patients
- Sickle cell
- Malnourished

Respiratory red flag signs in children >5 years and adults

- Central cyanosis.
- Chest in-drawing.
- Altered level of consciousness.
- Oxygen saturation <90%.

Diagnosis

As with paediatric presentations, diagnosis is primarily clinical, and can be based on a combination of symptoms (cough, localized chest pain) and signs (fever, tachypnoea, decreased breath sounds, focal crepitations). A chest X-ray is not usually necessary, though pulmonary ultrasound may soon be more useful for certain findings (e.g. pleural effusion or pneumothorax).

Management

- Outpatient:
  - Amoxicillin orally 1 g two times a day × 5 days.
  - If no improvement, add azithromycin orally on day 1 500 mg, then 250 mg days 2–5.
  - If worsening, refer for inpatient treatment.
- Inpatient—for patients with red flags or failed outpatient treatment:
  - Ampicillin IV 1 g 3 three times a day for 7 days or ceftriaxone IV/IM daily for 7 days.
  - If no improvement, strongly consider TB and testing for HIV.
  - If good improvement after 3 days of IV medications, can change to oral amoxicillin to finish 7 days of treatment.

Bronchiolitis

Definition
A viral illness that causes inflammation of small airways (bronchioles) in children <2 years of age and presents with URI symptoms followed by wheezing and/or crackles.

Epidemiology
- Most commonly caused by viruses, including respiratory syncytial virus, rhinovirus, parainfluenza, adenovirus, etc.
- Risk factors: prematurity <37 weeks, immunodeficiency (including HIV+ve or HIV exposure), or other cardiac/pulmonary diseases.

Presentation (signs/symptoms)
- Low-grade fever: usually not higher than 38.5°C.
- Upper respiratory symptoms predominate in first few days—rhinorrhoea, profuse nasal secretions.
- Lower respiratory symptoms can follow URI symptoms—tachypnoea, cough, in-drawing, wheezing, and crackles
- Pay attention to the age-specific vital signs and respiratory warning signs to screen for patients with severe illness.

Diagnosis
- As with LRTIs, the diagnosis is based on clinical findings. The classic findings of URI symptoms followed by lower respiratory symptoms can help identify those patients with isolated bronchiolitis. However, once these children develop lower respiratory signs, it can be difficult to differentiate between bronchiolitis and LRTIs.
- Chest X-rays are usually unhelpful as they can have non-specific and variable findings, and rarely change management.

Management
- Outpatient—for children without respiratory warning signs:
  - As needed nasal irrigation with 0.9% NaCl.
  - Small frequent feeds.
  - Antipyretics.
  - No need for antibiotics.
- Inpatient—for patient with respiratory warning signs or in whom severe pneumonia cannot be ruled out:
  - Nasal irrigation, oxygen as needed, small feeds.
  - Bronchodilators: unlikely to help, but a one time-trial is OK.
  - Steroids: not helpful.
  - Antibiotics: theoretically not necessary for isolated bronchiolitis, however, in some settings, it may be hard to differentiate between bronchiolitis and severe pneumonia. Given the high mortality of severe pneumonia, it may be prudent to give IV antibiotics to some patients. Your best judgement as a clinician is necessary.

Bronchiolitis is highly contagious through direct contact, so there is a need to use proper infection control in hospitals, especially hand washing.

Asthma

Definition
Chronic airway inflammatory disease marked by intermittent recurring symptoms, reflecting bronchoconstriction, inflammation, airflow limitation, and hyper-responsiveness of the airways.

Epidemiology
- Up to 334 million people worldwide, most people affected in LIC and MIC. There are typically two peaks, at 10–14 years and 75–79 years old.
- Pathophysiology: the incidence of asthma is related to a combination of inherited and environmental factors.
- Risk factors: include viral URI, exercise, second-hand tobacco smoke, and inhaled allergens (dust mites, animal fur).

Presentation (signs/symptoms)
- Variable respiratory symptoms: wheezing, dyspnoea, chest tightness, and cough.
- Patients are unlikely to have access to peak flow meters, so the severity of each attack should be evaluated according to the clinical assessment parameters discussed later in this section.

Diagnosis
Clinical diagnosis is based mainly on episodic respiratory symptoms *and* responsiveness to bronchodilator therapy:
- Spirometry is usually unavailable (and not recommended for children <5 years of age). However, if available, an increase in FEV_1 (forced expiratory volume in 1 second) >12% post-bronchodilator usage supports the diagnosis.
- Peak flow meters, if available, should not be used for diagnosis, but rather for evaluating the severity of an exacerbation relative to each patient's personal best.
- Association with personal or familial history of atopic diseases increases risk of asthma.

Acute asthma exacerbation
See Table 37.1 for clinical assessment and management of acute asthma.
Note: chest X-ray is not usually recommended or needed unless there is suspicion of pneumomediastinum/pneumothorax or consolidation, or in life-threatening asthma, failure to adequately respond to treatment, or patient requires ventilation. It should never delay treatment!

Acute management
Asthma attacks require *rapid treatment*.

Mild/moderate
- Salbutamol two to four puffs via spacer, review after 20 minutes. If needed, repeat every 20 minutes for 1 hour. If not improving, treat as severe. Observe for 1 hour after attack resolves.
- Children: prednisolone 1 mg/kg/day PO or dexamethasone 0.5 mg/kg once daily PO for 1–3 days.
- Adults: prednisolone 40–50 mg/day for 5 days.

Table 37.1 Acute management of asthma attacks

	Mild/moderate	Severe	Life-threatening
Appearance	Speaking in sentences	Inability to complete a sentence in one breath Respiratory distress/accessory muscle use/subcostal recession Lethargy	Reduced consciousness or collapse Exhaustion Cyanosis
Vital signs	RR <25 PR <110 Oxygen saturation (if available) >94%	RR ≥25 PR ≥110 <6 years: PR >140, RR >50 6–10 years: PR >120, RR >30 10–15 years: PR >110, RR >25 Oxygen saturation 90–94%	Poor respiratory effort, soft/absent breath sounds Variable pulse and respiratory rate Oxygen saturation <90%

PR, pulse rate (beats /minute); RR, respiratory rate (breaths/minute).

Severe/life-threatening
- Give salbutamol 4–12 puffs via spacer (or nebulizer), repeated every 20 minutes for 1 hour.
- Ipratropium bromide can be added if poor response to salbutamol.
- Start systemic steroids: oral prednisolone as above, *or* hydrocortisone IV every 6 hours (children 5 mg/kg/dose and adults 100 mg).
- Consider magnesium sulfate IV over 20 minutes (children 50 mg/kg once, adults 2 g once).
- Start oxygen if available when oxygen saturation <90%.
- Organize transfer to hospital.

Note: chest X-ray is not usually recommended or needed unless there is suspicion of pneumomediastinum/pneumothorax or consolidation, or in life-threatening asthma, failure to adequately respond to treatment, or patient requires ventilation. It should never delay treatment!

Chronic management

For asthma to be considered well controlled, it requires:
- use of a beta agonist two times or less a week
- night-time asthma symptoms two times or less per month
- almost no limitation of daily activities
- no severe exacerbation (i.e. requiring oral steroids or admission to hospital) in the past month
- if available, peak expiratory flow rate 80% of predicted.

If the answer is no to any of the above, consider stepping up treatment according to the following steps:
Step 1. Inhaled salbutamol as required (PRN).

Step 2. Inhaled salbutamol PRN + low-dose inhaled corticosteroid: e.g. beclometasone, starting with 100 mcg once or twice daily for children and 100 mcg twice daily for adults.

Step 3. Inhaled salbutamol PRN + increased dose inhaled corticosteroid, e.g. beclometasone 200 mcg or 400 mcg twice daily.

Step 4. Inhaled salbutamol PRN + inhaled corticosteroid + long-acting beta agonist, e.g. salmeterol 50–100 mcg twice daily if >6 years old.

Step 5. Inhaled salbutamol PRN + inhaled corticosteroid + long-acting beta agonist + oral prednisolone in lowest dose possible to control symptoms. Consider specialist referral if at all possible.

Note: remember that inhaled corticosteroids and leukotriene inhibitors are frequently unavailable due to cost. In addition, though some private clinics prescribe theophylline, it has fallen out of favour due to its high risk:benefit ratio. These limitations mean that the above steps need to be adapted to each patient and each setting.

At each step, check patient's adherence to treatment and observe their inhaler technique. Review asthma control minimally every 3–6 months.

Making a spacer in the field—soft drink is everywhere! Use a small soft drink bottle, and cut a hole in the bottom to fit a puffer snuggly. You can tape it in place if the patient will always use it like this. The patient breathes through the mouth of the bottle.

Note: parasitaemia (*Strongyloides stercoralis*) can cause wheezing and other respiratory symptoms. In settings where this is a possibility, consider treating with albendazole 400 mg twice a day for 3 days, a cheap and effective treatment for those who have not been treated for parasites within the past year.

Pertussis

Definition

A highly contagious bacterial pneumonia caused by *Bordetella pertussis*, spread through respiratory droplets.

Epidemiology

- In spite of an effective vaccine, in 2008 there were >16 million cases and 195,000 deaths, mostly in developing countries.[1]
- Pertussis is spread through respiratory droplets from the start of the catarrhal phase until the third week of the paroxysmal phase.
- Pertussis epidemics can occur when vaccination rates drop below 90% for a population. Common risk factors are population displacements and a dysfunctional public health system, such as during conflicts. Older children and adults have mild disease, but can act as a source of infection for young infants, in whom the disease is considerably more serious.
- Providers should be vigilant for suspected cases and inform the local MOH office so that proper laboratory confirmation and outbreak investigation can be done. Conversely, public health officers should track vaccination rates to assess if either catch-up campaigns (no confirmed cases) or reactive campaigns (after confirmed cases) should be considered.

Presentation

- Incubation: 7–10 days.
- Catarrhal phase: 1–2 weeks—like a viral syndrome, usually including a mild cough.
- Paroxysmal phase: 1–6 weeks—increasing cough with classic coughing fits, where the patient coughs repeatedly without breathing, then takes a deep breath ('whoop').
- Convalescent phase: weeks to months—slow decrease of cough over weeks to months.
- Atypical presentation: especially in children <6 months and partially vaccinated persons, can present with eye bulging, apnoea, cyanosis, or absent whoop.

Clinical assessment

Providers should follow the local epidemic definitions for *suspect*, *probable*, and *confirmed* patients. In particular, one should suspect cases in those patients:

- <3 months old: regardless of vaccine status if persistent, if un-improving respiratory symptoms, especially if there are family members with prolonged cough or there is a confirmed local pertussis outbreak.
- >3 months: mainly unvaccinated or incompletely vaccinated persons who present with persistent cough and URI symptoms >1 week, classic whoops, and especially if there are family members with prolonged cough or there is a confirmed local pertussis outbreak.

Diagnosis

- Individual patients will depend upon a clinical diagnosis. There is no need to have a declared outbreak before empirically treating suspect patients.
- Outbreak confirmation will need laboratory testing. Options include culture, reverse transcriptase polymerase chain reaction (RT-PCR), and serology. Ask the local MOH or a regional reference laboratory for their specific protocols. (See ➔ p. 644 for outbreak prevention and management.)

Management

<3 months

- Hospitalize patients.
- Supportive treatment (hydration, nutrition, oxygen).
- Azithromycin oral × 5 days (erythromycin/co-trimoxazole oral × 5 days can be alternative treatment).

>3 months

- Can be treated as outpatients if clinically stable.
- Supportive care ensuring proper hydration and nutrition.
- Azithromycin oral × 5 days (erythromycin/co-trimoxazole oral × 5 days can be alternative treatment).

Outbreak prevention and management

- Ensure proper reporting and communication with the MOH.
- Post-exposure prophylaxis can be offered to all close contacts and high-risk persons in the community (including infants aged <6 months, pregnant women, and immunocompetent patients). Post-exposure prophylaxis antibiotics are the same as the dosages and duration as the treatment regimen.
- Patient isolation:
  - Home: all patients with pertussis should stay home from school and be kept away from unvaccinated persons and infants until they complete 5 days of antibiotic treatment.
  - Hospitals: try to group patients with pertussis together.
  - A vaccination campaign can be considered if vaccination rates are <90%. However, as many communities are highly suspicious of vaccination campaigns, public awareness should be raised and anxieties addressed to alleviate concerns.

Other key respiratory issues

Malaria

- Malaria is the most common non-primary pulmonary cause of respiratory distress. This is especially common in children and pregnant women with severe malaria.
- Respiratory involvement is due to a complex mix of severe anaemia, metabolic acidosis, non-cardiogenic pulmonary oedema, and superimposed bacterial infection.
- As above, part of respiratory triaging should include both a rapid malaria test and Hb to determine if either of these could be contributing to the patient's respiratory distress. Targeted treatment of either of these problems is the appropriate first step.
- Studies of patients with overlapping malaria and pneumonia presentations show a final diagnostic co-prevalence of <20%.[2,3] Unfortunately, there are frequently no clinically available tools to differentiate between these two diseases in real time, especially in HIV+ve or exposed patients. Consequently, it then becomes a clinical judgement on the appropriateness of adding antibacterial medication.

Tuberculosis

- TB is one of the ten leading causes of death in LIC.
- TB should be considered whenever a patient fails to improve on standard pneumonia therapy, has prolonged symptoms, is HIV+ve or exposed, has known contacts with patients with TB, or comes from a high-risk setting, such as refugee camps and prisons.

HIV pulmonary infections

- Bacterial infections (e.g. *Streptococcus pneumoniae* and *Haemophilus influenzae*) and viral infections are still highly common.
- Other common infections are pulmonary TB and *Pneumocystis jirovecii*.
- Consider non-infectious causes such as Kaposi's sarcoma, non-Hodgkin's lymphoma, and bronchogenic carcinoma.

References

1. World Health Organization. Immunization, Vaccines and Biologicals: Pertussis. 2011. ℬ http://www.who.int/immunization/topics/pertussis/en/
2. Ukwaja KN, Aina OB, Talabi AA. Clinical overlap between malaria and pneumonia: can malaria rapid diagnostic test play a role? J Infect Dev Ctries 2011;5(3):199–203.
3. Bassat Q, Machevo S, O'Callaghan-Gordo C, Sigaúque B, Morais L, Díez-Padrisa N, et al. Distinguishing malaria from severe pneumonia among hospitalized children who fulfilled integrated management of childhood illness criteria for both diseases: a hospital-based study in Mozambique. Am J Trop Med Hyg 2011;85(4):626–34.

Further reading

How to make a field-based CPAP system. ℬ http://journals.plos.org/plosone/article?id=10.1371/journal.pone.0086327 and ℬ https://www.youtube.com/watch?v=B0rGMRdZiOY
MSF clinical guidelines and smart-phone app. ℬ https://medicalguidelines.msf.org/viewport/MG/en/guidelines-16681097.html
Partners in Health. Manual of Ultrasound for Resource-Limited Settings. 2011. ℬ https://www.pih.org/practitioner-resource/manual-of-ultrasound-for-resource-limited-settings
World Health Organization. Pocket Book Of Hospital Care For Children: Guidelines for the management of common childhood illnesses. 2nd ed. Geneva: WHO; 2013. ℬ http://www.who.int/maternal_child_adolescent/documents/child_hospital_care/en/

Gastrointestinal illness

Ingo Hartlapp

Introduction

Clinical presentations involving the gastrointestinal (GI) tract are extremely common globally. Annual deaths from diarrhoeal diseases (1.3 million), viral hepatitis (1.2 million from liver cirrhosis and 0.8 million from hepatocellular carcinoma), and cancer (of which approximately 25% originates from the GI tract) belong to the top ten causes of mortality worldwide. Further, diarrhoea is still a leading cause of under-five mortality, second only to respiratory tract infections.

Significant progress has been made though, and mortality from infectious diarrhoeal diseases has declined over the past decade from 2.6 million in 1990 to 1.3 million in 2013, primarily due to a combination of advances in medical management and public health interventions. Further, as diseases such as HIV/AIDS and TB have witnessed a recent expansion in diagnostic and treatment options, specifically applicable in low-resource environments, similar advances are also anticipated to reach GI diseases which have a global impact.

It can be a challenge to diagnose and manage such conditions in humanitarian settings but this chapter aims to provide doctors who practise in low-resource settings with the guidance to implement more specialized GI medicine. We have attempted to give a general overview of the most important GI pathologies in the field from typical clinical presentation to specific diagnosis and treatment, although would advise providers to always seek expert advice for further questions.

Gastrointestinal cancer

GI cancers deserve an important mention as they collectively make up 25% of all cancers and oesophageal, liver, and stomach cancer are much more frequent in the less developed countries. It is estimated that the number of cancer cases around the world will almost double within the next 25 years. It is very possible that clinicians in the field will encounter patients presenting with GI cancers; however, as with all types of cancers, these can be quite challenging to address in low-resource environments.

While formal diagnosis and management of GI cancers would be beyond the capacity of this handbook, it is important for providers to recognize such presentations, and to recognize that GI cancers which may have a lower incidence in their home countries, can be much more common in less developed countries. These include:

Oesophageal cancer

81% of cases occur in less developed countries, primarily squamous cell carcinoma with the highest incidence in Asia and Africa (top five incidence in Malawi, Turkmenistan, Kenya, Mongolia, and Uganda).

Stomach cancer

71% of cases occur in less developed countries with the highest incidence of stomach cancer in Asia, Latin America, and the Caribbean (highest rates in Korea, Mongolia, Japan, Guatemala, and China).

Liver cancer

83% of cases occur in less developed countries (highest incidence in Mongolia, Laos, Gambia, Egypt, Vietnam, and Korea) and are linked with endemicity of hepatitis B.

Signs and symptoms more specific for GI cancers

- Jaundice: this can be caused by mechanical cholestasis (e.g. pancreatic cancer, portal lymph nodes) or liver metastasis.
- Pallor/anaemia: can be due to chronic blood loss or if abundant present with haematemesis, melena.
- Vomiting/abdominal distension: the earlier after food intake, the higher the obstruction. Immediate regurgitation suggests oesophageal cancer; regurgitation after >2 hours suggests gastric cancer with gastric outlet obstruction.
- Left-sided supraclavicular lymph nodes suggest gastric cancer.
- Palpable epigastric mass.
- Enlarged and hard liver may suggest liver metastasis or hepatocellular carcinoma.
- Variceal bleeding due to increase in portosystemic pressure gradient from hepatocellular carcinoma or portal vein thrombosis.
- Signs of hepatic decompensation, including ascites, icterus, and encephalopathy (evolution can be rapid with portal vein thrombosis).

If GI cancers are suspected, the provider should be aware of what options for treatment may exist in the context in which they are working. Lack of formal management pathways may necessitate supportive measures.

Hepatitis B, hepatitis C, and hepatitis E

Liver-related mortality is among the top ten causes worldwide, this includes deaths from:
- liver cirrhosis: 1.22 million (roughly chronic hepatitis B (CHB) = chronic hepatitis C (CHC) = alcohol)
- hepatocellular carcinoma: 820,000 (CHB = CHC > alcohol)
- acute fulminant hepatitis: 137,000 in 2013 (acute hepatitis B > acute hepatitis E > acute hepatitis A).

Hepatitis B and C are clinically distinct infections, with some significant differences—primarily that hepatitis B virus (HBV) infection can be prevented by vaccination and specific antiviral therapy is usually lifelong, whereas for hepatitis C virus (HCV) there is no vaccination available but therapy is of limited duration and the potential for cure with new antiviral therapies is >90%. The clinical presentation and symptomatic management options, however, are sufficiently similar to warrant joint coverage as follows.

Epidemiology

Hepatitis B
- The prevalence of CHB is >10% of the population in South-East Asia, China and sub-Saharan Africa where it is the primary case of liver-related mortality due to liver cancer, complications of liver cirrhosis, and acute liver failure.
- Transmission in highly endemic countries can be:
  - vertical (mother to child)
  - horizontal (spread in early childhood through playmates and close household contacts)
  - by sexual contact, blood transfusions, or contaminated needles.
- The chance that acute infection will become chronic is dependent on the maturity of the immune system and is 70–90% for perinatal (vertical) infection, 20–50% for early childhood (<5 years) infection, and only 1–3% in immune-competent adults (higher rates in HIV patients!).

Hepatitis C
- The worldwide prevalence of CHC is about half that of CHB, however mortality is about the same.
- After acute infection with hepatitis C, 70% remain asymptomatic (and undiagnosed), 20–30% show hepatitis symptoms such as jaundice, fatigue, flu-like symptoms, and dark urine, and only 1% develop fulminant acute hepatitis with liver failure.
- Symptoms typically occur 6–8 weeks after exposure (often unknown) and last for about 2–12 weeks.
- Whereas HBV is more oncogenic, HCV infections are more likely to become chronic (50–80%) and to progress to cirrhosis (20–30%).

Hepatitis E
- This is an acute hepatitis. Genotypes 1 and 2 are seen in humanitarian settings, transmitted via the faecal–oral route (i.e. contaminated water, poor sanitation) and can present with outbreaks in camps.
- There are an estimated 20 million cases worldwide/year; incubation is 2–9 weeks and most cases are self-limiting within 2–6 weeks (with

an excretion period up to 4 weeks). Of these cases, only 3 million are symptomatic, with an overall case fatality rate of 1%.

- If symptomatic, clinical signs include jaundice, fatigue, anorexia, nausea, arthralgia, fever, tender hepatomegaly, splenomegaly, dark urine, clay-coloured stool, and abdominal pain.
- Fulminant acute hepatitis is a dreaded complication in pregnant woman with 20% mortality and >50,000 deaths/year.
- Disease course is usually self-limiting. Specific treatment (ribavirin, sofosbuvir) or immunization (HEV 239 vaccine) is not available in the field. Supportive measures (rest, hydration, nutrition) and avoidance of alcohol and hepatotoxic medication such as paracetamol is advised. Hospitalize pregnant women.

Clinical assessment of chronic hepatitis

History
In addition to standard history, inquire about hepatotoxic drugs (as alternative explanation for (a) elevation of liver enzymes, (b) acute liver failure); e.g. RHZ (rifampicin (R), isoniazid (H) and pyrazinamide (Z)), clavulanic acid in co-amoxiclav, nevirapine/efavirenz, etc.

Signs/symptoms
Check for signs of chronic liver disease or acute hepatitis, which include:
- cachexia (typical: contrast between thin extremities and increased abdominal girth due to ascites)
- ascites (determine clinically or via ultrasound)
- spider naevi= telangiectasia in the décolleté
- palmar erythema, Dupuytren's contractures, caput medusa
- icterus (if available confirm elevated bilirubin)
- multiple haematomas as sign of coagulopathy (lab: prothrombin time)
- splenomegaly
- extrahepatic manifestations of hepatitis C which can include autoimmune conditions, e.g. glomerulonephritis, cryoglobulinaemia, neutropenia/thrombocytopenia, arthralgia/arthritis, hypothyroidism, and vasculitis.

In developing countries, the typical patients with complicated cirrhosis or hepatocellular carcinoma are young adults as complications arise about 30 years after perinatal infection. It is not rare to see young man or pregnant women with icterus and decompensated ascites.

Diagnosis

Hepatitis B
- A detailed stepwise diagnostic algorithm is illustrated in Fig. 38.1.

Hepatitis C
- There is no serological marker for acute HCV infection and a combination of elevated ALT+ anti-HCV+ HCV RNA is needed to establish diagnosis; infectivity as well as CHC are defined by persistence of HCV RNA.
- Assessment of severity of liver disease is not generally feasible in low-resource settings and typically requires hospital-level referral.

Stepwise diagnosis of stage of hepatitis B infection

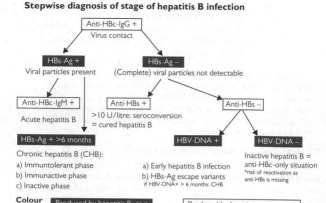

Fig. 38.1 Stepwise diagnosis of stage of hepatitis B infection.

Young adults with decompensated liver cirrhosis due to perinatal transmission are typical patients in large parts of Africa and Asia where abdominal TB is present as well. Ascites in this setting is not always a sign of abdominal TB; in fact clinical probability for ascites due to liver cirrhosis is much higher. This misconception might ultimately lead to inadequate treatment of patients with advanced liver cirrhosis with potentially hepatotoxic drugs such as isoniazid and RHZ.

Treatment

Hepatitis B

- Effectively treated with combination of tenofovir and lamivudine (TDF/3TC), generally lifelong. These medications are used in HIV treatment, so always assess HIV co-infection before starting hepatitis B treatment to avoid creating resistance.
- In resource-poor settings, priority for treatment is for:
  - those with signs of advanced cirrhosis (icterus, ascites, increased coagulopathy/haematoma). If blood count is available, marked thrombocytopenia <100/nl due to splenomegaly is also a good marker of relevant portal hypertension.
  - pregnant women (to prevent mother-to-child transmission)
  - HIV co-infected patients.

Hepatitis C

- Direct antiviral agents are HCV protease or polymerase inhibitors, which have been available since 2012. Advantages of these oral drugs include high cure rates (>95%), shorter treatment courses (generally 8–12 weeks, although longer for cirrhosis), and few side effects.

- Although costs are still high (~€40,000/12-week course), they are expected to decrease over time, similar to the evolution of HIV treatments, which will increase availability in the future. MSF has recently started a hepatitis C pilot project in Karachi (Pakistan) where some patients are treated with sofosbuvir.

Prevention

Hepatitis B

- Vaccination is indicated for health workers, pregnant women, children at birth, and those with other chronic liver diseases.
- WHO recommends vaccinating all children at birth.
- A schedule of 0, 4, and 24 weeks offers >95% protection (in term infants and adults).
- If possible, all pregnant women should be screened for HBV (hepatitis B surface antigen (HBs-Ag)) and women with CHB and a high viral load put on TDF/3TC to prevent transmission.
- Children at birth should receive active immunization within 12 hours of birth.
- All blood donors should be screened.

Hepatitis C

Universal precautions (sexual transmission, needles, etc.).

Liver cirrhosis

- Most of the complications of liver cirrhosis are signs of advanced disease and prognosis is usually very poor.
- While options are limited in low-resource settings, there are treatments with a proven impact on mortality.

Hepatic encephalopathy

- Treat underlying infection or dehydration.
- Treat with lactulose 10–20 mL 1–3×/day (aim at 2 soft stools/day).
- Treat with non-absorbable antibiotics such as neomycin or rifaximin (expensive).

Decompensated ascites

- Spironolactone/furosemide: normal starting dose in abundant ascites is *100 mg/40 mg*; ratio should be kept fixed and is dose adjusted to therapeutic goal of weight loss of 500–1000 mg per day.
- If diuretics alone are insufficient, or if there is painful abdominal distension or suspicion of infected ascites (spontaneous bacterial peritonitis), large volume paracentesis is indicated.
- If albumin is available, substitute 6 g albumin/litre of ascites otherwise paracentesis volume should be <5 litres to avoid deterioration of renal function or a small volume (500 mL) of plasma expander should be given after paracentesis.

> Even if coagulation is reduced, it is safe to perform paracentesis in both lower quadrants of the abdomen or ultrasound guided with a fine needle to aspirate ascites for analysis. Just keep in mind that a potentially enlarged spleen has to be avoided.

Spontaneous bacterial peritonitis

- Presents with fever, abdominal pain, deterioration of hepatic encephalopathy, abdominal tenderness, icterus, and paralytic ileus.
- Ceftriaxone or ciprofloxacin are the antibiotics of choice (in case of treatment failure consider intrinsically cephalosporin-resistant enterococci).

Acute variceal bleeding

- Prognosis is poor; up to 50% die within 6 weeks of first episode.
- While gastroscopy with banding is the treatment of choice, additional pharmaceutical treatment has proven benefit:
  - Vasoactive drugs (i.e. terlipressin) before endoscopy achieve haemostasis in 50%, but may only be available at the referral level.
  - Antibiotic prophylaxis with ciprofloxacin/ceftriaxone for 5 days.
  - Non-selective beta blockers as propranolol (starting dose 3 × 10 mg) can be used to prevent a second episode.
  - Proton pump inhibitor (PPI), e.g. pantoprazole 80 mg IV, then 2 × 40 mg (even in patients with liver cirrhosis, other causes of upper GI bleeding (peptic ulcer disease) are an important differential diagnosis).
  - Lactulose 3 × 20 mL to prevent encephalopathy (also via enema or NG tube).

Peptic ulcer disease and *Helicobacter pylori* infection

- *Helicobacter pylori* is found in more than half of the world's population, with a significantly higher prevalence in developing countries (e.g. Ethiopia, Nigeria, Bangladesh, India about 90%).
- Transmission is oral–oral or faecal–oral and linked to poor socioeconomic conditions with lack of proper sanitation.
- Chronic *H. pylori* infection can cause dyspepsia, peptic ulcer disease (10–20%), gastric cancer (1%) and gastric MALT lymphoma (<1%), but most of the carriers (80%) are asymptomatic.

Clinical assessment

The leading symptoms of peptic ulcer disease are:
- chronic epigastric/periumbilical pain aggravated 1–4 hours after food intake by gastric acid production (gastric ulcer) or
- pain at night/at fasting (duodenal ulcer) alleviated by eating (neutralization of gastric acid by alkali production in duodenum).

> Whereas in developed countries the typical patient with peptic ulcer is >65 years, the typical patient in developing countries is a young man (tobacco, alcohol) with chronic epigastric pain.

Diagnosis

Diagnosis in resource-poor settings is usually made on clinical grounds. Despite high prevalence, *H. pylori* as a public health problem will only be solved if therapeutic vaccination becomes available.

Treatment

- Due to side effects, and lack of universal effectiveness (contributing to increased resistance), only symptomatic patients especially with complications (peptic ulcer disease, upper GI bleeding, gastric surgery, or family history of gastric cancer) need treatment.
- There are multiple regimens for *H. pylori* eradication, chosen depending upon resistance rates and antibiotic accessibility; for all regimens longer treatment improves eradication rate.
  - *French triple therapy*: amoxicillin 2 × 1 g, clarithromycin 2 × 500 mg, PPI 2× standard dose for 7–14 days.
  - *Italian triple therapy*: amoxicillin 2 × 1 g, metronidazole 2 × 500 mg, PPI 2 × standard dose for 7–14 days.
  - *Quadruple therapy*: PPI 2 × standard dose, bismuth subcitrate 4 × 120 mg, tetracycline 4 × 500 mg, metronidazole 4 × 375 mg for 10–14 days (first line if high probability of clarithromycin resistance or after failure of triple therapy).
  - *Concomitant quadruple therapy*: PPI 2 × standard dose, amoxicillin 2 × 1g, clarithromycin 2 × 500 mg, metronidazole 2 × 500 mg for 7–10 days (first line if clarithromycin resistance >20%).

Diarrhoea

Context

- There are about 2 billion cases of diarrhoeal disease worldwide every year and it is still the second leading cause of death in children <5 years (after pneumonia).
- Incidence and mortality of acute diarrhoea is highest in children <5 years especially in the months after weaning from exclusive breastfeeding.
- About 5000 children die from diarrhoea each day and 78% of these deaths occur in Africa and South East Asia.

> From a pathophysiological point of view, there are two main mechanisms causing diarrhoea:
>
> - Osmotic diarrhoea is caused by problems in re-absorption of water and electrolytes (large bowel can only compensate up to 50% loss of small bowel function), it improves/stops with food pause: e.g. food intolerance (lactose), laxative abuse.
> - Secretory diarrhoea is caused by excessive secretions, it does not improve/stop with food pause: e.g. invasive infections, structural damage such as in inflammatory bowel disease (IBD).
>
> Inflammatory diarrhoea is present in most infections and is a combination of both mechanisms.

Assessment

- Most acute diarrhoea is mild and self-limiting and can be treated with ORS and zinc alone.
- The probability of a non-infectious (or parasitic) cause increases almost linearly with duration of symptoms (>3 weeks).
- It is important to identify those patients at risk of a fatal course:
  - Young children or very old patients with severe dehydration.
  - Abundant diarrhoea without improvement after 48 hours.
  - Malnutrition and immunosuppression (HIV/AIDS).
  - Those with clinical suspicion of cholera or typhoid fever (perforation).
  - Situations with epidemic potential (cholera, shigellosis, typhoid fever)
  - Non-infectious diarrhoea as a symptom of an underlying disease that needs further diagnosis and treatment

The following content focuses primarily on infectious causes of diarrhoea most commonly seen in humanitarian settings, although a list of non-infectious causes to consider can be found online.

Signs and symptoms

Acute diarrhoea is defined as at least three liquid (semisolid) stools per day for <2 weeks.

There are two clinical types of acute diarrhoea:

- *Simple diarrhoea without blood*, caused by viruses in 60% of cases.
- *Dysentery or bloody diarrhoea*, caused by bacteria (*Shigella* in up to 50% of the cases), or parasites (*Amoeba*).

Clinical examination

Assess for the following:

- Clinical signs of dehydration. In children, classify level of dehydration according to WHO integrated management of childhood disease.
- Temperature to identify systemic inflammation/invasive pathogen (fever >38.5°C).
- Abdominal examination. Tenderness/local rigidity can be seen in perforation; distension/palpable resistance in obstruction.
- Visual stool examination is very important. Look for blood, pus, and volume/consistency.
- Signs of other infections. Particularly in children, other illnesses (e.g. malaria, pneumonia, measles, and UTI) can present with diarrhoea.
- Main symptoms to help you to narrow down a potential diagnosis are shown in Table 38.1.

Diagnosis

- For acute diarrhoea, maintaining adequate hydration and correcting fluid and electrolyte loss are more important than identifying the causative agent.
- Acute bloody diarrhoea can usually be treated empirically. Presence of visible blood in febrile patients generally indicates infection due to invasive pathogens, such as *Shigella, Campylobacter jejuni, Salmonella*, or *Entamoeba histolytica*.
  - Stool leucocytes proves invasive colitis and usually establishes the necessity for antibiotic treatment (differential diagnosis IBD!).
- Stool cultures are usually unnecessary for immune-competent patients who present with watery diarrhoea, but may be necessary when there is clinical suspicion of a cholera outbreak or dysentery.
- In resource-poor settings it is very important to identify a cholera outbreak (case definition, special transport medium) and chronic diarrhoea/malabsorption caused by parasites (*Amoeba, Giardia, Ascaris, Schistosoma*). Usually stool microscopy for parasites is available and local expertise is quite high.
- Non-pathogenic amoebae are often detected in stool microscopy and get wrongly treated. Need for treatment is demonstrated only by phagocytosis of erythrocytes by amoeba.

Treatment

- Prevent/treat dehydration. Use:
  - oral rehydration with ORS by mouth
  - NG tube is preferred to IV and contraindications to NG tubes are only hypovolaemic shock and somnolence with reduced airway reflexes
  - be very careful with fluid overload in malnourished children.
- Give zinc sulfate for 10 days to children: 20 mg/day in those aged 6 months–5 years, 10 mg/day in those <6 months to reduce duration and reoccurrence.
- Prevent malnutrition: breastfeeding, local food, Plumpy'Nut® (frequent meals 6 ×/day to prevent hypoglycaemia and hypokalaemia).
- Multivitamins/minerals: if recommended by national protocol.
- Do not use antibiotics in acute watery diarrhoea!
- Do not use antiemetics (sedation impedes oral rehydration!) or loperamide in children or bloody/invasive diarrhoea!

See Table 38.2 for specific treatment.

Table 38.1 Diagnosis of diarrhoea

Symptom	Viruses (rotavirus, norovirus)	Food poisoning	Cholera	Typhoid fever	Dysentery	Parasites
Vomiting	+	+	++	+	–	–
Fever	+	–	– (mild in children)	+	+	–
Blood/pus	–	–	–	+/–	+	–
Watery diarrhoea	+	+	+++	+/–	–	Giardiasis, cryptosporidiosis, strongyloidiasis
Acute onset/ chronic diarrhoea >14 days	Acute	Acut	Acute	Acute ileocolitis, typhoid fever more protracted	Acute (Shigella, EHEC) Chronic (Amoeba, Schistosoma, Clostridium difficile)	Chronic
Abdominal pain/cramps	+	+	Painless!	++ both lower quadrants Rigidity if perforated!	++ (tenesmus)	+
Special remarks	Children: epidemics in cold season	Preformed exotoxines from Staph aureus Bacillus cereus Clostridium spp.	Shock, renal failure, prostration	Splenomegaly, rose spots, bradycardia, perforation	Salmonella, Campylobacter can be both mild watery or bloody	Malnourished children and HIV patients

Table 38.2 Specific treatment

Cause	First choice		Alternative		Comment
	Adults	Children	Adults	Children	
Cholera	D: 300 mg once	100 mg once	A: 1g once	20 mg/kg once	10–15 litres /first day; Ringer's lactate better than NaCl; risk of hypokalaemia if patient does not restore eating
Shigellosis	C: 2 × 500 mg (3 days) or 2g once	Not recommended	Cef: 1 × 2 g (3 days) or 2–4 g once	1 × 50–100 mg/kg (3 days)	
Typhoid fever	C: 2 × 500 mg (5–7 days)	Not recommended	Cef: 1 × 2g (7 days)	50–100 mg/kg (7 days)	Other alternatives: aminopenicillins or chloramphenicol
Giardiasis	M: 3 × 250 mg (5 days)	3 × 5 mg/kg	T: 2 g once	1 × 50 mg/kg (3 days)	Note: treat only if cysts/ trophozoites are found in stool and diarrhoea persists >14 days
Amoebiasis Note: treat only invasive forms	M: 3 × 750 mg (5–10 days)	3 × 10–15 mg/kg	T: 2 g once	1 × 50 mg/kg (3 days)	Note: ideally following M/T treatment diloxanide or nitazoxanide should be added to get rid of the cysts
Campylobacter	A: 1 × 500 mg (3 days)	30 mg/kg once	C: 2 × 500 mg (3 days)	Not recommended	Note: increase of quinolone-resistant strains around the world especially in Asia

A, azithromycin; C, ciprofloxacin; Cef, cefriaxone; D, doxycyline; M, metronidazole; T, tinidazole.

Although theoretically desirable, the implementation of new vaccines for cholera and rotavirus is not without controversy. Some proponents argue that preventative measures have been largely successful, reducing mortality from 2.6 to 1.3 million between 1990 and 2013 (data from the Global Burden of Disease project). There is concern that the high cost of these new vaccines could potentially channel developing countries' limited health budgets from these preventative measures into the pockets of big pharmaceutical companies. The newest vaccines are expensive: just three vaccines (rotavirus, pneumococcal, hepatitis B) account for 86% of the total cost to vaccinate a child (Humanitarian Congress Berlin 2015). Furthermore, for rotavirus vaccines, loss of protection after 2 years, serotype replacement by more virulent strains, vaccine costs, delivery/cold chain, side effects such as intussusception, and sustainability after the end of industry-funded initiatives are of great concern.

Gastrointestinal pathologies in HIV

The spectrum of GI pathologies in HIV patients as other opportunistic infections or AIDS-defining diseases is strongly dependent on the immune status. The following list is not comprehensive, but covers many of the common GI complaints which may be the presenting features of patients with HV (HIV-associated mucosal Kaposi sarcoma and anal cancer are covered elsewhere). At times, the advanced diagnostics necessary to formally diagnose some of these conditions may not be available. Presumptive treatment will therefore require discretionary judgement, with considerations including clinical suspicion and severity of symptoms.

Thrush/oral candidiasis
- Most common and often first opportunistic infection in HIV.
- >40% of untreated HIV patients show clinical evidence of thrush.
- Treatment is with fluconazole 100 mg PO for 7 days or mucoadhesive miconazole.

Candida oesophagitis
- *Candida* oesophagitis is an AIDS-defining disease requiring the start of ART.
- Main symptoms are dysphagia and retrosternal chest pain, but up to 50% are asymptomatic.
- 30% do not show oral thrush.
- Treatment: fluconazole 200 mg for 2 weeks.

Oral hair leucoplakia
- Local EBV replication in the lateral edge of the tongue.
- Unlike thrush, it is not removable but indicates the need to start ART.

Lymphoma
- HIV patients have approximately a 160-fold increased risk of mostly aggressive non-Hodgkin lymphoma and a 15–20-fold increased risk of Hodgkin lymphoma.
- Extranodal manifestations are common (80%) and among these, GI manifestations mostly in the stomach and rectum predominate.
- Clinical symptoms include B-symptoms, lymphadenopathy (not painful!), GI bleeding, and GI obstruction.
- Diagnosis generally requires gastroscopy or rectoscopy.
- Treatment: poor 5-year survival in resource-limited settings; treatment is mostly palliative with steroids plus available chemotherapeutic agents (vincristine, cyclophosphamide, etoposide, doxorubicin).

Viral oesophagitis
- Can present with pain while eating/drinking, local lymphadenopathy.
- Endoscopy finding of ulcerative panoesophagitis, histology is needed to distinguish herpes simplex virus 1 from CMV (owl's eye cells: *in situ* PCR).
- Herpes simplex virus esophagitis is suspected if CD4 <250/μL with treatment of aciclovir 5 × 400 mg PO or 3 × 500–750 mg IV for 1–2 weeks.
- CMV oesophagitis usually occurs only with CD4 <100/μL and treatment is ganciclovir 2 × 5 mg/kg IV or valganciclovir 2 × 900 mg PO for at least 3 weeks.

HIV enteropathy

- Presents with consecutive malabsorption and chronic diarrhoea.
- Diagnosis difficult to confirm (differential diagnosis: stool microscopy for parasites).
- Treatment: ART (usually presumptive) leads to villous regeneration and healing of *Cryptosporidium* infection (meanwhile symptomatic treatment with loperamide up to 16 mg/day if massive diarrhoea).
- Differential diagnosis: microsporidium—albendazole 2 × 400 mg for 2–4 weeks.
- *Cystoisospora belli* (previously known as *Isospora belli*): high-dose co-trimoxazole 800 + 160 mg 2–0–2 (10 days) → 1–0–1 (3 weeks) → secondary prophylaxis.
- *Note:* protease inhibitors frequently cause diarrhoea themselves!

CMV colitis

- Massive bloody diarrhoea (up to 20 × /day).
- CD4 count usually <100/µL.
- Diagnosis: multiple ulcers on endoscopy, positive CMV PCR in biopsies or significant viral load in the blood. These may not be available in low-resource settings so consider presumptive treatment if clinical suspicion is high, especially if low CD4 count.
- Treatment with ganciclovir 2 × 5 mg/kg for 3 weeks as mentioned earlier. Presumptive treatment especially if low CD4 count (<100/µL) and other manifestations of CMV infection: retinitis, esophagitis, CMV pneumonia (X-ray).

Salmonella septicaemia

- Recurrent non-typhoidal *Salmonella* septicaemia is an AIDS-defining infection, in Africa and Asia most common bacteria found in blood cultures of HIV patients.
- Clinical symptoms: fever, chills, diarrhoea not obligatory (!), septic shock, complications: osteomyelitis, empyema, lung abscess, pyelonephritis, and meningitis.
- Treatment: IV ciprofloxacin 2 × 500 mg or ceftriaxone 1 × 2 g for at least 14 days (!).
- Note: high risk of relapse in HIV patients with poor immune status: continue with oral ciprofloxacin or co-trimoxazole (800 + 160 mg 2–0–2 → 1–0–1 (if toxicity)) for a total of 4–6 weeks.

Helminthiasis

Strongyloides stercoralis is the only worm that can increase parasite burden in the human host due to an autoinfection cycle. This can be massive in HIV/immunosuppressed patients leading to a hyperinfection syndrome with numerous larvae in all organs and >90% fatality. Presentation:

- Asthma-like symptoms (lung migration), eosinophilia, skin rash.
- Abdominal pain, nausea, vomiting, diarrhoea, intestinal obstruction.
- Mucosal ulceration, massive haemorrhage, subsequent peritonitis.
- Bacterial sepsis, meningitis (larvae that penetrate intestinal wall can carry gram- bacteria).

Diagnosis: stool enrichment microscopy.

Treatment: *ivermectin*, in a single dose, 200 mcg/kg orally for 2 days *or* if not available, albendazole 2 × 400 mg for 3–7 days; presumptive screening/treatment of at-risk patients.

Visceral leishmaniasis (kala-azar)

- 12 million cases worldwide, 350 million people live in endemic regions.
- The core clinical signs are fever (generally in late afternoon/evening), pancytopenia, weight loss, cough, epistaxis, and hepatosplenomegaly. Lymphadenopathy is common in Africa.
- Abdominal distension and watery diarrhoea are also common.
- In Asia, the clinical course is less severe than in Africa and can progress for many months, whereas in Africa, untreated kala-azar can be fatal within weeks after clinical presentation.
- In HIV patients the course of kala-azar is particularly aggressive and will relapse again and again and eventually become unresponsive to all treatments.
- Diagnosis: Giemsa stained smears of spleen aspirates > bone marrow > lymph nodes or buffy coat (diagnostic yield of material) gold standard and test of cure, serological tests: rK39 antigen-based rapid tests (ELISA: only one manufacturer's test works in Africa!) and direct agglutination tests are used in low-resource settings.
- Treatment: IV pentavalent antimony, sodium stibogluconate (SSG) or meglumine antimoniate (MA), paromomycin (PM), amphotericin B (AmB), and miltefosine (MF) are used in different combinations, doses, and durations according to the region (Asia or Africa) and HIV status of the patient.
- Possible options for low-resource settings:
  - *Africa*: SSG 20 mg/kg/day + PM 15 mg/kg/day for 17 days (quite toxic, ensure good hydration, contraindicated in HIV).
  - *Asia*: where AmB is available: AmB 10 mg/kg in a single dose; Where AmB is not available: MF 100 mg (divided in two doses) + PM 15 mg/kg/day for 10 days each.
- HIV coinfection:
  - AmB 30 mg/kg (5 mg/kg on day 1, 3, 5, 7, 9, 11) + MF 100 mg (divided in two doses) for 14 days (Asia) or 28 days (Africa).

Inflammatory bowel disease and tuberculosis

Context

- IBD comprises two disease entities Crohn's disease and ulcerative colitis with both overlapping and distinct clinical and pathological findings.
- Always consider an infectious cause (e.g. acute: *Campylobacter, Yersinia*, chronic: *Leishmania, Giardia*) before diagnosing IBD.
- While there is generally a lower prevalence in developing countries the main challenge is to distinguish abdominal TB and Crohn's disease as steroid treatment in unrecognized TB can be fatal.

See Table 38.3 for differentiating features of Crohn's disease and TB.

Recommendations

- In HIV patients with poor immune status (<100/µL CD4) or patients under severe immunosuppression, consider CMV colitis (bloody diarrhoea).
- In diarrhoea (usually watery) after antibiotic treatment, consider *C. difficile* colitis.
- Always attempt the most to rule out TB in areas with high prevalence before starting steroids—do at least chest X-ray, abdominal US, sputum with microscopy plus TB-PCR plus TB-culture (if available).
- If in doubt initiate TB treatment and observe therapeutic effect for at least 2–4 weeks.
- Antibiotic therapy improves disease activity in many IBD patients—temporary improvement dose not prove infectious cause.
- IBD usually improves with steroids (prednisolone 1 mg/kg body weight) within 1 week.

Table 38.3 Key differentiating features of Crohn's disease and TB

	Crohn's disease	TB
Time course	History of remissions/relapses	Continuous course
Clinical presentation	Diarrhoea and abdominal pain from onset, fever often absent	Fever/weight loss from onset, then abdominal pain, diarrhoea is a late symptom
	Often seen: fistula, perianal disease, abscesses; perforation	Often: ascites and hepatosplenomegaly
History	History of IBD	History of TB/TB family contact
Diagnosis	US (mesenteric lymph nodes <1 cm)	US (mesenteric nodes >1 cm with calcifications)
	Normal chest X-ray	Abnormal chest X-ray
		TB microscopy, TB-PCR, TB culture

Gastrointestinal bleeding

Context

- As in developed countries, upper GI bleeding is much more common (85%) than lower GI bleeding (15%).
- Upper GI bleeding in developing countries is mostly due to gastroduodenal ulcers, varices, erosive gastritis, and reflux esophagitis.
- In regions where schistosomiasis is endemic, bleeding from oesophageal varices is the most common cause of upper GI bleeding.

Signs and symptoms

- Melaena stool and haematemesis are signs of upper GI bleeding.
  - Haematemesis usually indicates a higher intensity whereas melaena stool for several days before presentation usually indicates a lower intensity of GI bleeding.
- Haematochezia is usually a sign of lower GI bleeding but can indicate a massive upper GI bleeding.
- Vomiting first and then vomiting blood is the typical history of Mallory–Weiss lesion (heals spontaneously).

Ask patient about:
- epigastric pain aggravated by food—suggests a gastric ulcer
- epigastric pain while hungry which is alleviated by food—suggests a duodenal ulcer.

Signs of severe GI bleeding include:
- haemoglobin <9 g/dL
- pulse >100/min (reflecting loss of >25% of total blood volume)
- systolic BP <90 mm Hg (reflecting loss of >50% of total blood volume)
- thirst, nausea, restlessness, fever, altered consciousness, positive shock index
- diarrhoea as blood itself is a strong laxative.

In acute GI bleeding, haemoglobin does not change until interstitial fluid is redistributed to the intravascular space and/or IV fluids are given, so measuring initial haemoglobin often underestimates the severeness of the GI bleeding (pulse and BP are more useful). Due to further haemodilution, haemoglobin might drop by 1–2 g/dL in the next 24 hours even if GI bleeding has stopped.

It is important to look for clinical signs of liver cirrhosis/portal hypertension, malignant disease (cachexia), or renal insufficiency as all these conditions have an increased risk for severe GI bleeding.

Treatment

- Assess haemodynamic parameters and insert two large volume IV catheters:
  - Take blood for compatibility testing, prepare whole blood transfusion if required and available.
  - Start IV fluids +/- volume expander.

- In suspected peptic ulcers, give acid suppression: give PPI 2 × standard dose IV e.g. pantoprazole 2 × 80 mg/dL, 2 × 40 mg (days 2–5) PO.
- Gastroscopy (oesophagogastroduodenoscopy) is gold standard if available in severe GI bleeding. If gastroscopy is not available or not successful in variceal bleeding, use haemostatic NG tube (Sengstaken/Linton) for 24 hours to stabilize patient or before transport into a bigger health facility.
- Vitamin K 2–10 mg IV and whole blood (containing coagulation factors) or plasma. In variceal bleeding, early administration of vasoactive drugs (terlipressin 2 mg or glyceryl trinitrate 80 mg slowly IV) and antibiotics (ciprofloxacin 2 × 500 mg or ceftriaxone 2 g IV to be continued for 5 days) has been shown to lower mortality.

Tropical diseases that can present with acute abdomen

Ascariasis

- The most prevalent human helminth; >1 billion people infected worldwide.
- A heavy worm load causes intestinal obstruction with 20,000 deaths annually.
- Good sanitation to prevent faecal contamination of soil is key.

Clinical presentation

- *Ascaris* generally live in the small bowel, but can also migrate to biliary tree and other orifices (mouth, rectum). Three phases of *Ascaris* may be present:
  1. Pulmonary with hypersensitivity (larvae).
  2. Intestinal (adult worms). May cause intestinal colic, vomiting, in- tussusception, volvulus, obstruction, appendicitis, appendicular perforation, anaemia, and malabsorption. Perforation with eggs released into the peritoneum may cause granulomas resembling TB peritonitis.
  3. Hepatobiliary. Worms in the biliary tree/liver can cause hepatic abscess, biliary colic, recurrent cholangitis, and acute cholecystitis/ pancreatitis.
- Diagnostic clues include history of passage of worms via mouth or rectum, microscopic identification of worm eggs in the faeces, anal pruritus, eosinophilia, and plain abdominal images (X-ray) with distended small bowel with air-fluid levels and shadows of round worms; typical ultrasound image of round worms can confirm diagnosis.

> Gastrografin® is used to diagnose complete intestinal obstruction or to relieve the partial obstruction by hyperosmolar properties dragging liquid to the intestinal lumen and separating and perhaps shrinking the worms.

Management

- Early presentation with no fever, slight distension, and mild diffuse tenderness can be managed conservatively with NG tube, IV fluids correcting dehydration, hypertonic saline enema or liquid paraffin and anthelmintic agents (mebendazole 500 mg, albendazole 400 mg, pyrantel pamoate in pregnancy).
- Paralysing vermifuges (e.g. pyrantel pamoate, piperazine, ivermectin) *should be avoided* in patients with complete or partial intestinal obstruction since the paralysed worms increase the size of the worm bolus and may cause further complications.
- Late presentation with high fever, dehydration, signs of peritonitis and above-mentioned signs not improving after 48 hours of conservative management generally need laparotomy.

Amoebic colitis

Clinical presentation
- Diarrhoea with blood and mucus, slight tenderness of colon, cramps in the form of tenesmus, sometimes tender mass in right iliac fossa.
- Amoebic liver abscess or amoebic perforation can be late stage complications requiring urgent definitive intervention.

Management
- Metronidazole 500 mg three times daily IV for 7–10 days.
- Ultrasound-guided drainage of amoebic liver abscess if >6 cm in diameter.
- Failure to respond within 48 hours indicates transmural disease and may require urgent surgery.

Ileocaecal tuberculosis

Clinical presentation
Subacute obstruction, wasting, mild colics getting worse over weeks, abdominal distension ± ascites (quantity is usually less than in liver cirrhosis and is an exudate with protein >30 g/l (Rivalta's test positive)), palpable mass in right lower quadrant.

Management
Check for systemic signs of TB, consider chest X-ray and abdominal ultrasound, and other tests to rule out differential diagnosis (HIV, CHB + CHC, stool microscopy depending on clinical situation), then start RHZE (rifampicin (R), isoniazid (H) and pyrazinamide (Z), and ethambutol (E)) (response usually within 2 weeks).

Pigbel disease (clostridial necrotizing enteritis)

Clinical presentation
Acute abdomen due to necrotizing enteritis from toxins of *Clostridium perfringens* following a large meal, classically of pork meat.

Epidemiology
More common in children/young adults especially if malnourished, carrying heavy *Ascaris* infestation, or on a diet rich in sweet potatoes, the latter two are associated with high levels of trypsin inhibitors preventing intestinal proteases from degrading the toxin.

Management
IV antibiotics (penicillin or chloramphenicol), fluid resuscitation, *Clostridium perfringens* type C antiserum (if available), urgent surgery in peritonitis, ileus or shock, conservative therapy of milder forms with bloody diarrhoea (NG tube, start oral food after 24–48 hours).

Prevention
Immunization with type C toxoid.

Chapter 39

Neurology

Aaron L. Berkowitz

Context

Neurological diseases cause an estimated 17% of the yearly global burden of mortality.[1] Neurological diseases can also cause major disability, and can lead to severe stigma that can affect familial, social, and professional aspects of life.

A common misconception is that diagnosis of neurological conditions is heavily dependent on laboratory tests such as MRI, electroencephalography (EEG), and electromyography (EMG), leading to a neurological nihilism in humanitarian settings where such diagnostics are often inaccessible. However, neurological diagnosis is ultimately highly clinical, relying on specific clues in the history and physical examination to develop and refine a differential diagnosis.

As of 2014, LIC had on average 0.03 neurologists per 100,000 population compared to 5.14 per 100,000 population in HIC.[2] Patients with neurological disease in humanitarian settings therefore often present to generalist providers or mental health practitioners. In these settings, diagnostic tests such as neuroimaging, EEG, EMG, and cerebrospinal fluid (CSF) analysis may be unavailable (or inaccessible/unaffordable) to many patients in humanitarian settings.

In spite of these resource limitations, a logical approach to clinical diagnosis in neurology can significantly narrow the differential diagnosis between many of the leading causes of death and disability due to neurological disease.

Diagnosis in neurology

Diagnosis in neurology relies on two aspects:
- The localization within the nervous system that explains the patient's symptoms.
- The time course over which symptoms have arisen and evolved.

Localization in neurological diagnosis

The nervous system can be divided into the central nervous system (CNS—brain, brainstem, cerebellum, and spinal cord) and the peripheral nervous system (PNS—nerve roots, peripheral nerves, neuromuscular junctions, and muscles).

Brain
- Diseases affecting the brain can cause deficits in any cognitive function (e.g. language, memory, and attention), weakness, and/or alterations in sensation (most commonly somatosensory or visual).
- Symptoms caused by brain lesions depend on the size and location of the lesion(s):
  - *Focal* lesions of the brain (e.g. stroke, tumour, and abscess) that cause weakness or sensory changes tend to affect one side of the body (the side contralateral to the lesion).
  - Processes that affect the brain *globally* (e.g. systemic infections, drug intoxications, metabolic disturbances, and encephalitis) generally lead to altered consciousness and/or cognition (e.g. confusion, coma), although focal signs may also be present.
- If both sides of the body are affected with weakness and/or sensory changes *without* alteration in consciousness, this makes a brain disorder less likely.

Brainstem
- The brainstem contains the descending motor pathways, ascending sensory pathways, and the cranial nerve nuclei that control functions above the neck (e.g. eye movements, facial strength and sensation, hearing, taste, swallowing, and speaking).
- Lesions of the brainstem commonly affect one or more cranial nerves, leading to symptoms such as eye movement abnormalities and facial weakness.
- Since nearly all cranial nerves project from the brainstem to the same side of the head, but the motor and sensory pathways for the extremities project to and from the opposite side of the body, brainstem lesions may cause *crossed signs*: ipsilateral dysfunction in the face with contralateral dysfunction in the extremities.

Cerebellum
- The cerebellum controls coordination. Lesions of the cerebellum lead to uncoordinated movements (*ataxia*).
- Cerebellar lesions may also cause nausea, vomiting, vertigo, dysarthria, and/or nystagmus.
- Cerebellar lesions do *not* cause weakness or sensory changes in the limbs.

Spinal cord
- The spinal cord only controls motor and sensory functions of the trunk and limbs.
- Spinal cord lesions often cause bilateral symptoms/signs: weakness and/or sensory changes in all four limbs if there is a lesion at the level of the cervical spine; weakness and/or sensory changes in both legs if there is a lesion at the level of the thoracic or lumbar spine.
- Bowel and bladder function is commonly affected with spinal cord lesions.

Nerve roots
- Nerve root lesions cause pain radiating from the neck into the arm(s), or back into the leg(s).
- If several lumbosacral nerve roots (*cauda equina*) are affected together, this may cause asymmetric bilateral leg weakness and bowel/bladder dysfunction in addition to pain.

Peripheral nerves
- Peripheral nerves may be affected individually (mononeuropathy), or diffusely and symmetrically (polyneuropathy). Less commonly, several individual nerves are affected in sequence (mononeuropathy multiplex).
- A mononeuropathy causes motor and/or sensory dysfunction in a limited region supplied by the nerve (e.g. pain and sensory changes in the lateral hand and thumb weakness with median neuropathy in carpal tunnel syndrome; foot drop and lateral shin numbness in peroneal neuropathy).
- Polyneuropathy causes diffuse symmetric weakness and/or sensory dysfunction (sensory loss, paraesthesias, and/or pain).

Neuromuscular junction
Diseases of the neuromuscular junction (e.g. myasthenia gravis) cause fluctuating, fatigable weakness.

Muscle
Diseases of muscle (e.g. myopathies, muscular dystrophies) cause symmetric proximal weakness.

Time course in neurological diagnosis
Once a patient's symptoms and signs are localized to a particular region of the nervous system, the time course of symptom onset and evolution narrows the differential diagnosis (Table 39.1).

Table 39.1 Diagnosis of neurological conditions by time course

	Brain	Brainstem	Cerebellum	Spinal cord	Nerve roots	Peripheral nerves	Neuromuscular junction	Muscle
Sudden onset	Stroke (ischaemic or haemorrhagic) Intoxication/drug toxicity Trauma Metabolic disturbance Seizure Migraine			Trauma Disc herniation Haemorrhage	Disc herniation	(Uncommon)		Rhabdomyolysis
Acute	Bacterial or viral meningitis Viral encephalitis Acute demyelination Intoxication/drug toxicity		Post-infectious cerebellitis (children)	Transverse myelitis Epidural abscess Disc herniation	Disc herniation Viral radiculitis	Guillain–Barré syndrome	Botulism	
Subacute	Fungal or tuberculous meningitis Tumour Paraneoplastic syndromes		PML	Pott's disease Vitamin B12 deficiency	Disc herniation	Vitamin B12 deficiency Drug-induced neuropathy		Drug-induced myopathies
Chronic	Dementia Parkinson's disease HIV-associated neurocognitive disorders		Alcohol-related cerebellar degeneration Spinocerebellar ataxias	Degenerative disease of the spine HTLV-1 (tropical spastic paraparesis) HIV-associated vacuolar myelopathy	Degenerative disease of the spine	HIV neuropathy Vitamin B12 deficiency Diabetes-associated neuropathy	Myasthenia gravis Lambert–Eaton syndrome	Muscular dystrophies Polymyositis/dermatomyositis

Symptom-based approach to neurological diagnosis

Confusion

Primary neurological disorders that cause confusion include:
- hyper-acute (sudden onset): seizure and/or post-ictal state; diffuse embolic strokes
- acute: meningitis, encephalitis, acute disseminated encephalomyelitis
- subacute: brain tumour (primary or metastatic), chronic subdural haematoma, paraneoplastic limbic encephalitis
- chronic: neurodegenerative dementia (e.g. Alzheimer's disease), tertiary syphilis, HIV-associated dementia.

Systemic disorders that cause confusion include:
- metabolic disturbances (vitamin deficiencies, uraemia, hepatic failure)
- systemic infections
- medication or drug toxicities.

Confusion may also be seen in psychiatric disorders, but this is a diagnosis of exclusion.

> Wernicke's encephalopathy is characterized by confusion accompanied by abnormal eye movements and gait dysfunction. It is caused by thiamine (vitamin B1) deficiency. Although this condition is commonly associated with chronic alcohol use, malnutrition can also cause the disorder. When administering glucose in malnourished patients, thiamine should always be given simultaneously to avoid potential precipitation of Wernicke's encephalopathy.

Coma

- Primary brain lesions that cause coma include head trauma, intracranial haemorrhage, meningitis, encephalitis, seizures with post-ictal state or non-convulsive seizures, and elevated intracranial pressure.
- Systemic conditions that cause coma include drug overdose, hepatic encephalopathy, uraemic encephalopathy, hypoxia, hypercarbia, hypoglycaemia, and hyperglycaemia.

Coma due to a primary brain lesion

- For coma to arise due to primary brain disease, there must be a lesion in the brainstem or both cerebral hemispheres, or elevated intracranial pressure with herniation.
- Coma with focal features (e.g. asymmetric pupils, asymmetric motor responses) is suggestive of focal brain pathology, though a large focal brain lesion causing herniation may produce a symmetric clinical picture.
- A post-ictal state following seizure can produce coma. If a patient recovers from coma with no specific intervention, consider unwitnessed seizure with post-ictal state.
- Non-convulsive seizures can produce coma with subtle findings (e.g. subtle twitching of the eye lids or eyes, gaze deviation) or with no findings beyond altered level of consciousness. The diagnosis can only

be made with EEG, which is often unavailable in humanitarian settings. In patients with unexplained coma who have epilepsy, an intracranial lesion, or active brain infection, if the level of consciousness improves with a trial of benzodiazepine, this may suggest non-convulsive seizures.

Coma due to systemic conditions

- *Myoclonus* (brief jerking movements throughout the body) can be a clue that coma may be due to metabolic causes (e.g. uraemia, hepatic encephalopathy), cardiac arrest with hypoxic-ischaemic brain injury, or drug intoxication.
- Family members should be asked what medications/drugs may be available to the patient and a toxicology screen should be performed if possible.

Headache

Headache can be classified as primary or secondary:

- *Primary*: no underlying structural or systemic cause.
- *Secondary*: due to underlying structural or systemic cause. Secondary causes of headache include pathology of any of the structures of the head and/or neck including the brain/meninges (e.g. tumour, haemorrhage, infection), eyes (e.g. visual strain, glaucoma), nose/sinuses (e.g. sinusitis), teeth/jaw (e.g. dental disease), neck (e.g. carotid or vertebral artery dissection), and systemic conditions such as hypertension, systemic infections, and giant cell (temporal) arteritis.

Secondary headaches

'Red flags' that suggest a serious underlying cause of headache related to the brain include:

- sudden-onset headache (suggests vascular cause)
- new-onset and/or progressive headache in an adult (suggests intracranial mass)
- headache worse in the supine position, with coughing, or with straining (suggests elevated intracranial pressure)
- headache in patient with cancer (suggests metastases)
- headache in a patient with HIV or other cause of immunocompromise (suggests opportunistic CNS infection)
- headache accompanied by fever (suggests intracranial infection)
- papilloedema on funduscopy (suggests elevated intracranial pressure)
- focal neurological signs (suggests focal brain lesion).

If 'red flags' concerning an underlying structural brain lesion are present, neuroimaging with CT or MRI is usually obtained. Where neuroimaging is unavailable, neurosurgeons able to intervene on tumours are often also unavailable. Therefore, if neuroimaging is unavailable in a patient with one or more 'red flags' for a serious underlying aetiology, empiric treatment of potentially treatable conditions based on the patient's HIV status and CD4 count may be considered. In a patient with a progressive, intractable headache and progressive neurological deficits in whom there is concern for a brain tumour, empiric steroids may decrease tumour-related oedema and palliate tumour-related headache and neurological deficits if neurosurgical intervention is not available.

Primary headache syndromes

The features and treatment options for the most common episodic primary headache syndromes are listed in Table 39.2.

Vertigo

Dizziness versus vertigo

Dizziness is an imprecise term that may refer to vertigo, light-headedness, or unsteadiness. Vertigo refers to a false sense that the world (or the patient) is moving, and often has an underlying neurological aetiology. Non-vertiginous dizziness has many causes including cardiac disease, medications, anaemia, and anxiety.

Localization of the cause of vertigo

Causes of vertigo can be classified as peripheral or central based on the location of the underlying pathology:
- *Peripheral:* inner ear or vestibulocochlear nerve.
- *Central:* brainstem or cerebellum.

Although both peripheral and central causes of vertigo can cause nausea, vomiting, and gait unsteadiness, clinical features that aid in localization include the following:
- Peripheral aetiologies of vertigo cause nystagmus in which the fast phase is *in the same direction* in all directions of gaze.
- Central aetiologies of vertigo tend to cause nystagmus in which *the fast phase changes direction* depending on the direction of gaze (e.g. left-beating on left gaze, right-beating on right gaze), and may be associated with focal neurological deficits such as eye-movement abnormalities and/or ataxia (though not always).

Peripheral causes of vertigo
- Inner-ear causes of vertigo include:
  - benign paroxysmal positional vertigo: intermittent brief spells of vertigo provoked by head turning; diagnosed by the Dix–Hallpike manoeuvre and treated with the Epley manoeuvre
  - Meniere's disease: recurrent unprovoked episodes of vertigo, hearing loss, tinnitus, and ear fullness; treatment is with low-salt diet and diuretics.
- Vestibulocochlear nerve causes of vertigo include:
  - acute vestibular neuritis: usually post-infectious; may be treated with brief course of steroids.

Central causes of vertigo

Central causes of vertigo include any cause of a lesion in the brainstem or cerebellum (e.g. stroke, demyelinating lesion, tumour).

Seizures

Seizures are caused by abnormal brain activity that may be either focal or generalized. Focal seizures cause focal symptoms (e.g. rhythmic movements affecting one side of the body), whereas generalized seizures cause bilateral symptoms and/or alteration in level of consciousness.

Distinguishing seizures from other spells of altered consciousness

Seizures must be distinguished from other episodes of altered consciousness such as syncopal episodes and psychogenic non-epileptic spells. This

Table 39.2 Primary headache syndromes

	Clinical features	Acute treatment	Prophylactic treatment (if 4 or more headaches per month and/or disabling headaches)
Migraine	Pulsating Unilateral Severe Photo/phonophobia Nausea/vomiting 20–25% have associated aura	NSAIDs[a] Paracetamol (acetaminophen) Sumatriptan[b] Antiemetics Ergots[b,d]	Propranolol Amitriptyline Topiramate[c] Valproate[c]
Tension	Tight feeling Generalized Moderate	NSAIDs[a] Paracetamol	Amitriptyline
Cluster	Sharp Unilateral Often associated with eye tearing, nasal discharge	Oxygen	Verapamil Lithium[c]

[a] Avoid in first and third trimesters of pregnancy.
[b] Avoid in patients with cardiovascular disease.
[c] Avoid in pregnant women and women of childbearing age.
[d] Avoid in pregnancy.

requires eye-witness accounts of events, though distinction can be difficult even with such accounts:

- Generalized convulsive seizures cause bilateral synchronous rhythmic movements, inability to respond to external stimuli, altered consciousness following the event (post-ictal state), and often incontinence and/or self-injury (e.g. tongue biting). The eyes are often open and may be deviated laterally or upward during generalized seizures.
- Syncope does not usually cause incontinence, but may cause self-injury if the patient hits their head. Patients may have brief, non-sustained twitching with syncope (i.e. a few jerks), but do not have prolonged tonic–clonic movements. Patients return rapidly to normal after the event. Patients may report feeling faint or light-headed immediately prior to a syncopal episode.
- Psychogenic non-epileptic spells usually cause erratic, non-synchronous, bilateral movements. During the event, eyes are often closed and patients may respond to external stimuli. There is often a history of psychological trauma or psychiatric disease.
- Despite these generalizations, if the clinician does not witness the event, it can be challenging to accurately distinguish between these entities. To make matters more complicated, some patients have both epileptic seizures and non-epileptic spells.

- EEG can only determine aetiology of spells if obtained *during an event* (which usually requires prolonged EEG monitoring in the hospital). A normal inter-ictal EEG (i.e. when the patient is in a normal state between events) does *not* exclude the possibility that one or more events were seizures (insensitive test), and an abnormal inter-ictal EEG does *not* prove that one or more events were seizures (non-specific test). Where EEG is unavailable (and even where it is available), clinicians should use their best judgement as to whether to try treatment for epilepsy in clinically ambiguous cases.

Provoked seizures, unprovoked seizures, and epilepsy
A seizure may be provoked or unprovoked:
- *Provoked seizures* are caused by acute reversible pathology (e.g. hypo- or hyper-glycaemia, hyponatraemia, alcohol withdrawal, acute head trauma, drug toxicity, systemic or nervous system infection, eclampsia).
- *Unprovoked seizures* occur spontaneously without reversible provoking factors (e.g. idiopathic/genetic epilepsy syndromes and brain lesions such as tumour or prior stroke, trauma, infection).
- Epilepsy refers to recurrent unprovoked seizures. Epilepsy generally requires long-term antiepileptic therapy (See ➔ 'Epilepsy' pp. 685–8).

Evaluation of seizures
- Seizures require evaluation for an underlying cause: serum electrolytes and blood sugar, evaluation for infection (including HIV), medication history (drugs that can cause seizure include isoniazid, quinolones, imipenem, bupropion, tramadol), alcohol/drug history (and toxicology screen if available), and consideration of neuroimaging (if available).
- If seizure has been provoked and the underlying cause is identified and reversed (e.g. acute hypoglycaemia; acute alcohol withdrawal), long-term antiepileptic therapy is generally not necessary.
- For causes of seizures that will take time to treat and may cause persistent brain lesions (e.g. neurocysticercosis), long-term antiepileptic treatment is generally warranted.

See ➔ 'Epilepsy' pp. 685–8 for management of acute seizures.
See ➔ Chapter 42 for emergency management of eclampsia.

Weakness

The two key clinical features used to localize the cause of weakness are:
- the *pattern* of weakness
- *physical examination findings* such as reflexes and muscle tone.

Patterns of weakness and most common localization
- Weakness affecting one entire side of the body including the face: brain (Fig. 39.1A).
- Weakness affecting one side of the face and the other side of the body: brainstem (Fig. 39.1B).
- Symmetric bilateral weakness: spinal cord (Fig. 39.1C), peripheral nerves (Fig. 39.1D), or muscles.
- Weakness affecting one region of one limb: root(s), nerve(s), or muscle(s) (Fig. 39.1E).

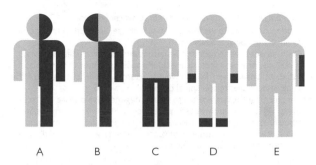

Fig. 39.1 Patterns of weakness and most common localization.

Physical examination findings in the localization of weakness

Weakness due to CNS lesions (brain, brainstem, spinal cord; *upper motor neuron*) are distinguished from peripheral nervous system lesions (nerve root, peripheral nerve; *lower motor neuron*) on physical examination:

• *Upper motor neuron signs* include hyper reflexia, clonus, increased tone (spasticity), and Babinski's sign.
• *Lower motor neuron signs* include hypo-reflexia or areflexia, decreased tone, muscle atrophy, and fasciculations.

Upper motor neuron signs take time to emerge and may not be present in acute CNS lesions (e.g. acute stroke, acute spinal cord injury). However, sudden-onset conditions are more common in the CNS (e.g. stroke) than in the peripheral nervous system.

A common cause of mixed upper and lower motor neuron signs in humanitarian settings is vitamin B12 deficiency.

Paraplegia

Paraplegia (bilateral lower extremity paralysis) or *paraparesis* (bilateral lower extremity weakness) is a common presenting pattern of weakness in humanitarian settings.

Paraplegia is most commonly caused by diseases of the spine. When bilateral leg weakness is rapid in onset, Guillain–Barré syndrome should also be considered in the differential diagnosis along with spinal cord disease. Acute spinal cord diseases is more likely to cause bowel/bladder dysfunction, and continued progression of symptoms in the legs without affecting the arms would also favour spinal cord disease as the aetiology of paraplegia rather than Guillain–Barré syndrome (i.e. Guillain–Barré most often causes upper extremity symptoms in addition to lower extremity symptoms as it progresses).

Differential diagnosis of paraplegia due to spinal cord disease

- Sudden onset: acute vertebral or disc collapse, acute spine trauma, or rarely acute spinal cord infarct.
- Acute onset (over hours to days): transverse myelitis (inflammatory, infectious, or post-infectious), epidural abscess, acute schistosomiasis.
- Subacute onset (over days to weeks): vitamin B12 deficiency, TB of the spine, metastases to the spinal column.
- Chronic onset (over months to years): degenerative disease of the spine, HTLV-1 (tropical spastic paraparesis), HIV vacuolar myelopathy, tabes dorsalis (syphilis), tumour of the spine (primary or metastatic; usually over months rather than years), hereditary spinal cord diseases (e.g. hereditary spastic paraplegia).

Common scenarios, symptoms, and signs beyond time course that aid in diagnosis of common causes of paraplegia/paraparesis in resource-limited settings:

- Profound sensory dysfunction (sensory ataxia, loss of vibration/proprioception) with mixed upper and lower motor neuron signs in the setting of bilateral lower extremity weakness is highly suggestive of vitamin B12 deficiency. If vitamin B12 level cannot be assessed, elevated mean corpuscular volume is an important clue, though neurological manifestations of vitamin B12 deficiency may be present with normal mean corpuscular volume.
- Visible spine deformity correlating with vertebral collapse on X-ray in a patient with paraplegia and no history of trauma is suggestive of TB of the spine (Pott's disease) where TB is common. Patients may not necessarily have a history of pulmonary TB.
- Acute onset of paraplegia in patients who swim in a fresh water lake is suggestive of schistosomiasis in endemic regions.

In humanitarian settings, infections and vitamin B12 deficiency are two of the most common—and two of the most treatable—aetiologies of non-traumatic paraplegia. If there is radiographic evidence of vertebral damage without a history of trauma, TB of the spine (Pott's disease) is the most likely treatable diagnosis (metastases are another possibility but less likely to be treatable in humanitarian settings). In cases of paraplegia with normal X-ray or CT where MRI is unavailable, empiric treatment for locally endemic parasitic infections and empiric vitamin B12 repletion should be considered.

Facial weakness

Facial weakness can be caused by lesions of the brain/brainstem or lesions of the seventh cranial nerve:

- A lesion of the seventh cranial nerve causes weakness in the upper face (inability to close eye or raise eyebrow on one side) *and* lower face (inability to smile on one side) (Fig. 39.2A):
  - Differential diagnosis of seventh nerve palsy includes HIV seroconversion (may cause unilateral or bilateral facial weakness), Guillain–Barré syndrome (usually bilateral and accompanied by extremity symptoms), sarcoidosis, and Lyme disease (in endemic regions).

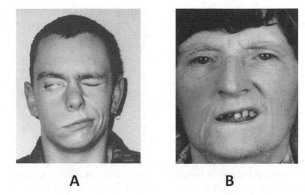

A   **B**

Fig. 39.2 Facial weakness. Reproduced with permission from Donaghy, Michael Brain's Diseases of the Nervous System (12 ed.), Oxford University Press (2009).

Idiopathic facial nerve palsy (*Bell's palsy*) is more common in the third trimester of pregnancy and in patients with diabetes. Bell's palsy is generally treated with a short course of oral prednisone.
- If facial weakness affects the ability to close the eye, the eye must be protected with a patch to avoid keratitis.
• A lesion in the brain only causes weakness in the lower face (i.e. the ability to smile) *without* affecting the upper face (preserved ability to close eye and raise eyebrow) (Fig. 39.2B):
  • Differential diagnosis of facial weakness caused by a lesion in the brain includes any cause of brain lesion (e.g. stroke, tumour, infection).

Sensory changes

Sensory loss or altered sensation (e.g. paraesthesias, pain) can be caused by dysfunction anywhere in the central or peripheral nervous system. The patterns of symptom distribution used to localize are the same as for weakness (see ➲ Fig. 39.1 p. 679). Sensory loss/changes accompanied by upper motor neuron signs suggests central pathology, whereas sensory loss/changes accompanied by lower motor neuron signs suggests peripheral neuropathy.

Ataxia

Ataxia refers to incoordination. Ataxia may be due to:
• *cerebellar* dysfunction
• *proprioceptive* dysfunction (*sensory ataxia*), which may be caused by pathology in the spinal cord or peripheral nervous system.

Cerebellar ataxia causes a tremor brought out and worsened by movement that is commonly perpendicular to the direction of movement, and may be accompanied by gait and/or truncal instability and nystagmus:

- Unilateral cerebellar ataxia suggests a focal cerebellar lesion (stroke if sudden in onset; progressive multifocal leucoencephalopathy (if HIV+ve patient with CD4 <100 or exposure to immunosuppressant medications) or tumour or if subacute to chronic in onset).
- Bilateral cerebellar ataxia suggests a toxic effect (e.g. chronic alcoholism, chronic phenytoin use), an inflammatory condition (e.g. acute post-infectious cerebellar ataxia, paraneoplastic cerebellar degeneration), vitamin E deficiency, or a degenerative condition (e.g. spinocerebellar ataxia).

Acute-onset symmetric cerebellar ataxia in children can be a post-infectious phenomenon (most commonly after a viral infection (commonly varicella)). Most cases resolve within 1–2 weeks without treatment.

Sensory ataxia causes uncoordinated movements that lack the regularly oscillating tremulous quality of cerebellar ataxia, and may be accompanied by loss of proprioceptive and vibration sense as well as hyperreflexia if due to spinal cord pathology, or hyporeflexia/areflexia if due to peripheral nervous system pathology. A classic sign of proprioceptive dysfunction is *Romberg's sign*: the patient is asked to stand with their feet together and their eyes closed; the test is considered positive for proprioceptive dysfunction if the patient becomes unstable and takes a step when the eyes are closed.

An important cause of sensory ataxia in humanitarian settings is vitamin B12 deficiency. In vitamin B12 deficiency, there is commonly a mix of both upper motor neuron signs and lower motor neuron signs. An elevated mean corpuscular volume is suggestive corroborating evidence, but may not be present in all cases.

Diagnosis and management of neurological disease in humanitarian settings

Stroke

Diagnosis of stroke

Stroke refers to sudden-onset neurological deficits caused by either:
• cerebral ischaemia or
• intracerebral haemorrhage.

These two aetiologies of stroke can be distinguished by CT (Fig. 39.3):
• Intracerebral haemorrhage: *hyper*density (Fig. 39.3A).
• Ischaemic stroke: normal acutely, *hypo*density after 6–12 hours (Fig. 39.3B).

> CT is often unavailable in humanitarian settings. The following signs at stroke onset (in addition to acute-onset focal deficits) are suggestive of intracerebral haemorrhage rather than ischaemia as the cause of stroke headache, nausea/vomiting, coma, diastolic BP >110 mmHg.[3]

Management of stroke

General acute supportive treatment for both ischaemic stroke and intracerebral haemorrhage includes:
• prevention of aspiration
• maintenance of euglycaemia and euthermia
• prevention of deep venous thrombosis (pharmacological prophylaxis is safe immediately after ischaemic stroke and as soon as 24 hours after intracerebral haemorrhage)
• treatment of seizures if they occur
• early mobilization.

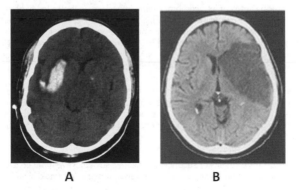

A   **B**

Fig. 39.3 CT of stroke. A. Hemorrhagic Stroke. B. Ischemic Stroke

Image A reproduced from Warrell, David A., et al. Oxford Textbook of Medicine 5e (2010);
Image B reproduced from Manji, Hadi, Oxford Handbook of Neurology 2e (2014), with permission from Oxford University Press.

Two key parameters differ between acute management of ischaemic stroke and intracerebral haemorrhage:

- BP:
  - Ischaemic stroke: BP generally allowed to auto-regulate (as high as 220/110 mmHg) for first 24 hours after onset, then lowered gradually.
  - Intracerebral haemorrhage: BP controlled (at least <180 mmHg systolic; appears safe to go as low as 140 mmHg, but of uncertain benefit)
- Coagulation:
  - Ischaemic stroke: thrombolysis or antiplatelets administered (though thrombolysis generally not available/feasible in humanitarian settings)
  - Intracerebral haemorrhage: coagulopathy reversed (though reversal agents are typically not available in humanitarian settings), and aspirin/anticoagulants withheld.

If CT is unavailable to determine if stroke is ischaemic versus haemorrhagic, decision analysis modelling suggests that if stroke is clinically thought to be ischaemic, it may not be unreasonable to administer aspirin after 24 hours.[4]

Beyond acute management of stroke, hospitalization focuses on determining the underlying aetiology for secondary prevention, supportive care, and rehabilitation. Evaluation for aetiology of ischaemic stroke involves:

- determining if the patient has modifiable risk factors: hypertension, diabetes, hyperlipidaemia, and/or smoking
- echocardiography (if available) to look for valvular lesions or thrombus
- cardiac monitoring to look for atrial fibrillation
- imaging of the arteries of the head and neck with ultrasound, CT angiogram, or magnetic resonance angiogram (if available) to look for stenotic vessels (if there are local surgeons capable of intervening on such vascular lesions).

Common causes of intracerebral haemorrhage are uncontrolled hypertension, trauma, vascular malformation, anticoagulant use, and, in the elderly, amyloid angiopathy. Evaluation for underlying vascular malformation can only be undertaken with angiography (CT, magnetic resonance, or digital subtraction) and such malformations require advanced neurosurgical care often unavailable in resource-limited settings.

Beyond traditional cardiovascular risk factors, endocarditis, chronic meningitis (TB or fungal), meningovascular syphilis, sickle cell anaemia, and hypercoagulable states should be considered as causes of stroke, especially in patients who are young and/or without cardiovascular risk factors.

Secondary prevention of stroke

- Important elements of secondary ischaemic stroke prevention: control of hypertension, diabetes, and cholesterol, and quitting smoking and aspirin.
  - Long-term, daily low-dose aspirin (70–100 mg) is an effective secondary prevention medication, unless the patient has atrial fibrillation, which requires anticoagulation where feasible. If atrial fibrillation

is discovered and anticoagulation is not feasible due to resource limitations (often the case in humanitarian settings), low-dose aspirin should be administered (no clear benefit—and increased bleeding risk—with higher aspirin doses).

- The most important element of secondary prevention of intracerebral haemorrhage is control of hypertension.
- Where CT is unavailable to determine the underlying aetiology of stroke (i.e. ischaemic vs haemorrhagic), decision analysis modelling suggests that the secondary prevention benefits of long-term low-dose aspirin may outweigh the potential risks of haemorrhage recurrence.[5]

Epilepsy

Epilepsy refers to recurrent unprovoked seizures, which may be due to:
- underlying irreversible structural brain lesion (e.g. congenital brain malformation; prior stroke, head trauma, or CNS infection)
- idiopathic/genetic epilepsy syndrome.

Diagnosis and psychosocial aspects of epilepsy in humanitarian settings
Epilepsy is a clinical diagnosis: it has been effectively diagnosed and managed *without* EEG in resource-limited settings.

- Epilepsy is a highly stigmatized disease, leading some patients not to seek treatment. Community case finding is therefore an essential component of epilepsy care. Patients with epilepsy may present to mental health practitioners or traditional healers and so clinicians should collaborate with such providers in the treatment of epilepsy.
- Psychiatric comorbidities of epilepsy are common and should be regularly screened for in collaboration with mental health practitioners.
- Patients with epilepsy in humanitarian settings frequently suffer injury or death due to burns, traffic accidents, and drowning. Patients and their families must be counselled on safety: working near a fire or at heights, swimming/bathing alone, and driving should be completely avoided until seizures are well controlled for at least 6 months.
- Patients and family members should be educated about epilepsy: it is caused by brain dysfunction not by a curse or other spiritual affliction, it is treatable, and treatment must be maintained daily with no missed doses even if/when seizures stop.

Management of epilepsy in humanitarian settings
The four most commonly available antiepileptic drugs (AEDs) in resource-limited settings are phenobarbital, phenytoin, carbamazepine, and valproate (valproic acid) (Table 39.3).

- Carbamazepine is particularly effective for focal seizures, but may worsen paediatric absence seizures and other paediatric idiopathic epilepsy syndromes.
- Of the four AEDs just listed, carbamazepine is the safest in pregnancy. Valproate has the highest risk of teratogenicity and should be avoided in women of childbearing age.
- Of the four AEDs just listed, valproate is the most effective for paediatric absence seizures.
- AEDs commonly interact with other medications:
  - Due to effects on oral contraceptives, the barrier method is recommended in patients on AEDs and oral contraceptives.

Table 39.3 Common antiepileptics

	Phenobarbital		Phenytoin		Carbamazepine		Valproate	
First line	(Broad spectrum)		(Broad spectrum)		Partial seizures Women of childbearing age/pregnant		Absence epilepsy Idiopathic generalized epilepsy syndromes *Avoid in women of child bearing age or pregnant women*	
Dosing	Once daily at night		Once daily at night		Twice to three times daily		Twice daily	
	Adult	Child	Adult	Child	Adult	Child	Adult	Child
Starting dose	60 mg daily	3 mg/kg daily	300 mg	5 mg/kg	200 mg twice daily	5 mg/kg (divided: 2.5 mg/kg twice daily)	200–250 mg twice daily	15 mg/kg/day (divided: 7.5 mg/kg twice daily)
'Step' of titration (Amount to increase total daily dose each month)	30 mg	2 mg/kg	50 mg	2–5 mg/kg	200 mg total If appears to 'stop working' at 6 weeks, increase dose by one step	5–10 mg/kg	500 mg	5–15 mg/kg
Maximum dose	180 mg	8 mg/kg	600 mg	300 mg/day	1600 mg daily (total)	30 mg/kg (divided: 15 mg/kg twice daily)	2500 mg (total) daily	30 mg/kg/day

Toxicities	Serious	All: rash, liver failure, blood count abnormalities: If *rash* patient must be told to stop medication immediately. Carbamazepine car also cause hyponatraemia			
	Common	All: fatigue, dizziness, nausea/vomiting, incoordination, double vision. Valproate also causes tremor			
Monitoring		LFTs, CBC	LFTs, CBC	LFTs, CBC, sodium	LFTs, CBC
Effect on oral contraceptives		Decreases efficacy	Decreases efficacy	Decreases efficacy	No effect
In pregnancy		Do not initiate. If patient already taking, make sure on folic acid 4 mg daily; if increased seizures, may need higher dose	Second choice of these four agents in pregnancy/childbearing women	First choice of these four agents in pregnancy/childbearing women	Do not initiate. If patient already taking, make sure on folic acid 4 mg daily; if increased seizures, may need higher dose
		FOR ALL: if increased seizures during pregnancy, may need higher dose. Give folic acid 4 mg four times daily through pregnancy			
Antiepileptic drugs and antiretrovirals[6]		Patients receiving phenytoin may require a lopinavir/ritonavir dosage increase of about 50% to maintain unchanged serum concentrations			Patients receiving valproic acid may require a zidovudine dosage reduction to maintain unchanged serum zidovudine concentrations

CBC, complete blood count; LFTs, liver function tests.

- Valproate can increase the levels of other medications and attention needs to be given to those on ARTs.
- All antiepileptics carry a risk of Stevens–Johnson syndrome, a potentially fatal condition that begins with a rash. Therefore all patients (and family) should be counselled to stop antiepileptic medications immediately if a rash develops.
- Hepatic dysfunction and bone marrow suppression are potentially life-threatening toxicities and so hepatic function and complete blood count should be assessed at baseline and followed at regular intervals.

After starting a single AED at the lowest dose, the patient should be followed regularly and assessed for any change in seizure frequency, side effects, and if patient is taking the medication consistently/properly.

- If seizure control is incomplete but no side effects occur on the initial dose of a medication, the medication dose should be up-titrated.
- If side effects are intolerable, a different medication should be tried.
- If a maximal dose (or maximally tolerated dose) is reached with only partial control of seizures, a second AED may be added and slowly up-titrated.
- If seizures are recalcitrant to therapy (and patient is taking medication(s) properly), and imaging is not available, one can consider empiric treatment of neurocysticercosis in endemic regions where CT is unavailable to evaluate for this condition.

Management of status epileptics in humanitarian settings

Status epilepticus refers to continued seizures for >5 minutes or repeated seizures without return to consciousness between them. Treatment of status epilepticus involves three parallel aspects:
- Medical management of the 'ABCs'.
- Assessment for an underlying aetiology (e.g. electrolyte abnormality, drug toxicity, alcohol withdrawal, antiepileptic medication withdrawal in patient with epilepsy, intracranial infection).
  Treatment of status epilepticus proceeds in several steps:
- Treatment of seizures.
- Begin with serial doses of IV benzodiazepine, monitoring respiratory status; glucose and thiamine are generally administered in parallel in case of hypoglycaemia.
- If seizures continue, load with IV phenytoin 15–20 mg/kg (no faster than 50 mg/minute). If unavailable, can load with IV phenobarbital 15–20 mg/kg (no faster than 50 mg/minute). Continuously monitor respiratory status and BP.
- If seizures continue, can give additional smaller load of IV phenytoin (10 mg/kg) or IV phenobarbital (10 mg/kg) (or load with agent not used in previous step if both available), continuously monitoring respiratory status and BP.
- If seizures continue, the next step is to intubate the patient and medically induce a coma. This option is often not available in humanitarian settings, so treatment of seizures must be carefully balanced with respiratory status and BP parameters when administering antiepileptic medications at the doses generally recommended for treatment of status epilepticus.
- Initiate a daily antiepileptic medication (see p. 686).

Neurological infections

Meningitis

Clinical features and diagnosis of meningitis

- Meningitis is most commonly caused by bacteria, viruses, fungi, and TB, and causes headache, neck stiffness, fever, and/or altered mental status. Seizures may also occur.
- Bacterial and viral meningitis are typically acute in onset, and viral meningitis tends to be less severe. Fungal and tuberculous meningitis are typically more subacute to chronic in onset.
- Cranial nerve palsies and strokes are common in cryptococcal and tuberculous meningitis, leading to focal neurological deficits.
- CSF analysis in bacterial, fungal, and tuberculous meningitis demonstrates elevated white blood cell count, elevated protein, and decreased glucose, with the most extreme values seen in bacterial meningitis. Elevated WBC count and elevated protein with normal glucose in the setting of meningitis suggest a viral aetiology. Definitive microbiological diagnosis is often challenging to obtain in humanitarian settings.

Treatment of meningitis in humanitarian settings

- If there is suspicion for acute bacterial meningitis, treatment should be initiated immediately to cover for the most common pathogens (*Streptococcus pneumonia* and *Neisseria meningitidis*) with ceftriaxone (and vancomycin, where available); in patients >50 years of age and/or immunosuppressed, ampicillin should be added to cover *Listeria*.

- Antibiotics should not be delayed while awaiting lumbar puncture when bacterial meningitis is suspected, since delays in antibiotic initiation can lead to poorer outcomes.

- TB culture from CSF is insensitive. TB meningitis should be treated empirically in patients who do not respond to treatment for bacterial meningitis and/or who have a subacute/chronic-onset meningitis.
- In HIV+ve patients with CD4 <200, treatment for cryptococcal meningitis should be considered if there is no response to treatment for bacterial and/or tuberculous meningitis.
- In cryptococcal meningitis, patients may be highly sensitive to changes in intracranial pressure, becoming obtunded over hours after lumbar puncture. Repeated lumbar puncture may be needed during the acute period of treatment.

Encephalitis

- Encephalitis is most commonly viral, and causes headache, fever, altered mental status, and/or seizures.
- Of all of the many causes of viral encephalitis, only herpes simplex virus encephalitis and varicella zoster virus encephalitis are treatable (with IV aciclovir). Therefore, if there is concern for viral encephalitis, empiric aciclovir should be administered.

Cerebral malaria

Cerebral malaria causes altered mental state progressing to coma, often accompanied by seizures.

- Most common in children in endemic regions, but can affect adult travellers without acquired immunity.
- Funduscopic examination revealing retinal haemorrhages, retinal vascular abnormalities, and whitening of the retina is highly suggestive of the diagnosis of cerebral malaria.
- Treatment involves treatment of malaria, treatment of seizures, and supportive care.
- Mortality is high and many surviving patients have neurological deficits and/or epilepsy.

Neurocysticercosis

Neurocysticercosis causes up to 30% of epilepsy cases in endemic regions. It is caused by *Taenia solium*, acquired by eating undercooked pork. Neurological manifestations of cysticercosis are due to consuming the eggs passed in stool, which are transmitted by faecal–oral route (meaning that pork need not be consumed to develop neurocysticercosis).

If available, CT can show the various identifiable stages of neurocysticercosis which can help guide the need for treatment with steroids and antiparasitics.

- Vesicular stage (spherical hypodense cystic lesion(s) with central hyperdensity) (Fig. 39.4A) and colloidal stage (cysts with surrounding oedema (hypodensity) and contrast enhancement): treated with antiparasitics and corticosteroids (and AEDs, if seizures are present).
  - If innumerable cysts are seen (neurocysticercotic encephalitis; most commonly occurs in young women), patients should be treated with steroids only; antiparasitics can cause diffuse cerebral oedema and should not be administered.
- The calcified stage (punctate hyperdensities on CT (Fig. 39.4B) may cause seizures and/or headache. Seizures should be treated with AEDs, but antiparasitic therapy is not indicated.

Where CT is not available, empiric treatment of neurocysticercosis may be considered in patients with repeated seizures who do not respond readily to treatment with AEDs at reasonable doses.

Tuberculosis of the spine

- TB can affect the spine in one of three ways: involvement of the vertebral bodies (Pott's disease), spinal meningitis/arachnoiditis, and/or tuberculoma of the spinal cord.
- Presentation is generally with back pain followed by progressive paraplegia and bowel/bladder dysfunction.
- Pott's disease often causes a palpable spinal deformity (*gibbus deformity*), and vertebral collapse can generally be visualized on a radiograph of the spine.
- See Chapter 31 for information on treatment.

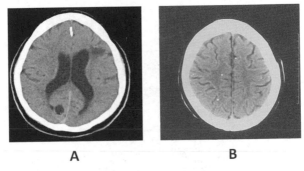

Fig. 39.4 CT of neurocysticercosis. Image B reproduced from Warrell, David A., et al. Oxford Textbook of Medicine 5e (2010), with permission from Oxford University Press.

Neuroschistosomiasis
Schistosomiasis can affect the spinal cord (leading to acute-onset paraplegia and bowel/bladder dysfunction), or less commonly the brain (causing seizures and/or focal deficits). Neuroschistosomiasis as an aetiology of paraplegia should be suspected in patients who swim in fresh water lakes and develop acute-onset bilateral leg weakness. Treatment is with steroids and praziquantel.

Leprosy
Leprosy is one of the most common causes of peripheral neuropathy worldwide, typically causing sensory and/or motor deficits in the distribution of multiple individual nerves (mononeuropathy multiplex), with the ulnar nerve of the medial arm and hand commonly affected The great auricular nerve (just beneath/ behind the ear) or the ulnar nerve (at the medial elbow) may be palpable (Fig. 39.5). See ➔ Chapter 30 for more information.

Neurology of HIV
Neurological manifestations of HIV can be caused by HIV itself, opportunistic infections, or treatment-related neurotoxicity. The neurological manifestations of HIV infection can occur at seroconversion or late in the disease:
• At seroconversion: Guillain–Barré, acute facial palsy, acute meningitis.
• Late in the disease: HIV neuropathy, HIV dementia, HIV-associated vacuolar myelopathy.

Neurological opportunistic infections can be divided into those causing global syndromes and those causing focal symptoms. Note that diffuse multifocal lesions can cause a generalized encephalopathy and global syndromes such as cryptococcal meningitis can also cause focal features such as cranial nerve palsies or strokes.
• Global neurological syndromes: cryptococcal meningitis (CD4 <200), CMV encephalitis (CD4 <50).
• Focal neurological syndromes: toxoplasmosis (CD4 <100), progressive multifocal leucoencephalopathy (CD4 <100), primary CNS lymphoma due to EBV infection (CD4 <200), CMV radiculitis (CD4 <50).

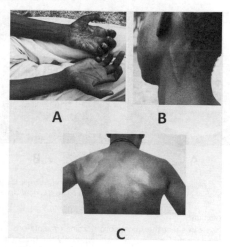

Fig. 39.5 Signs of leprosy. Reproduced from Warrell, David A., et al. Oxford Textbook of Medicine 5e (2010), with permission from Oxford University Press.

Complications related to ART include the following:
- *Distal neuropathy* with development of pain, sensory loss, and/or gait dysfunction, usually beginning in the feet (caused by didanosine, stavudine, zalcitabine). A change in antiretroviral regimen is necessary to avoid progression. Note that neuropathy may worsen briefly after discontinuation of therapy.
- Neuropsychiatric effects caused by efavirenz.
- *Immune reconstitution inflammatory syndrome (IRIS):* a clinical worsening may be seen after re-establishment of the immune system with ART. If a patient presents with a neurological infection and is found to have a new diagnosis of HIV, ART may be deferred until neurological infection is adequately treated to avoid IRIS. If IRIS occurs, steroids are used to treat this condition.

Movement disorders

Movement disorders are classified as:
- *hyperkinetic* (excess movement): examples include tremor and chorea or
- *hypokinetic* (decreased movement): parkinsonism.

Tremor

Tremor is rhythmic oscillation of a body part, most commonly one or both hands, although the jaw or head may be affected with some types of tremor.
- Bilateral symmetric tremor suggests a systemic condition (e.g. hyperthyroidism), medication effect (e.g. lithium, AEDs), enhanced physiologic tremor (e.g. due to anxiety), or essential tremor (an inherited condition).

- Unilateral tremor suggests unilateral cerebellar lesion or idiopathic Parkinson's disease. These can be distinguished:
  - A cerebellar tremor is typically not present at rest and emerges with action.
  - A parkinsonian tremor is typically present at rest and disappears with action.

Chorea

Chorea refers to continuous, irregular, non-purposeful, dance-like movements. Chorea can be caused by:

- *drugs* such as cocaine
- systemic conditions such as lupus
- *prior infection* such as following streptococcal infection (*Sydenham's chorea*)
- pregnancy (chorea gravidarum)
- structural lesions in the basal ganglia, e.g. stroke or toxoplasmosis
- hereditary neurodegenerative disorders, e.g. Huntington's disease.

Chorea in a child is commonly post-infectious (commonly post-streptococcal) and generally resolves on its own.

The most common inherited cause of chorea is Huntington's disease, which also causes neuropsychiatric symptoms. Chorea in this condition may be treated with tetrabenazine or antipsychotics.

Unilateral chorea suggests a structural lesion, and toxoplasmosis should be considered in HIV+ve patients with CD4 <100 due to its propensity for the basal ganglia region. HIV should be tested in all patients who present with unilateral chorea. Rarely, hemichorea can occur in the setting of severe hyperglycaemia.

Parkinsonism

Parkinsonism refers to the combination of the following features:

- Slowing of movements (bradykinesia).
- Resting tremor that resolves with action (most commonly in the hands).
- Cogwheel rigidity: when the examiner moves the affected limb(s) passively through their range of movement, the joints appear to 'click' through the movement rather than move smoothly.
- Postural instability.

Parkinsonism may be caused by:

- *neurodegenerative disease*, most commonly Parkinson's disease
- chronic cerebrovascular disease (vascular parkinsonism)
- *medications (drug-induced parkinsonism)*: antipsychotic, dopamine-blocking antiemetics (e.g. metoclopramide), or alpha- methyldopa; drug-induced parkinsonism is commonly bilateral but may present unilaterally or bilaterally but asymmetrically; drug-induced parkinsonism may improve when the offending agent is withdrawn (if medically feasible).

Diagnosis and management of Parkinson's disease in humanitarian settings
In Parkinson's disease, rest tremor, bradykinesia, and rigidity typically begin unilaterally (or asymmetrically) but often become bilateral as the disease progresses. Parkinson's disease is a clinical diagnosis and no ancillary testing is required.

Parkinson's disease generally responds to dopamine replacement with levodopa/carbidopa or dopamine agonists (levodopa/carbidopa preparations are the most commonly available agents in humanitarian settings).

- These are symptomatic treatments and are not disease modifying, so are only indicated in patients with disability from symptoms. These medications may lose their effectiveness as the disease progresses, requiring change in dose and/or frequency of medications.
- One medication is generally started at the lowest dose and up-titrated as necessary and as tolerated.
- A lack of response to dopamine replacement should cause one to question the diagnosis of idiopathic Parkinson's disease, as this condition almost always responds to dopamine replacement.

Peripheral neuropathy

Peripheral neuropathy may cause weakness and/or sensory disturbance (sensory loss, paraesthesias, and/or pain). Reflexes are decreased or absent in affected limbs. Peripheral neuropathies can be classified as follows:
- *Mononeuropathy*: one individual nerve affected, leading to symptoms isolated to one region of one limb. This is most commonly caused by compression or trauma (e.g. carpal tunnel syndrome affecting the median nerve).
- *Mononeuropathy multiplex*: several individual nerves affected in sequence leading to several isolated regions of dysfunction that are usually asymmetric between the two sides of the body. This pattern may be seen in leprosy, vasculitis, HIV, and hepatitis C.
- *Polyneuropathy*: all nerves affected symmetrically. Polyneuropathies can be divided into those that affect axons verses myelin:
  - Axonal neuropathies are typically caused by toxic or metabolic aetiologies and tend to affect the longest nerves first, causing a length-dependent pattern: the feet are affected and symptoms generally have ascended to the mid-shin before affecting the hands.
  - Demyelinating neuropathies are commonly immune-mediated or chronic inflammatory neuropathies affecting all nerves simultaneously, causing a non-length dependent pattern.

Chronic peripheral polyneuropathy
Common treatable causes of chronic peripheral neuropathy include:
- vitamin B12 deficiency (may be accompanied by myelopathy; see ➜ p. 680)
- diabetes
- multiple myeloma
- HIV
- leprosy
- drug-induced neuropathy
- chronic alcohol use

Treatment of the underlying aetiology (or discontinuation of the causative drug) may prevent worsening rather than improvement in the neuropathy.

Acute peripheral polyneuropathy: Guillain–Barré syndrome

Guillain–Barré syndrome is an acute-onset demyelinating polyneuropathy that most commonly emerges after an infectious illness:

- Guillain–Barré syndrome most commonly presents with weakness and/or sensory changes beginning in the lower extremities and evolving to the upper extremities, cranial nerves, and/or respiratory muscles. Autonomic instability is common.
- Diagnosis is supported by elevated protein with no or minimal WBCs on CSF analysis, though CSF may be normal initially.
- If WBCs are elevated in the spinal fluid in a patient with Guillain–Barré syndrome, HIV seroconversion should be considered.
- As treatments with IV immunoglobulin or plasma exchange are generally unavailable in resource-limited settings, steroids are sometimes considered when no other options are available (and if there is considered to be little risk of latent parasitosis or TB that could worsen with steroids).

References

1. GBD 2015 Neurological Disorders Collaborator Group. Global, regional, and national burden of neurological disorders during 1990–2015: a systematic analysis for the Global Burden of Disease Study 2015. Lancet Neurol 2017;16:877–97.
2. World Health Organization and World Federation of Neurology. Atlas: Country Resources for Neurological Disorders. 2nd ed. Geneva: World Health Organization; 2017.
3. Runchey S, McGee S. Does this patient have a hemorrhagic stroke? Clinical findings distinguishing hemorrhagic stroke from ischemic stroke. JAMA 2010;303:2280–6.
4. Berkowitz AL, Westover MB, Bianchi MT, Chou SH. Aspirin for acute stroke of unknown etiology in resource-limited settings: a decision analysis. Neurology 2014;83(9):787–93.
5. Berkowitz AL, Westover MB, Bianchi MT, Chou SH. Aspirin for secondary prevention after stroke of unknown etiology in resource-limited settings. Neurology 2014;83(11):1004–1.
6. Birbeck GL, French JA, Perucca E, Simpson DM, Fraimow H, George JM, et al. Antiepileptic drug selection for people with HIV/AIDS: report of the Quality Standards Subcommittee of the 5. American Academy of Neurology and the Ad Hoc Task Force of the Commission on Therapeutic Strategies of the International League Against Epilepsy. Neurology 2012;78(2):139–45.

Urology

Axel Bex

Context

The demographic burden of urological diseases on any healthcare system is immense. It has been estimated that every second human being will require urological care during their lifespan. It is therefore very likely that you will encounter urological diseases that require medical attention during any humanitarian crisis, but the primary aim of relief operations is the alleviation of acute distress and life-threatening conditions. As a consequence, you will not have the time and resources to diagnose and treat chronic conditions which characterize most of the genitourological diseases. It is important for providers to rely on clinical skills for the differentiations of the varying urological presentations. Within the context of humanitarian relief operations, most urological presentations will be of acute conditions.

Approach to urological conditions

Most urological emergencies are straightforward and history, symptoms, and clinical examination will most often allow proper diagnosis. While imaging is an important part of diagnostic procedures in urology, advanced imaging modalities are often unavailable in the field. Portable ultrasound devices are an exception and especially helpful to visualize obstructive uropathy, retention, collections, and blood clots.

The handling of endoscopic instruments, even if available, should be left to those with formal specialist training to avoid injuries to the patient or yourself. Likewise, IV contrast urography or urethrogram should generally be avoided by the untrained.

Urethral catheterization can be performed for both diagnosis and therapy, and catheters, stents, and drains are an essential part of urological equipment. In situations of low resources, if urinary catheters are unavailable, inventive use of other rubber tubes, infant feeding tubes, or infusion drips can be alternatives.

For normal catheterization 14–18 French (Fr) sizes are used. 1 Fr is 0.33 mm in diameter (e.g. 18 Fr = 6 mm diameter).

- Larger 20–24 Fr catheters are preferred to remove blood clots and irrigate the bladder.
- Catheters come with or without inflatable balloons and a limb for inflation, straight or curved or with an additional limb for bladder irrigation. Curved catheters (Coudé or Tiemann tip) help to negotiate the S-shaped male bulbar urethra and strictures. More commonly, straight catheters (Foley or Nelaton) are used for long-term bladder drainage.

Non-traumatic clinical conditions

Acute urinary retention

Definition
Inability to void urine.

Acute urinary retention is not a single disease entity but is caused by a variety of underlying diseases and is frequently seen in low-resource countries. Common causes are:

- benign prostatic hyperplasia (BPH)
- urethral strictures
- urinary stones
- malignancies such as prostate cancer
- bladder clot due to gross haematuria (see ➔ 'Gross haematuria' pp. 700–1)
- urethral injury.

> Note: BPH is a chronic disease and often requires surgical open or trans-urethral resection once acute urinary retention has ensued and been treated by catheterization. This however, will not be within the limits of humanitarian contexts. The same applies for urethral strictures.

Presentation
A typical presentation shows a patient in distress and unable to void.

Diagnosis
- Physical examination is usually sufficient for diagnosis and will reveal a tender lower abdomen with a palpable bladder mass.
- Additional physical examination should aim to establish the diagnosis of an underlying cause. Digital rectal examination of the prostate is mandatory.
- Patient history and inability to place a transurethral indwelling catheter may point towards a urethral stricture.
- Urethral injuries have a typical presentation and history.

Treatment
- Catheter drainage will be the primary treatment and often the only option under field conditions.
- Urethral injury can be an exception to this approach.

Transurethral catheterization
- Normally, the transurethral route is the preferred method of catheterization unless the patient's history suggests complex urethral strictures (i.e. younger age, genital trauma, sexually transmitted diseases (STDs)). In these instances, transurethral catheterization should be carefully attempted but if impossible, suprapubic catheters should be preferred.
- Although transurethral catheterization does not require great skill, it can be difficult even for the experienced:
  - The catheter should never be forced through resistance as a false route may ultimately cause more damage.
  - Never use internal metal rods to stiffen silicone catheters if you are inexperienced.
  - If attempts at transurethral catheterization fail, revert to the suprapubic approach early.

Suprapubic catheterization
- In acute urinary retention, the bladder will often contain a large amount of urine which increases the safety of suprapubic catheterization.
- Start with physical examination of the lower abdomen. If the bladder can be palpated above the pubic bone, access should be straightforward.
  - Due to the retention of large amounts of urine in the bladder the peritoneal fold and bowel is being pushed upward and the extraperitoneal part of the bladder will be exposed above the pubic rim (see Fig. 40.1).
- Current suprapubic catheterization sets provide an access sheath and the catheter that is placed in the access sheath.
  - The skin should be anesthetized with intra- and subdermal injection of 2–5 mL of 1–2% lidocaine in the midline roughly 2 cm above the pubic bone.
  - If a long enough needle is used, the same syringe can be used to move the tip of the needle perpendicular to the pubic bone at an angle of 80–90° into the bladder until urine can be aspirated. This confirms safe access to the bladder.
  - With a finger on the needle before pulling it, out the depth of the bladder can be estimated.
  - Then a small skin incision is made to allow introduction of the access sheath.
  - With gentle pressure the sheath is introduced into the bladder with correct placement usually confirmed by urine extravasation.
  - The catheter is then introduced into the bladder and the balloon inflated.
  - If no suprapubic catheter set is available, a transurethral, indwelling catheter should be placed through a *sectio alta* (cystostomy) of the bladder, a more advanced surgical procedure requiring a specialist. (See Fig. 40.2.)

Ethical considerations
Although catheterization is a successful treatment of acute urinary retention, treatment of the underlying cause is essential. Under conditions of humanitarian medicine, resources are inadequate to treat BPH or urethral strictures. Chronic indwelling catheters need care and neglect can cause urinary tract infection (UTI), discomfort, urinary septicaemia, and potentially death. Leaving patients with catheters in an environment without resources at the end of a humanitarian project is an ethical dilemma.

Gross haematuria
Definition
Visible blood in urine.

Aetiology
Can be caused by several benign or malignant diseases. Gross haematuria can be due to bladder or prostate cancer in the elderly. In younger patients, causes include trauma, stone disease and infectious diseases, bacterial UTI, or parasites.

Presentation
Generally painless haematuria, but a frequent complication is obstructive uropathy due to coagulation of blood clots in the bladder. If not evacuated, clot formation and organization may require specialist care.

(a) When the bladder is empty abdominal content will fill the pelvis

(b) A full bladder will push the abdominal content upwards allowing safe placement of a suprapubic catheter 2 cm above the pubic bone

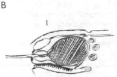

Fig. 40.1 Suprapubic catheterization.

Diagnosis

Visualization of gross haematuria is usually sufficient. Examination should focus on identifying an underlying cause.

Treatment

- In uncomplicated cases, increase fluid intake and observe.
- In case of blood clot obstruction or organized blood clot formation, transurethral bladder irrigation via catheter is recommended:
  - Irrigation catheters have an extra access for a saline irrigation drip. Preferably, use irrigation catheters with a wide lumen (20 Fr and above). Alternatively, place a standard catheter with a wide lumen and irrigate manually at intervals as described below.
  - A bladder syringe is used to create a strong vacuum for clot extraction. To avoid the bladder wall being sucked against the lumen of the catheter, vary the position of the catheter by pushing or pulling it up and down in the bladder. If clot extraction is unsuccessful, a clot may effectively have obstructed the catheter, irrigate with 30–50 mL of saline using the bladder syringe to free the catheter from the clot and allow evacuation.
  - Once the clots are removed, continuous irrigation may lead to co-agulation and decrease in haematuria. If an irrigation catheter is not available, irrigate manually with a standard catheter.
  - If unsuccessful, the patient needs endoscopic transurethral treatment under anaesthesia at a higher-level centre, if available.

Gross haematuria, especially with clot formation, often signifies serious underlying disease which will be difficult to diagnose and treat with the available resources. Even if clot evacuation was successful, resources for continuous irrigation of the bladder may not be available. If saline is not available, an alternative to consider is copious amounts of water (boiled and then cooled) by gravity-drips. If not a specialist or in the absence of transurethral endoscopic equipment, a *sectio alta* of the bladder may be straightforward to gain access to the bladder and prostate with the potential source of bleeding but aggravates the disease if bladder cancer is the cause. (See Fig. 40.2.)

(a) Anatomical borders for *sectio alta* showing the umbilicus, pubic bone, lateral borders and the limits of the bladder retention. The bladder dome may be as cephalad as the umbilicus.

(b) After the midline skin incision expose the rectus fascia and perform a midline incision between the two rectus muscles

(c) After incision of the fascia the distended bladder wall will often bulge into the wound

(d) Place stay sutures of 2–0 vicryl and open the bladder wall in the midline over a length of 2–3 cm, slightly lifting up the wall with the stay sutures

(e) Insert a 18–20 F balloon catheter into the bladder

(f) Inflate the balloon and close the bladderwall around the catheter with a purse string suture

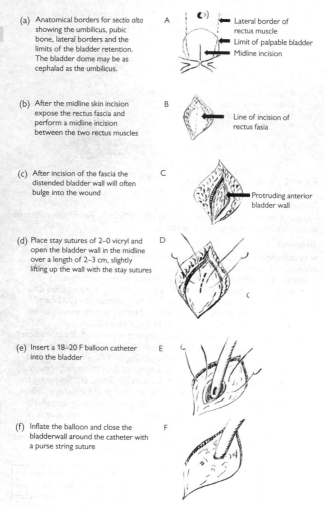

A — Lateral border of rectus muscle
— Limit of palpable bladder
— Midline incision

B — Line of incision of rectus fasia

C — Protruding anterior bladder wall

Fig. 40.2 Sectio alta and suprapubic, indwelling catheterization.

Acute scrotal pathology

Testicular torsion

Definition
Reduced or absent circulation of the testicle due to torsion of the spermatic cord.

Presentation
Acute onset of excruciating pain in the affected testicle is usually the clinical leading sign.

Diagnosis
- Clinical examination by palpation of the scrotal content is often impaired by pain and retraction of the testicle close to the inguinal canal.
  - Typically the cremasteric reflex that can be provoked by tickling the inside of the thigh is absent.
- Another condition causing severe scrotal pain is a torsion of a hydatid cyst. This can often not be differentiated from testicular torsion by physical examination and if in doubt scrotal exploration is indicated.
- Ultrasound is not absolutely required but is helpful to exclude other pathology with potentially similar clinical presentation such as epididymitis, abscess, or cancer but should *not* be used to confirm the diagnosis to justify scrotal exploration.

Treatment
- Occasionally manual detorquation can be successful without a surgical intervention. As torsion is an inward rotation of the testicle, the correct procedure is to manually rotate the testicle outward. Acute pain relief usually indicates that the procedure was successful.
- Typically, emergency scrotal exploration within 6 hours of onset of complaints is necessary and indicated to restore circulation. (See Box 40.1.)

Box 40.1 Procedure for scrotal exploration

This is an emergency procedure and can be performed with basic surgical skills if timely referral is not an option. Some familiarity with the scrotal layers is helpful but not essential.

Scrotal exploration is through a midline scrotal incision through which the tunics of the affected testis should be opened first. The testis together with the spermatic cord is easily exposed. The torsion is manually repositioned by outward rotation after which the testicle should be suture-fixed to the fibrous subcutaneous scrotal layer, repeated as a preventive measure for the contralateral testicle.

If the torsion was >6 hours, a decision has to be made to remove the testicle. This will depend largely on the appearance during surgery after release of the torsion. If the testicle fails to regain 'colour' it should be removed to prevent secondary scrotal infections or abscess from necrosis.

Testicular cancer

Definition

Malignancy deriving from testicular germ cells.

Presentation

Often, but not always, the testicle is enlarged and the patient presents with a painless scrotal swelling. If not concerned by the swelling, patients may present with symptoms due to late-stage metastasis (i.e. loss of performance, weight loss, dyspnoea, upper urinary tract obstruction).

Diagnosis

• Physical examination may reveal a stony hard mass.
• Ultrasound if available should be used to confirm an intratesticular mass and may help to examine the retroperitoneal lymphatics.

Treatment

• Basic surgical skills are required for an inguinal orchiectomy and surgery can be performed under simple conditions.
• Testicular cancer does have a fast growth rate and early metastatic spread to the retroperitoneal lymph nodes which can only be cured with chemo- or radiotherapy.
• Ideally, a patient should be referred to a nearby healthcare system with the capacity to provide pathology, imaging, laboratory analysis, and systemic therapy. With orchiectomy prior to full workup, the loss of the pathological specimen may deprive the patient of life-saving treatment decisions based on proper diagnosis. If the above workup is not available within a reasonable time frame (i.e. 2 months), orchiectomy should be performed as in cases of locally confined testicular cancer, removal of the primary tumour may be curative in conditions where chemo- or radiotherapy are not available.

Epididymitis

Definition

Inflammation of the epididymis.

Aetiology

STD, urethral strictures in the young, BPH in the elderly.

Presentation

The scrotum may be painful, swollen, red, and warm (dolour, rubor, calor, tumour). Pyrexia may be present

Diagnosis

• Diagnosis is usually clinical with painful scrotal contents and swollen epididymis (distinguished from a painless testicle).
• If the condition persists, epididymo-orchitis may develop involving the testicle and eventually the scrotal skin. In some instances, a scrotal abscess may develop.
• On rectal examination the prostate may be painful. In older men, UTI due to residual volume is the most common cause for epididymitis. In younger men, STDs such as chlamydia are more frequent.
• Scrotal ultrasound, urinalysis, and STD test kits are helpful but are not essential for diagnosis and treatment.

Treatment

- Treatment is generally non-surgical except for a scrotal abscess.
- Tissue-penetrating antibiotics (i.e. ofloxacin or levofloxacin) over 2–4 weeks are the treatment of choice but the classic antibiotics to treat UTI (i.e. trimethoprim-sulfamethoxazole or ciprofloxacin) are alternatives.
- If STD is suspected, treatment with a cephalosporin should be considered.
- If painful, the patient may be instructed to take rest and elevate the scrotum with a rolled up towel to release traction on the inflamed scrotum (See Fig. 40.3.)
- Tight underwear or swimming gear to support the scrotum is helpful once the acute inflammation is controlled. NSAIDs are preferred for pain relief.
- The patient should be instructed that although the acute inflammation can be controlled quickly, the inflammatory induration may take a long time to resolve. Residual swelling is often a reason to continue antibiotics unnecessarily beyond 6 weeks.
- If the swelling increases despite antibiotics and especially when the scrotal skin is involved, an abscess should be suspected (see following section).

Scrotal abscess

- Suspected if prolonged treatment for epididymitis is unsuccessful (see ➔ 'Epididymitis' pp. 704–5).
- If an ultrasound is unavailable, a needle aspiration may help to establish the diagnosis.

> ### Treatment of scrotal abscess
> - The abscess is treated by a small scrotal incision and evacuation of pus.
> - In large abscesses, a forceps may be introduced through the skin incision so that another incision can be made through the opposing side of the abscess wall. A drainage can be pulled through both openings and externally bend into a loop fixed with suture material to prevent loss of the drain and allow for continuous drainage until clean.
> - If the abscess will not heal, consider TB or scrotal (testicular) malignancy as a rare underlying condition.

Orchitis

Definition

Inflammation of the testicle.

Isolated orchitis is a rare viral inflammation. Orchitis is most frequent in combination with epididymitis. see ➔ 'Epididymitis' pp. 704–5.

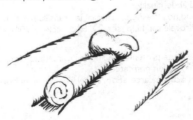

Fig. 40.3 A rolled up towel can be used to support the scrotum in case of inflammation. This enhances lymphatic flow and reduces swelling.

Non-acute scrotal swellings

The patient is often unaware how long the scrotal swelling has been present and may consider non-acute conditions an emergency. Likewise, some scrotal swellings may erroneously be considered as acute conditions by healthcare providers unfamiliar with the specific clinical signs and symptoms.

Hydrocele

Definition
Fluid collection within the tunica vaginalis.

Presentation
Painless scrotal swelling.

Diagnosis
In a shaded or darkened room, a light source such as a simple electrical torch can be used to transilluminate the scrotal content. In a hydrocele, light will shine through the contralateral skin.

Treatment
- Usually not required.
- In some rare instances, the size of the hydrocele may cause local symptoms:
  - Definitive treatment consists of resecting the tunica.
  - Tapping the hydrocele leads to only temporal relief and may cause infection or haematoma. Although tempting, it is a therapeutic misadventure.

Scrotal hernia

Definition
Herniation of abdominal content through the patent inguinal canal into the scrotum.

Presentation
Although a scrotal hernia may exceptionally present with acute abdominal pain, nausea, and vomiting, it is usually a chronic condition with a painless scrotal bulging lump which may vary in size. The swelling and a feeling of heaviness may cause the patient to present.

Diagnosis
- Physical examination reveals a scrotal bulging lump which may be repositioned abdominally.
- If in doubt and no ultrasound is available, transillumination to distinguish it from a hydrocele can help (see ➔ 'Hydrocele' p. 706).

Treatment
- This is not an acute presentation and as incarceration is uncommon, herniation may be left untreated.
- With signs of acute incarceration, surgery has to be performed.

Varicocele

Definition

Varicose enlargement of the venous plexus surrounding the testicle.

This is often due to incompetence of venous valves on the left side where the spermatic vein drains at a right angle into the renal vein.

Presentation

A chronic scrotal swelling of varying size. The swelling and a feeling of heaviness may lead to the presentation.

Diagnosis

Physical examination with classical clinical signs:

- With the patient supine the varicocele often disappears.
- When asked to increase the abdominal pressure or when in upright position, the veins fill up and yield the classical 'sac of worms' sign.

Treatment

Not required under field conditions or in humanitarian conflicts.

Spermatocoele

Definition

Cystic enlargement of a tubule of the epididymis.

Presentation

A chronic, painless scrotal swelling. Concern may cause the patient to present.

Diagnosis

- At physical examination the swelling is on top of the testicle or lateral to it.
- Ultrasound or transillumination with a flash light reveals the cystic character.

Treatment

Not required under conditions of humanitarian conflict.

Acute genital pathology

Paraphimosis

Definition
Swelling and oedema of the retracted foreskin constricting the glans.

> Paraphimosis is often caused by health professionals having retracted the foreskin for examination or catheter placement. Do not forget to bring the preputium back into its natural position afterwards.

Diagnosis
Clinical by inspection revealing the oedema of the foreskin and marked swelling of the glans.

Treatment
Manually compress the glans and oedematous foreskin to reduce the engorgement, then try to push the glans through the constricting ring. If unsuccessful, a dorsal slit in the foreskin or circumcision has to be performed. Basic surgical skills are sufficient.

Priapism

Definition
A prolonged painful erection of >4 hours unrelated to sexual arousal.

Aetiology
• There are multiple causes, including sickle-cell anaemia, malignancy, and a coagulation disorder.
• 95% of cases are ischaemic and an emergency. Hypoxia and acidosis of 12–24 hours cause irreversible damage. Intervention later than 14 hours may reduce pain but has no effect on erectile recovery.

Diagnosis
The painful erection of several hours with a typically flacid glans leads to immediate diagnosis.

Treatment
• Aspirate blood from the cavernous tissue first. Use a 20 mL syringe with a 21 G needle, placed into one of the cavernous corpora lateral to avoid the urethra. After aspiration irrigate with 0.9% sodium chloride using the syringe. Repeat this a few times, disconnecting the syringe from the needle without removing it from the corpora cavernosa.
• If the erection does not resolve, inject alpha-adrenergic drugs diluted in 1 mL 0.9% sodium chloride in the corpora. The doses are maximum doses per injection, not per millilitre. Control BP.
  • Epinephrine (adrenaline): 10–20 mcg.
  • Phenylephrine: 100–500 mcg.
  • Ephedrine: 50–100 mg.
  • Norepinephrine (noradrenaline): 10–20 mcg.

Genitourinary infections

Patients with acute urological infections usually present with fever, pain, and with signs of infection which may be general or localized. Differentiating the sources, however, is essential as the therapeutic approach may differ significantly.

Acute pyelonephritis, pyonephrosis, and renal abscess

Definition
Inflammation of the renal pelvis and adjacent renal parenchyma.

Aetiology
Generally, an ascending UTI is the most common pathogenesis. Pathogens involved are most commonly of the Enterobacteriaceae family (*Escherichia coli, Klebsiella, Enterobacter, Proteus, Pseudomonas, Serratia, Citrobacter*).

Presentation
The triad of acute-onset fever, chills, and flank tenderness that distinguish pyelonephritis from lower UTIs which have dysuria, urge, and frequency in common.

Diagnosis
- The diagnosis is clinical with flank pain as the leading sign.
- Urinalysis and Gram stain are helpful but not essential
- In acute-onset flank pain, ultrasound may help to identify underlying causes such as obstructive uropathy.
- Uncommon renal abscess is difficult to diagnose but generally distinguished from acute pyelonephritis by:
  - symptoms for >5 days prior to hospitalization
  - fever for >5 days once appropriate antibiotics are started.

Treatment
- Assuming susceptibility testing is not available, use antibiotics directed against Gram-negative bacteria (ampicillin, aminoglycosides, third-generation cephalosporins, ofloxacin, ciprofloxacin and classical antibiotics to treat UTIs such as trimethoprim–sulfamethoxazole).
- Duration of therapy should be 14 days.
- Persistent fever and flank pain in the first days after start of antibiotics are common. If persistent beyond 5 days, suspect an underlying cause such as upper urinary tract obstruction or abscess.
- If ultrasound to distinguish an underlying cause is not available, seek to refer the patient for imaging rather than switching the antibiotic.

Acute prostatitis and prostatic abscess

Definition
Acute inflammation of the prostate.

Aetiology
- Generally caused by pathogens of the Enterobacteriaceae family (see ➋ 'Pyelonephritis' p. 709).
- BPH may be an underlying cause.
- If untreated, a prostatic abscess may develop.

Presentation
- Patients have acute-onset fever, chills, and signs of UTI with frequency, urge dysuria, and even lower urinary tract obstruction due to oedema of the prostate.
- Patients feel acutely ill and may complain about perineal and suprapubic pain.

Diagnosis
Clinical presentation leads to the diagnosis in most cases.

Treatment
- Acutely ill patients require IV antibiotics. If IV antibiotics are not available, oral antibiotics can be used. Ciprofloxacin is preferred in this situation due to good pharmacodynamics and tissue penetration.
- In situations where susceptibility testing is not available, start with classical antibiotics to treat UTIs such as trimethoprim–sulfamethoxazole or antibiotics directed against Gram-negative bacteria (ampicillin, aminoglycosides, third-generation cephalosporins, ofloxacin, ciprofloxacin).
- Patients generally respond rapidly and treatment should be continued for 30 days.
- Consider using an oral antibiotic if the patient has been afebrile for 48 hours.
- Avoid prostatic massage or urethral catheters as this may cause septicaemia. Be aware of acute urinary retention. In these instances, a suprapubic catheter should be placed.

Fournier gangrene
Definition
A form of necrotizing fasciitis involving perineal and genital tissues with infection of deeper subcutaneous tissue down to and including the muscle.

Aetiology
A rare disorder with a classic presentation typically caused by staphylococcal and streptococcal strains or Gram-negative and anaerobes in immunocompromised patients (i.e. diabetes, malnutrition, HIV, consuming diseases such as cancer).

Presentation
Due to the rapid course of the disease, the clinician is more likely to observe the fully developed disease with high fever, red cellulitic perianal and genital skin, with lymphoedema extending towards the skin of the lower abdomen.

Diagnosis
- Diagnosis is by physical exam.
- An early sign may be a red cellulitis-like plaque with red streaks of lymphangitis.
- The skin is hypoaesthetic with blisters containing yellow fluid.

Treatment

This is an emergency with no time for referral. Although more than basic surgical skills are required, a delay or decision not to intervene will dramatically reduce the patient's chance of surviving. Immediate wide surgical debridement of all involved tissues with simultaneous IV penicillinase-resistant antibiotics and metronidazole followed by a second look debridement if the patient recovered is necessary. Although the debridement is in the perineal region, most structures are superficial and necrosis readily identifiable which reduces the risk of arterial bleeding from deeper large vessels. The wound is left open and plastic reconstruction is of secondary concern if the patient survives.

Acute bacterial cystitis

Definition

Acute inflammation of the bladder most commonly caused by pathogens of the Enterobacteriaceae family (see ➋ 'Pyelonephritis' p. 709).

Presentation

Clinical presentation with frequency, urge, and dysuria.

Diagnosis

Diagnosis is clinical and urinalysis and Gram stain are helpful but not essential.

Treatment

- Start with oral classical antibiotics to treat UTI such as trimethoprim monotherapy, or if no allergy is present in combination with sulfamethoxazole (TMX).
- Patients usually respond rapidly to therapy and a 3-day course of 300 mg trimethoprim/day is effective in the majority of patients.

Epididymitis

(See ➋ 'Acute scrotal pathology' pp. 704–5.)

Acute epididymitis and scrotal abscess

(See ➋ 'Acute scrotal pathology' p. 705.)

Stone disease

Stone disease is an important cause of morbidity and mortality in LIC. It affects all age groups and the most dangerous consequence is acute kidney injury, especially in children.

Presentation
- Most stones cause severe paroxysmal colics, ± nausea and vomiting.
- Haematuria and fever may be present, especially in obstructive uropathy.
- Depending on the location of the stone, the pain may be located in the flank (renal pelvis), the groin (mid ureter), or in the scrotum or labia (distal ureter).

Diagnosis
Clinically the diagnosis is often straightforward but other diseases such as appendicitis or diverticulitis are part of the diagnostic spectrum. In long-standing obstructive uropathy, clinical signs may be absent.

Treatment
- Stone disease may cause a therapeutic dilemma under field conditions due to the very restricted tools available for diagnosis and treatment.
- Fortunately, 80% of urinary stones pass spontaneously. IV fluids (saline) and pain relief assist spontaneous passage. Stones >5 mm will have a lower probability to pass spontaneously.
- Most patients benefit from IM or IV morphine (10–15 mg) and hyoscine butylbromide 10–20 mg.
- Ultrasound and plain abdominal film are minimum requirements for assessing the likely passage of a stone and course of the disease, including uropathy and hydronephrosis. If imaging is not available consider referring the patient if this is an option.
- An obstructed kidney due to urolithiasis may rapidly cause acute life-threatening septicaemia. If appropriate IV antibiotics fail, percutaneous or open nephrostomy may be a life-saving intervention.

Chapter 41

Reproductive health

Marianne Stephen

Introduction to reproductive health

The UN's Sustainable Development Goals are a set of 17 goals aiming to 'end poverty in all its forms' by 2030 and includes *improving maternal health, achieving gender equality*, and *combating HIV/AIDS*.[1] The goals encompass maternal health and universal access to sexual and reproductive health (SRH) services.

Although there will be regional variations, the fundamental principles of SRH care remain largely the same. Taking this into account, services therefore have to be individually tailored to a population's needs, easy to access/implement, and provided without discrimination in a safe environment. This means maintaining respect, confidentiality, privacy, and dignity of the people who attend at all times.

In addition, 22 million abortions are performed unsafely each year leading to death in 47,000 women and disability in around 5 million.[2] Most of these could be prevented by safe methods and providing post-abortion care. It is essential to make abortion services safe and accessible with good family planning follow-up and SRH education.

Cultural considerations for reproductive health in humanitarian settings

Whether overt or subtle, the importance of considering cultural perspectives is fundamental to establishing effective services. For example, over the years, there have been countless well-intentioned organizations and programmes aiming to increase awareness of family planning methods or widespread distribution of condoms. However, these campaigns do not always address the reality that many women do not have the voice or power in their relationships to negotiate contraceptive use.

It is important to acknowledge the restricted reproductive health rights and the challenges that women face. This can range from governmental policies which make family planning difficult to obtain, or the requirement of a husband's consent for reproductive treatments or procedures. Even beyond this, there are direct experiences with patients who have had procedures performed, without their consent or even knowledge. These key development issues have important implications in the humanitarian context.

Establishing services

There are multiple strategic frameworks and recommendations for developing a gender-based violence (GBV) and reproductive health programme in a humanitarian setting. The common features of these plans include partnership, coordination, treatment, and prevention among actors and organizations working in the humanitarian setting. In most acute crises, the UN will develop a multi-cluster system to coordinate an overall approach, though the UN agencies may be absent in some settings. In most cases, a GBV cluster will be formed to bring together the actors and organizations and to coordinate activities and resources. It is important that the plan recognizes the different phases of the humanitarian crisis and includes plans for the emergency (crisis) phase and the stabilization (post-crisis) phase.

Minimal Initial Service Package

The Minimal Initial Service Package (MISP) for Reproductive Health in Crisis Situations represents a collaborative effort between UN agencies, governmental organizations, and NGOs. It is a set of priority activities implemented during the early stages of an emergency to reduce morbidity and mortality among populations affected by crisis and/or displacement. Key objectives include:
- coordination and implementation
- prevention of GBV and assistance to survivors of GBV
- reducing transmission of STIs and HIV
- reducing maternal morbidity and mortality
- planning for provision and integration of comprehensive reproductive health services.

Various reproductive health kits are available through UNFPA with contents tailored for intended use.

Sexually transmitted infections: a syndromic approach

Sexually transmitted infections (STIs) present an enormous medical burden and there are around 498 million new cases of curable STIs occurring globally each year. Morbidity and mortality worldwide from STIs disproportionately affect women, and are almost always due to a lack of access to appropriate healthcare. In this section, guidance on treatment of STIs is simplified as much as possible, although diseases endemic to specific areas must be taken into account when implementing guidelines for treatment, as should any observed antimicrobial resistance.

In low-resource setting where diagnostic tests are expensive, limited (i.e. lack the sensitivity and specificity to be diagnostic), or perhaps simply unavailable, a syndromic approach can be used for suspected STIs. This relies on good history taking and examination, and the subsequent analysis of signs and symptoms in order to choose the most appropriate treatment option. Important points to note:

• Treatment at initial consultation—don't delay waiting for results. Patients may be unable to attend for follow-up.
• Partner treatment! It is pointless treating a patient if they will be immediately re-infected. Partner testing may require careful counselling, especially in contexts, for example, where women are marginalized.
• If treatment for STI is implemented, sexual abstinence should be advised for at least 7 days.
• Condom promotion is essential as they are only effective if used correctly. Don't assume patients will know how to use them. Obstacles to condom use include cultural beliefs and lack of access to supplies.
• Patients with STIs should be counselled for HIV testing.

STIs: the usual suspects

Bacteria
• *Neisseria gonorrhoea* leading to gonococcal infections.
• *Chlamydia trachomatis* leading to chlamydial infection and in some cases lymphogranuloma venerum (buboes or abscesses in the groin).
• *Treponema pallidum* causes syphilis (early syphilis divided into primary with ulcer/chancre and secondary with rash/condylomata lata/ mucocutaneous lesions/generalized lymphadenopathy, late syphilis with *gummatous/neurological/cardiological* features.
• *Klebsiella granulomatis* causes granuloma inguinale/donovanosis (painless, progressive, ulcerative lesions with lymphadenopathy).
• *Haemophilus ducreyi* causes chancroid (infected, painful ulcers).
• Bacterial vaginosis is a polymicrobial clinical syndrome in the vagina.

Viruses
• HIV and subsequent AIDS infection.
• Herpes simplex virus type 2 and increasingly type 1 causes genital herpes (blister like lesions).
• Human papilloma virus (HPV) causes genital warts—subtypes 16 and 18 are especially associated with cervical cancer (painless clusters, 'cauliflower' appearance or macules).
• Hepatitis B: leading to liver inflammation and possibly cancer.

Parasites
- *Trichomonas vaginalis*: flagellated protozoan, may cause 'strawberry appearance' cervix. Produces thin, frothy, greyish-yellow discharge.
- *Candida albicans*: diploid fungus, causes thrush, presenting with white 'curd-like' discharge and itching.

Taking a history

Pay special attention to the following:
- Presenting complaint and duration.
- Presence of genital ulcer: check onset/pain/recurrence.
- Presence of inguinal bubo (localized enlargement of lymph node).
- Presence of discharge:
  - Men: check dysuria/frequency/scrotal pain or lump.
  - Women: check dysuria/frequency/abnormal vaginal bleeding/lower abdominal pain/dyspareunia (pain on sexual intercourse).
- Past medical history including STIs (type, treatment, response, and test results), childbirth history in women, menstrual cycle and where they currently are in the cycle, last menstrual period.
- Menstrual history in women as this may alter diagnosis and management, e.g. in pelvic pain, ectopic pregnancy is a potential diagnosis. Enquire about dysmenorrhoea and menorrhagia.
- Medications and allergies including current contraception in use.
- Sexual history:
  - Last sexual intercourse: date and whether barrier contraception used.
  - Previous sexual intercourse.
  - Whether with a new partner within last 3 months.
  - Presence of partner symptoms.
  - History of possible sexual assault.
- Risk assessment perform if:
  - cervicitis suspected in women with abnormal vaginal discharge
  - urethral discharge in partner
  - consider in the context of sexual violence or prostitution
  - new partner or more than one partner in preceding 3 months.
- Neonatal symptoms: check for the presence if applicable, e.g. presence of eye infection with possible chlamydia infection (ophthalmia neonatorium).

Examination

Examination must be performed maintaining dignity and with respect for local culture. Ensure that the patient understands the process, through translation if necessary, and has given informed consent. Examine in a private area with the use of a chaperone if at all possible. Use a sheet to cover the patient during the examination to minimize unnecessary exposure.

For women
- Check vital signs (tachycardia/pyrexia indicating infection).
- Supine abdominal and pelvic palpation checking for pain, masses, scars.
- External genitalia looking for ulcers, discharge (colour, amount, smell), excoriation, bleeding.

- Bimanual palpation of uterus and adnexa performing simultaneous digital vaginal examination and pelvic palpation to identify size, position, and mobility of the uterus and any adnexal masses/tenderness.
- Examination with Cusco's speculum with visualization of the vagina and cervix, looking for cervical discharge, bleeding, appearance of the cervix. Swabs can be taken if possible at this point from the endocervix and high vagina.

For men

- Supine examination with abdomen exposed and trousers/underwear lowered. If no couch is available, it may be possible to examine the patient standing up although this is suboptimal and it is important to ensure that the patient is comfortable with this and understands the examination process.
- Inguinal palpation for lymphadenopathy and presence of buboes.
- Scrotal palpation feeling for testes, spermatic cord, and epididymis.
- Examination of the penis for sores or rash, retracting the foreskin to look at the glans and urethral meatus.
- Looking for urethral discharge (colour, amount, smell), milking the urethra if discharge absent. If discharge is produced this can then be swabbed and disposed of carefully.

Criteria for effective STI treatment

- Close to 95% effective.
- Low cost.
- Acceptable in toxicity and tolerance.
- Unlikely to result in antimicrobial resistance.
- Single dose and oral route if possible.
- Acceptable for use in pregnant or lactating women.
- Non-judgemental and supportive.
- Advice to attend follow-up if not improved.
- Advice for partner treatment if not already dispensed.

Flowcharts for a syndromic approach to reproductive health

This approach excludes treatment based on history only if the symptoms are observed by the healthcare provider. However, a good history may still warrant treatment in the absence of verifiable symptoms

Urethral discharge

See Fig. 41.1.

Treatment options for men and non-pregnant women
- Chlamydia: azithromycin 1 g PO single dose or doxycycline 100 mg PO twice daily for 7 days.
- Gonorrhoea: ceftriaxone 250 mg IM single dose or cefixime 400 mg PO single dose plus azithromycin 1 g PO single dose or spectinomycin 2 g IM single dose (poor efficacy against pharyngeal infections).

Treatment options for pregnant women
- Chlamydia: azithromycin 1 g PO single dose or erythromycin 1 g PO twice daily/500 mg four times daily for 7 days.
- Gonorrhoea: ceftriaxone 500 mg IM single dose[3] or cefixime 400 mg PO single dose.

> *Important*: worldwide there is concern regarding antimicrobial resistance to gonococcal infections,[4] with resistance already reported to penicillins, sulfonamides, tetracyclines, quinolones, and macrolides (including azithromycin). This is due to the rapidly evolving gonococcal gene which undergoes continual mutation. Beware of resistance and advise the patient to take medications as prescribed, and to return if no improvement is observed within 1 week. Report occurrence and use an alternative regimen if available, such as gentamicin 240 mg IM single dose + azithromycin 1 g PO single dose.

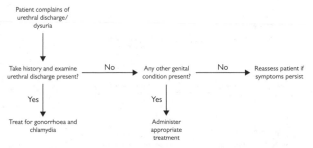

Fig. 41.1 Urethral discharge flowchart.

Vaginal discharge
See Fig. 41.2.

Treatment of bacterial vaginosis
Metronidazole 500 mg PO twice daily for 7 days *or* tinidazole 2 g PO once daily for 2 days *or* tinidazole 1 g PO once daily for 5 days.

Treatment of trichomoniasis
Metronidazole 2 g PO single dose *or* tinidazole 2 g PO single dose *or* metronidazole 500 mg PO twice daily for 7 days.

Treatment of vulvovaginal candidiasis
• Clotrimazole 500 mg pessary per vagina (PV) single dose *or* clotrimazole 100 mg pessary PV nightly for 7 days *or*
• Nystatin 100,000 IU pessary PV nightly for 14 days.

Metronidazole gel and clindamycin cream are other alternatives but will rarely be available in a resource-poor setting. Metronidazole is safe in pregnant and lactating mothers, but avoid tinidazole.

Genital ulcers
Consider differential diagnosis of lymphogranuloma venereum, syphilis, herpes, or granuloma inguinale. (See Fig. 41.3.) The frequency of certain conditions differs by geographical area and population but usually genital herpes is the most prevalent. Genital ulcers can also have more than one aetiological cause.

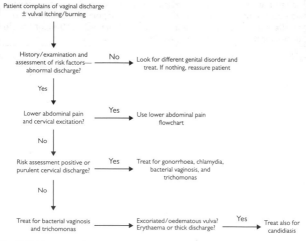

Fig. 41.2 Vaginal discharge flowchart.

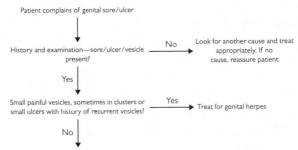

Patient complains of genital sore/ulcer

History and examination—sore/ulcer/vesicle present? →No→ Look for another cause and treat appropriately. If no cause, reassure patient

Yes↓

Small painful vesicles, sometimes in clusters or small ulcers with history of recurrent vesicles? →Yes→ Treat for genital herpes

No↓

Treat for syphilis and chancroid. In endemic areas also treat presumptively for lymphogranuloma venereum and/or donovanosis. May need referral for further treatment and investigation

Fig. 41.3 Genital ulcers flowchart.

Treatment of genital herpes
First episode

Aciclovir 400 mg PO three times daily for 7–10 days *or* aciclovir 200 mg PO five times daily for 7–10 days.

Recurrent infection

Aciclovir 400 mg PO three times daily for 5 days *or* aciclovir 800 mg PO twice daily for 5 days *or* aciclovir 800 mg PO three times daily for 2 days.

Episodic infection

Consider prolonged treatment with aciclovir 400 mg PO twice daily.

Severe infection: in disseminated infection, pneumonitis, or hepatitis
- Aciclovir 5–10 mg/kg IV three times daily for 2–7 days or until improvement.
- Encephalitis may require 21 days of treatment.
- Reduce dose if renal impairment.

> Herpes simplex virus in pregnancy can be a risk to the fetus if there is a primary infection near to time of delivery or there are active lesions at the time of delivery. If primary infection is near the time of delivery, caesarean section is recommended.[5]

Treatment of syphilis
Primary and secondary stages
- Adult: benzathine benzylpenicillin 2.4 million units IM single dose.
- Children: benzathine benzylpenicillin 50,000 units/kg IM single dose.

Tertiary stage

Adult: benzathine benzylpenicillin 7.2 million units as three divided doses of 2.4 million units IM at 1-week intervals.

Neuro- and ocular disease
Aqueous crystalline benzylpenicillin 18–24 million units/day as 3–4 million units IV every 4 hours or as continuous infusion for 10–14 days or procaine benzylpencillin 2.4 million units IM once daily + probenecid 500 mg PO four times daily both for 10–14 days.

> There is limited data for penicillin alternatives in syphilis. In primary and secondary stages, *ceftriaxone 1–2 g daily IM or IV for 10–14 days* can be considered. All penicillin regimens are considered appropriate in pregnancy. Clinical and serological evaluation should be undertaken if at all possible at 6 and 12 months after treatment.

Treatment of chancroid
- Azithromycin PO 1 g single dose or ceftriaxone IM 250 mg single dose or ciprofloxacin PO 500 mg twice daily for 3 days or erythromycin 500 mg PO three times daily for 7 days.
- Fluctuant lymph nodes may be aspirated (not incised and drained) through healthy skin.

Treatment of lymphogranuloma venereum
- Doxycycline PO 100 mg twice daily for 21 days or erythromycin PO 500 mg four times daily for 21 days.
- Fluctuant lymph nodes may be aspirated (not incised and drained) through healthy skin.

Treatment of donovanosis
- All treatment regimens are for 3 weeks or until lesions have completely healed.
- Azithromycin 1 g PO once per week or 500 mg daily or doxycycline 100 mg PO twice daily or ciprofloxacin 750 mg PO twice daily or erythromycin 500 mg PO four times daily or trimethoprim–sulfamethoxazole 160 mg/800 mg PO twice daily.

Lower abdominal pain in women
Important points
- Is the patient of childbearing age and if so, pregnant?
  - Regardless of the history, all women of childbearing age must be assumed to be pregnant until excluded by a negative pregnancy test. Local circumstances and supply will dictate availability of pregnancy tests. Beware of a possible false-negative pregnancy test, especially when suspecting ectopic pregnancy.
- Is it associated with abnormal vaginal bleeding?
  - Amenorrhoea, intermenstrual bleeding.
- Does the abdomen feel peritonitic with guarding and rebound or pain in adnexal regions?
- Is there pyrexia?
- Is there cervical motion tenderness and/or abnormal vaginal discharge?
- Is there dyspareunia (pain on sexual intercourse)?

If the pain is following delivery or abortion seek specific obstetric/gynae-cological advice. However, if any combination of the above-listed signs and symptoms are present in the non-pregnant woman, pelvic inflammatory disease should be suspected and treatment commenced. Pelvic inflammatory disease can involve any part of the female upper genital tract, including the uterus, tubes, and even the peritoneal cavity. In cases of complicated infection (peritonitis, sepsis, or abscess), hospitalization, consultation with a surgical colleague, and IV antibiotic treatment should be considered without delay.

Management
- Remove any intrauterine contraceptive and offer a suitable contraceptive replacement.
- Provide analgesia (paracetamol plus NSAID would be appropriate).
- Partner treatment for chlamydia and gonorrhoea even if asymptomatic is essential.
- Default to ambulatory (outpatient) treatment as follow-up can be difficult to organize and patients may be reluctant for admission.
- Criteria for inpatient treatment include pregnant women and those with systemic signs of sepsis or who are immunocompromised.

Ambulatory treatment of pelvic inflammatory disease
Cefixime PO 400 mg single dose or ceftriaxone IM 500 mg single dose + doxycycline PO 100 mg twice daily for 14 days + metronidazole PO 500 mg twice daily for 14 days.

Hospital treatment of pelvic inflammatory disease
Cefotetan 2 g IV every 12 hours + doxycycline 100 mg PO or IV every 12 hours *or* cefoxitin 2 g IV every 6 hours + doxycycline 100 mg PO or IV every 12 hours *or* clindamycin 900 mg IV every 8 hours + gentamicin loading dose IV or IM, 2 mg/kg then maintenance dose 1.5 mg/kg every 8 hours.

Anogenital warts
90% of anogenital warts are HPV subtypes 6 or 11; however, there are at least 100 subtypes of HPV infection and persistent oncogenic HPV infection is the strongest risk factor for the development of HPV-associated pre-cancer and cancer. Patients can be asymptomatic but can also present with itching, burning, pain, and discomfort. Treatment depends on size and location—warts can be flat and papular or pedunculated. Genital warts can increase in pregnancy and in rare cases lead to severe peripartum bleeding, but on the whole, usually do not need to be treated and regress after delivery. It is important to check that patients are tested for concurrent HIV infection.

Treatment of external warts <3 cm and vaginal warts
Patient-administered options:
- Podophyllotoxin 0.5% solution applied locally with a cotton bud, sparing surrounding healthy skin and allowing to air dry. Vaginal warts will need application via speculum and allowed to air dry before withdrawal. Apply twice daily, 3 consecutive days per week for up to 4 weeks. Contraindicated in breastfeeding and pregnancy. Do not apply to cervical, intra-urethral, rectal, oral, or extensive warts, *or*
- Imiquimod 3.75% or 5% cream, *or*
- Sinecatechins 15% ointment.

Provider-administered options:
Cryotherapy with liquid nitrogen or cryoprobe *or* surgical excision/curettage *or* trichloroacetic acid solution.

Treatment of external warts >3 cm, cervical, intraurethral, rectal, and oral warts
Surgical excision, cryotherapy, or electrocoagulation. These methods may not be available in remote settings or peripheral community clinics. They are suitable for pregnant and breastfeeding patients.

Contraception

Planned pregnancy has importance on multiple levels in humanitarian settings. Many people are not financially able to support large families. This can lead to children leaving school to work, in addition to having a direct impact on the quality of life of the family members. In terms of pregnancy itself, a great deal of obstetric risk is attributed to grand multiparity (having more than five births) and also to pregnancy very early in reproductive years, before a girl is physically and mentally ready.

Choice of contraceptive in a remote humanitarian setting is difficult. It is important to take into account the lack of gender equality and autonomy many women face with regards to their health choices. Furthermore, cultural traditions and beliefs of the population and in some cases, national laws, impact choice. Respectfully challenge those with authority if the outcome is of benefit to the patient. It is also important to involve male partners in the education and application of contraception as this may improve uptake and acceptance.

Methods must be simple and easy to administer. Remember that patients may find it difficult to come for follow-up injections or comply with daily oral medication. Make sure they understand the purpose of the treatment given to them and any side effects they may experience.

Reinforce the need for barrier contraception as the only method preventative against STIs. SRH education is paramount. If a patient does not understand why they are using a condom or taking a tablet, they are less likely to be compliant. It is also worth thinking of what methods are available locally, i.e. through local NGOs or MOH routes, as these organizations will prevail long after a project is finished. Temporarily introducing new and less available methods will only have a short-term effect.

Options

- See Table 41.1 for contraceptive methods.
- Emergency contraception can be provided in the form of levonorgestrel ('morning after pill') taken as a 1.5 mg stat dose up to 120 hours post unprotected sexual intercourse although efficacy will decline after 72 hours. A copper intrauterine contraceptive device (IUCD) or a levonorgestrel IUCD can also be inserted up to 120 hours after unprotected sexual intercourse or within 5 days of expected ovulation for a copper IUCD. Counsel the patient regarding sexual risk and long-term methods of contraception.
- Patients who have completed their family may wish to undergo a permanent method of contraception such as bilateral tubal ligation—either by cutting and tying off tubes, or insertion of a clip or ring onto the tube to prevent passage of an egg.[6] This can be done as a mini-laparotomy or basic single-port laparoscopic procedure but requires facilities with an operating gynaecologist.
- Male vasectomy is a simple outpatient procedure which can be done under local anaesthetic[6] but requires a skilled operator and may not be seen as culturally acceptable in some settings. It is a safe and effective option.

Table 41.1 Contraceptive methods

Contraceptive method	Mode of action	Efficacy and complications
Barrier contraception: male and female condoms, diaphragms, and cervical caps	Physical barrier to conception. If used correctly also prevent STIs	Male condoms 98% effective if used correctly, but with typical use, are 82% effective
		Correct use of female condoms 95% effective, cervical caps 96%, and diaphragms 92% with similar failure rates with typical use to male condom
		Use caps and diaphragms with spermicide—these do no reduce rates of HIV/STI or cervical intraepithelial neoplasia (CIN)
Combined oral contraceptive (COC) pill	Inhibits ovulation by acting on the hypothalamic–pituitary–ovarian axis and inhibiting follicle stimulating hormone and luteinizing hormone. Alters cervical mucous	99.7% effective with correct use, but typical use (including inconsistent and incorrect use) 91% effective
	Once-daily pill for 21 days then 7 days' break or placebo pills, inducing withdrawal bleed.	Not suitable with breastfeeding, migraine, hypertension, or venous thromboembolism. Increases background risk of breast cancer but decreases risk of ovarian and endometrial cancer
	Start on first day of menstrual cycle	Extra precautions are no longer advised with antibiotic use unless diarrhoea or vomiting is present
	24-hour window before pill is 'missed' (48 hours after last pill was taken)	If a pill is missed, refer to specific instructions for precautions but as a rule use a barrier method
Progestogen-only pill (POP)	Acts mainly by altering cervical mucus. 40% of cycles will be ovulatory	99.7% effective with correct use, 92% with typical
	Pill taken daily with shorter window of 3–12 hours before 'missed' (27–36 hours after last pill was taken) depending on brand	20% of women will be amenorrhoeic, 40% will have regular bleeding, and 40% will have irregular bleeding. Also can lead to altered mood and depression
		POP can be used during breastfeeding, immediately postpartum and in cases of previous breast cancer, venous thromboembolism, and hypertension

Table 41.1 (*Contd.*)

Contraceptive method	Mode of action	Efficacy and complications
Intrauterine contraceptive device (IUCD) Copper bearing: Cu-IUCD Levonorgestrel releasing: LNG-IUCD	T-shaped device inserted into the uterus. Positional effect blocks contraception in both devices plus progesterone released by LNG-IUCD has additional contraceptive properties and can also help with benign dysfunctional uterine bleeding Can be inserted immediately after surgical abortion and in first 48 hours after medical abortion, otherwise 4 weeks after. Can be inserted 4 weeks postpartum	98–99% effective but insertion must be under aseptic conditions by an experienced operator as there is a 0.2% risk of uterine perforation. *In situ* for 5, 8, or 10 years depending on individual device Devices may 'migrate' into the abdomen, check threads from cervix and by ultrasound or X-ray Risk of ectopic pregnancy is no higher than without contraception but if pregnancy occurs with IUCD *in situ*, there is a slightly raised risk of ectopic pregnancy from other methods. Ongoing intrauterine pregnancy with IUCD *in situ* carries risk of second trimester loss. If first trimester, then removal should be attempted
Progestogen-only injectable contraception	3-monthly injection administered in the upper outer quadrant of the buttock	99.6% effective. May lead to a delay in return of fertility up to 1 year Amenorrhoea in 11.4%, irregular bleeding in 52.1%, and prolonged bleeding in 33.5%. Also may cause weight gain
Progestogen-only implant	Subdermal rod, usually inserted under local anaesthetic into the underside of the upper arm, 3–5 years duration depending upon brand	99.9% effective if inserted correctly (most pregnancies result from incorrect insertion or timing of sexual intercourse on insertion/removal). Acts by preventing ovulation, serum levels are sufficient 8 hours after insertion. Fertility regained 3 weeks to 3 months after removal. Women may experience irregular menstrual bleeding after insertion

Cervical cancer

Cervical cancer results in 270,000 deaths annually, 85% of which are in developing countries, according to the WHO. It mainly affects women of childbearing age although any immunosuppressed woman, most commonly HIV+ve, will be at increased risk.

HPV and vaccination

- Cervical cancer is linked to HPV, specifically types 16 and 18, which confer a 400× and 250× increased risk respectively.
- Two types of HPV vaccine are available: a quadrivalent licensed in 2006 and a bivalent in 2007. Used in Western countries, it has been shown that vaccinating girls before their sexual debut can decrease cervical cancer over a period of time by preventing transmission of the oncogenic types responsible for 70% of cervical cancer.
- Global cost-effectiveness analysis suggests vaccinating pre-adolescent girls is usually cost-effective, especially in resource-poor settings where access to cancer screening, prevention, and treatment is limited.
- The WHO recommends inclusion into national immunization programmes, both bivalent and quadrivalent, and there are various ongoing delivery strategies, campaigns, and outreach projects. Considerations include compatibility with 'cold chain' facilities (ability to transport and store vaccines at the correct temperature), affordability, and level of coverage. At present, WHO does not consider male vaccination a priority.
- Health education and condom promotion are required as increased exposure to unprotected sex with multiple partners is a risk factor.

Screening

There is an increasing need to set up cervical screening in humanitarian settings despite the challenges this may present. 'Screening' implies that all women would be regularly called up for examination but in reality, it may be done more on an opportunistic basis in some settings, e.g. approaching women when they present with a medical issue.

VIA (visual inspection with acetic acid) and VILI (visual inspection with Lugol's iodine) are the general method used in low-resource settings as it can be done by a less experienced operator and under direct vision. VIA relies on the principle that abnormal cervical tissue turns white when vinegar is applied. When iodine is then applied, pre-cancerous cells turn a mustard colour, squamous epithelium black, and columnar epithelium pink. Average sensitivity of VIA is 77% and specificity 86% for detecting pre-cancerous cells, with VILI up to 92% sensitive and 85% specific.

Management

Methods for removing precancerous cells of any CIN grade include electro-cautery loop excision, cryotherapy, or 'cold knife' cone biopsy, all of which should be performed by an experienced operator. Any carcinoma *in situ* or invasive disease would need referral to a tertiary centre with the capacity for gynaecological surgery. At field level any necessary supportive measures would be appropriate, such as analgesia, antibiotics, and blood transfusion, in addition to palliative care and emotional support.

Bartholin's cyst and abscess

Bartholin's glands are located to either side of the vaginal introitus, and if a mass is palpable, it will be located on the inner aspect of the labia minora, sometimes bulging into the vagina if very large. The normal function of the Bartholin's gland is to produce mucous which aids with lubrication. A Bartholin's abscess or cyst may present with pain and swelling, and may be discharging if ruptured. For differentiation between a Bartholin's abscess and a cyst, see Table 41.2.)

If the presentation is of an abscess then it is reasonable to commence an oral antibiotic to try and minimize progression, although this is unlikely to cure an infected collection. Co-amoxiclav or a cephalosporin + metronidazole are good choices.

Surgical management of Bartholin's cyst is only recommended if the patient is very symptomatic as it is common for bleeding to occur from the bed of the excised cyst. Otherwise manage conservatively. Surgical management of both a cyst and an abscess can be achieved under local anaesthetic and this procedure requires only a basic level of surgical skill. Beware, however, of excising hard, inflamed tissue—this may only be cellulitis of the area and incision will not yield any fluid or pus.

Table 41.2 Bartholin's abscess and cyst

Abscess	Cyst
Gland is enlarged and fluctuant	Gland is enlarged and fluctuant
Erythema present	Erythema absent
Surrounding tissue inflammation and cellulitis	Surrounding tissue not inflamed and cellulitis absent
Pyrexia possibly present ± tachycardia	No pyrexia
Raised white blood cell count (lab tests may be unavailable)	No raise in white blood cell
Bacteria and white blood cells present in pus contained within gland	No bacteria or white blood cells in serous fluid within cyst

Excision of a Bartholin's gland cyst

- Infiltrate subcutaneously with local anaesthetic making sure not to inject intravenously (draw back on the syringe before injecting). A good choice would be lidocaine, 1% 5–10 mL subcutaneously around the mass, causing a 'bleb' of the skin but being careful not to enter the cavity of the mass, therefore rupturing it.
- Make an incision over the mucosa of the cyst (medial aspect of the labia minora). This is preferable to the outer vulval skin as dissecting the cyst wall from the outer skin is more likely to tear it. An opening through the outer skin may result in a permanent fenestration.
- Bluntly dissect out the cyst with a finger/scalpel handle or with dissecting scissors if necessary. Try not to rupture the cyst—if it is removed intact without leaving any capsule behind this may reduce the risk of recurrence or a residual nodule. If the capsule is ruptured, it may be possible to peel it from the cyst bed.
- Ensure haemostasis at the base of the cavity with mattress sutures if needed, using a delayed absorbable suture such as Vicryl®. Do not suture too tightly as this may cause necrosis.
- Marsupialization may be required to keep a tract open and allow drainage of the gland, although it is most useful in chronic or recurrent abscesses. This technique involves cutting a slit into the cyst/abscess and suturing the edges to form a continuous surface from the exterior surface to the interior surface of the cyst/abscess. See Fig. 41.4.
- Again under local anaesthetic with an incision in the same position as the cyst over the fluctuant point.
- The contents (pus) are drained and it is possible to irrigate the cavity with sterile water or saline. Break down any internal loculations with blunt finger dissection as pockets of pus will allow the abscess to re-accumulate.
- It is rarely possible to remove any capsule from an abscess, instead the internal cavity lining is everted and approximated to the vaginal mucosa with interrupted 3.0 delayed absorbable sutures. This will leave the incision open and create a tract, allowing the contents to drain, minimizing recollection
- A formal drain or pack is not needed but the site should be kept clean and the course of antibiotics complete.

(a)

(b)

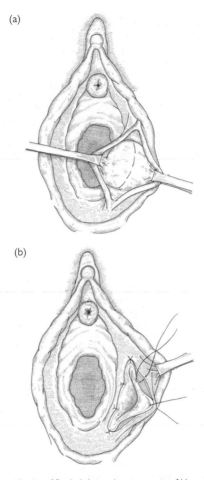

Fig. 41.4 Marsupialization of Bartholin's cyst. Image courtesy of Hannah Megee 2013.

Female genital mutilation

Female genital mutilation (FGM) or cutting is defined as all procedures involving partial or total removal of the external female genitalia or other intentional injury to the female genital organs, whether for cultural or other non-therapeutic reasons. There are no medical benefits. UNICEF estimates that worldwide 125 million women and girls have undergone FGM and that it is a traditional practice in 29 African countries—the top five are currently Somalia (98%), Guinea (96%), Djibouti (93%), Egypt (91%), and Eritrea (89%). FGM is also practised in Yemen, Iraq, Kurdistan, Malaysia, and Indonesia, and other countries. These procedures are commonly carried out on girls between the age of infancy and 15 years, often by a local practitioner or elder under unsanitary conditions and without pain relief. See ➲ Chapter 5 for more information.

The British Journal of Obstetrics and Gynaecology explored the 'significant, negative psychophysical outcomes' of this practice in a recent 2014 article. The paper identified 'key knowledge gaps in the clinical care of women with FGM' and focused on obstetric outcomes, surgical interventions, and the skills and training of health care professionals involved in preventing and managing FGM.[7]

Types of FGM

- *Type 1: cliteroidectomy*—partial or complete removal of the clitoris and/ or prepuce.
- *Type 2: excision*—partial or total removal of the clitoris and labia minora and/or excision of the labia majora.
- *Type 3: infibulation*—narrowing of the vaginal orifice with creation of a covering seal by cutting and opposing the labia minora and/or the labia majora, with or without excision of the clitoris.
- *Type 4:* pricking, piercing incising, scraping, and cauterizing not for medical purposes.

Complications of FGM

Immediate complications can include:

- haemorrhage
- infection: bacterial, tetanus, risk of HIV transmission if shared tools/ instruments
- urinary retention and renal failure
- death of the girl/woman.

Long-term complications can include:

- haematocolpos (filling of the vagina with menstrual blood due to blocked outflow)
- abscess formation and fusion of tissues
- chronic vaginal infection and painful sexual relations
- rape and sexual assault due to inability to penetrate the vagina
- complications during childbirth and the postpartum period for both mother and baby, including neonatal death. The more anatomically destructive the mutilation, the greater risk of obstetric sequelae
- infertility
- death of the girl/woman.

Management

Infibulation may be reversed by *defibulation* (removal of this physical barrier) in a sterile surgical setting antenatally, in the first stage of labour, during delivery itself, or perioperatively after caesarean section (if planned defibulation is deferred due to mode of delivery becoming caesarean).

Defibulation prior to delivery

A catheter is placed if possible prior to procedure and an incision made along the vulval excision scar. Diathermy incision can be useful to prevent bleeding. The incised edges are sutured with absorbable suture material and antibiotic prophylaxis given (cephalosporin + metronidazole).

If vaginal access is adequate, defibulation may occur naturally at delivery or can be carried out by an experienced professional then. A useful guide is that if the urethral meatus is observed or if two fingers can be inserted into the vagina without discomfort, the infibulation is unlikely to impede the process of labour. When performing defibulation in labour it is better to use scissors just prior to crowning of the head. Lidocaine without adrenaline may be infiltrated and an episiotomy is often also required due to scarring of the vaginal introitus. *Cutting excessive or multiple episiotomies to expedite labour is not a substitute for defibulation in a case of obstructed labour due to FGM.*

Women may request reinstatement of infibulation postpartum, however, there is no ethical or medical reason to perform this procedure and medical staff working with a humanitarian organization should never do so. There could be serious implications for medicalizing and thus legitimizing this procedure. There is no evidence that performing it in medicalized, sanitary circumstances reduces complications in the long term.[8]

General approach

Medical and psychological management of the consequences of FGM is paramount in both acute and chronic settings. Any real change in the practice of FGM will come from education, research, and development. A global strategy has been implemented by the WHO in order to help communities abandon FGM practices.[9]

When discussing FGM, consider the local cultural practices and traditions—the role of women within the society. Woman may have few decision-making abilities so early dialogue is needed during antenatal appointments so that an agreement and plan can be put in place. An explanation of policies and guidelines may be helpful, and take the opportunity to dispel any misconceptions and give education.

Termination of pregnancy

The purpose of this section is to talk about the specific practice and methodology for surgical and medical abortion, in addition to discussing the implications for setting up and safely running such a service in a field or humanitarian setting, and what kind of realistic legacy to leave when a project finishes. Healthcare services are often first to suffer in a crisis situation where infrastructures may be threatened or have broken down. Access to adequate healthcare services is a fundamental human right but, sadly for many people, not a reality.

The debate over abortion is not new, but whether it is deemed right or wrong, it is a part of all cultures and societies, albeit often marked by stigma and secrecy. As medical practitioners we are obliged to offer care without discrimination, and although many people would not choose to be part of a termination of pregnancy it is undeniably an essential part of any SRH service. This is because it can be life-saving, either as abortion or post-abortion care. The context may be complicated by underlying issues such as sexual and gender-based violence and unwanted pregnancy. Unsafe abortion is associated with significant maternal mortality.

The more women are marginalized for seeking abortion services, the more likely they are to receive them from unsafe and unsanitary sources. Any abortion service set-up must have clear objectives and provide a safe and confidential environment for surgical and medical terminations, in accordance with current guidelines, either international such as WHO or specific to an organization. Often a combination of these will be appropriate. Tragically, if abortion is not offered in safe conditions, women will source it elsewhere through desperation. Subsequently, they present with serious complications such as sepsis and organ damage. Each year, 21.6 million women experience unsafe abortion worldwide with 18.5 million of these occurring in developing countries. Annually, 47,000 women die from the complications of unsafe abortion with deaths related to this contributing to around 13% of maternal deaths.

An in-depth analysis of the local context is required which needs to include national law, customary law, practicalities of setting up clinical services in communities, and educational platforms.

General guidance for termination of pregnancy care

Counselling

Patient should be clear in their decision and not coerced in any way. They should receive practical information on the procedure and risks, in addition to worsening advice about post-procedure complications and also a comprehensive plan for family planning follow-up.

Consent

A simple method of consent should be taken. This could be a confidential register with the patient's details, signature or thumb print for those who cannot write as consent, and method of abortion marked as complete or incomplete post procedure (this will help identify those who need additional medical management or proceed to surgical management). This helps with record keeping and data collection. Also record the method of family planning administered to keep data on uptake rates and methods.

Medical termination

- Pregnancy up to 63 days (9 weeks): use mifepristone (progesterone receptor antagonist) 200 mg PO followed by misoprostol (prostaglandin) 24–48 hours later, PV, sublingually or bucally 800 mcg, PO 400 mcg. Between 7 and 9 weeks, do not use an oral preparation.
- First trimester pregnancy 63–84 days (9–12 weeks) and second trimester 1–24 weeks: mifepristone 200 mg PO followed by misoprostol 800 mcg PV 36–48h later. Subsequent doses of misoprostol 400 mcg 3-hourly PV until expulsion up to four doses.
- >24 weeks' gestation: decrease the dose of misoprostol to 200 mcg as the uterus becomes more sensitive to prostaglandins. Beware of the risk of uterine rupture in a previous uterine scar, therefore careful observation is necessary.

Surgical termination

- Manual vacuum aspiration (MVA) is recommended over traditional dilation and curettage (D&C) as it is safer and easy to perform in outpatient settings. It involves a plastic suction curette inserted into the dilated cervix which is connected to a large syringe.
- This should only be performed by an experienced operator. It is useful for incomplete medical abortion and presenting septic or failed abortions performed elsewhere.

Pre-termination care

- Ultrasound is not absolutely necessary prior to abortion in a low-resource setting, although can be useful if available in differentiating ectopic and molar pregnancies. Beware of incomplete abortion with scanty products expelled in the presence of localized iliac fossa pain. If products appear unusual (grape-like clusters or vesicles), it could indicate possible molar pregnancy or choriocarcinoma, which has a higher incidence in Asian populations and carries a risk of bleeding. This requires referral to a tertiary centre and appropriate follow-up.
- For surgical procedures, the cervix should be prepared with misoprostol 400 mcg PV, sublingual, or buccal routes to aid cervical dilation at any gestational age and regardless of parity. Surgical terminations should also have antibiotic prophylaxis—ceftriaxone 1 g IM just prior to procedure then doxycycline 100 mg PO twice on the day of procedure or ofloxacin 400 mg PO twice on the day of procedure.[2]
- Pain management includes non-steroidal anti-inflammatories and paracetamol. For surgical procedures performed without general anaesthetic, a tranquillizer such as diazepam may be helpful or a stronger analgesic such as tramadol, PO or IM routes. Infiltration of local anaesthetic to the cervix is also an option.

Post-termination care

- Determine family planning methods prior to the patient's departure.
- No routine follow-up is needed but the patient must be aware of possible post-procedure complications such as bleeding, infection, and incomplete abortion, and to re-present if any symptoms occur.
- Check rhesus blood type incompatibility. Any rhesus negative patients undergoing medical abortion >9 weeks or any surgical procedure should have anti-D immunoglobulin injection within 72 hours of completion. Medical terminations <9 weeks do not require anti-D. Offer STI screening including HIV test.[2]

Dysfunctional uterine bleeding

The menstrual cycle is measured from the first day of a bleed to the first day of the next bleed. A mean cycle is 28 days with the bleeding period lasting 3–8 days. The upper limit of menstrual blood loss is ~60–80 mL. The pattern changes with age. The cycle length decreases, the duration of a period decreases, and the bleeding becomes more irregular and erratic towards the menopause (the perimenopausal stage). Menopause is usually a retrospective diagnosis when a woman has at least 1 year of amenorrhoea, typically between the age of 45–50 years, although it can be difficult to give a firm diagnosis due to irregular bleeding.

- *Menorrhagia*: abnormally heavy menstrual bleeding.
- *Intermenstrual bleeding*: irregular bleeding between periods.
- *Dysmenorrhoea*: lower abdominal/pelvic pain related to periods, prior to and during menstruation.

A comprehensive history is needed

- Current age, age at menarche, age of possible menopause (if relevant).
- Obstetric history: number of children and mode of delivery, miscarriages, terminations. Test for pregnancy to exclude intrauterine or ectopic.
- Usual bleeding pattern: cycle length (from day 1 of bleed to day 1 of next bleed), duration of bleeding, regularity, intermenstrual bleeding, heaviness ('flooding' would be described as soaking through clothes/ pads), last menstrual period.
- Contraceptives currently in use.
- Useful to know if they have ever had cancer of ovary/breast due to association although this information might not be available.
- Current symptoms: heavy bleeding, irregular bleeding, pelvic pain (when in relation to cycle?), dyspareunia, postcoital bleeding, urinary or bowel symptoms (could be a result of large uterine fibroids).
- Any medical conditions including thyroid problems, haematological disorders, e.g. von Willebrand disease—these may be difficult to diagnose in field settings.

Examination

- Observations including pulse, temperature, BP, general demeanour, presence of pallor, or shortness of breath.
- Abdominopelvic examination checking for pain, adnexal masses, palpable uterine fundus. The uterus should not be palpable outside of pregnancy but can be sized in comparison. A fundus felt at the level of the pubic symphysis is classified as a bulky '12-week' uterus, at the level of the umbilicus it is '20–22 week' size.
- Bi-manual examination digitally with two fingers in the vaginal fornix and the other hand palpating abdominally. Adnexal masses may be balloted between two hands. Check uterine size, position (anteverted it will be falling forward in the abdomen, retroverted it will lie towards the back). Check if the uterus feels mobile or fixed, bulky or irregular. Note if palpation elicits pain.
- Speculum examination to check for abnormal-looking cervix or cervical polyp as a cause of bleeding.

Menorrhagia and intermenstrual bleeding

Causes
- Uterine fibroids: benign tumours of the myometrium, more prevalent in African women.
- Uterine or cervical polyps.
- Less commonly endometriosis: growth of the lining of the uterus (endometrium) outside the uterine cavity.
- Thyroid or blood disorders such as von Willebrand disease: these may be difficult to diagnose without laboratory investigations.
- Endometrial dysplasia: less common prior to menopause. In postmenopausal women, any bleeding must be investigated with endometrial biopsy, usually by dilation of the cervix and curettage of the endometrial lining (D&C) under anaesthetic. Sample is sent for histopathological examination if possible.
- Cervical neoplasia (see ➡ 'Cervical cancer' p. 728).

Treatment
- First-line treatment of benign menorrhagia or intermenstrual bleeding (not due to haematological or endocrine disorders) is usually hormonal. It is reasonable to commence oral combined or progestogen-only contraceptive in order to regulate bleeding. A levonorgestrel IUCD (progestogen-secreting intrauterine device) is an effective way of treating heavy menstrual bleeding and can shrink fibroids in some cases. Tranexamic acid (a fibrinolytic) can also be used at a dose of 1 g four times daily maximum PO daily.
- Surgical management should be undertaken by an experienced gynaecologist and includes myomectomy (surgical excision of fibroid lesions), polypectomy (removal of cervical or endometrial polyp) or hysterectomy (removal of the uterus).

Dysmenorrhea

Causes
- *Primary dysmenorrhoea* indicates no underlying pathology and may be due to release of prostaglandins leading to increased uterine tone and myometrial ischaemia. It could also be due to an imperforate hymen
- *Secondary dysmenorrhoea* has an underlying pathology and usually a later onset. Causes include adenomyosis (presence of endometriosis within the uterine myometrium), cervical stenosis post procedure, congenital malformations, endometrial polyps, fibroids, IUCD present, pelvic inflammatory disease (see ➡ 'Lower abdominal pain in women' pp. 722–3), ovarian tumour—symptoms.

Treatment
- Conservative measures for primary dysmenorrhoea include advice on stress reduction, smoking cessation, and reduced alcohol intake.
- Remove an IUCD if present and a possible source of pain. Use of NSAIDs such as ibuprofen are effective if no contraindications.

- The combined oral contraceptive pill may be used as treatment of hormonal and cycle-related dysmenorrhoea.
- Cervical stenosis may be treated by dilation of the cervical canal under anaesthetic. Likewise, removal of any polyp may relieve symptoms. Adenomyosis and fibroids may be treated hormonally as previously described, and pelvic inflammatory disease must be treated with antibiotics as per protocol. Any surgery will require referral to the appropriate specialist.

Fistula

An obstetric fistula usually results from a prolonged second stage of labour (the woman is fully dilated) when the pressure of the baby's head erodes through the vaginal wall to form a connection with the bladder (vesico-vaginal), the rectum (recto-vaginal), the cervix (cervico-vaginal), or the uterus (utero-vaginal). Vesico-vaginal fistula is most common, then recto-vaginal, and fistulas can occur at multiple sites simultaneously.

It is important to take into account psychosocial factors. The defect often means that women will leak urine or faeces into the vagina. This can cause an odour and can lead to stigmatization, embarrassment, shame, and social exclusion. Sexual relationships and marriages are also affected and a woman may be rejected by society. In societies where obstetric fistulas are prevalent, there are often inadequate medical services during childbirth, and women are left without correct treatment of their subsequent condition.

Risk factors for complicated labour and subsequent fistula

- Short stature which may lead to obstructive delivery.
- Prolonged second stage of labour (full dilatation) ranging from 4 hours to several days.
- Lack of access to safe obstetric care, e.g. caesarean section in obstructed labour.
- Lack of family planning and antenatal care.
- Early marriage and young age at delivery.
- Practices such as FGM.

Prevention of obstetric fistula hinges on good care in and around childbirth—access to appropriate services, including operative vaginal delivery, and identifying signs of obstructive delivery using the WHO partograph (see ➡ Chapter 42). If an obstetric fistula is suspected, precautions should be taken immediately—it may be possible for a small defect to close if given time to heal (15–20%).

Management of obstetric fistula

- Check for faecal or urinary soiling, dermatitis, or ulceration of genitalia due to ammonia.
- Check for genital trauma.
- Check for signs of UTI or renal stones secondary to dehydration.
- Insert a size 16 or 18 Foley catheter if suspicious of vesico-vaginal fistula. This may be *in situ* for up to 6 weeks, although if there is no evidence of urine vaginally after 14 days it may be removed.
- Perform vaginal speculum examination as soon as possible and remove any damaged/necrotic tissue. A defect may not be immediately apparent. If possible, use methylene blue dye, inserted into the bladder by means of the catheter, clamped off for 30 minutes to allow the bladder to fill. Perform speculum examination to check for the presence of blue dye in the vagina, indicating a vesico-vaginal defect.
- Twice-daily cleaning of the vagina with saline solution.
- Encourage the woman to drink fluids—women with fistulae tend to dehydrate themselves as they are fearful of passing urine and smelling.
- Prophylaxis against UTI may be considered and any revealed infection should be treated.

Any proven fistula that requires repair, fresh or old, must be referred to the appropriate facility for surgical management as this is highly specialized. Patients will require an in-depth explanation of their condition and are likely to need additional support such as counselling, including on implications for future pregnancies.

References

1. United Nations. Sustainable Development Goals. ℘ http://www.sustainabledevelopment. un.org
2. World Health Organization, Department of Reproductive Health and Research. Safe Abortion: Technical and Policy Guidance for Health Systems. 2nd ed. Geneva: WHO; 2012. ℘ http://www.who.int/reproductivehealth/publications/unsafe_abortion/9789241548434/ en/
3. Barry PM, Klausner JD. The use of cephalosporins for gonorrhoea: the impending problem of resistance. Expert Opin Pharmacol 2009;10(4):555–77.
4. Gonococcal Isolate Surveillance Project (GISP). ℘ http://www.cdc.gov/std/gisp/gisp-protocol-feb-2015_v3.pdf
5. Mertz GJ, Rosenthal SL, Stanberry LR. Is herpes simplex virus type 1 (HSV-1) now more common than HSV-2 in first episodes of genital herpes? Sex Transm Dis 2003;30(10):801–2.
6. Royal College of Obstetricians and Gynaecologists. Sterilisation for Women and Men: What You Need to Know. London: RCOG; 2004. ℘ https://www.rcog.org.uk/globalassets/documents/ patients/patient-information-leaflets/gynaecology/sterilisation-for-women-and-men.pdf
7. Abdulcadir J, Rodriguez MI, Say L. Research gaps in the care of women with female genital mutilation: an analysis. BJOG 2015;122(3):294–303.
8. World Health Organization, Department of Reproductive Health and Research. Eliminating Female Genital Mutilation: An Interagency Statement, OHCHR, UNAIDS, UNDP, UNECA, UNESCO, UNFPA, UNHCR, UNICEF, UNIFEM. Geneva: WHO; 2008. ℘ http://www.who. int/reproductivehealth/publications/fgm/9789241596442/en/
9. World Health Organization. Global Strategy to Stop Health-Care Providers from Performing Female Genital Mutilation. UNFPA, UNHCR, UNICEF, UNIFEM, WHO, FIGO, ICN, MWIA, WCPA, WMA. Geneva: WHO; 2010. ℘ http://www.who.int/reproductivehealth/publications/fgm/rhr_10_9/en/

Further reading

Médecins Sans Frontières. Genitourinary Diseases. In: Clinical Guidelines: Diagnosis and Treatment Manual. Paris: MSF; 2010.
World Health Organization. Comprehensive Cervical Cancer Control: Programme Guidance for Countries. Geneva: WHO; 2011.

Obstetrics

Benjamin Oren Black and Susan Ann O'Toole

Context of obstetrics

Maternal health in humanitarian settings

Women living in humanitarian settings suffer disproportionately from complications of pregnancy and childbirth. The burden of poor health is higher in certain groups of women, such as refugees and displaced persons. Globally, an estimated 303,000 maternal deaths occurred in 2015; however, 185,000 (61%) of these occurred in countries considered to be vulnerable to natural disasters, conflict, or with ongoing humanitarian crises.

Overall, the global maternal mortality ratio (MMR) in 2015 was 216 maternal deaths per 100,000 live births. This MMR is not evenly distributed in the world, as the rates in developing regions are approximately 15 times higher than in developed regions. Fragile states, or those affected by humanitarian crises, had an estimated MMR of 417 maternal deaths per 100,000 live births. In addition, for every woman who dies in childbirth, a further 20–30 suffer injury, infection, or disability.

The WHO defines maternal death as 'the death of a woman while pregnant or within 42 days of termination of pregnancy, irrespective of the duration and site of the pregnancy, from any cause related to or aggravated by the pregnancy or its management but not from accidental or incidental causes'. The principal causes are shown in Fig. 42.1. Almost all deaths occurred in developing countries (99%), with almost two-thirds in countries deemed fragile or with humanitarian crises.

The practice of obstetrics varies widely across the globe. Decisions on when and how to intervene in pregnancy depend on local norms, experience, and context.

This chapter aims to lay out the general strategies for the health provider to reduce maternal mortality and morbidity in the humanitarian setting. Readers with experience in other settings will notice there are important differences in decision-making and thresholds for interventions, in particular when to perform a caesarean section (CS).

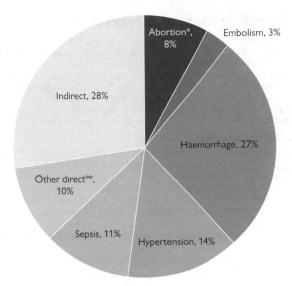

Fig. 42.1 Causes of maternal death globally.

* Nearly all (99%) abortion-related deaths are from unsafe termination of pregnancy.
** Includes deaths resulting from obstructed labour or anaemia.
Data sourced from: Say L et al., 'Global causes of maternal death: a WHO systematic analysis'
Lancet Global Health. http://dx.doi.org/10.1016/S2214-109X(14)70227-X, May 6, 2014.

Addressing maternal mortality

Nearly all maternal deaths are avoidable, so what is it that causes there to still be so many? Economic, political, and sociocultural factors all play into the attention and efforts needed to effectively prevent maternal deaths. Maternal mortality can be viewed as a symptom of inequality and poorly functioning systems. In order to truly address the problem, these underlying issues will ultimately need addressing too. In the humanitarian context, the first priority is to save life, this means initially responding to the direct causes of death, and then working to find more sustainable solutions.

Availability of obstetric services

Most maternal deaths occur during the intrapartum period and first 24 hours postpartum making access to services and close attention during this time a priority. Obstetric services are divided into basic (typically primary health centre) and comprehensive (hospital) obstetric and newborn care. These should both be available 24 hours per day, 7 days per week, with clear referral and communication pathways from basic to comprehensive.

Signal functions of basic and comprehensive obstetric services

Basic emergencsssy obstetric and newborn care (BEmONC)
- Administration of parenteral antibiotics, oxytocics, and anticonvulsants.
- Manual removal of placenta.
- Removal of retained products of conception (manual vacuum aspiration).
- Assisted vaginal delivery (vacuum delivery).
- Neonatal resuscitation (bag and mask).

Comprehensive emergency obstetric and newborn care (CEmONC)
Includes the above-listed components of BEmONC plus the following:
- Surgery with anaesthesia (caesarean delivery/laparotomy).
- Blood transfusion.

Access to safe maternity care is one part of the wider sexual and reproductive health needs of a population, including those in the humanitarian setting. Attempts to ensure access to the other components (family planning, prevention and treatment of STIs (including HIV), gender-based violence, safe care for termination of pregnancy, and services for adolescents) should begin from the earliest possible time in order to provide the recognized minimum standards. More information on providing the Minimum Initial Services Package (MISP) for reproductive health in crisis situations can be found at ℘ http://iawg.net.

Delays with access to care

Reducing maternal morbidity and mortality requires ensuring early recognition of danger signs, planned facility birth or swift referral to a facility with a skilled birth attendant when complications arise, and quality care during admission to the facility. Community engagement, communication, and education are all key interventions for achieving this.

Unavailable, inaccessible, unaffordable, or poor quality care increases the risk of preventable maternal deaths. Factors such as these, prolong the interval between the onset of obstetric complications and accessing care. They have been described as the 'three delays'[1]:

- Delay in the decision to seek care.
- Delay in arrival at a health facility.
- Delay in provision of adequate care.

Strategies to address the three delays

First delay

- Conduct community-level information campaigns on the importance of pregnancy care and delivery with a skilled attendant.
- Educate pregnant women and the community about danger signs in pregnancy, childbirth, and the postnatal period.
- As the reputation of the health facility and poor staff attitudes can contribute to this delay, focus on improving perception of quality of care in the facility.

Second delay

- Encourage antenatal birth planning.
- Address transportation challenges. Disseminate information on available services, and consider transport alternatives when appropriate. These could include construction of two or three stretchers mounted on two bicycle wheels to be made available for selected remote communities, or establishing contacts/contracts with local car/truck owners.
- Offer a maternity waiting home close to the facility for those approaching their due dates.

Third delay

- Ensure a sufficient number of skilled birth attendants and maintain an adequate supply of essential drugs and materials.
- Establish a culture of positive interactions between staff and patients and set and enforce quality of care standards including establishing *a sense of urgency* in managing complications.
- Promote a culture of learning from adverse events, such as regular morbidity and mortality reviews.

Delays in the humanitarian setting

The nature of humanitarian contexts often exacerbates these delays and barriers to seeking healthcare for women. Whether this is due to decreased security, loss of infrastructure, destruction of facilities and transport networks, or healthcare workers leaving the area, these changes tend to increase the vulnerability of pregnant women to poor outcomes, particularly where previously available coping mechanisms are no longer possible or acceptable.

Antenatal care

Antenatal care is intended to provide disease prevention, identification, and management of medical conditions and pregnancy complications. It is also an opportunity for more general health promotion. The WHO recommends eight antenatal care visits—timed around 12, 20, 26, 30, 34, 36, 38, and 40 weeks. Increase according to specific needs.

Screening and treatment

- Screening for anaemia, asymptomatic bacteriuria (UTI), diabetes, syphilis, and HIV should be routinely offered.
- In endemic areas, preventative anthelminthic treatment and malaria prevention should be offered.
- Malaria is a major cause of maternal morbidity and mortality, prevention should include encouragement (and supply) of insecticide-treated bed nets, advice on prevention of mosquito bites, and intermittent preventative therapy (sulfadoxine–pyrimethamine (SP) from second trimester until delivery at least 1 month apart, ideally a minimum three doses. Each dose = 3 tablets of 500 mg/25 mg SP).
- At each visit the woman should be screened for hypertensive disorders (i.e. BP and proteinuria).
- All women should be checked for tetanus immunity and given tetanus toxoid vaccination as required to avoid neonatal tetanus (see Table 42.1).
- Antenatal care is also an opportunity to optimize nutritional education and supplementation; in undernourished populations, balanced energy and protein supplementation should be offered. Consumption of alcohol, smoking, and substance use should be asked about, and general health promotion given.

Table 42.1 Tetanus toxoid immunization schedule for women of childbearing age and pregnant women without previous exposure to TT, Td, or DTP

Dose of TT or Td according to card or history	When to give	Expected duration of protection
1	At first contact or as early as possible in pregnancy	None
2	At least 4 weeks after TT1	1–3 years
3	At least 6 months after TT2 or during subsequent pregnancy	At least 5 years
4	At least 1 year after TT3 or during subsequent pregnancy	At least 10 years
5	At least 1 year after TT4 or during subsequent pregnancy	For all childbearing age years and possibly longer

Box 42.1 Clean delivery kit

The kit should be clearly labelled and packaged. It is intended for single use and not to be opened until time of delivery.

Contents

- Plastic sheet (approx. 1 metre × 1 metre) to provide a clean delivery surface.
- Soap bar: for the assistant to wash their hands and to clean the perineum.
- Two pieces of clean string: for tying the umbilical cord after delivery.
- Clean razor blade: for cutting the cord.
- Single-use examination gloves: for assistant.
- Pictorial guide: explaining how to use the kit.

Further guidance on making and using clean delivery kits can be found at ℗ https://www.path.org/publications/files/RH_dk_fs.pdf

---

Intimate partner violence increases during pregnancy. Always consider enquiring about intimate partner violence, and where there is capacity, offering support.

Fetal assessment

The extent of fetal assessment will depend on context and available skills. Check for presence of fetal movements and presence of fetal heart sounds. Palpation and measurement of the abdomen will depend on local skills. If an ultrasound machine is available, determining the viability, gestational age, and number of fetuses in the second trimester is of great value. Placental location should not be confirmed until after 36 weeks.

Birth preparedness

Antenatal care gives an opportunity for the woman and their healthcare worker to make a birth plan. This is of high importance in the humanitarian setting, particularly when conditions may be volatile or change rapidly. Taking into account the woman's specific needs, resources available, travel conditions, and local context, a plan should be in place for birth and complications or emergencies. This should include access to (or saving) emergency funds, location of health centre, and available transport options. Delivery at a well-functioning health facility is encouraged as most complications during childbirth are unpredictable. If unlikely to be able to reach healthcare, consider providing clean delivery kits (see Box 42.1).

For more information on WHO antenatal care standards refer to ℗ http://www.who.int/reproductivehealth/publications/maternal_perinatal_health/anc-positive-pregnancy-experience/en/.

Approaching obstetric emergencies and complications

Obstetric care is often considered a specialist field, hence many clinicians will not have experience managing pregnant and postpartum women. In the humanitarian setting, these divisions are less apparent and there are many generic and transferrable skills. Knowing one's limitations is paramount. However, do not be afraid to get involved as it could mean the difference between life and death. As a general rule, the mother's life comes first. If a mother dies, her newborn and pre-existing children also have a dramatically increased risk of dying during childhood.

ABC (including fetal heart rate)

As with any other medical emergency, a structured approach should be used for obstetrics, with small modifications:

Airway + left tilt

Is the patient conscious? Ensure airway is open and unobstructed. Tilt the body to the left, or manually displace the gravid uterus, to relieve aortocaval compression if >22 weeks pregnant.

Breathing

Rapidly assess breathing, consider oxygen, measure respiratory rate and oxygen saturation levels.

Circulation

Pulse, BP, and level of consciousness/confusion. Check for evidence of bleeding.

Fetal heart rate (FHR)

Is the fetus alive? If the fetus is dead or the FHR abnormally high (>160 bpm) or low (<110 bpm), this could indicate maternal instability. Consider significant blood loss (including concealed internal haemorrhage), sepsis, and hypertensive complications.

Key interventions

- Rapidly assess and check vital signs, including temperature.
- Ensure good IV access early. Two large-bore cannulas for haemorrhage: check Hb and blood group.
- Resuscitate with IV fluids, unless pre-eclampsia/eclampsia (see ➋ p. 755).
- If sepsis is suspected, begin IV antibiotics early; in endemic areas, always check and treat for malaria.
- In most obstetric emergencies an indwelling urinary catheter will be useful for monitoring response to resuscitation, treating complications, and preparing for possible surgery.

Prepare for the unexpected

Approximately 15% of pregnant women will have a potentially life-threatening complication and the majority are unpredictable. Preparing for complications will reduce time and stress when they happen.

- Have clearly labelled emergency boxes ready with drugs, materials (IV set, catheter, syringes, etc.), and protocols inside. These could include haemorrhage, eclampsia, symphysiotomy, and CS preparation.
- Run practice drills of emergencies in the department to train and assess response. This will help familiarize protocols, awareness of where to find equipment, build confidence, and highlight areas for improvement.

Caesarean section

When to do a caesarean?

Decision for CS (or laparotomy) is often difficult and can be ethically challenging. A CS can be life-saving for the mother and/or baby but has both immediate surgical risks (haemorrhage, infection, organ damage) and long-term complications for future pregnancies including risk of uterine rupture, placenta praevia, and placenta accreta, all of which can be life-threatening. Consideration should therefore be given to both her current and future circumstances, particularly if she is likely to continue having poor or delayed access to healthcare.

CS decision-maker's responsibilities

- See and examine the patient yourself, be sure CS is indicated.
- Confirm the fetus is alive.
- Consider alternatives (see ➜ below "Procedures to avoid CS").
- Consent for procedure, including discussion of sterilization (bilateral tubal ligation) where appropriate (e.g. repeat CS, uterine rupture, or multi-parity).
- Remember that labour is dynamic and circumstances can rapidly change; in theatre, prior to beginning surgery re-examine to ensure vaginal delivery is still not possible and confirm that the fetus is still alive.
- Pre-empt complications: someone present to resuscitate neonate, drugs for postpartum haemorrhage (PPH), relatives/donors needed for blood.
- Documentation of assessment, indication, complications, and recommendations for future pregnancy. Including contraceptive/birth spacing recommendations.

Procedures to avoid CS

Managing labour correctly and utilizing alternative delivery methods in a timely manner can prevent the need for a CS. The following interventions should be considered prior to a CS:

- If delay in progress of labour, appropriate use of membranes rupture, oxytocin augmentation, emptying the bladder (urinary catheterization), correct dehydration, treatment of infections, mobilization, and change in birthing positions.
- If delay in second stage of labour, assess for instrumental delivery, symphysiotomy, destructive delivery/craniotomy.
- Malposition/malpresentation attempt: external and/or internal version, manual rotation.
- Psychological support and encouragement of the mother during labour and expulsive efforts.

Absolute indications: CS/laparotomy
- Uterine rupture
- Uncontrolled antepartum haemorrhage (placenta praevia, abruption with haemodynamic compromise).
- 'Obstructed labour' feto-pelvic disproportion where other interventions failed or contraindicated.
- Malpresentation that cannot be corrected (transverse lie, brow, shoulder or mento-posterior face presentation).
- Cord prolapse with a live fetus that cannot be rapidly delivered vaginally.
- Three or more previous CSs.
- Uncontrolled PPH.
- Extrauterine (ectopic) pregnancy.

Relative indications: CS/laparotomy
- Previous CS with breech presentation.
- Previous uterine rupture/classic caesarean/obstetric fistula.
- Multiple pregnancy when first fetus breech, and second cephalic.
- 'Fetal distress' that is continuing and other form of delivery not possible. Fetus confirmed alive *just* prior to CS, and repeat vaginal examination to ensure not fully dilated and possible to deliver vaginally. True fetal hypoxia is difficult to diagnose or quantify, delivery on this indication alone should be with due attention to the specific case and context.

Further indications will depend on the specific context, obstetric experience, and population expectations.

Technique
CS technique and complications change according to the indication, stage of labour, lie of fetus, and gestation. If you are not obstetrically trained but have the surgical skills required and you anticipate that you will be expected to perform CS in the field, it is highly advised to spend time with experts before departure.

In almost all circumstances a transverse incision to the lower uterine segment should be used. This has a lower rate of complications and results in significantly less risk of uterine rupture in future pregnancies.

Referral
If working in a facility without surgical or blood transfusion capability, ensure that referral systems are clear, including means of transport. Early referral is life-saving in obstetrics. If a complication is anticipated it is better to refer before it happens or worsens. When it is logistically not possible to refer, stabilize the patient, stay calm, get help, and intervene if you are confident to do so.

Early pregnancy complications

- Bleeding in the first trimester is common. Differential diagnoses include miscarriage, termination of pregnancy (TOP), ectopic pregnancy (EP), molar pregnancy, and non-pregnancy-related causes (e.g. cervical bleeding from cervicitis, cervical polyps, and cancer).
- Any woman of reproductive age with bleeding, pelvic pain, or having collapsed should have pregnancy excluded. Use a catheter to obtain urine sample in unconscious patients.
- See Table 42.2 for diagnosis and management of common causes.

> Terminology can be confusing and change according to context. We refer to spontaneous pregnancy loss as miscarriage and intentional loss of pregnancy as TOP. Abortion can be used in reference to either. In general, 'safe abortion care' refers to safe access and aftercare of TOP.

General approach for first-trimester bleeding

- Follow an ABC approach. Treat signs of shock with rapid IV infusion.
- Blood loss can be difficult to estimate, particularly in EP.
- A urinary pregnancy test should be taken at the earliest opportunity.
- If there is access to ultrasound, location and viability of pregnancy can be confirmed. Evidence of haemoperitoneum can also assist with diagnosing a ruptured EP. Beware: ultrasound is only as good as its operator, in unqualified hands there is potential for misdiagnosis and dangerous decisions. An empty uterus could indicate complete miscarriage, early viable pregnancy, or EP. Use as an adjunct to full clinical picture.
- In the humanitarian context, access to contraception and control of fertility wishes can be markedly reduced. TOPs, including unsafe practices, increase in these circumstances. Any woman presenting with suspected miscarriage should be sensitively asked if she has sought or attempted to end the pregnancy, and what method was used. Where there is suspicion, treat as unsafe TOP and ensure antibiotic cover is given. If pregnancy is ongoing, offer safe TOP.
- Suspected EP should be stabilized and transferred to a surgical facility, ideally with relatives for blood transfusion.
- If available, offer anti-D immunoglobulin prophylaxis to women with a rhesus negative blood group following heavy bleeding or medical/surgical intervention.
- As with after any pregnancy, all women should offered contraception as part of their treatment before discharge.

Management of miscarriage

Conservative
Patient is stable, miscarriage is in progress or near completion. Observe patient for blood loss, sepsis, or incomplete miscarriage.

Medical
Inevitable or incomplete miscarriage, give misoprostol 600 mcg PO as a single dose. If heavy bleeding, MVA may be required.

Surgical

MVA is the first-line surgical method in the humanitarian context. The procedure can be done in remote locations with simple analgesics; sterility must be maintained. Guidance on how to perform MVA can be found in the manuals listed at the end of this chapter (➲ 'Practical manuals' p. 786) or videos online (e.g. ♫ https://vimeo.com/71366227).

Table 42.2 Diagnosis and management of first-trimester bleeding

	Diagnosis	Management
Threatened miscarriage	Light PV bleed ± cramping Cervical os closed Ultrasound: viable intra-uterine pregnancy	Reassure
Inevitable miscarriage	Heavy PV bleeding + cramping pain Cervical os open Ultrasound: POC within uterine cavity (incomplete)	Resuscitate. Manage according to patient haemodynamic status and wishes.
Septic abortion (usually post unsafe TOP)	Fever and severe pelvic pain ± PV bleeding/pus Evidence of vaginal injury, uterine perforation, foreign bodies. Sensitively ask if TOP was attempted Ultrasound: terminated or viable pregnancy	Resuscitate, broad-spectrum IV antibiotics for at least 24 hours before MVA Provide tetanus cover (vaccination or immunoglobulin) Refer to surgical facility if uterine perforation/internal organ injury suspected
Molar pregnancy	Heavy PV bleeding with passing of vesicles Uterus size larger than should be for date and soft Ultrasound: typical 'snowstorm' appearance	Resuscitate, evacuation of uterus ideally in surgical facility. Risk of heavy bleeding—have blood ready for transfusion (see ➲ notes on p. 753)
Ectopic pregnancy	Light or no PV bleed Severe pain, often unilateral to side of ectopic Evidence of haemoperitoneum: guarding, diarrhoea, shoulder-tip pain, fainting Cervical os closed Ultrasound: empty uterus, adnexal mass, free fluid in pouch of Douglas	Resuscitate and refer to surgical facility Blood in peritoneum can be autotransfused back to the patient providing sterile circuit is maintained (scoop blood into transfusion bag, pass through gauze to remove clots, and return to patient via IV line). No compatibility or transfusion-transmitted infection testing required

MVA, manual vacuum aspiration; POC, products of conception; PV, per vaginam.

Incomplete miscarriage in second trimester

Definition
Partial expulsion of products of conception.

Management
First-line treatment is to attempt to complete evacuation with a mifepristone/misoprostol regimen, with the same doses as for a first trimester miscarriage. If placenta remains retained, removal using fingers may be possible ± MVA for small fragments. If unsuccessful or facilities/skills not available, refer patient ASAP.

Be aware that brisk bleeding may follow complete evacuation of the uterus. If this occurs:
- First try bimanual compression of the uterus.
- Administer oxytocin 5 units IV or 10 units IM.
- Follow PPH guidance (see p. 777).

Safe TOP

If available, mifepristone 200 mg taken 36–48 hours prior to misoprostol increases effectivity of medical TOP. MVA is a safe surgical method for TOP before 14 weeks' gestation. (See also pp. 751–3.)

Molar pregnancy

Definition
Overgrowth of histologically abnormal trophoblastic tissue.
- IV oxytocin 20 IU in 1 litre of crystalloid run over 2 hours, given during uterine evacuation reduces risk of haemorrhage and uterine perforation.
- Retention of molar vesicles is not uncommon which can cause a risk of a persistent mole and bleeding. If still bleeding 2 weeks post evacuation, repeat MVA.
- At 8 weeks, a pregnancy test should be negative. If positive, refer to tertiary level to exclude persistent trophoblastic disease and ongoing treatment. If referral impossible, repeat MVA. If negative, repeat pregnancy test every 8 weeks for 6 months.
- Advise to avoid pregnancy for at least 1 year

Preterm labour

Overview

Definition

Onset of labour before 37 weeks' gestation.

Presentation

Painful or painless dilatation of the cervix, may present as vaginal bleeding, rupture of membranes, or with uterine contractions.

Management

Give consideration to the likelihood of fetal survival, if there are no facilities for the care of a very pre-term or low-birthweight infant, attempts to save the pregnancy may be futile. In the humanitarian setting it is important to consider the wider patient and facility needs; explain what is happening clearly to the patient and involve paediatric and local colleagues in decisions.

Management

- Bed rest.
- Perform speculum examination to confirm if membranes have ruptured or dilatation of cervix.
- If ultrasound available, confirm viability of pregnancy (fetal heart activity and gestation), presentation of fetus, position of placenta, and number of fetuses.
- Check for and treat any predisposing condition, especially malaria and UTI.
- Give corticosteroids for fetal lung maturation if pregnancy is assumed to be <34 weeks. Betamethasone 12 mg IM, two doses 12 hours apart, or dexamethasone 6 mg IM, four doses 6 hours apart. Caution in patients who appear overtly septic or have underlying infection (e.g. TB) as steroids may precipitate an immunocompromised state.
- Contractions can be stopped using nifedipine, this is only beneficial to give time for corticosteroid administration or transfer of patient. It is not a treatment in itself.
- Give loading dose of nifedipine 20 mg PO, followed by 10–20 mg three to four times daily according to uterine activity. Stop after 48 hours.
  - Do not stop contractions if signs of chorioamnionitis, bleeding, or rupture of membranes. Allow labour to continue, the body is attempting to remove a source of sepsis or potential placental abruption.

Hypertensive disorders

Definitions

Hypertension in pregnancy
Mild = 140–149/90–99 mmHg; moderate = 150–159/100–109 mmHg;
severe >160/110 mmHg (medical emergency).

Chronic hypertension
↑BP before 20 weeks' gestation or prior to pregnancy.

Gestational hypertension
New ↑BP diagnosed after 20 weeks without proteinuria.

Pre-eclampsia (previously known as pre-eclamptic toxaemia)
New ↑BP diagnosed after 20 weeks with proteinuria.

Eclampsia
Convulsions associated with pre-eclampsia (medical emergency).

Management of hypertensive disease in pregnancy

In general, aim to keep BP within safe range to avoid maternal complications, but not too low that there is placental hypo-perfusion. 130–149/
80–99 mmHg is usually adequate. IV route can be used in severe cases not responding to PO medication. See Table 42.3 for anti-hypertensive medications.

Severe pre-eclampsia and eclampsia

Severe pre-eclampsia and eclampsia are life-threatening medical emergencies. Symptomatic treatment is to control BP and prevent convulsions. The
only definitive treatment is to deliver the pregnancy—this should be by the
safest method possible (normally vaginal delivery).

Diagnosis can be difficult; presentation can be rapid and unpredictable.
Occasionally eclamptic seizures present before changes in BP or proteinuria
arise, 40% of seizures occur in the postpartum period. Any convulsions in pregnancy or postpartum should be treated as eclampsia until proven otherwise.

Signs and symptoms
• BP >160/110 mmHg.
• Significant proteinuria (>3+ on test strip).
• Headache, visual disturbances, right upper quadrant/epigastric pain,
  nausea/vomiting, confusion/agitation.
• Facial oedema, hyper-reflexia, clonus >3 beats.
• Blood results: ↑urea, ↑creatinine, ↑ALT/AST, ↑urate, ↑lactate
  dehydrogenase, ↓platelets, ↑clotting time.

Management
• ABC approach.
• Magnesium sulphate (MgSO₄) is first line for treatment and prevention
  of seizures. Do not use diazepam as a substitute. Commence MgSO₄
  protocol ASAP (see Box 42.2).
• Urinary catheter to begin strict in/out measurement.
• Deliver: give corticosteroids if mother is stable and fetus <34 weeks'
  gestation.

Rupture membranes and augment labour. Aim for delivery within 24 hours of
severe pre-eclampsia or 12 hours of eclampsia. CS if vaginal delivery impossible.

Table 42.3 Antihypertensive medications in pregnancy

Medication	Dose	Notes
Methyldopa	250 mg twice daily – 1 g three times daily	Post-natal use associated with depression. Change when possible.
Nifedipine	10 mg twice daily – 30 mg three times daily	Use modified release to avoid rapid ↓BP
Labetalol	100 mg twice daily – 600 mg four times daily	Avoid in asthma
Atenolol	50–100 mg once daily	Avoid in asthma
Hydralazine (IV)	5 mg over 2–4 minutes. Repeat each 20 minutes until BP <150/90. Maximum of 4 doses (20 mg)	Caution: can cause rapid and profound hypotension. Consider bolus of fluid if rapid BP drop. Can be given IM if IV impossible.
Labetalol (IV)	20 mg over 1 minute, after 10 minutes if still ↑BP repeat 20 mg. If still ↑BP after further 10 minutes give 40 mg, after another 10 minutes give 80 mg if still not responding.	Continue every 10 minutes until adequate response. Maximum cumulative dose: 300 mg

Box 42.2 MgSO$_4$ protocol

Warning: MgSO$_4$ comes in different concentrations always check vial.
- *Loading dose:* 4 g of 20% MgSO$_4$ slow IV injection 15–20 minutes (if 20% MgSO$_4$ unavailable, dilute 4 g of 50% MgSO$_4$ in 100 mL of 0.9% NaCl), then 5 g of 50% MgSO$_4$ + 1 mL 2% lidocaine by deep IM injection in each buttock (10 g MgSO$_4$ IM total).
- If further seizures after 15 minutes give 2 g MgSO$_4$ by slow IV injection.
- If still having convulsions give diazepam.
- *Maintenance:* 5 g of 50% MgSO$_4$ + 1 mL 2% lidocaine by deep IM injection into buttock every 4 hours (alternate buttocks).
- Continue for 24 hours after delivery or after last seizure, whichever is latest.

Monitoring

MgSO$_4$ is toxic. Close attention must be paid to signs of toxicity:
- Confusion, absent reflexes, respiratory depression, hypotension, arrhythmia, and cardiac arrest.
- MgSO$_4$ is renally excreted: urine output <30 mL/hour increases risk of toxicity. If oliguric, halve or stop maintenance. Do not give fluid challenge.
- If toxic, stop MgSO$_4$ and give 10 mL of 10% calcium gluconate (1 g) IV over 10 minutes.
- Fluid management: there is a high risk of fluid overload with pulmonary oedema. Keep patient nil by mouth and restrict to a total of 80 mL/hour (1 litre/12 hours).

Antepartum haemorrhage

Overview

Definition
Vaginal bleeding after 24 weeks' gestation, with or without pain.

Management
Rapid ABC assessment and approach (see ⊃ p. 748). For all antepartum haemorrhages, blood loss can be massive, easily under-estimated, or concealed. Anticipate need for blood transfusion; in all cases request relatives and send with patient if transferring.

Placenta praevia

Definition
The placenta partially or completely covers the cervical os.

Presentation
Suspect with painless vaginal bleeding, though can also present with contractions.

Management
- Vaginal examination should be avoided if placenta praevia is suspected as disturbing the placenta can cause catastrophic bleeding.
- Ideally ultrasound should be used to confirm the location of the placenta. If not possible, speculum examination can be carefully performed; this should reveal blood flowing from the cervical os.
- If significant vaginal bleeding and not in a surgical facility, attempt to transfer the patient; regardless of whether or not you are able to confirm the diagnosis, suspicion alone is enough.

Once placenta praevia is suspected, the management will depend on your location:

BEmONC unit
- Resuscitate (ABC approach) and if possible transfer patient to a surgical facility with relatives.

Emergency procedure in BEmONC unit: if transfer is totally impossible and the woman is in advanced active labour (almost fully dilated) with heavy vaginal bleeding, the following can be attempted as a last resort in order to try and stop the bleeding and save maternal life:

- This is only possible for a partial placenta praevia with membranes bulging. Rupture the membranes and augment labour. The descending presenting part will tamponade the placental edge and augmentation (consider giving oxytocin) encourages dilatation. Deliver the fetus and placenta as soon as possible, then aggressively treat for PPH. In breech presentation, the legs can be grasped and pulled through the os so that the buttocks tamponade the placenta.
- This is an 'extreme measure' for saving of maternal life if no alternative or possibility of transfer is available. In such a situation the mother is already likely to have lost significant amounts of blood and may be unconscious, perimortem CS can also be considered to arrest the bleeding in extremis.
- Resuscitation and transfer to a CEmONC unit remains the fastest and safest approach.

CEmONC unit

- Resuscitate. Assess haemodynamic status to decide if immediate surgery is needed. Check blood group and test relatives for compatibility.
- If bleeding has settled and she is pre-term, administer corticosteroids and optimize Hb (iron and nutrition). Keep admitted, or in a nearby location, until around 38 weeks then perform CS.
- If unstable or term, deliver by CS. Be prepared for PPH and the possibility of needing to perform emergency hysterectomy.

Placental abruption

Definition
Separation of the placenta from the uterine wall.

Presentation
Uterus is hard and tender. There may be little or no vaginal bleeding when the haemorrhage is 'concealed' behind the placenta. The amount of bleeding seen may not represent the haemodynamic state of the patient. The fetus may be dead or alive depending on degree of placental separation and blood loss.

Management
Resuscitate and stabilize patient. Transfer to a CEmONC unit with relatives.

- Stabilize maternal haemodynamic status with fluids and try to deliver the baby vaginally as soon as possible by active management of labour: rupture of membranes, oxytocin, and vacuum extraction. Anticipate PPH.
- If haemorrhage is heavy or progress of labour slow, do not delay emergency CS, even if fetus is dead.
- There is a high risk of PPH and DIC with placental abruption. Be as prepared as possible for major haemorrhage. Treat aggressively, hysterectomy may be required.

- Prepare for transfusion with fresh, whole blood if possible.
- Decision on mode of delivery can be difficult: in general, vaginal delivery is preferred and usually safer, but CS can be performed quickly which can be life-saving.
- All possible factors should be taken into account, e.g. availability of blood, haemodynamic status of patient, progress of labour, and experience of the surgeon.

Uterine rupture

Definition
Complete or partial opening of the uterine muscle. Suspect in women with previous CS (particularly classical, vertical, scar), prolonged labour or un-safe use of uterotonics (e.g. administered in community).

Presentation
- Pain, cessation of contractions, loss of presenting part. Fetus may be easily felt under abdominal skin if expelled from uterus.
- Maternal shock. Fetus is usually dead, but not always. Vaginal bleeding may be present, but not representative of overall blood loss.

Management
- Resuscitate and transfer to a CEmONC unit with relatives.
- At surgical facility, prepare patient for laparotomy; if a clean rupture, repair is usually safer. If anatomically not possible, or there is a long delay in reaching the surgical facility (evidence of tissue necrosis), proceed to sub-total hysterectomy. Always check for posterior wall rupture, bladder injury, and broad ligament haematoma.
- There is a risk of uterine rupture in future pregnancy. If possible, take consent for bilateral tubal ligation prior to surgery, otherwise counsel carefully and provide long-acting contraception.

Labour and delivery

Childbirth is an everyday event, and while it can be straightforward there can also be life-threatening complications for both mother and child. Early recognition and prompt management of these are vital in reducing morbidity and mortality.

Labour is diagnosed by coordinated uterine contractions that increase in frequency and strength, resulting in progressive dilatation of the cervix and delivery of fetus (or fetuses) and the placenta. In insecure settings, women may present very late in labour when complications have already escalated. However, the opposite may also occur, with women presenting early, even before labour begins, to avoid difficult travelling conditions.

Monitoring progress: stages of labour

- *Latent phase:* the cervix dilates from 0 to 3 cm, there is no time limit for this and it is not considered to be true labour.
- *First stage:* once 4 cm dilated, a woman is considered to be in 'active' labour and the clock begins. The partograph (see ➔ p. 761) is the recommended tool for detecting delay in progress; begin documenting from diagnosis of active labour. Progress of dilatation from this point should be monitored, slowing or stopping of progress may indicate obstruction or other complications. Progress of <2 cm in 4 hours should raise concerns, or slowing down of progress in a multiparous woman.
- *Second stage:* full cervical dilatation (no cervix can be felt). During the second stage the fetus (or fetuses) is delivered. As a general rule, the second stage should not last beyond 3 hours in a primiparous woman or 2 hours in a multiparous woman. Expulsive efforts signify an 'active' second stage, a primip should deliver within 2 hours and multip 30–60 minutes. Delay during the second stage must be recognized and resolved in the safest way for mother and baby, either through assistance for vaginal delivery or CS (see ➔ pp. 749–50 on decision for CS).
- *Third stage:* from delivery of baby until completion of delivery of placenta and membranes. WHO recommends an active third stage through routine administration of oxytocin 10 IU IM after delivery of the last baby (always check that it is not a multiple pregnancy before injecting!). See Third Stage Complications and PPH sections for more details.

> A *partograph* (see Fig. 42.2) is a chart for recording FHR, uterine contractions, maternal vital signs, clinical interventions, cervical dilatation, and descent of the presenting part. The alert and action lines signal when labour progress is less than adequate and that patient transfer and/or medical interventions are indicated.

Labour support

- Encourage the woman to mobilize and take whichever position is comfortable to her, providing it is safe to her and the healthcare worker.
- Local practices may include delivery in various positions, such as lying on her side, squatting, or on all fours.
- Complicated deliveries (e.g. breech or multiple births) are usually easier to assist in lithotomy. Perform instrumental delivery in lithotomy.

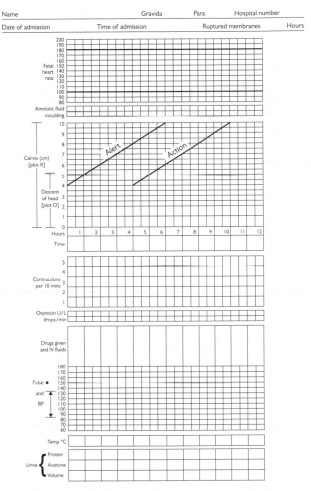

Fig. 42.2 The modified WHO partograph. Reproduced with permission from WHO, Managing Complications in Pregnancy and Childbirth, 2000, pC-67.

Malposition and malpresentation

The presenting (lower most) part of the fetus must be either cephalic (head) or breech (buttocks) with a longitudinal lie to deliver vaginally, any other presentation needs to either be corrected to cephalic/breech or delivered by CS. Diagnosis of the fetal position in a cephalic presentation is through feeling for the anterior and posterior fontanelles; if the head is low the fetal ears may also be palpable. The fetal head is egg-shaped, therefore different positions will present with varying diameters. The optimal fetal position is with the posterior fontanelle palpated anteriorly (i.e. the baby is looking down towards the mother's rectum).

Malposition is a common cause of poor labour progress. This can be corrected by changing maternal position, mobilizing, and increasing uterine contractions strength thereby assisting with fetal rotation. General options include the following:

- Try all fours (hands and knees), pelvic rocking, kneeling, or any position in which the woman feels comfortable.
- Weak uterine contractions do not facilitate rotation of the fetal head and so improving uterine contractions may help achieve a more optimal presentation. Before starting oxytocin examine the patient for signs of obstruction, particularly in a multiparous woman; if concerned, refer to a surgical facility for possible CS.

Face/brow presentation
Diagnosis
Can be difficult to distinguish from breech, feel the presenting part carefully for landmarks.
- Face: orbital ridges, nose, mentum, mouth and gums (may feel the fetus suck on the examination finger).
- Brow: anterior fontanelle, frontal sutures, orbital ridges and root of nose, presenting part will remain high.

Management
- Follow the same principles as for normal cephalic presentation. The majority of brow/face presentations will flex during the course of labour to a more favourable position.
- Vaginal delivery with persistent face presentation is only possible if mento-anterior (fetal chin at maternal pubic-symphysis). Persistent brow or face (mento-posterior) cannot deliver vaginally, do not attempt assisted delivery. The woman should be referred for CS.
- If CS is impossible manual flexion and rotation of fetal head to a more favourable presentation can be attempted. This is a last-resort measure, which comes with risk of uterine rupture, cord prolapse, and injury to fetus.

Breech presentation and delivery
- The fetal buttocks/feet present in a longitudinal lie. The fetal head can usually be palpated at the fundus. Where possible, ultrasound should be used to confirm presentation of fetus and placenta.
- Vaginal breech delivery is possible; the diagnosis may be made when already in active labour or pre-labour. As usual, the long- and short-term risks and benefits of CS must be balanced against those of vaginal delivery.

- Breech presentation should be delivered in a surgical facility, in case CS is required. However, as women can present in late labour, all facilities should be prepared to manage this presentation.

Types of breech
- Extended breech (majority): buttocks present, with both legs extended with feet by head.
- Flexed breech: buttocks and feet present, legs flexed at knees.
- Footling breech: foot presenting, one or both legs extended below the breech. Increased risk of cord prolapse and unsuccessful vaginal delivery, likely to need CS.

Management of breech delivery
Pre-labour
- If term, external cephalic version can be attempted. Using the palm of hands push the breech up out of pelvis and roll the fetus forward until cephalic presentation, using hands to control the fetal breech and head.
- If forward roll unsuccessful, backwards roll can be attempted. Do not use excessive force, if the breech is not rotating or procedure causing maternal pain, stop.

Vaginal breech labour and delivery
- If possible, confirm diagnosis with ultrasound and manage in a CEmONC facility.
- Avoid rupture of membranes, increased risk of cord prolapse.
- Progress of labour should be normal; any delays should raise concern of fetal/pelvic disproportion and a warning sign of later complications.
- Ensure that cervix is fully dilated before active pushing begins.

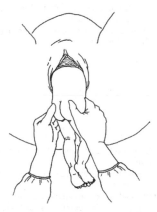

Fig. 42.3 Position for holding breech. Reproduced with permission from WHO, Managing Complications in Pregnancy and Childbirth, 2000, p-38.

Delivery of breech baby

- Episiotomy may be required, have delivery set, local anaesthetic, and episiotomy scissors ready
- Breech babies are more likely to need resuscitation—have space and equipment prepared before delivery
- Delay maternal expulsive efforts until breech is low, ideally with the buttocks visible.
- Encourage maternal effort, do not touch or pull on the breech as this can cause the fetus to extend the neck and cause head entrapment.
- Fetal back should remain upwards (anterior), if rotating round gently steer back to upwards position. (See Fig. 42.3.)
- Once the scapulas are visible, the arms are brought down by hooking the index finger at the fetal elbow and drawing the arm downwards.
- If the arms are stretched upwards and not easily reachable use 'Lovset's manoeuvre'. (See Fig. 42.4.)
- Allow body to hang, placing hands underneath in case of rapid delivery.
- Once nape of neck is visible, the head should either spontaneously deliver or assistance will be needed. Place the fetal body on the right fore-arm, put two fingers from right hand over the maxilla, and two fingers of the left over the back of fetal head (occiput), with maternal effort flex and deliver the head (see Fig. 42.5). This should be a smooth, controlled motion. No pulling.
- If the fetal head fails to deliver, do not panic. Use McRobert's position (see ➋ 'Shoulder dystocia' pp. 773–5), ensure bladder is empty (pass catheter if unsure), and ask an assistant to give suprapubic pressure on fetal head to assist with flexion while repeating above-described manoeuvre.
- If head remains entrapped, forceps (if trained), emergency CS, or symphysiotomy assuming fetus is still alive.
- If fetus dies and remains entrapped, destructive delivery may be more appropriate. See ➋ pp. 769–70

Transverse and oblique lie

Presentation

Fetal head is on one side of the mother's abdomen and the buttocks/legs on the other.

Management

- The fetus must either be rotated to a cephalic or breech presentation or be delivered by CS.
- If diagnosis is made before labour begins, the patient should be referred to a CEmONC facility.
- If the fetus is transverse, back down, CS can be difficult. Consider a classical (vertical) uterine incision.
- If fully dilated with a dead fetus, destructive delivery can be attempted depending on available practitioner skill and experience (see ➋ 'Practical manuals' p. 786 for procedure details).

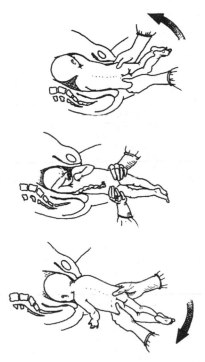

Fig. 42.4 Loveset's manoeuvre. Reproduced with permission from WHO, Managing Complications in Pregnancy and Childbirth, 2000, p-39.

Delivery of fetal head

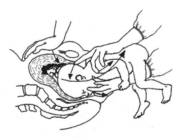

Fig. 42.5 Mauriceau–Smellie–Veit manoeuvre. Reproduced with permission from WHO, Managing Complications in Pregnancy and Childbirth, 2000, p-41.

Multiple birth

In the humanitarian setting, women may present either in labour or before with no knowledge of how many fetuses they are carrying. Suspicion may be raised by a large uterus, difficulty palpating the lie, or auscultation of more than one FHR.

- Ultrasound is the gold standard for diagnosis, and confirming the number and presentation of the fetuses.
- Multiple births have an increased risk of complications and should be managed in a CEmONC facility whenever possible.
- In labour, insert IV access and prepare for delivery of appropriate number of babies, call for assistance.
- If leading fetus is cephalic, vaginal delivery should be attempted. If breech, consider CS due to risk of inter-locking twins.
- After delivery of first baby:
  - Stabilize the second baby into a longitudinal lie and deliver as cephalic or breech (using an oxytocin infusion if required to restore regular contractions).
  - If the second twin is transverse, attempt external version to cephalic or breech presentation. If not possible, internal podalic version (grabbing one or both feet and bring fetus into pelvis as a breech presentation) should be undertaken. The operator may need to deflect the head upwards with one hand on the abdomen, while applying steady traction on the feet.
  - Avoid rupture of membranes until feet are in the vagina.
  - If second fetus remains transverse proceed to immediate CS.
- Second fetus has increased risk of needing neonatal resuscitation so have equipment ready.
- Multiple births have an increased risk of PPH, prepare for an active third stage and further management as required. Always check there is not another fetus before giving oxytocin IM.

Obstructed labour

Definition

Obstructed labour cannot be diagnosed until active labour has been established (i.e. cervix dilated at least 4 cm and adequate contraction pattern).

Presentation

Obstructed labour has risks to both mother and fetus, including uterine rupture, obstetric fistula, sepsis, and maternal and fetal death.

The partograph is used to alert the clinician to a delay in progress of labour which may indicate obstruction.

Management

- Monitor the mother and fetus closely.
- Consider the use of oxytocin to augment labour if labour progress is slow due to inadequate contractions.
- See section on CS (see ➔ pp. 749–50) for further interventions
- Transfer patient to a CEmONC facility if obstruction requiring surgical intervention is suspected, or if the skills for other measures are not available locally.

- If the woman has reached full dilatation with cephalic presentation, and the fetus is alive, but the fetus has failed to deliver after 1–2 hours despite maternal pushing, the management is based on descent of the fetal head:
  - If the fetal head is not palpable above the symphysis pubis (0/5) and ≤ ischial spines: assisted vaginal delivery (forceps or vacuum depending on user competence).
  - If at least 3/5 of the fetal head is descended into the pelvic cavity (<1–2/5 palpable above symphysis): symphysiotomy.
  - If less than 3/5 of the fetal head is descended into the pelvic cavity (>3/5 palpable above symphysis): CS.
- In case of prolonged obstructed labour with intrauterine fetal demise, if possible avoid CS, especially where women's access to an emergency obstetric and newborn care facility in future is uncertain. CS should be for maternal indication only.
  - Cervix >7 cm dilated and station 2/5 or lower: attempt destructive delivery (see pp. 769–70).
  - Cervix <7 cm dilated or station 3/5 or higher: CS.

Symphysiotomy

Definition
An increase of pelvic diameter (by about 2 cm) through division of fibrocartilaginous symphysis pubis.

Indication
Moderate obstructed labour; failure (or anticipated failure) of instrumental delivery; severe shoulder dystocia; entrapped after-coming head of breech.

Prerequisites
Live fetus, fully dilated, fetal head ≤ −2 ischial spines or ≤ 3/5 palpable above symphysis pubis, appropriate equipment, sterility, competent provider, and assistance. It can be performed with local anaesthetic but should be ideally performed at CEmONC level, however, it can be safely performed at a BEmONC unit, providing sterility, analgesia, and aftercare are provided.

Symphysiotomy and destructive procedures are rarely performed in modern medical practice. However, in the resource-poor setting, where timely access to healthcare during pregnancy is unlikely, they are life-saving and relatively simple procedures that avoid a uterine CS scar. Both are likely to be performed after a prolonged labour, which increases the risk of PPH, infection, and obstetric fistula. These complications should be pre-empted, prepare for their prophylactic and active management (should include secondary prevention of obstetric fistula).

Procedure
- Clean the area for incision and infiltrate anterior, superior, and inferior aspects of symphysis with local anaesthetic (e.g. lidocaine)
- Place in lithotomy position; have an assistant holding each leg at no more than 45° abduction from the midline (Fig. 42.6). The assistants must continue to support the legs throughout the delivery.

- Pass a rigid catheter into the bladder (metal or plastic), empty bladder, and keep catheter in place to identify urethra. Place a finger in the vagina and displace (push the catheter) the urethra away from midline (Fig. 42.7).
- Using the other hand, make a stab incision with thick, firm scalpel 1 cm below the upper edge of the symphysis, cut downwards until the pressure of scalpel can be felt by vaginally placed finger, do not cut into vagina.
- Remove the scalpel, rotate blade, re-insert and cut upwards to top of symphysis. The full length of symphysis should now be divided. Normally the separation of pubic bone will be felt to approximately a thumb's width (Fig. 42.8).
- Remove the catheter and deliver the baby using a vacuum extractor; early episiotomy is recommended to reduce tension and trauma.
- After delivery, re-catheterize with indwelling Foley. Keep in place until the patient is mobilizing (or longer if fistula prevention is indicated).
- Suturing of stab incision is usually not required, unless bleeding.
- Give broad-spectrum antibiotic prophylaxis and adequate analgesia.
- Apply plastic strapping across the front of the pelvis from one iliac crest to the other, this stabilizes the pelvis and reduces pain. Treat patient with bedrest, nursed on her side as much as possible until mobile (usually around day 3).
- Mobilize with support from an assistant, frame, or back of a chair. If available request physiotherapy input. Ensure good analgesia during recovery time. Advise to avoid heavy work/lifting for 3 months.

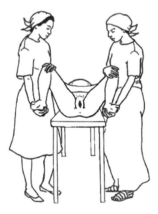

Fig. 42.6 Position for symphysiotomy. Reproduced with permission from WHO, Managing Complications in Pregnancy and Childbirth, 2000, p-54.

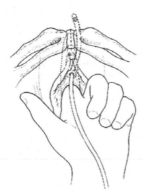

Fig. 42.7 Push urethra away from midline. Reproduced with permission from WHO, Managing Complications in Pregnancy and Childbirth, 2000, p-55.

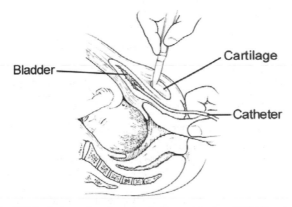

Fig. 42.8 Divide the cartilage. Reproduced with permission from WHO, Managing Complications in Pregnancy and Childbirth, 2000, p-55.

Destructive delivery

Definition

To assist in the vaginal delivery of a dead fetus through reduction of the fetal size.

Destructive procedures are life-saving, however the operator, assistants, and patient must be counselled appropriately on what can be a distressing operation for those involved. There are several destructive procedures, depending on the presentation. Procedure for craniotomy is described here; however, for decapitation, cliedotomy (cutting of clavicles), and evisceration (for transverse lie) refer to ➲ 'Practical manuals' p. 786.

Indication

Obstructed labour with intrauterine fetal death; fully dilated (can be attempted from ≥7 cm); uterine rupture not suspected or imminent; appropriate sterility, analgesia, equipment, and assistance. If at all possible transfer patient to a CEmONC facility, where anaesthesia (ideally general anaesthesia) can be given and early recourse to laparotomy made if required (failed procedure or uterine rupture).

Procedure

- Lithotomy position, broad-spectrum IV antibiotics, insert urinary catheter, and empty bladder.
- Have an assistant stabilize the uterus and fetus, this is done by placing both palms to the fetal head (from over the maternal abdomen) and applying downward pressure to the pelvis. This is to stop the fetus moving upwards during the procedure, risking uterine rupture.
- Make a cruciate (cross) incision on the fetal scalp.
- Open the cranial vault via a fontanelle using large, sharp scissors or heavy, blunt forceps/clamp. If face presentation, perforate through the orbits.
- Open and close within the cranium several times to allow the intracranial contents to drain out
- Grasp edges of the skull with several heavy-toothed forceps (e.g. Kocher's) and pull downwards to deliver, make an episiotomy.
- After delivery, gently examine for any evidence of uterine rupture, vaginal, or cervical trauma.
- Repair any tears and episiotomy.
- Leave catheter in place, fistula prevention will most likely be indicated.
- Trapped after-coming head of breech: same as above, except:
  - Make incision at base of neck and perforate through occiput, open and close as widely as possible.
  - Apply traction to fetal body.

Perineal trauma and repair

Perineal injury is common during childbirth; timely recognition and appropriate repair reduce the risk of immediate and later complications.

Reducing risk

There remains a lack of evidence on methods to minimize trauma, however, the following have been suggested:

- Control the speed of delivery: direct the woman in the final stages of the delivery on when to push and when to stop. As the presenting part crowns, use a hand to control the speed (allowing time for tissues to stretch). Support the perineum with either a hand or material (e.g. sanitary pad) pushing the tissues up and inwards as the presenting part delivers.
- Episiotomy: routine episiotomy is to be discouraged. However, when the perineum is tight, or rapid delivery required (e.g. fetal distress or instrumental delivery), episiotomy may be indicated to reduce uncontrolled perineal tearing.

- Episiotomy should be performed after infiltration of the perineal tissue with lidocaine 0.5%, the cut should be made at a 60° right medio-lateral angle (see online video: ♫ https://youtu.be/XSRv3FdyL8g) as the presenting part is delivering.

Identification of trauma

The perineum should be examined after every delivery, this should include both vaginal and rectal examination; ensure there is appropriate lighting and explain to the woman what is being done.

Classification of perineal tear

- First degree: vaginal mucosa and perineal skin only.
- Second degree: vaginal mucosa and perineal muscles.
- Third degree: involvement of the anal sphincter.
- Fourth degree: disruption of the rectal mucosa.

Repair

- Perineal tears should be repaired as soon after deliver as possible.
- Ensure appropriate analgesia, lighting, and explanation. Maintain sterility; consider repairing in the operating theatre (e.g. third-degree, fourth-degree, or complex tears).
- See Fig. 42.9 for repair of episiotomy (same technique as for second-degree tear). Consult ➔ 'Practical manuals' p. 786 for more detailed techniques, or the following online video: ♫ https://youtu.be/XSRv3FdyL8g.
- Bleeding tends to originate from the top of the tear, tying a knot just above the apex is vital in all repairs in order to gain haemostasis.
- The objective is to restore anatomy, when uncertain return to this point.
- Occasionally bleeding can persist despite repair, either due to DIC or multiple grazes and lacerations; applying pressure can be helpful either intermittently or with a sterile pack for 12 hours.
- Always count instruments and swabs before a repair, and check that this is the same after (i.e. leave nothing behind).
- Patients should be educated on perineal hygiene and care after any repair to avoid infection and complications.

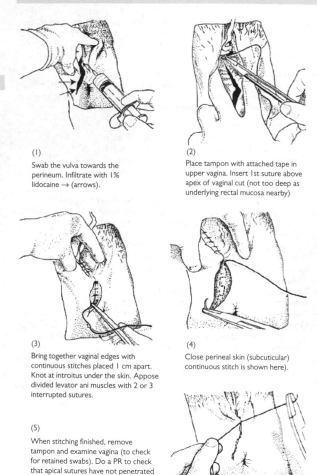

(1)

Swab the vulva towards the perineum. Infiltrate with 1% lidocaine → (arrows).

(2)

Place tampon with attached tape in upper vagina. Insert 1st suture above apex of vaginal cut (not too deep as underlying rectal mucosa nearby)

(3)

Bring together vaginal edges with continuous stitches placed 1 cm apart. Knot at introitus under the skin. Appose divided levator ani muscles with 2 or 3 interrupted sutures.

(4)

Close perineal skin (subcuticular) continuous stitch is shown here).

(5)

When stitching finished, remove tampon and examine vagina (to check for retained swabs). Do a PR to check that apical sutures have not penetrated rectum.

Fig. 42.9 Episiotomy repair. Reproduced from Collier J, Longmore M, Brinsden M. (2006). Oxford Handbook of Clinical Specialties, 7th edn. Oxford: OUP. By permission of Oxford University Press.

Intrapartum and postpartum emergencies

Maternal collapse

- Follow an ABC approach.
- In the unconscious pregnant woman always consider eclampsia, could she be in a post-ictal state? If still pregnant, stabilize the mother and deliver by safest and quickest means possible.

Cord prolapse

The umbilical cord presents below the fetal presenting part, resulting in occlusion of fetal blood supply, hypoxia, and possible death. This is one of the few clear indications of CS for fetal distress.

Management

If the woman is fully dilated, assist a rapid vaginal delivery (e.g. instrumental delivery):
- If imminent vaginal delivery is not possible and fetus is alive, proceed to emergency CS.
- If the cord has prolapsed out of the vagina, gently replace in order to reduce vasospasm due to exposure and cold.
- If fetus is dead, allow labour to progress and deliver vaginally. CS for maternal indications only (e.g. transverse lie).
- To check if fetus is alive either auscultate the FHR, or if not possible, gently palpate the cord for pulsations (avoid repeatedly touching the cord as this can cause vasospasm). If alive, attempt to displace the presenting part upwards to relieve cord compression, this is done by either:
  - putting the patient in 'knees to chest' position
  - manually pushing the presenting part upwards with a hand
  - filling the bladder: insert a urinary catheter, using a giving-set infiltrate 500–700 mL of saline into the bladder and clamp the catheter. This is particularly effective when patient transfer or delay in getting to theatre is likely. REMEMBER to unclamp the catheter prior to CS otherwise there is a high risk of bladder injury!!
- In theatre re-check that the FHR is still present prior to beginning the CS.

Shoulder dystocia

This occurs when the fetal shoulder impacts against the pubic symphysis. It is diagnosed when the head delivers but remains tightly applied to vulva, retracts, or the shoulder does not deliver with normal traction. This is an unpredictable emergency and should be anticipated at any delivery.

Management

- Call for help.
- Evaluate for episiotomy, to allow for space to perform manoeuvres, not to relieve the obstruction.
- Get the woman into McRobert's position (Fig. 42.10); on her back pulling knees as far up to the chest as possible. This will relieve the majority of shoulder dystocia.

If this fails, proceed to:
- Ask an assistant to apply suprapubic pressure with heel of hand to disimpact the shoulder under the symphysis.
- Deliver the posterior arm: gently reach in (patient should stop pushing) and feel for the posterior arm, flex the elbow and sweep the arm over the fetal chest to deliver it, then apply gentle traction on the arm to encourage rotation of the shoulders. The fetus should then deliver. (See Fig. 42.11.)

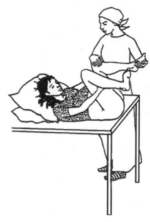

Fig. 42.10 McRobert's position. Reproduced with permission from WHO, Managing Complications in Pregnancy and Childbirth, 2000, pS-84.

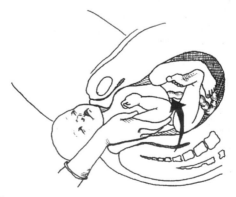

Fig. 42.11 Delivery of the posterior arm. Reproduced with permission from WHO, Managing Complications in Pregnancy and Childbirth, 2000, pS-85.

- If still not possible attempt to rotate one or both shoulders using your fingers, change maternal position (all fours), repeat from the beginning. If the fetus is still alive and nothing has worked consider symphysiotomy or fracturing the fetal clavicle.
- After delivery, prepare for neonatal resuscitation, PPH, and perineal repair. Debrief the mother on the events of the delivery.

Retained placenta

The placenta should deliver within 30 minutes after birth. Retained placenta increases the risk of haemorrhage and infection; it should be dealt with promptly.

Management

- Ensure there is IV access, the bladder is empty, and unclamp the cord to allow the fetal blood to drain out. If not given administer oxytocin and attempt controlled cord traction, if this is unsuccessful a manual removal of placenta (MROP) will be required. (See Fig. 42.12.)
- MROP requires aseptic conditions and adequate analgesia/anaesthesia.
- With the non-dominant hand stabilize the uterine fundus and push it downwards. Insert the lubricated dominant hand gently, but firmly, through the cervix and reach up to the placenta.
  - Try to find the placental edge and shear it away from the uterine wall.
  - Use the non-dominant hand to keep the uterus stable and massage the fundus to create contraction.
  - Attempt to remove the placenta in one piece, always check the cavity is empty and remove any small pieces left inside.
- Anticipate PPH, have all drugs ready, and administer prophylactic antibiotics.

Uterine inversion

Uterine inversion is a rare complication in which the uterus turns inside out during or with delivery of the placenta.

Suspect if there is sudden maternal collapse or shock, severe pain, or haemorrhage. On examination there may be loss of the fundus abdominally, a mass in the vagina, or the uterus visible beyond the introitus.

Management

This is an emergency requiring immediate recognition and response; the longer left untreated, the more difficult replacement becomes.

- ABC resuscitation (consider giving atropine in cases of unresolving bradycardia).
- If placenta is still attached leave alone. Remove after uterus has been replaced.
- If possible, move quickly to theatre and give anaesthesia.
- Attempt to manually replace the uterus: under sterile conditions, firmly push uterus back into vagina and then up through the cervix back into position. Hold the uterus in place with one hand inside and the other abdominally.
- Only now give oxytocin (not earlier), manually remove placenta if still attached and treat PPH. (See Fig. 42.12.)

- Give broad-spectrum IV antibiotics.
- Leave urine catheter in place to monitor urine output and recovery from shock.
- If manual replacement is impossible, consider using hydrostatic pressure or abdominal surgery.

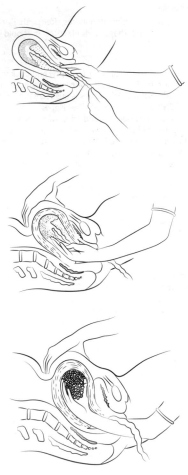

Fig. 42.12 Manual removal of placenta. Reproduced with permission from WHO, Managing Complications in Pregnancy and Childbirth, 2000, pp. 77–78.

Postpartum haemorrhage

Definition

Blood loss of 500 mL or more from the genital tract occurring within 24 hours after birth.

> PPH is the leading cause of maternal death in LIC, and the primary cause of approximately 25% of cases globally. The majority are avoidable with prophylactic uterotonics (oxytocin) and prompt management. For prophylaxis, all women should be offered uterotonics during third stage of labour. Oxytocin 10 IU IM is first line. When unavailable use other injectable uterotonics (see Table 42.4) and misoprostol 800 mcg PO/sublingually.

Management

Early recognition is key, call for help as soon as PPH is suspected.
Repeat vital signs regularly to monitor haemodynamic state. (See Table 42.4.)

Systematic approach

- Ask an assistant to give oxygen if available, insert two wide-bore IV lines, commence fluid resuscitation, blood transfusion, and blood products as required and insert Foley urine catheter. Check Hb and blood group (full blood count, clotting, urea and electrolytes, and liver function tests if available).
- Rub uterine fundus (massage) to stimulate a contraction. Uterus should feel hard (like a cricket ball) after delivery; if atonic begin medical treatment and ensure bladder is empty to encourage contraction.
- Check that the placenta is complete. If in doubt or placenta is undelivered, proceed to MROP (see ➔ 'Retained placenta' p. 775). Ensure uterus is empty of clots and placenta.
- Perform bimanual compression of the uterus: non-dominant hand on uterine fundus pushing down, dominant hand in vagina pushing up. Aim to compress the uterus between both hands. (See Fig. 42.13.)
- Check for trauma: use a speculum to visualize the cervix; with sponge holding forceps work around the cervix clockwise. If there is a tear that is bleeding, ligate the apex and close. If there is a tear that is not bleeding, leave it alone. Check vagina and perineum, any bleeding tears should be sutured; always take the apex first and work down. (see ➔ 'Perineal trauma and repair' pp. 770–1)
- Continued bleeding will need surgical intervention. This will largely depend on where you are, and the skills and facilities available. If in a remote setting, aortic compression or a non-pneumatic anti-shock garment can be used as a temporizing measure. Intrauterine balloon tamponade should be the first-line measure (see Box 42.3); this can be performed in both BEmONC and CEmONC facilities.
- Keep the patient warm (hypothermia reduces clotting capacity).

Surgical steps

- Examine under anaesthesia, check for trauma and uterine contents. Consider: intrauterine balloon, uterine brace suture, uterine devascularization (arterial ligation or embolization). If previous CS, check for uterine rupture.

- Hysterectomy: in ongoing PPH, especially when there are limited resources, a decision should not be delayed. Sub-total hysterectomy is quicker, safer, and technically easier (see ➲ 'Practical manuals' p. 786).
- Consider clotting disorders/DIC: transfuse fresh, whole blood.

Aftercare
Monitor for secondary PPH, check Hb, debrief, and advise future delivery in a CEmONC facility.

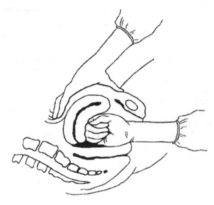

Fig. 42.13 Bimanual compression of the uterus. Reproduced with permission from WHO, Managing Complications in Pregnancy and Childbirth, 2000, pS-84.

Table 42.4 Medical management of postpartum haemorrhage

Medical treatment	Administration	Notes
Oxytocin 5 IU slow IV injection	Do not give as IV bolus	
Oxytocin infusion: 20 IU in 1 litre crystalloid	Run at 60 drops/minute	Maximum 3 litres
Ergometrine 0.2 mg IM or slow IV injection	If required repeat after 15 minutes, maximum of 5 doses	Avoid in ↑BP/pre-eclampsia/heart disease
Carboprost 0.25 mg IM	Repeat every 15 minutes, maximum of 8 doses	Avoid in asthma
Misoprostol 800 mcg sublingual	If sublingual route not possible give 1000 mcg rectally	
Tranexamic acid 1 g IV	Second dose after 30 minutes if continued bleeding	

Box 42.3 Intrauterine balloon tamponade

Indication

Atonic PPH not responding to conservative/medical measures.

There are several balloon tamponades available (e.g. Bakri® Balloon). The device can also be easily replicated using a Foley catheter (largest size available) and male latex condom, this is invaluable in the resource-poor setting.

- The woman should already be catheterized, with available uterotonics given and in lithotomy position.
- Unroll the condom and open the Foley catheter. Using a suture (string if no suture available), tie the condom to the top (bladder end) of the catheter.
- Insert the condom and catheter through the cervix and into the uterine cavity.
- Inflate the condom (via the catheter) with saline using a large syringe or giving-set. Stop when resistance is felt, or at 500 mL, and clamp catheter.
- A vaginal pack (or large swab) can be used to keep the balloon in place. Broad-spectrum IV antibiotic cover should be given.
- The patient can be transferred with the balloon *in situ*.
- If there is no further bleeding, gradually deflate and remove the balloon after 24 hours.

Sepsis

Sepsis is a major cause of maternal and newborn morbidity and mortality globally. In the humanitarian setting where patients may present late or with multiple complications, there must be fast recognition and rapid response to the signs of sepsis.

Diagnostic criteria for sepsis

Sepsis is a systemic response to infection, and a medical emergency that can deteriorate rapidly. Two or more general features signify sepsis; a drop in BP signifies septic shock. Additional features assist in quantifying severity of the inflammatory response, tissue hypo-perfusion, and organ damage.

Indicators of sepsis

General features
- Temperature <36°C or >38°C.
- Pulse >90 bpm.
- Respiration >20 breaths/minute.
- Reduced conscious level/confusion.
- Significant oedema/positive fluid balance.
- Hyperglycaemia in absence of diabetes mellitus >7.7 mmol/L.
- Skin discoloration/bruising suggests late fasciitis.

Inflammatory markers
- White cell count <4 or >12 × 10^9/L.
- C-reactive protein >7 mg/L.

Tissue perfusion
- Systolic BP <90 mmHg or ↓ >40 mmHg.
- Mean arterial pressure (MAP) <70 mmHg.
- Lactate ≥4 mmol/L.
- ↓ Capillary refill/skin mottling.

Organ dysfunction
- Urine output <0.5 mL/kg/hour with adequate fluid.
- Creatinine ↑ >44.2 μmol/L.
- Creatinine level >176 μmol/L (severe sepsis).
- Abnormal clotting.
- Platelets <100 × 10^9/L.
- Total bilirubin >70 μmol/L.
- Absent bowel sounds/ileus.

Management
- ABC approach.
- Give oxygen.
- IV access (depending on resources take bloods for: full blood count, urea and electrolytes, liver function tests, clotting, lactate, C-reactive protein, glucose, and culture).
- Rapid fluid resuscitation guided by BP/pulse/urine output.

- Broad-spectrum IV antibiotics according to local protocol (in absence of protocol consider: co-amoxiclav 1.2 g three times daily or metronidazole 500 mg three times daily + amoxicillin 1 g four times daily + gentamicin 3–5 mg/kg once daily).
- Urinary catheter (check urine for UTI).
- In endemic areas always check and treat for malaria.

Search for the source

Pregnant women are exposed to all the same risks of infection as the general population. Work from head to toe in a systematic manner.

Pregnancy specific

- Chorioamnionitis: suspect if membranes are ruptured or uterus tender. Treat as above-mentioned and expedite delivery of fetus and placenta.
- Post CS: check scar for cellulitis or dehiscence, if peritonitic consider bowel perforation.
- Post vaginal delivery: check vagina and perineum for infected episiotomy/tear. Perineal abscess. Retained swabs or foreign bodies.
- Mastitis: check breasts for evidence of cellulitis, blocked ducts and abscess.
- Endometritis: the most common cause of puerperal sepsis, treat on suspicion particularly when delivery conditions may not have been ideal. If retained products of conception (either from delivery, miscarriage, or TOP) are suspected, perform MVA/MROP once sepsis treated.
- Appendicitis: the appendix is displaced upwards by the growing uterus, hence presentation is often atypical and diagnosed late.
- HIV/AIDS: a leading cause of maternal death, consider opportunistic infections and treat aggressively
- Venous thromboembolism: pregnancy and puerperium are high risk for venous thromboembolism; presentation has similar signs to sepsis and should be considered as a differential diagnosis.

For further guidance, see the Royal College of Obstetricians and Gynaecologists guidelines.[2,3]

Intrauterine fetal death

Intrauterine fetal death is a common occurrence in the humanitarian setting. Intrauterine fetal death may occur before labour or intrapartum.

Diagnosis is ideally made with ultrasound visualization of the fetal heart. Reliance on fetal heart auscultation or fetal movements should be taken with caution as there is a wide margin for error. If uncertain and mother is stable, do nothing and re-check in 1 week.

Pre-labour

- Providing the mother is stable (e.g. no sign of sepsis, pre-eclampsia, or placental abruption) and membranes intact, there is no rush to deliver. Allow time for her to understand and discuss the diagnosis.
- Either allow time for labour to begin spontaneously (may take several weeks), or commence induction of labour.
- Induction: mifepristone 200 mg PO + metoclopramide 10 mg PO.
- 36–48 hours after give misoprostol 25 mcg PO every 2–4 hours (dissolve 200 mcg in 40 mL water; 5 mL = 25 mcg).
- If mifepristone is not available, misoprostol can be used alone.
- If membranes rupture, give IV broad-spectrum antibiotics.

Extra care must be taken if previous CS due to risk of uterine rupture.
- If available, give mifepristone 600 mg PO once daily for 2 days.
- If required, begin misoprostol as above after 36–48 hours from last dose.
- Reduce misoprostol dose if necessary (e.g. administer 6-hourly).

Intrapartum

Allow labour to progress normally and deliver vaginally.

Post-delivery

- Ensure that the woman has a chance to ask questions and offer her psychological support.
- Provide lactation suppression: cabergoline 1 mg within 48 hours after delivery.
  - If cabergoline is unavailable, provide analgesia, avoid expressing milk (though if she is extremely uncomfortable with engorgement she may express small amounts of milk for relief of immediate pain).
  - Consider breast binding: open the seams of a pillow case, or use a piece of material of similar size, and use the cloth as a breast binder; wrap it snugly—but not uncomfortably tight—and tie or pin it in place; milk will generally be dried up in a week's time.
  - Follow local customs regarding management of stillborn.
  - Offer contraception before discharge.

Trauma, sexual violence, and epidemics

Pregnant women living in areas of instability and humanitarian context are exposed to the same risks as the general population. It is important to consider the response to them and their specific needs:

Trauma

- Trauma may be blunt or penetrating. Changes in the fetal heart pattern (rapid, slow, or absent) can indicate internal bleeding due to hypoperfusion of the placenta.
- Observe pregnant women with trauma to the abdomen for signs of placental abruption, uterine rupture, and pre-term labour. If in doubt, admit and monitor for changes in vital signs or development of contractions/vaginal bleeding.
- Penetrating injury to the abdomen will usually require a laparotomy. If the uterus is intact and there is no other indication for CS, leave alone and allow normal delivery to take place with spontaneous labour.

Sexual violence

- Pregnant women who have been sexually assaulted should still be offered post-exposure prophylaxis for HIV, tetanus, and STIs. Doxycycline should be substituted with azithromycin 1 g PO stat.
- Pregnancy, delivery, and the postnatal period can be particularly challenging for survivors of sexual violence. Avoid vaginal examinations where possible.
- If feasible, try to have continuity of care with a health worker who can build a rapport of trust with the patient (see ➲ Chapter 5).

Epidemics

- Pregnant women can be particularly vulnerable to complications of disease outbreaks (e.g. measles, hepatitis E, viral haemorrhagic fevers).
- As far as possible, keep infected pregnant women isolated away from other pregnant women and neonates.
- Pre-term labour and miscarriage are common, as is the risk of haemorrhage. Provide supportive treatment, monitoring response closely.
- Remember that the mother's life comes first; do not deny potentially life-saving treatment of a disease for theoretical risks to the pregnancy.
- Effective health education advising pregnant women to avoid contact with those infected is an important part of the community engagement.

Famine

- In situations of famine, pregnant and breastfeeding women should be identified and provided with nutritional supplementation. This should include balanced energy and protein-rich foods in order to avoid immunocompromise, stillbirth, and low-birthweight neonates.
- Vitamins and minerals should also be provided depending on the context, particularly to avoid anaemia, night blindness, and complications of deficiency.

Postnatal care

Approximately 40% of maternal deaths occur in the postnatal period, defined as the first 6 weeks after delivery. The first 24 hours after delivery is the period of highest risk.

- In developing countries, if postnatal care was provided with the same dedication as antenatal care, it is estimated that around 90% of postnatal maternal deaths could be avoided.
- Like antenatal care, postnatal care can be scheduled according to patient convenience. Ideally there are two postnatal consultations—one within 8 days of delivery and one at 4–6 weeks postpartum.
- In some cultures, the practice of a so-called lying-in period (for 40 days following childbirth), during which time mothers and their babies are not allowed to leave the home, is cited as a major constraint. Measures to overcome this include encouraging community elders to give permission to attend postnatal care during this period or having an outreach team visit women in their homes with referral for those with complications.
- Offer all women contraception postpartum. Encourage long-acting forms.

Depression

Common during pregnancy and the postpartum period, this has an even higher frequency in humanitarian settings.

- Separation from family and support structures, intimate partner violence, and a history of mental illness are important contributing factors.
- Presentation can vary from mild to severe with suicidal intentions.
- Women should be routinely asked about possible symptoms of depression or if they are struggling to cope.
- Offer psychosocial support and refer to appropriate services for ongoing care and possible antidepressant treatment.

Puerperal psychosis

- Occurs in approximately 1–2/1000 women within the first month postpartum. Previous psychiatric history (bipolar affective disorder) or first-degree relatives with a similar history is a significant risk factor.
- This is a medical emergency—the woman may be acutely paranoid, hallucinating, or violent. There is significant risk of harm to both herself and the baby.
- Admit the woman, avoid leaving her alone or unobserved with the infant, and seek expert help if possible.

Breastfeeding

- Breastfeeding is the best option for infant feeding; it is cheap, readily available, and clean. Breastfeeding should be initiated immediately after birth (i.e. within 1 hour). Colostrum, a thick yellow fluid produced in first days postpartum, is beneficial to the baby's immune system and gut maturation.

- Mothers should be advised on exclusive breastfeeding (breast milk only, with no water, other fluids, or solids) for the first 6 months, with supplemental breast feeding continuing for 2 years and beyond.
- Instruct mothers to wash their hands before handling the breasts, and to stay well hydrated by drinking plenty of water.

The same advice applies to women who are HIV+ve unless there is a safe option for replacement feeding. Mixed feeding, i.e. breastfeeding plus formula/liquids/food, carries the greatest risk (e.g. diarrhoeal disease, HIV transmission). It is thought that this is due to damage of the baby gut by the other foods/liquids which then allows easier transmission of the virus. Mothers must be clearly educated about this point. Breastfeeding does not increase rate of hepatitis B virus infection. See ➲ Chapter 31 for more information.

Insufficient milk supply
- Virtually all mothers can produce enough milk. If the baby is well hydrated and passing dilute urine and milk can be expressed from the breasts, then milk is likely sufficient. If not, provide feeding assistance.
- In newborns too weak or too ill to breastfeed, milk should be expressed by hand and fed to them, e.g. by dripping the milk directly from the nipple into the baby's mouth, dribbling it by spoon, or use of a narrow feeding tube.
- Ensure the mother is herself well hydrated and receiving adequate nutrition (provide supplements, such as Plumpy'Nut® if concerned). A short course of a dopamine antagonist can be useful, e.g. metoclopramide 10 mg three times daily for 10 days.

Nipple pain
- Usually caused by improper positioning during feeding. Assist during feedings until proper latch-on is achieved by the mother independently.
- Rinse nipples with water before and after feeding; manage pain with mild analgesic and warm compress.

Engorgement
- Engorgement (hard, painful breasts) is benign and typically develops around postpartum day 3 or 4 and lasts from a few days to 2 weeks.
- Management includes more frequent nursing, ensuring appropriate latch, complete emptying of breasts at each feeding, warm compress, and gentle expression of a small amount of milk as needed to relieve pressure.

Practical manuals

The following manuals and guidance have been referred to in the preparation of this chapter. They explain how to perform obstetric procedures in the resource-poor setting, and manage complications. They are invaluable assets for preparation and while in the field:

Botton M. Primary Surgery. Vol 1: Non-Trauma. Global Help 1990 (updated 2016). ℘ http://global-help.org/products/primary-surgery/

Médecins Sans Frontières. Essential Obstetric and Newborn Care. 2015 edition. ℘ http://refbooks.msf.org/msf_docs/en/obstetrics/obstetrics_en.pdf

van den Broek N. Life Saving Skills Manual: Essential Obstetric and Newborn Care. London: Royal College of Obstetricians and Gynaecologists; 2007.

WHO, UNFPA, UNICEF, World Bank, Managing Complications in Pregnancy and Childbirth: A Guide for Midwives and Doctors. 2nd ed. Geneva: WHO; 2017. ℘ http://www.who.int/maternal_child_adolescent/documents/managing-complications-pregnancy-childbirth/en/

References

1. Thaddeus S, Maine D. Too far to walk: maternal mortality in context. Soc Sci Med 1994;38(8):1091–110.
2. Royal College of Obstetricians and Gynaecologists. Bacterial Sepsis in Pregnancy. Green-top Guideline No. 64a. April 2012. ℘ https://www.rcog.org.uk/globalassets/documents/guidelines/gtg_64a.pdf
3. Royal College of Obstetricians and Gynaecologists. Bacterial Sepsis following Pregnancy. Green-top Guideline No. 64b. April 2012. ℘ http://www.rcog.org.uk/globalassets/documents/guidelines/gtg_64b.pdf

Further reading

Collins S, Arulkumaran S, Hayes K, Jackson S, Impey L (eds). Oxford Handbook of Obstetrics and Gynaecology. Oxford: Oxford University Press; 2013.

Royal College of Obstetricians and Gynaecologists. Green-top guidelines, a series of evidence-based guidance for obstetrics and gynaecology. ℘ https://www.rcog.org.uk/guidelines

Global Library of Women's Medicine. ℘ http://www.glowm.com

World Health Organization. Inter-Agency Field Manual on Reproductive Health in Humanitarian Settings. 2010. ℘ http://www.who.int/reproductivehealth/publications/emergencies/field_manual/en/

World Health Organization. Reproductive Health Library, guidelines. ℘ https://extranet.who.int/rhl/guidelines

World Health Organization. Sexual and Reproductive Health Publications, including manuals and guidelines. ℘ http://www.who.int/reproductivehealth/publications/en/

Chapter 43

Neonatology

Jonathan Spector and Marie Claude Bottineau

Neonatal care and common problems

While vast regional disparities persist, significant reductions in under-five child mortality took place in the decade preceding expiration of the Millennium Development Goals in 2015. As child mortality rates fell, however, the percentage of child deaths attributable to neonates (aged 0–28 days) rose steadily, to 44% globally according to 2014 estimates. This epidemiological shift underscores the difficulty of impacting newborn harm at scale, a challenge which derives from the complexity of safeguarding the well-being of individual babies in low-resource and conflict/post-conflict settings.

Nearly 3 million neonatal deaths occur annually, primarily from infection, intrapartum-related problems, and prematurity. Most neonatal deaths take place in the first week of life, and most of those in the first 24 hours. Newborns are an exceedingly vulnerable population at baseline because of their susceptibility to environmental conditions, weak immune systems, high caloric needs for growth, and absolute reliance on caregivers. These risks are magnified in the context of humanitarian emergencies where access to antenatal services, skilled assistance at delivery, and adequate postnatal care is insecure.

Care of the newborn begins before birth through high-quality maternal care, and continues at the time of delivery by ensuring a baby's healthy transition to *ex utero* life. Since complications in newborns are unpredictable, at least one skilled attendant who is capable of providing routine and emergent newborn care should be present at every birth. A full assessment of every baby, which includes consideration of risk factors known to be linked with potential health problems, should take place in the first minutes and hours after birth and then periodically thereafter. Unique to the approach of caring for newborns relative to other populations is the urgency with which health problems must be recognized and addressed; even conditions as seemingly minor as hypothermia (low body temperature) can cause a baby's clinical status to quickly deteriorate and spiral downwards. Most neonatal deaths are completely avoidable with timely identification and proper management of health problems.

Establishing field capacity for newborn care

Defining the level of neonatal care that can reasonably be delivered will depend on the context and reliable availability of human resources, medications, equipment, and supplies. A framework for establishing neonatal services generally follows three tiers:

An essential package of neonatal care

Should be available everywhere babies are born, typically with midwifes or nurses as first-line health workers who are trained to provide basic maternal care, newborn resuscitation, and essential newborn care. Components include the following:
- A clean, hygienic birth environment.
- A designated neonatal resuscitation area outfitted with standard equipment including a cleanable bulb syringe plus bag-and-mask.
- Skin-to-skin care (also known as kangaroo mother care) for thermal management of newborns weighing <2000 g.
- Breastfeeding support for new mothers.
- Neonatal health promotion during the first week of life, possibly by CHWs.

An intermediate package of neonatal care

Should be available in health centres or equivalent health structures with midwifes, nurses, and/or assistant physicians as first-line health workers. Components include the essential package as previously mentioned and:
- essential medicines, including antibiotics, and IV fluids
- oxygen, pulse oximetry, and IV access
- a small-baby unit to care for not sick low birth weight babies, including caffeine citrate to guard against apnoea of prematurity
- alternative feeding methods (such as NG feeds) for newborns that cannot breastfeed
- phototherapy to treat newborn jaundice.

A comprehensive package of neonatal care

Should to be implemented wherever it is feasible but specifically in district and reference hospitals with midwifes, nurses, and doctors or paediatricians as first-line health workers. Components include the intermediate package as previously mentioned and:
- advanced newborn resuscitation, including chest compression, capacity for intubation, epinephrine (adrenaline), and fluid boluses
- incubators to provide warmth for unstable babies or those too fragile for skin-to-skin care
- case management of main neonatal diseases and sick premature babies
- respiratory support, including continuous positive airway pressure or ventilators
- pain management and palliative care
- simple neonatal surgery.

Newborn resuscitation

- At least one attendant at every birth should be capable of providing basic newborn resuscitation. A standard training course for use in austere settings is the 'Helping Babies Breathe' programme (⅋ http://www.aap.org). (See Fig. 43.1.)
- All babies should be dried immediately and kept warm at birth. The vast majority of newborns (80–90%) require no specific intervention to transition normally.
- Suctioning with a cleanable bulb syringe should be done only if the mouth or nose has secretions that could block the airway. Routine nasal or oral suction is not recommended for babies born through clear amniotic fluid who breathe spontaneously since this could provoke a vagal response and induce apnoea.
- Approximately 10% of babies require assistance to begin efficient breathing. It is crucial that an apnoeic (not breathing) or gasping baby receive assistance immediately within the first, 'golden minute' of life.
- Most apnoeic or gasping babies will respond to stimulation administered by firmly rubbing the back up and down two or three times.
- If a poorly breathing baby fails to respond to drying and stimulation, then the single most important intervention is *positive pressure ventilation* (PPV) with a self-inflating bag-and-mask.

Positive pressure ventilation

- For PPV, the mask must properly fit the mouth and nose.
  - Oxygen is not immediately recommended; positive pressure should initially be delivered with air alone. Oxygen can be added after 30 seconds of efficient PPV if available and needed (SpO$_2$).
  - Note: there is no substitute for PPV with a bag-and-mask; no new-born resuscitation guidelines suggest that mouth-to-mouth resuscitation could be used as a backup.
- To deliver PPV, the baby's head should be in the 'sniffing' position, which is slight extension of the neck (hyperflexion or hyperextension of the neck will block the trachea and prevent air movement). PPV should be given at 40–60 breaths per minute.
  - Good chest rise signals effective ventilation.
  - If good chest rise is not achieved, briefly cease ventilation and rapidly correct any of the following: improper 'sniffing' position, poor seal of the face mask over the baby's mouth and nose, or secretions in the nose or mouth that may block the airway.
- Only if PPV is effectively delivered without results should advanced resuscitation measures be delivered.

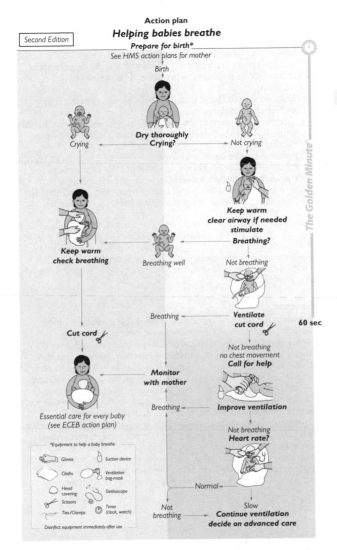

Fig. 43.1 Action plan for newborn resuscitation. Reproduced with permission from helping Babies Breathe, 2nd edition, American Academy of Paediatrics (www.aap.org/en-us/advocacy-and-policy/aap-health-initiatives/helping-babies-survive/Pages/Helping-Babies-Breathe-Edition.aspx).

Advanced resuscitation

- Less than 1% of newborns require advanced resuscitation techniques including chest compression and epinephrine.
- If the baby's heart rate remains <60/minute after 30–60 seconds of adequate PPV, begin chest compressions at 90 per minute (3:1 ratio with breaths).
  - Ensure a firm surface is under the baby's back in order to effectively deliver chest compressions.
  - Compress one-third of the anterior–posterior diameter of the chest at the lower part of the baby's sternum, just below the line connecting the nipples.
- Infants who require significant resuscitation must be monitored closely in the post-resuscitation period, on-site if possible or transferred to a reference hospital when not feasible.
- If there are no signs of life (heart beat or respiratory effort) after 10 minutes of resuscitation, the resuscitation effort may be stopped.

If the baby's heart rate remains <60/minute after 30 seconds of both effective PPV and chest compressions, give IV epinephrine 0.1–0.3 mL/kg of a 1:10,000 dilution followed by saline flush (e.g. a 3 kg baby would receive somewhere between 0.3–0.9 mL of epinephrine).

If the baby is hypovolaemic, also give 10 mL/kg of isotonic saline over several minutes.

IV access

- Generally, an umbilical venous line is the quickest reliable method for obtaining intravascular access in newborns and, faced urgently with a severely distressed baby, probably remains the approach of choice despite the risks of introducing infection. Nevertheless, the umbilical catheter should be removed as soon as IV line can be secured (maximum few hours). If this route is chosen, the skin and umbilicus should be sterilized and umbilical ties placed. The catheter should be placed approximately 2–4 cm below the skin surface. Confirmation of access is made when blood return is noted after insertion.
- The intraosseous route is also possible but in the case of resuscitation it is poorly studied and may take too long for epinephrine to travel centrally following administration in a limb. If this route is chosen, the skin should first be sterilized. The needle should be placed in the tibial plateau approximately 1 cm below the knee joint. Confirmation of access is made by infusion of normal saline without resistance.

Routine newborn care

A systematic assessment of every baby and a core set of essential practices should be performed at every birth. A standard training course for use in austere settings is the 'Helping Babies Survive: Essential Care for Every Baby' programme (an updated version of WHO's older 'Essential Newborn Care' programme).

- 'Late' cord clamping (1–2 minutes after birth) is recommended for all births while initiating simultaneous essential newborn care.
- Dry the newborn with warm dry sheets or blankets and then remove wet cloths. Well-appearing babies should be kept in skin-to-skin contact with their mothers after birth to maintain warmth, promote breastfeeding, and support bonding.
- Encourage initiation of breastfeeding as soon as the baby shows signs of readiness, at least within the first hour after birth. Colostrum is nutritious for the baby and should not be discarded. Breastfeeding also helps the mother by stimulating the uterus to contract thereby decreasing the likelihood of postpartum bleeding.
- Apply a 1 cm ribbon of 0.5% erythromycin or 1% tetracycline ophthalmic ointment (or alternative medicine, according to national guidelines) in both eyes to prevent serious bacterial conjunctivitis.
- To expose a baby's eye safely, wash hands with soap and water first and then gently pull down the lower lid of the eye.
- Administer 1 mg of vitamin K (usually supplied as an ampoule) IM in the anterolateral aspect of the thigh to prevent haemorrhagic disease of the newborn.
  - Give 1 hour after birth.
  - Swab skin with isopropyl alcohol prior to injection.
  - For newborns that weigh <1500 g, the adjusted dose is 0.5 mg of vitamin K.
- The umbilical cord should be kept clean and dry.
- Daily application of 7.1% chlorhexidine digluconate (4% chlorhexidine) solution or gel to the umbilical cord stump in settings with high risk of infection may be recommended to decrease the risk of infection.
- Examine the baby to assess for potential problems including danger signs (see ⮕ p. 794).
  - A well baby should have a non-cyanotic skin tone; breathe comfortably at 40–60/minute; have an axillary temperature of 36.5–37.5°C; lay with arms and legs flexed when at rest; have no drainage or bleeding from the umbilical cord; and have no obvious abnormalities of the head, face, mouth, palate, chest, abdomen, genitalia, anus, limbs, or skin.
- Weighing babies is important to identify those at higher risk of complications:
  - Babies <2500 g may require special care to maintain warmth.
  - Babies <2000 g should receive prolonged skin-to-skin care and may need nutritional support.
  - Babies <1500 g usually require advanced care for thermal, nutritional, and respiratory needs.

- Provide antiretroviral medications for HIV-exposed babies, according to national guidelines.
- Delay bathing for at least 24 hours to decrease the risk of hypothermia.
- If not possible due to cultural factors, encourage delay of bathing for a minimum of 6 hours.
- Give immunizations according to national guidelines.
- These usually include hepatitis B (0.5 mL IM given in the anterolateral aspect of the thigh), bivalent oral polio (2 drops on the tongue), and BCG (0.05 mL intradermal in the arm).
- Newborns and their mothers should receive close postnatal care monitoring for at least 24 hours after birth. Monitor for danger signs (see Table 43.1).
  - Home visits in the first week of life are recommended.

Danger signs

- See Table 43.1 for newborn danger signs.[1] A baby with one of the following danger signs is very sick and at risk of death. Danger signs are caused by infection or another serious problem.
- A newborn with a danger sign should be treated emergently with antibiotics and receive advanced care.

General antibiotic recommendations

- The recommended antibiotics are ampicillin IM (50 mg/kg every 12 hours) and gentamicin IM (First week of life: 5 mg/kg every 24 hours if normal birth weight; 3 mg/kg every 24 hours if low birth weight).
- If suspected meningitis or alternatively, give ampicillin IM and cefotaxime IM (First week of life: 50 mg/kg every 8 hours if normal birth weight; every 12 hours if premature).

Table 43.1 Newborn danger signs

Fast breathing and/or cyanosis	Respiratory rate > 60/minutes
	There may be blue colour to the skin or inside the mouth, representing cyanosis
	May result from pneumonia or bloodstream infection
Chest indrawing (retractions)	Spaces between, above, or below the ribs indent with each breath
	There may be a blue colour to the skin or inside the mouth, representing cyanosis
	May result from pneumonia or bloodstream infection
Temperature too low or too high	Axillary temperature <35.5°C or >37.5°C that does not respond to re-warming
	Re-warming should be attempted by restarting or improving skin-to-skin care, increasing room temperature and avoiding drafts, ensuring the baby has dry clothing and a hat, and adding a layer of clothing, socks, and an additional blanket (for additional information, see ➜ p. 788)
Not feeding or abdominal distension	Poor suck, swallow, or interest in feeding
	Vomits large quantities of each feeding
	Abdominal distension with poor/absence emission of stools
	Healthy babies usually feed every 2–4 hours and feed 8–12 times daily
No movement, hypotonia, lethargy	No spontaneous movement or no movement when stimulated
Convulsions	Rhythmic movements of the limbs that do not stop with holding
	May also result from low blood sugar (see ➜ p. 796)
	Jitteriness is not a convulsion, and can usually be stopped by gently holding the limb
Omphalitis	Red skin around the umbilicus

Key problems and interventions in neonatology

Hypothermia

Definition
- Axillary temperature <35.5°C.
- Hypothermia results in cellular dysfunction.

Common causes
- Common causes are environmental (particularly at night-time), prematurity, hypoglycaemia, and sepsis.
- Systematically check vital signs looking for sepsis and control for glycaemia before treating for environmental cause.

Management
- Warm the baby immediately by using a hat and socks, and providing skin-to-skin contact including wrapping of the mother and the baby jointly.
- If unsuccessful:
  - Use an external heat source.
  - Feed the baby to increase blood glucose.
  - Consider wrapping the newborn in a survival blanket (in some cultures, skin-to-skin contact is not accepted, although it should be encouraged as the first-line option).
- Have close surveillance. If a cold baby is difficult to re-warm then begin treatment with antibiotics for presumed sepsis.

Hypoglycaemia

Definition
- Blood glucose level <2.5 mmol/L (45 mg/dL).
- Profound or prolonged hypoglycaemia can result in neurological impairment.

Common causes
- Prematurity, small or large for gestational age, hypothermia, sepsis, and following resuscitation/critical care.

Signs/symptoms
- Many hypoglycaemic babies will be asymptomatic.
- Signs of hypoglycaemia, when they occur, include jitteriness, tremors, altered mentation and seizures; hypothermia; hypotonia, apnoea, and tachypnoea; poor feeding; bradycardia; and cyanosis.

Management
- The best treatment for mild hypoglycaemia is to ensure adequate feeding. Breastfeeding is always the preferred method. When that is not possible, replacement feeds can be given.
- Asymptomatic hypoglycaemia can be treated with feeding 5 mL/kg of 10% oral glucose solution, and re-evaluation.

- Treat symptomatic hypoglycaemia, or persistent asymptomatic hypoglycaemia, immediately with an IV bolus of 2–4 mL/kg of 10% glucose solution:
  - Give a second bolus and/or subsequent continuous IV infusion as needed.
  - Check glucose level 20 minutes after the treatment and then before each meal until normal two times successively, and then at three to four intervals as needed.

Bacterial sepsis and meningitis

Definition
Systemic infection by bacteria; in newborns, sepsis can rapidly progress to meningitis since the newborn's blood–brain barrier is weak.

Common causes
- Early-onset (within the first 7 days) infection is often caused by Gram-negative enterics (*Escherichia coli*, *Klebsiella*, *Serratia*, *Pseudomonas*, and *Salmonella*) or group B *Streptococcus* (GBS).
- *Streptococcus* causes a high proportion of late-onset (after 7 days) infection.

Risk factors
- Major risk factors are maternal peripartum fever (> 37.9°C or 100.4°F), chorioamnionitis (perineal infection in the mother), prolonged membrane rupture (>18 hours), and maternal GBS colonization.
- Minor risk factors include prematurity, low birth weight (<2000 g), and birth resuscitation with bag-and-mask.

Signs/symptoms
- Sepsis and meningitis are difficult to distinguish clinically.
- Signs of disease can take many forms including lethargy (poor movement on stimulation), poor feeding, fast breathing (>60/minute), chest in-drawing, hypothermia, hyperthermia, convulsions, and/or a bulging fontanelle (late sign).

Management
- Cerebrospinal fluid is ideally obtained before treatment but should not delay the immediate administration of antibiotics.
- First-line treatment is as listed previously for danger signs, with ampicillin plus cefotaxime.

Duration of treatment is generally 10–14 days for sepsis and 14–21 days for meningitis.

Congenital syphilis

Definition
- Transmission of spirochete *Treponema pallidum* from a pregnant woman to her fetus.

Cause
- Syphilis in newborns can be acquired by transplacental transmission, or less commonly, through direct contact with an infectious lesion during birth.

- 1.5 million women are infected with syphilis each year and half are untreated.[2]
- Every woman should be routinely screened in pregnancy with an RPR test at the first prenatal visit. Women at particularly high risk should be screened again at 28 weeks' gestation and at the time of delivery. Proper maternal treatment reduces transmission from 70–100% to 1–2%.
- Adverse birth outcomes include early fetal loss, still-birth, neonatal death, low birth weight, and neonatal infection.

Signs/symptoms
- Infected newborns are often symptomatic at birth. Signs include low birth weight; syphilitic rhinitis ('snuffles'); hepatomegaly and splenomegaly; jaundice; and anaemia.
- Cutaneous lesions are initially maculopapular with small pink spots, or bullous. They typically evolve to crusting and peeling and then dusky lesions. Fissures may be present in mucocutaneous and anal areas.

Management
- If the maternal RPR test is positive during pregnancy, treat the mother with 2.4 million units of benzathine benzylpenicillin IM (administered as two injections at different sites) to decrease the risk of transmission to the newborn (if the mother has a penicillin allergy, than alternatively give erythromycin 500 mg PO every 6 hours for 15 days). Also, treat the newborn with 50,000 units/kg of benzathine benzylpenicillin IM (single dose).
- If a baby is born with suspected congenital syphilis, do a VDRL (Venereal Disease Research Laboratory) test.
- Treat symptomatic infants with 50 mg/kg of procaine benzylpenicillin IM once daily for 10 days. Alternatively, give 30 mg/kg of benzylpenicillin IV every 12 hours for the first week of life followed by 30 mg/kg IV every 8 hours for 3 additional days.
- Any time a woman or baby is confirmed to have syphilis, be sure to treat the mother's partner for syphilis and check for other possible sexually transmitted diseases.

Severe jaundice

Definition

Jaundice of the face <24 hours after birth or jaundice of the palms or soles at any time.

Cause

Jaundice results from elevated levels of bilirubin in the blood. Bilirubin is released from RBCs as they are normally broken down after birth. Pathological hyperbilirubinaemia frequently results from isoimmunization with maternal blood causing increased RBC haemolysis in the newborn. Other risk factors for jaundice include breastfeeding; certain medicines (notably oxytocin and diazepam); Asian or Native American ethnicity; gestational diabetes; birth trauma resulting in cephalohaematoma or bruising; polycythemia; and prematurity. Severe neonatal hyperbilirubinaemia can lead to acute encephalopathy (called kernicterus) which results in permanent neurological impairment.

Signs/symptoms
In dark skinned-babies, it may be difficult to appreciate.
- Detect by pushing a finger against the forehead and observing if the skin is yellow after releasing pressure.
- Severe forms are also associated with fever or last >14 days at term or 21 days in premature neonates.[3]

Management
- Severe jaundice requires treatment with phototherapy and may require exchange transfusion.
- It is standard practice to protect a newborn's eyes with the use of a mask when administering phototherapy.
- Filtered sunlight (using special canopies that filter out ultraviolet light and some heat) was found to be non-inferior to conventional phototherapy for treatment of neonatal hyperbilirubinaemia in a study in Africa.[4]
- Dehydration is a risk factor for newborns that receive phototherapy. Fluid intake should be increased as needed to maintain normal fluid output.

Neonatal tetanus

Definition
Infection by *Clostridium tetani*.

Cause
- Occurs from infection of the umbilicus in a baby whose mother was poorly immunized against tetanus (less than two doses).
- Poor hygiene during delivery and harmful traditional community practices (such as rubbing dirt or dung on the umbilicus) can contribute to disease risk.

Note that clinical infection of the cord may not be evident.

Signs/symptoms
Typical onset is at 3–21 days after birth.
- Early signs are irritability and feeding difficulties. Rigidity and muscle spasms then set in.
- The life-threatening complications of tetanus result from the baby's inability to feed and paralysis of respiratory function.
- Birth asphyxia or sepsis can be associated.

Management
- Neonatal tetanus is extremely challenging to treat, even in high-resource settings. Mortality ranges from 10% to 60% globally.
- Hospitalize the baby in a dark and quiet room (external stimuli aggravate spasms) but ensuring close surveillance, secure the airway, give IV fluids and/or NG feeds as needed, administer 500 IU human tetanus immunoglobulin IM (split the volume and administer at two different sites), and systemic antibiotics with IV metronidazole for 14 days (loading dose 15 mg/kg administered over 60 minutes, then 24 hours later begin a 7.5 mg/kg/dose every 12 hours).

To treat muscle spasms well, babies should be intubated and ventilated when possible. In this circumstance, give IV diazepam emulsion (0.1 mg/kg/dose every 2 hours as needed), and/or other anesthetics and muscle relaxants as needed.

After recovery, give tetanus vaccine to the baby and complete the mother's vaccination.

Omphalitis

Definition

- Infection of the umbilical stump and possibly also the skin around the umbilicus.
- Omphalitis, which can develop in the first days after birth, can rapidly progress to bacterial sepsis.

Signs/symptoms

- Signs include redness, tenderness, and purulent and sometimes foul-smelling discharge.

Risk factors

- Risk factors are the same as for sepsis plus home delivery, poor hygiene during delivery, and improper cord care after birth.

Management

- Treat with IV/IM cloxacillin for 10 days (50 mg/kg every 8 or 12 hours in the first week of life; every 6 or 8 hours in weeks 2–4) and gentamicin for 5 days.
- If progressive, add metronidazole or change IV cloxacillin for IV clindamycin. Metronidazole should have a loading dose of 15 mg/kg administered over 60 minutes, then 24 hours later begin 7.5 mg/kg/dose every 12 hours
- Use with 4% chlorhexidine topically three times daily as needed.

References

1. American Academy of Pediatrics. Helping Babies Survive: Essential Care for Every Baby. ℘ https://www.aap.org/en-us/advocacy-and-policy/aap-health-initiatives/helping-babies-survive/Pages/Essential-Care-Every-Baby.aspx
2. Department of Reproductive Health and Research, WHO. Investment Case for Eliminating Mother-to-Child Transmission of Syphilis. WHO; 2012. ℘ http://www.who.int/reproductivehealth/publications/sexual_health/9789241504348/en/
3. Brent A, Davidson R, Seale A. Oxford Handbook of Tropical Medicine. Oxford: Oxford University Press; 2014, p. 23.
4. Slusher TM, Olusanya BO, Vreman HJ, Brearley AM, Vaucher YE, Lund TC, et al. A randomized trial of phototherapy with filtered sunlight in African neonates. N Engl J Med 2015;373(12):1115–24.

Further reading

American Academy of Pediatrics. 'Helping Babies Breathe' and 'Helping Babies Survive: Routine Care for Every Newborn' educational courses. ℘ http://www.helpingbabiesbreathe.org
Lawn JE, Blencowe H, Oza S, You D, Lee AC, Waiswa P, et al. Every newborn: progress, priorities, and potential beyond survival. Lancet 384(9938):189–205.
World Health Organization. Pregnancy, Childbirth, Postpartum and Newborn Care: A Guide for Essential Practice. Geneva: WHO; 2015.

Chapter 44

Ophthalmology

William Mapham

Global context for ophthalmology

While eye conditions can seem daunting to health workers with little ophthalmology training, recognizing and treating ophthalmological conditions in the field is particularly important due to their prevalence and the availability of treatment options to prevent the lasting disability of blindness.

As an external organ, the eye is particularly affected by environmental factors, poor hygiene, infections, and poor nutrition. People with eye conditions living in areas without access to medical services are likely to present with advanced progression of curable disease, leading to permanent vision loss. This is further compounded by the general lack of rehabilitation or support services in low-resource areas.

Most causes of blindness globally are either preventable or treatable and the main cause of permanent disability is often the lack of available and accessible medical resources (see Fig. 44.1). With a relatively few number of medications and surgical procedures, it is possible to both save and restore vision for many people. This is particularly true for group 1 conditions, which are only found in the tropics and are easily preventable. Once blindness has occurred, however, treatment is difficult or impossible. Causes of blindness in group 2 and 3 conditions largely require specialized equipment for evaluation and treatment.

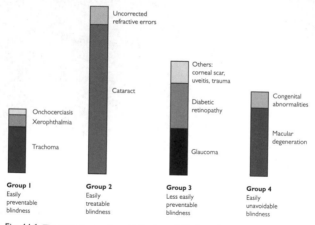

Fig. 44.1 The main causes of world blindness divided into four groups. The size of each column gives an impression of how many people are blind from this particular cause.

Approach to eye care in a humanitarian setting

Eye conditions in humanitarian settings require special care, but there are usually treatment options even in low-resource settings.

Trained professionals and task shifting

In a poorly resourced setting, it is better for eye care to be given by a 'specialist' trained in ophthalmology who is not a doctor, than by a doctor with very little special training in ophthalmology. This results in a higher quality of care from skill development. This can be done by training one or two health workers who can see all ophthalmology cases. When this is not feasible, there are still a variety of approaches which can be used depending upon the setting and resources.

Minimum services

Basic eye health training for all clinical staff. Common conditions can be treated on site and all other cases referred for specialist opinion and/or surgery.

Outreach care

Patients with eye conditions can attend the health facility on a specific day when an ophthalmologist is present.

- *Tele-ophthalmology*: photographs, combined with visual acuity and patient information, are being used for diagnosis and treatment of eye conditions. In the absence of specialized telemedicine technology, smartphones with secure referral apps can be used. See Box 44.1 for recommendations.

Recommended equipment for a humanitarian setting

Ophthalmology is a speciality where the tools you use are very important (and in which you can honestly blame your tools for not being able to do your job). In order to offer an ophthalmology service, you can prioritize your requests for equipment with the following lists. At the most basic level, you will only have the contents of your pocket to work with.

Minimum: outreach, community, home-based care, or emergency care settings
In this setting, the best you can often do is obtain a history, conduct an examination, possibly take a photo, and get an opinion from a specialist at a later date. The specialist can help teach you case by case how urgently the patient needs to be seen at an appropriate health facility.

- Camera or smartphone with a camera.
- Torch or smartphone with a light source.
- Smartphone app to enable communication with a specialist.

Basic: controlled environments such as a clinic, or day hospital
Here you will likely have access to more equipment and basic ophthalmic medications. This will enable you to identify most ocular pathology and either treat or refer correctly to a specialist.

- Chart for testing visual acuity, e.g. Snellen chart.
- Fluorescein drops or impregnated strips.

Box 44.1 Ophthalmology apps
Community Eye Health Journal—readers' choice (2015):
- *Medscape* (iOS, Android, Kindle Fire): drug references, evidence-based disease and condition reference, medical news, continuing medical education courses. ℘ http://www.medscape.com/public/mobileapp
- *Eye Hand Book* (iOS, Android): comprehensive smartphone treatment reference and specialist diagnostic settings for use by eye care professionals. ℘ http://www.eyehandbook.com
- *Vula Eye Health* (iOS, Android): set up your own referral system for faster better ophthalmology referrals from health workers to specialists. Also includes basic eye conditions library and chat function. ℘ http://www.vulamobile.com

- Local anaesthetic eye drops, e.g. benoxinate (oxybuprocaine) 0.4%.
- Quick-acting, short-lasting mydriatic for dilating the pupil, e.g. tropicamide.
- Miotic agent for constricting the pupil, e.g. pilocarpine.
- Ophthalmoscope.

Advanced: outreach ophthalmology service
The first step in providing a screening service and giving patients access to a comprehensive service is to provide an outreach ophthalmology linked to a more comprehensive service.
- Slit lamp.
- Lenses to enable views of the retina.
- Gonioscopy lens for viewing the angle in the anterior chamber.
- Tonometer for measuring intraocular pressure.

Additional technology suitable for a humanitarian setting
- Smartphones can aid an ophthalmology examination with visual acuity tests, provide clinical information, and provide contact with specialist referral systems.
- Retinal photos can be taken using devices that can be clipped onto smartphones. The best ones offer a wide field of view (see Fig. 44.2).

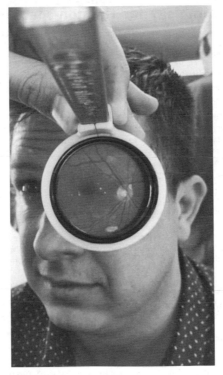

Fig. 44.2 Retinal photograph taken through a dilated pupil with a smartphone and clip-on device. A person with no healthcare training can take the photograph. You will see that the retinal image is rotated through 180°.

Ophthalmology for the non-specialist

When working in a high-pressure environment or faced with an overwhelming number of patients, patients should be screened with prioritization given to those with pain or acute loss of vision.

Preliminary information

Prior to the formal ophthalmic examination, you can triage patients with eye conditions by gathering preliminary information. This includes:

Visual acuity

Visual acuity is the best indicator of how well the eyes are functioning. Any loss of vision, either recent or long-standing, must be investigated. Test the eyes separately with a physical chart or electronic version (phone, tablet, or computer).

Chart testing

• Process: the patient reads each letter on the chart and the vision can be recorded from the notation on the side. Normal vision is recorded as 6/6 (metric notation), which means that at 6 metres the patient sees what a normal person sees at 6 metres.

• Illiterate population or children: if available you can use the tumbling E test that only uses the capital E, but rotated in four directions. Patients indicate the direction of E. The vision can be recorded from the notation on the chart.

• Extreme vision loss: in many humanitarian settings the patient's visual impairment may mean that he/she will not be able to read the largest letter on the chart.

  • You can then check if the patient can identify the number of your fingers held 3, 2, or 1 metre away; e.g. record this finding as 'count fingers' at 1 metre.

  • Failing this, wave your hand 15 cm away from the patient. Record this as 'hand movements' vision.

  • The final test is the light perception test. Preferably use the ophthalmoscope, a small torch, or the light on your phone. Shine the light on and off the eye. Record the vision as either 'light perception' or 'no light perception'.

If the eye appears essentially normal, but the vision is poor, there may be a refractive error, which means that vision can be improved with spectacles. Check for a refractive error by using an occluder with a pinhole to see if vision improves. You can construct your own occluder with a pinhole by making a 1.5–2 mm hole in a piece of dark card or paper. Ask the patient to hold the card and look through the hole. An improvement in visual acuity indicates a refractive error. An exception is with severe refractive errors, where there will be no improvement.

Pupil reactions to light

Test and record the pupil reactions of both eyes separately with a light source. You can use an ophthalmoscope, a small torch, or the light on your phone.

Always check for a relative afferent pupil defect which can indicate optic nerve abnormality (e.g. advanced glaucoma) or retinal pathology:

• A normal test is when both pupils react equally when light is shone into either eye.
• If one pupil dilates when you shine the light into the other eye then this is a relative afferent pupil defect.

Pupil dilation

If the visual acuity has decreased, there is no refractive error, and no findings on examination of the cornea or lens, then there could be retinal or optic nerve pathology. Dilating the pupils will facilitate further examination:

• First check that the *eclipse test* is negative prior to attempting this.
• To do the eclipse test, shine the light from the temporal side of the eye:
  • Normally the entire iris is illuminated.
  • If there is a shadow on the nasal side of the iris, creating the appearance of a half-moon, this indicates that the iris is bulging forward centrally.
  • In these cases, there is a contraindication for dilation due to the risk of inducing iatrogenic acute angle-closure glaucoma.

Ophthalmic history and examination

History

Presenting complaint: the patient will complain of one or a combination of pain, loss of vision, and/or an unusual appearance. Pain and a sudden loss of vision are most likely emergencies and should be prioritized over a long-standing abnormal appearance or a slow loss of vision

Ophthalmic history:

record any previous ocular complaints, conditions, treatments, and surgeries.

Family history:

a family history of eye conditions can indicate a genetic cause for the eye condition.

Medical history:

e.g. diabetes, TB, HIV, or syphilis can all have a negative effect on the eye. Record any treatments the patient is using.

Examination

The ophthalmic examination can be easily remembered by simply going from the front to the back of the eye. Start with the skin around the eye and the lids, then examine the rest of the eye in order: conjunctiva, cornea, anterior chamber, iris, lens, vitreous, and retina. The examination of the retina can include a description of the macular, the vessels, and the optic nerve.

Simple tool

If the eyelids are swollen or closed you can construct your own mini eyelid retractors with a pair of paperclips. The paperclips do not need to be sterile, but must be cleaned and washed with before and after use. Open the paperclips to form an 'S' shape. Fold each paperclip one-quarter back. Use topical local anaesthetic drops and insert the hooked ends under the upper and lower eyelids. (See Fig 44.3.) Gently pull to enable an examination of the eye.

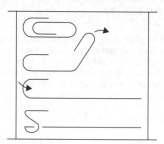

Fig. 44.3 How to fold a paperclip

Children

Paediatric ophthalmology is a specialized skill. However, despite the difficulties, in the following situations an examination is mandatory and may result in vision-saving treatment:

- A new-born infant with a purulent discharge.
- Discharge obscuring the surface of the eye which indicates a risk of corneal ulceration.
- If there has been any trauma with a possible laceration of the eye.
- A report of a foreign body hitting the eye.
- No red reflex and a white pupil indicating possible cataract.
- Any history indicating a loss of vision.
- An infant whose mother says that he/she does not look at her, indicating lack of visual function.

Tips for examining a child

With an assistant, lay the child on a bed on top of a blanket. Cross the child's arms over the chest keeping them as straight as possible. Wrap the blanket around the child. Keeping the child on the bed your assistant can hold the blanket closed and keep the child as still as possible. A second assistant may be required to put his/her hands on either side of the head to keep it still while you are examining. You may require a further assistant to open the eyes with retractors in extreme cases.

Diagnosis and treatment of common eye-related conditions

WHO and the International Agency for the Prevention of Blindness (IAPB) launched a plan in 1999 called 'Vision 20/20: The Right to Sight' which aims for 'A world in which no one is needlessly blind and where those with unavoidable vision loss can achieve their full potential'. Their recommendation was to focus attention on a few diseases which cause nearly all avoidable blindness, which include the following:

- Cataract.
- Trachoma: associated with poor hygiene and inadequate access to water and sanitation. Typically in hot and dry areas it affects the most deprived within a community. Occurs in many equatorial regions as well as in pockets in South America and Australia.
- Xerophthalmia: a result of vitamin A deficiency, it occurs in developing countries, typically in children <9 years old.
- Onchocerciasis: 99% of those infected live in sub-Saharan Africa. Spread via infected flies that breed in rivers.
- Serious refractive errors.
- All other causes of childhood blindness as well as xerophthalmia.

The following section will outline the recognition and treatment of common conditions, including those just listed, categorized according to anatomical location.

Skin and eyelids

See Table 44.1 for conditions affecting the skin and eyelid.

Conditions involving the skin and eyelids do not require special equipment to be examined. However, basic surgical equipment will be required for some treatments.

Management for specific conditions

Herpes zoster ophthalmicus

- Aciclovir 800 mg five times per day PO for 10 days.
- Amitriptyline 25 mg at night PO for 3 months.
- Chloramphenicol ointment four times daily in affected eye.
- Dressing for wounds—treat as if they are burns.

Pre-septal cellulitis

- Oral antibiotics e.g. co-amoxiclav 250–500 mg/125 mg twice daily or three times daily; *or* 875/125 mg twice daily PO.
- Check tetanus status in cases following trauma.

Orbital cellulitis

- IV antibiotics, e.g. ceftazidime with oral metronidazole for 4 days, followed by 3 weeks of oral treatment.
- The abscess can be drained in severe cases under guidance from an ear, nose, and throat specialist as the primary infection is typically in one of the sinuses.

Conjunctiva

The conjunctiva has three parts that need to be examined:
- *Bulbar conjunctiva*: you can see directly.
- *Palpebral conjunctiva*: behind the eyelids.
- *Fornices*: where the other two parts meet.

To examine the palpebral conjunctiva and fornix of the upper lid use a cotton bud to lightly press on the top of the eyelid, hold onto the upper lid lashes, and gently fold back the eyelid. The palpebral conjunctiva of the lower lid can be examined by gently pulling the lid down and away from the eye. The inside of the lid should appear smooth. Common abnormalities in children include small bumps and redness, which indicate allergic and vernal conjunctivitis. You may also locate foreign bodies trapped under the eyelids. (See Table 44.2 for conditions affecting the conjunctiva.)

Management of conjunctivitis

Allergic
- Short term for relief of mild symptoms: antihistamine drops.
- Long term: add oral antihistamine, e.g. cetirizine.

Viral (watery discharge)
- Symptomatic with lubricating eye drops.

Bacterial (purulent discharge)
- Chloramphenicol 1% ointment four times a day for 5 days.
- *Or* for second-line therapy: ciprofloxacin 0.3% 4-hourly for 2 days, then four times a day for 5 days.
- *Or* ofloxacin 0.3% 4-hourly for 2 days, then four times a day for 5 days.

Gonococcal conjunctivitis (severe purulent discharge)
- Quinolone, gentamycin, chloramphenicol, or bacitracin 1–2-hourly *and*
- Systemic third-generation cephalosporins, e.g. ceftriaxone IM injection or IV.

For all infective conjunctivitis the following is advised:
- Irrigation to remove excessive discharge.
- Reduce risk of transmission with frequent hand washing and avoidance of towel sharing.
- Cease contact lens wear if applicable.

Cornea

One of the most common presentations of corneal injury in the humanitarian setting is chemical injury, and giving emergency treatment will likely be vision-saving. Other conditions such as foreign bodies, corneal ulcers, and trauma to the eye require treatment as soon as possible

Please see Table 44.3 for conditions affecting the cornea.

For a detailed examination, setting your ophthalmoscope to +10D converts it into a handheld magnifier. This can then be used to assist with examination, as well as a magnifying tool when removing a corneal foreign body.

Table 44.1 Summary of conditions affecting the skin and eyelid

Signs and symptoms			Most likely diagnosis	Treatment guide
Abnormal appearance	Pain	Loss of vision		
Single mass on eyelid (typically older person)	None	None	Carcinoma	Requires complete excision with histology to confirm borders
One or more likely many small bumps on the eyelids and periocular skin	None	None	Molluscum	Typically occur in children. May require sedation to excise
Smooth lump or small abscess in the eyelid	Yes, if active infection	None	Chalazion	Initially can be treated with warm compresses, topical and oral antibiotics. Incision and drainage for a non-responsive case
Macular popular vesicular rash typically covering upper half of the face and head	Yes. Neurological pain, responds best to amitriptyline rather	Eyelids can be extremely swollen obscuring vision Severe cases may have discharge and corneal ulceration	Herpes zoster ophthalmicus	In addition to treatment, in young people this indicates a low immune status. An HIV test is recommended (see ➋ p. 522)
Swollen lids No proptosis No swelling of conjunctiva	Pain from swollen eyelids No pain and no decrease in eye movements	Swollen lids obscure vision, but vision is normal if lids are retracted	Pre-septal cellulitis	Can be treated with antibiotics as an outpatient (see ➋ p. 809)
Swollen lids Proptosis Swelling of conjunctiva	Pain from swollen eyelids Decreased painful eye movements	In severe cases there will be signs of optic nerve dysfunction e.g. relative afferent pupillary defect (RAPD)	Orbital cellulitis	Requires inpatient treatment with IV antibiotics (see ➋ p. 809)

Table 44.2 Conditions affecting the conjunctiva

Signs and symptoms			Most likely diagnosis	Treatment guide
Abnormal appearance on gross examination	Pain	Loss of vision		
Rough appearance with large feeder vessels	Scratchy irritation with large lesions	Very rare in long-standing cases where the lesion covers the cornea	Squamous cell carcinoma	Requires excision and histology to confirm diagnosis. HIV testing recommended
Smooth wing-shaped growth from conjunctiva on to the cornea	Scratchy irritation with large lesions. Can be become mildly painful if inflamed	Can cause astigmatism and loss of vision	Pterygium	With poor resources, excise when vision is affected. Treat inflamed lesions with topical steroids
Red, bloodshot appearance	None	None	Subconjunctival haemorrhage	Reassure patient that condition will completely resolve in a few weeks
Red conjunctiva and watery discharge	Itchy sensation	None	Allergic conjunctivitis	Antihistamines. Topical and/or oral
Red conjunctiva. May have small raised bumps around the limbus and/or on the inner eyelids	Severe itchy sensation, often resulting in chronic rubbing of the eyes	Rubbing can result in corneal deformities in the long term, leading to a loss of vision	Vernal conjunctivitis	Associated with atopic conditions such as asthma. The itchy stimulus for chronic rubbing needs to be controlled to prevent damage to the cornea
Purulent or yellow/white discharge. Red, inflamed conjunctiva	Yes	Yes	Infectious conjunctivitis	Treat according to most likely infectious agent. See following suggested treatments in text

Table 44.3 Conditions affecting the cornea

Signs and symptoms Grossly abnormal appearance or seen with ophthalmoscope	Pain	Loss of vision	Most likely diagnosis	Treatment guide
History of chemical injury with pale conjunctiva and opaque cornea	Pain can be severe	Vision will be decreased	Chemical injury. An alkali injury has a worse prognosis than an acid injury	Requires emergency irrigation. See ➔ p. 814 for details
Black dot on cornea with metallic foreign bodies. Wooden foreign bodies also occur	Highly irritating and scratchy pain	Only if the foreign body is in the middle of the cornea and in the visual axis	Foreign body	Removal and prophylactic antibiotics for 1 week after removal. See ➔ pp. 814–16 for details
Laceration to cornea. May extend into the sclera. Iris tissue may extrude through the laceration. The lens may appear white	The level of pain will depend on the type and extent of the injury	Vision will be decreased due to the laceration. If the lens was involved in the injury, then the vision will be very poor	injury with laceration to cornea. The sclera and lens may also be involved	Requires protection to prevent further injury and complications. Give an immediate dose of an oral antibiotic. Ciprofloxacin has good ocular penetration. See ➔ p. 814 for surgical management
White area on cornea. May have a discharge. Red conjunctiva. The area will stain with fluorescein drops and can be best viewed using blue light from your ophthalmoscope	High level of pain, especially with larger lesions	Severe loss of vision if in the visual axis	Rounder lesions are likely bacterial corneal ulcer. The herpes simplex virus causes a dendritic pattern. A lesion, which has surrounding satellite lesions, is most likely fungal	

Management of specific conditions
Emergency irrigation of chemical wounds
- Chemical injuries to the eye are an emergency and common in certain humanitarian settings. The eye needs to be irrigated as soon and profusely as possible to prevent permanent damage.
- Alkali injuries (e.g. from cleaning agents containing ammonia and sodium hydroxide) are worse than acidic injuries and are more common.

In a busy humanitarian setting, a simple solution for eye irrigation is to use the small tubing attached to a butterfly needle (see Fig. 44.4):
- Take the tubing and remove the needle.
- Tie a knot at the end nearest where the needle was located.
- Create a loop with the tube and puncture the tubing many times along its length.
- The loop can be placed underneath the eyelids around the cornea. Chemicals and foreign matter are often trapped under the eyelids, so ensure the tubing is placed there.
- Attach a 1-litre saline drip to the tubing and let it run, then repeat with a second litre. The eye will be then irrigated, while freeing you to attend to other patients.

Foreign body

This is common in humanitarian settings, especially from wood or metal, and removal is necessary.

Foreign body removal procedure
- You can use the ophthalmoscope as a magnifier as described earlier to view the foreign body.
- First add topical anaesthetic to the eye.
- Start with a cotton bud to remove superficial items, otherwise use a needle with the bevel facing away from the patient to remove the foreign body from the corneal surface.
- If the item is embedded deep in the cornea, use a slit lamp if one is available, or refer to the nearest specialist ophthalmology unit.
- Discharge with antibiotic ointment for lubrication and infection prevention.

Protection of eye injuries

If there has been a traumatic injury to the eye, further damage can be done if pressure is exerted on the eye. The reason is that if the globe has been cut or ruptured, then pressure can cause extrusion of the contents. The aim is to prevent any rubbing or pressure on the eye before definitive surgical management becomes available. Therefore do not use an eye pad, rather place an eye shield and secure with tape. In the absence of formal equipment you can secure a large plastic bottle cap resting above and below on the orbital rim. The patient can then be worked up for surgical repair in a specialized centre, if available.

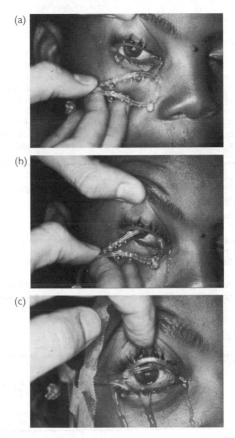

Fig. 44.4 Create an eye irrigation device using the tubing attached to a butterfly needle.

Corneal ulcer
- In a humanitarian setting without access to a laboratory to differentiate infectious agents, start with hourly antibiotics that cover both Gram-positive and Gram-negative organisms.
  - If the ulcer is suspected to be a fungal infection as the result of an injury with organic matter, it will not respond to first-line therapy. A topical antifungal eye drop should be administered.
- Suggested initial combination regimen:
  - Cefazolin 50 mg/mL every 5 minutes for 30 minutes, then every hour on the hour for 2 days.

- Tobramycin 14 mg/mL every 5 minutes for 30 minutes, then every hour on the half hour for 2 days.
- Preparation:
  - Cefazolin 50 mg/mL: add 2 mL water for injection to a 500 mg vial of cefazolin powder and shake well. Withdraw 1 mL of this solution and inject it into a sterile dropper bottle. Add 4 mL of Refresh Tears® to the dropper bottle. You now have 250 mg of cefazolin in 5 mL of watery Refresh Tears®. Label and date the mixture.
  - Tobramycin 14 mg/mL: withdraw 1.5 mL of Tobrex® from the commercial preparation and discard it. Now withdraw 1.5 mL of tobramycin for injection (80 mg/mL) from a 2 mL vial and add this to the remaining commercial Tobrex®. Label and date the mixture.

Anterior chamber

There are two conditions you may encounter in a humanitarian setting: angle-closure glaucoma (more common in elderly people) and uveitis (more common in younger patients) (see Table 44.4).

Management of angle-closure glaucoma
- The definitive initial treatment is a peripheral iridotomy to relieve the angle closure, however this requires specialist management.
- In a low-resource or primary setting, it is necessary to lower the pressure in the eye to reduce the corneal oedema and enable a clear view of the iris:
  - Start with a stat oral dose of a carbonic anhydrase inhibitor as well as a combination of topical drops that reduce the intraocular pressure, e.g. brimonidine, a beta blocker, and a prostaglandin derivative.

Table 44.4 Conditions affecting the anterior chamber

Signs and symptoms			Most likely diagnosis	Treatment guide
Abnormal appearance	Pain	Loss of Vision		
Red and severely inflamed conjunctiva. Opaque cornea. Poor red reflex. Positive eclipse sign	Severe pain	Severe loss of vision	Acute angle-closure glaucoma	See ➋ pp. 816–17 for initial medical therapy. Patient will require emergency referral to a specialist centre
Red, inflamed conjunctiva focused around the edge of the cornea	Common to have severe pain and photophobia (painful sensitivity to light)	Decreased vision	Uveitis. Common in young adults with syphilis, TB, and HIV-related viral infections. In children and older populations, it is likely related to an autoimmune reaction	This can be a difficult diagnosis to make for a non-specialist. A history of syphilis, herpes, HIV, and TB places a patient at higher risk and will require systemic treatment. Medical treatment involves topical steroids and atropine

- Add topical steroid drops to reduce inflammation, and potentially delay likely blindness until referral for an iridotomy can be done.
- Once the acute management has been completed, the cause for the angle closure will be found and treated.

Lens

Cataracts

- Cataract formation in the lens is the most common form of visual impairment and blindness. In an infant it is most likely congenital; in teenagers and adults is likely to be trauma related, and in elderly patients most likely age related.
- To aid your examination, hold the ophthalmoscope close to your eye and shine the light at the patient's eyes from 1 metre away:
  - In a normal eye you will see a red reflection from the retina.
  - The absence of a red reflex indicates pathology blocking the reflection from the retina. In the absence of other pathology, an absent or dim red reflex commonly indicates a cataract.
  - This will require surgery to restore vision. In children with congenital cataracts, the faster the surgery, the better the outcome.

Retina

A retinal examination and treatment of conditions are likely beyond the scope of a health worker in humanitarian settings. However, it is important to attempt an examination before referral for specialist care, especially for high-risk patients such as those with diabetes and decreased immune systems, e.g. HIV infection.

- At a minimum, a retinal exam will require an ophthalmoscope or pan-ophthalmoscope preferably through a dilated pupil.
- Identify the optic nerve first, and then look at the vessels.
- Examine the macular last because this is the most sensitive part of the retina and the bright light can be uncomfortable for the patient. Abnormalities will likely require referral to a specialist.

A common condition that affects the retina is diabetes. If you have a diabetic patient with deceased vision they are best referred to a specialist centre for treatment. Do consider tele-options for screening by sending the photos to a specialist (see Box 44.2) which can save transport costs for the patient, eliminate an overload on the referral centre, and ensure that the appropriate patients are prioritized for treatment.

Box 44.2 New technologies for humanitarian settings

In a humanitarian setting, new techniques are now available to aid retinal examination including an easy-to-use clip-on device that enables taking retinal photographs using a smartphone (see ➔ Fig. 44.2 p. 805). Email support@vulamobile.com to order one or to download the file on how to make one yourself using a three-dimensional printer.

Optic nerve

Open-angle glaucoma

Open-angle glaucoma is the most common condition affecting the optic nerve. This is difficult to diagnose in a humanitarian setting because it requires a measurement of the intraocular pressure, visual field testing, and a view of the optic nerve. Patients are likely to present late with a painless, slowly progressive loss of vision. Although it is a common cause of blindness, it is harder to set-up screening and treatment programmes than for other common causes such as cataracts and diabetes. It will require dedicated, specialist help and in a humanitarian setting will not likely be a priority.

Drug toxicities

Some medical treatments for TB, e.g. ethambutol, may be toxic to the optic nerve. If you have patients on treatment who start to lose vision, they will need an examination. Ethambutol toxicity is a diagnosis of exclusion and you need to confirm that there are no abnormalities on examination, except in long-standing severe cases with a paler optic nerve. The treatment is to discuss stopping the ethambutol with the health worker running the TB treatment service.

Further reading

Bowling B. Kanski's Clinical Ophthalmology. 8th ed. Philadelphia, PA: Elsevier; 2016.

Denniston AKO, Murray PI. Oxford Handbook of Ophthalmology. Oxford: Oxford University Press; 2014.

Rajak S, Stanford Smith J. Eye Diseases in Hot Climates. 5th ed. London: JP Medical Ltd; 2015.

Ear, nose, and throat

**Laurent Bonnardot, Olivier Malard,
Elisabeth Sauvaget, and Sarah Giles**

Context for ear, nose, and throat

Ear, nose, and throat (ENT) problems may be overlooked in humanitarian emergencies where gunshot wounds, infectious disease, and malnutrition seem the most pressing concerns. But ENT problems can be life-threatening and life-altering, so it is important to get the diagnosis and treatment right the first time.

ENT problems are intricately associated with the ability to breathe while also affecting patients' self-esteem and visual appearance. ENT complaints must be taken seriously as minor complaints may mask important life-threatening conditions.

Who and when to refer is then the key question in any ENT acute disorder.

Disorders of the ENT can be congenital, infectious, neoplastic, or acquired. As with all of medicine, the key to the diagnosis will almost always be in the history which, in the humanitarian setting, may require a skilled and patient interpreter.

Challenges in ENT conditions within humanitarian settings lie in the difficulty of confirming the diagnosis in a specialty that relies heavily on equipment likely to be unavailable, such as CT and fibreoptic scopes. In the humanitarian environment, diagnosis and management are mainly based on clinical findings. It may not be possible to cure many ENT ailments and some disorders can only be solved with complex specialized surgery that may not be available to your patients in the field. In those cases, your role is to try your best to access services for your patient and, failing that, provide high-quality pain control and palliation where required.

If a patient is not responding to a commonly effective cure, clinicians should consider zoonotic diseases paying special attention to where the patient has been, their living environment, their eating habits, and whether or not their immune system is compromised.[1]

Clinical assessment for ear, nose, and throat

Understanding the basic ENT anatomy is fundamental for both diagnosis and management. Knowing the anatomic terms helps to accurately describe the site of a lesion and to document examination findings. Common ENT problems encountered in the field can be considered in terms of anatomical location. (See Fig. 45.1 and Fig. 45.2.)

The ear

Outer, middle, and inner ear conditions.

- External canal (2.5 cm length): tympanic membrane (TM) (handle malleus, light reflex).
- Middle ear: equalization of air pressure on both side of TM by Eustachian tube (opened while swallowing).
- Inner ear with cochlea (hearing/tinnitus), labyrinth (balance system/ nystagmus)

The nose

Traumatic problems (epistaxis, nasal fracture, mid-face fracture) and atraumatic conditions (sinusitis).

The sinuses

Ethmoidal cavities are present at birth, maxillary bone appears after 3 years of age, frontal after 7–12 years, and sphenoidal sinusitis can be seen from 4 years. Maxillary, frontal, and ethmoidal anterior sinuses drain into middle meatus (ostiomeatal complex), ethmoidal posterior drain into upper meatus. The sphenoidal sinus has its own meatus.

The throat: oral cavity

Tongue, floor of mouth, cheeks, palate; pharynx (naso/oro/hypopharynx), retropharyngeal space larynx, thyroid, oesophagus, and lymph nodes.

- Ask key questions for ENT with key symptoms:
  - Ear: hearing loss, tinnitus, dizziness, discharge.
  - Nose: trauma, bleeding diathesis, discharge, swelling, pain on leaning forward, post-nasal drip, snorting of any substances.
  - Throat: pain on swallowing, cough, trouble breathing, swelling, need to clear throat, any history of choking.
- Ask patients about immunocompromise, immunization history, past history of ENT problems, any dental problems, pain.

Ear examination

- It is important to be systematic for all patients and to start on the 'good' side.
- Push on the mastoid to check for tenderness.
- Examine the pinna for signs of infection; a gentle tug on the pinna that causes pain can be a clue to otitis externa.
- To get a good view of the TM, hold your otoscope like a pen, pull on the pinna to straighten out the canal:
  - While gently inserting the otoscope, check the walls of the canal for redness, inflammation, and exudate.

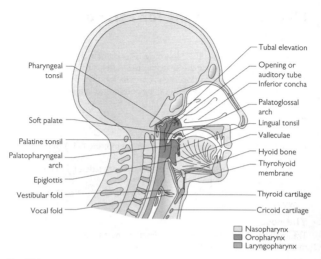

Fig. 45.1 Neck anatomy. Reproduced with permission from M E Atkinson, Anatomy for Dental Students, Fourth Edition, Oxford University Press.

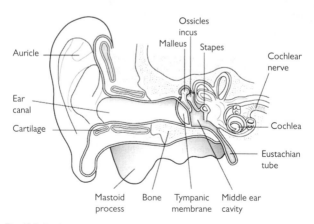

Fig. 45.2 Ear Anatomy. Reproduced from Perry, Michael, Head, Neck and Dental Emergencies, 2005 (OUP) Fig 10.1.

- If you cannot see the TM because of exudate, use a cotton-tipped applicator to soak up the liquid until you get a clear view.
- When examining the TM, look for small perforations, air–fluid levels, and exudate behind the TM.
- The ear has multiple sources of innervation, be sure to look for non-ear causes of pain by checking the teeth, cranial nerves, and pharynx.

Auditory examination
- While the gold standard examination for ear pain includes an audiogram, this is often not feasible in the field. You can grossly check hearing by rubbing hair on the side of each ear to see if hearing is intact and equal. It indicates hearing better than 20 db.
- Tuning forks are often unavailable in the field, but if found, differentiate conductive and sensorineural hearing loss (HL):
  - Weber test: hold it in the midline (forehead):
    —Sound heard equally both sides (centrally = normal hearing).
    —Louder on one side means HL. Sound lateralized to the deaf ear = conductive HL; sound lateralized to the normal ear = sensorineural HL.
  - Rinne test: compare bone conduction (BC): fork placed firmly on mastoid bone and air conduction (AC): fork held close to external auditory canal.
    —AC ≥ BC= normal or sensorineural HL.
    —BC > AC = conductive HL.

Nose examination

- View the nose from both sides to assess for symmetry and deformity. Check the nares for discharge (mucous, CSF, blood, vesicles).
- Lift the tip of the nose—look for deviation or polyps.
- Palpate the nasal bone for pain and swelling.
- Percussion the frontal and maxillary sinuses for tenderness.
- Look at the posterior pharynx for post-nasal discharge or bleeding.
- Use the otoscope and nasal speculum and a light to examine Kiesselbach's plexus (the most common site of anterior bleeding) and the septum for haematomas.

Throat examination (oral cavity, pharynx, thyroid, neck)

- Using a tongue depressor, look through the mouth, under the tongue, obtain a good view of the tonsils and posterior pharynx. Consider removing the tongue depressor if it is making the patient gag.
- Palpate (with gloves) the tongue (base in particular) and floor of the mouth (bidigital examination).
- Dental examination including four quadrants of teeth (percussion and vitality testing) and periodontal tissues should be systematic.
- Salivary gland—check for mass or stones; attempt to express saliva from ducts (parotid and submandibular):
  - The parotid duct (Stensen) is opposite to second upper molar.
  - The submandibular duct (Wharton) is on the anterior floor of the mouth.
- Check anterior and posterior cervical chains for lymphadenopathy.
- Palpate the thyroid for masses nodule (solitary/multiple), goitre (enlargement regular or irregular), tenderness, or asymmetry.
- Perform a swallow test: thyroid lobes should move upwards on swallowing.

Common ear disorders

Wax impaction

The ear is generally a self-cleaning organ, and there is generally no need to clean the external ear canal. Rinsing with shower spray water and drying afterwards is often sufficient for most people.

Definition

When cerumen has accumulated in the canal and prevents the TM from being seen.

Presentation

Patient complains of decreased hearing, dizziness, or recurrence of known problem. May obscure an infected TM of otitis externa.

Diagnosis

Yellow/brown cerumen obliterates view of TM.

Management

- If the wax is very dry, ask patient to put drops of mineral/vegetable oil in the ear twice daily for 3 days and then return.
- Warn patients that this procedure may cause them to feel dizzy and uncomfortable. Do not perform if TM is potentially ruptured.
- If wax is moist (or not—you can make it moist with ear bath), take a 60 mL syringe and attach the plastic portion of an 18 G angiocatheter. Cut the angiocath to about 1 cm in length. Using tepid water, flush the canal but direct the syringe to the roof of the canal. The water will eventually get behind the wax and push it out. Stop if the patient complains of pain. If the provider is proficient with its use, a curette can remove large chunks that are stuck to the canal wall. Do not touch the TM and proceed very carefully since the ear canal skin is very thin. For ears that have dried wax, diluted peroxide (50% water, 50% hydrogen peroxide) works extremely well in place of water.

Auricular haematoma

Definition

Laceration of the pinna, which may or may not include a haematoma.

Presentation

Traumatic context is usually clear.

Diagnosis:

Typically by visual inspection. Be aware of underlying basal skull fractures, closed head injuries, and traumatic TM rupture.

Note: with auricular haematoma, blood collection between cartilage and perichondrium can lead to cartilage infection and necrosis. Any exposed cartilage must be closed over quickly as the skin provides the blood supply to the cartilage.

Management
- Under general or local anaesthesia, evacuate any auricular haematomas and then close with stitches through the ear and over rolls of petroleum jelly gauze on each side to reapply skin on cartilage and prevent re-accumulation. Keep for 5 days with close follow-up.
- Use oral antibiotics. If a human bite, cover with co-amoxiclav and consider post-exposure prophylaxis for HIV and hepatitis B.
- Update tetanus and rabies vaccine if indicated.

Traditionally, lidocaine without epinephrine (adrenaline) is used for numbing the ear to avoid vascular complications but the evidence for this is lacking. Another approach is to perform an ear field block by injecting a total of 10–20 mL of lidocaine above and below the ear in a diamond-shaped block. Aspirate prior to injecting to avoid the temporal artery.

Traumatic tympanic membrane perforation

Definition
Hole or rupture in the TM.

Presentation
Traumatic context is usually clear (blow to head, foreign object in ear) and can present with sudden-onset ear pain, bleeding in the canal, hearing loss, vertigo usually after obvious trauma.

Diagnosis
TM perforation on otoscopy.

Management
- Most heal spontaneously within 2 weeks.
- Keep ear dry perfectly dry.
- If chronic requires a skilled ENT surgeon for myringoplasty which may not be available in the field.

Otitis externa

Definition
Bacterial or fungal infection of the ear canal.

Presentation
Pain in ear, discharge, usually without fever.

Diagnosis
Pain when the tragus or pinna is gently tugged, discharge in the canal, redness and swelling in the canal. If the canal is itchy and has white discharge, consider fungal infection.

Management
- Keep ear as dry as possible through frequent removal of exudate.
- If canal is very narrow, insert an ear wick to be placed so that drops can be put in ear.
- Ciprofloxacin eardrops two drops three times daily for a week is standard treatment for moderate to severe presentations. If ear is not clearing up after 3 days but the TM is still intact, consider using a hydrogen peroxide bath three times a day before instilling ear drops.

- Gentian violet drops 0.5% applied once daily is a treatment option for mild to moderate presentations if TM is confirmed to be intact.
- If no improvement with drops, oral antibiotics may be necessary.
- Fungal otitis media can present with pruritus and white, thick discharge. It can be treated with nystatin powder.

> Note: hydrogen peroxide 10% or ofloxacin drops can be given if TM is opened since they are harmless to the inner ear.

Otitis media (chronic/acute)

Definition

Inflammation in the middle ear whose mucosa lines not only the middle ear cavity but also mastoid air cells and the Eustachian tube. Eustachian tube dysfunction or obstruction is central.

Presentation

Ear pain with or without fever, common in children.

Diagnosis

Effusion behind the TM, decreased light reflex on the TM, TM retraction, and erythema.

Management

Uncomplicated otitis media

- Most otitis media is easily treated with oral antibiotics combined with several times a day nasal irrigation and topical drops (ofloxacin or 10% hydrogen peroxide); in case of purulent discharge (perforation), use topical drops.
- The vast majority of media otitis will heal without sequelae. In some cases, effusion can persist for >3 months, leading to non-suppurative chronic otitis media (persistent, painless discharge through a TM perforation where it can lead to HL), cholesteatoma (where the squamous cells in the middle ear can break down the surrounding bones and cause HL).
- Immunocompromised and malnourished patients are most likely to experience complications. One of the main severe complications, most common in children, is mastoiditis.

Mastoiditis

- Caused by infection of mastoid air cells complex and/or post-auricular abscess.
- Patients present with pain over mastoid process (behind pinna) with oedema and redness.
- Aggressive empiric antibiotic therapy with ceftriaxone IM for 10 days and ciprofloxacin PO for 14 days or, in higher-resource settings, vancomycin and ceftazidime or cefepime. Definitive treatment may involve surgery (mastoidectomy).
- Complications include risk of facial palsy and intracranial extension so if no clear improvement, consider referral if possible.

Chronic suppurative otitis media

Defined by a persistent infected discharge through a TM perforation, this is a common cause of hearing impairment in LIC.

- Instilling five drops of 50% peroxide solution in sterile water to clear the canal for 30 seconds prior to applying drops can help patients dry mop their own ears.
- 2% acetic acid irrigation or Burrow's solution (13% aluminium acetate), or povidone-iodine three times daily for 3 weeks can be extremely effective where topical quinolones three times daily for a week are not available or as an adjunct when they have failed.

Cholesteatoma

- Caused by formation of deep retraction pockets on the periphery of the TM. They should be considered when chronic suppurative otitis media does not resolve with maximal medical treatment.
- Can cause HL, seventh and sixth cranial nerve palsies, and venous thrombosis.
- Difficult to definitively diagnose without CT. Examination may show marginal/posterior or superior retraction pocket (looks like perforation) with white debris and crust.
- Surgical treatment required (temporal bone removal and mastoidectomy) and this may be impossible to access in the field.

Foreign body in ear

Presentation

Much more common in young children. Objects may be food, toys, insects, etc. May present with foul smelling discharge, ear pain, or foreign body sensation.

Diagnosis

Foreign object seen on otoscopy.

Management

- If the TM is intact, most objects can simply be flushed carefully by using a 60 mL syringe with an 18 G angiocatheter cut short and attached (this allows for a bit more pressure) and filled with tepid water. Collect the water that runs out of the ear with a kidney basin to collect the object as it falls.
- If the foreign body is a live insect, placing a few drops of 10% peroxide solution in the ear acts as a toxin to drown the insect, and allows for easy removal.

Hearing loss

Definition

In the field where audiometry is not available, it is often a patient's or parent's subjective sense that the patient's hearing has decreased.

Presentation

Can be sudden or gradual in onset, bilateral or unilateral, associated with trauma, infection, noise exposure, or congenital.

Diagnosis

Generally based on patient report, definitive diagnosis often requires testing not available in the field.

Management

Otoscopy to look for effusion behind TM, TM perforation, and wax.

- Tuning fork tests can help to test for sensory neural HL versus conductive HL; however, tuning forks are rarely found in the field and little can be done for HL that is not caused by foreign bodies, wax, or infection.
- When possible, treat obvious causes of HL. Sudden unilateral sensory HL (idiopathic sudden HL) may respond to rest (in low-noise environment) and steroids for 1 mg/kg for 7 days but be wary of this in immunocompromised patients. Definitive diagnosis and management is challenging in the field.

Common nose disorders

See Fig. 45.3 for anatomy of the sinus.

Fracture of the nose

Presentation

Most common facial fracture. Symptoms include swelling, deformity or deviation, skin injury, and epistaxis.

Diagnosis

Can be made clinically or with X-rays, consider mid-face fracture, head injury, and spinal injury in your differential.

Management

- Spinal precautions and head injury management if necessary.
- Control epistaxis (see ➔ p. 832).
- Check septum for haematoma. If present, incise and drain, pack, put patient on prophylactic antibiotics.
- Most fractures heal with minimal deformity and only cause aesthetic concerns. If there is a gross deformity or the airway is compromised, closed reduction can be attempted under general anaesthetic within 10 days of injury. After manipulation by an experienced practitioner, the nose should be packed for 3 days and an external plaster splint applied for 7 days.

Foreign bodies of the nose

Presentation

Often witnessed by caregiver, or unexplained, foul-smelling, unilateral nasal discharge in young children or adults with cognitive problems or unilateral nasal obstruction.

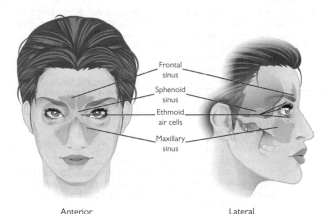

Anterior   Lateral

Fig. 45.3 Sinus anatomy. Reproduced from Openstax College, Anatomy & Physiology, Connexions, http://cnx.org under the Creative Commons Attribution-Share Alike 3.0 Unported license.

Diagnosis

Typically a diagnosis based on clinical suspicion.

Management

- Visible solid foreign bodies can be removed by placing any long, thin probe with a soft angulated tip at the end that goes in the nose behind the object and pulling forward.
- Soft foreign bodies can be removed with crocodile forceps.
- For objects that cannot be seen, while you obstruct one nostril, have a caregiver seal over the patient's mouth with their mouth and blow forcefully. This increase in intranasal pressure is often enough to force the object out or move it to a visible position.

Acute sinusitis

Definition

Inflammation of the paranasal sinus mucosa.

As sinuses are not yet fully formed in children <8 years old (except ethmoid cells), this is a presentation in older children or adults.

Presentation

After a viral rhinitis, an acute bacterial sinus infection can form, generally not diagnosed until symptoms have been present for at least 10 days. Symptoms include pressure in the regions of the maxillary and frontal sinuses, especially when leaning forward, fever, copious purulent nasal and post-nasal discharge, sore throat, dental pain, and feeling systemically unwell.

Diagnosis

Is made clinically, but differential diagnosis includes dental abscess, atypical facial pain, migraine, and trigeminal neuralgia.

Management

- Nasal irrigation with normal saline four times per day, decongestant.
- Oral antibiotics (amoxicillin or amoxicillin/clavulanic acid for 10 days) if no improvement with above-mentioned measures.
- Consider oral steroids if severe inflammation.
- Can develop into an intracranial abscess or periorbital sinusitis which may require referral if possible for sinusotomy.
- Consider fungal sinusitis (mucormycosis, aspergillus, and candida) in the immunocompromised patient and consider aggressive treatment with IV amphotericin.

Acute ethmoid sinusitis

Definition

- Inflammation of the ethmoid sinus.
- Occurs often after or during viral rhinosinusitis, mainly due to *Haemophilus influenza*, *Staphylococcus*, and *Pneumococcus*. This can have tragic consequences if not treated properly as it has risk for severe visual impairment from contiguous spread to orbit (lamina papyracea bone very thin in children).

Presentation
Upper eyelid swelling and erythema, pain, and high fever. No suppuration present (unlike conjunctivitis or dacryocystitis).

As CT scanning is most likely not available, careful examination will focus on the following:

Diagnosis
Clinical signs suggestive of neurological (meningitis) or orbital complications (orbital cellulitis, orbital or subperiosteal abscess) including:
• extrinsic and intrinsic ophthalmoplegia (low or non-reactive mydriasis), diplopia
• decreased visual acuity (at late stage)
• corneal anaesthesia (trigeminal nerve V1).

Management
• *If no sign* of these three above-listed complications: symptomatic treatment, start immediate IV antibiotics (amoxicillin + clavulanic or third-generation cephalosporin) then switch to oral treatment when patient afebrile for a minimum of 10 days.
• *If one sign* of orbital complication (see ➔ p. 831) is present, the gold standard treatment would be referral to an ENT surgeon for retrocanthal orbitotomy and drainage (high risk of visual loss) but this is not always possible in a humanitarian setting.

Epistaxis

Definition
Blood coming from the nasal cavities.

Presentation
• Bleeding from the nose that can range from trivial to life-threatening.
• May be spontaneous—most cases arise from the anterior nasal septum 'Little's area', follow trauma, or are related to underlying pathology such as thrombocytopenia or haemophilia. *Consider haemorrhagic fevers in endemic areas.*
• Blood may be seen at the nares or in the posterior pharynx.
• Patients may also vomit blood that they have swallowed.

Management
• Wear safety glasses and mask for all cases and consider full personal protective equipment for moderate to severe epistaxis.
• ABCs—consider the need for fluids, blood, antihypertensives, and analgesia.
• Anterior bleeding is much more common than posterior bleeding but posterior bleeding is more dangerous.
• Small anterior bleeds may stop with these basic measures. If that does not work try, try anterior nasal packing.
• If the bleeding is initially severe, coming out of both nares, or is high volume in the posterior pharynx, consider a posterior bleed. In these cases, patients may be more comfortable with suction in their mouth so they can spit out blood. Posterior nasal packing is necessary for a posterior bleed.
• See Box 45.1 for control of epistaxis.

Box 45.1 Steps for control of epistaxis

Basic measures

- If patient is stable, have them blow their nose to remove clots, lean forward, and suck on ice if available.
- Apply pressure to the bridge of the nose for 10 minutes.
- If available, cotton wool soaked in lidocaine and xylometazoline can be inserted to both nares to cause vasoconstriction and decrease discomfort. After 1 minute, examine the nasal cavity with a nasal speculum and light to look for the area of bleeding. Check posterior pharynx for the extent of bleeding.

Anterior nasal packing

- Ensure large-bore IV access.
- If possible, introduce in both nasal cavities topical analgesia (cotton with lidocaine and vasoconstrictor) to ease the examination.
- Insert a lubricated nasal tampon (5–7 cm in length) by introducing it *parallel* to the floor (*not* upwards towards the top of the head). Warn the patient that this is not comfortable.
- Help the tampon to expand by squirting some saline at the tip.
- Tape the strings to the side of the face.
- Place patient on prophylactic antibiotics to guard against toxic shock syndrome.
- Check posterior pharynx to make sure bleeding has truly stopped.
- Remove packing and stop antibiotics in 48–72 hours.
- If nasal tampons not available or nasal anatomy does not allow for its use, use 3 cm/1 inch-wide petroleum jelly-impregnated gauze.

Posterior nasal packing

- Ensure two large-bore IV access.
- Bilateral 10 cm lubricated nasal tampons may stop the bleeding but if this fails, either use a specially made epistaxis balloon or, more commonly in the field, insert a 10 Fr Foley catheter into the anterior nare and push it through the nose until you can see it in the posterior pharynx.
  - Inflate the bladder with 7–10 mL of saline and then pull the anterior aspect of the catheter through until the bladder is placing fluid at the site of the bleeding.
  - Place a clamp at the nose to stop the catheter from falling out of place.
  - Packing the anterior nares will increase your chances of haemostasis.
  - Admit the patient if possible.
  - Manage packing as per anterior packing (see earlier in this box); remove it after 48 hours of balloon packing.
- If bleeding does not stop, surgical ligation will be required but that is unlikely to be available in the field.
- Oral tranexamic acid may be considered in life-threatening cases.

Common throat disorders

Pharyngitis/tonsillitis

Definition
Viral or bacterial infection of the pharynx and/or tonsils.

Presentation
Sore throat, fever, pain on swallowing, ear pain, and cervical lymphadenopathy.

Diagnosis
Based on examination, different clinical features can be distinguished (see Fig. 45.4). Common presentations in the field are listed below, which help direct management.

Management principles
Analgesia, IV antibiotics if inability to drink or to eat properly (Fig. 45.5), and mouth wash with diluted iodine four to six times a day can be helpful.

Erythematous

- Presents with erythematous, enlarged red tonsils, sometimes covered by whitish purulent exudate.
- The most common feature, mainly due to virus (80%) followed by bacteria, in particular beta-haemolytic streptococci group A (SGA) which can cause rare (1%) but serious complications such as rheumatic fever or acute glomerulonephritis.
- See Box 45.2 for Centor scoring.
- If available, a positive rapid strep test confirms SGA infection and guides antibiotic therapy relevance. Test indicated for children >3 years old and for adults if Centor score >2 (SGA infection probability <5% if score £2).

Pseudomembranous

- Diphtheria presents with a pseudomembrane of grey sticky exudate on the tonsils and uvula. This is rare, but ~5000 cases occur per year in sub-Saharan Africa, India, and Indonesia.
- Complications can include infectious spread to larynx and airway compromise (10% of cases) or exotoxin-induced neurological impairment or myocarditis.
- Due to infectious potential, these patients need to be isolated.
- Treatment consists of diphtheria antitoxin and antibiotics (penicillin or erythromycin).
- Contacts should receive prophylactic antibiotics and a diphtheria booster.
- EBV presents with diffuse lymphadenopathy, impressive tonsillar exudate, low-grade fever, and possible splenomegaly.
- Treatment is supportive with possible oral steroids if obstructive tonsillar swelling

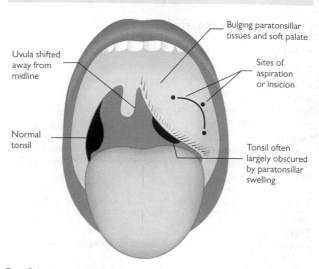

Bulging paratonsillar tissues and soft palate

Uvula shifted away from midline

Sites of aspiration or insicion

Normal tonsil

Tonsil often largely obscured by paratonsillar swelling

Fig. 45.4 Tonsillar anatomy. Reproduced with permission from Warner, Giles, et al, Otolaryngology and Head and Neck Surgery, 2009, OUP.

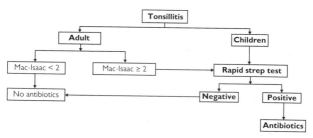

Fig. 45.5 Antibiotics in tonsillitis.

Box 45.2 A modified Centor score can help to determine which patients with SGA would benefit from antibiotics
- Age 3–14 years +1; age 15–44 years: 0.
- Age >45 years: −1.
- Exudate or swelling on tonsils: +1.
- Tender/swollen anterior cervical lymph nodes: +1.
- Fever? Temperature >38°C: +1.
- Cough absent: +1

Vesicular
- Herpangina due to Coxsackievirus: presents in ages 2–20 years, with similar symptoms to streptococcal pharyngitis but can also include vomiting and abdominal pain. There is a red halo at the posterior pharynx with vesicular lesions. The condition is self-limited and treatment is supportive
- Hand, foot, and mouth disease: presents with painful vesicles on the palms, soles of feet, and in the mouth and accompanied by fever. Mostly seen in young children. Treatment is supportive.

Ulcero-necrotic
- If unilateral: termed the Vincent tonsillitis, this occurs most commonly in young adults with poor oral hygiene.
- Presentation is with fatigue, often tonsillar ulcer.
- Standard treatment is with penicillin 10 days. Consider possibility of syphilitic chancre if in the context of STDs, in which case treatment should be as per genital disease or tonsil cancer if not healing or persistent.

Management
- Only bacterial infections require antibiotics.
- Analgesia, oral antibiotics (penicillin V or macrolide), IV treatment if inability to drink or to eat properly, mouth wash with diluted iodine four to six times a day can be helpful.
- Even with antibiotics, complications can occur, including peritonsillar abscess and retropharyngeal abscess:
  - Peritonsillar abscess occurs when pus accumulates outside of the tonsillar capsule. Also known as quinsy. Patients present with a very sore throat, 'hot potato' voice, trismus, drooling, and fever. On examination, the uvula is not mid-line.
  - Retropharyngeal abscess has similar symptoms to a peritonsillar abscess but one-third have normal oral examination, signs localize to the neck, and can mimic meningitis. It is most common in children <6 years and lateral X-rays can help with diagnosis. Admit the patient, treat with IV antibiotics (amoxicillin–clavulanic acid, third-generation cephalosporin).
- Indications of tonsillectomy:
  - Obstructive sleep apnoea (children).
  - Recurrent tonsillitis (more than three to five per year, 3 consecutive years) or phlegmonous.
  - More than one peritonsillar abscess.

Treatment of a peritonsillar abscess requires incision and drainage or aspiration. As the carotid artery lies beneath the area of incision, one must be cautious not to go too deep. Visualizing the area can be challenging: having an assistant or the patient depress the tongue with a laryngoscope with a functioning light or with the bottom half of a vaginal speculum while the doctor dons a head lamp may help. Spraying the area liberally with lidocaine helps with patient comfort before the procedure. A needle with the needle cover partially cut and put back on the needle or a rubber stopper from a lab test tube can be used to reduce the chance of penetrating too deeply. After incision and drainage, treat with clindamycin and oral steroids. Consider admission.

Lymphadenitis

Definition

Inflammation of a lymph node complicated by infection.

Presentation

- Inflamed cervical mass (>1 cm × 1cm) with fever. This is one of the most common presentations of mycobacterial disease.
- Most common in immunocompetent children <8 years but frequently seen in the immunosuppressed.
- Differential includes cat-scratch disease, toxoplasmosis, HIV and TB, lymphoma, and inflammation of congenital branchial cyst.
- Diagnosis: if possible, aspiration. This can assist with differentiation of purulence from infection from possible cancer.

Management

- Incision and drainage often leads to sinus formation. Surgical excision is the preferred treatment, however, 3 months of clarithromycin and rifabutin may be effective.
- See ➲ Chapter 31 for more information.

Congenital branchial cyst inflammation

Definition

Congenital epithelial cysts on the lateral neck.

Presentation

Single, painless, smooth, fluctuant mass that presents on the neck of a child or young adult. Only 2–3% are bilateral.

Diagnosis

Fine-needle aspiration can differentiate an abscess, but should be avoided if neoplasm is suspected. Do not aspirate a pulsatile mass as it may be a carotid body tumour!

Management

As long as no compressive symptoms are present, these benign cysts call for reassurance only. Any abscesses should be treated with antibiotics. If compressive symptoms are present, excision by an experienced surgeon may be considered.

Thyroid mass

Definition

Abnormal enlargement of the thyroid gland.

Presentation

- May be unilateral or bilateral, patients may present with barely palpable nodules or massive goitres. Patients may complain of difficulty swallowing or shortness of breath.
- Endemic goitre due to a lack of dietary iodine is common in the Himalayas, Andes, and parts of Africa.
- Obstructive symptoms are rare but endemic cretinism is common.

Diagnosis

Diagnosis is difficult in the field as thyroid-stimulating hormone (TSH), triiodothyronine (T3), thyroxine (T4), ultrasound, and scintigraphy are generally part of the work-up. The most common cause of goitre world-wide is endemic goitre.

Management

Endemic goitre can be treated with iodination of salt or drinking water or yearly IM or PO doses of iodine. If the patient is clinically hypothyroid, a trial of levothyroxine may decrease symptoms. Thyroidectomy can have significant morbidity and mortality and should be avoided.

Epiglottitis

Definition

Inflammation of the epiglottis.

Presentation

This is rarely seen in the richer countries due to the *Haemophilus influenza* vaccine but still present in areas not covered by vaccine. Most common in children aged 2–7 years but can be seen in adults. Presentation includes sudden-onset high fever, severe inspiratory dyspnoea, dysphagia, pain on talking, drooling of saliva, and muffled voice.

Diagnosis

Diagnosis is made clinically. *This can be a life-threatening emergency.* If the patient is very stable, an anteroposterior X-ray may show a classic 'thumbprint sign'.

Management

- Patients will place themselves in a tripod position—leave them there and keep them calm.
- If possible, arrange for urgent intubation by an anaesthetist in the operating room.
- Do not examine the child outside of the operating room as upset may lead to decompensation.
- In a low-resource environment, keep the child calm, and give humidified oxygen and nebulized epinephrine if available. Administer ampicillin 200 mg/kg/day and fluids. Consider sedation to help keep child calm. Despite interventions, this has a poor prognosis.

Laryngotracheobronchitis (croup)

Definition

Viral infection of the airway caused mostly by parainfluenza virus and respiratory syncytial virus, most common in children.

Presentation

Gradual onset >24 hours, harsh inspiratory stridor with barking cough worse at night, mild fever, and coryza. May be mild to life-threatening. Peak age 1–3 years old.

Diagnosis

Clinical diagnosis helped by the classic cough. Anteroposterior X-ray may show steeple sign. Differential includes foreign body and epiglottitis.

Management

Humidified oxygen or steam if not available, corticosteroids (prednisone 1–1.5 mg/kg PO once daily for 3 days or dexamethasone 0.6 mg/kg IM/IV for more severe causes), nebulized epinephrine, and intubation if available and if the patient shows signs of impending respiratory failure.

Paediatric airway problems/dyspnoea

Upper airway obstruction is characterized by an inspiratory dyspnoea that can be associated with swallowing difficulties and/or dysphonia. In-drawing at the xiphoid or supraclavicular regions are key clinical signs for localizing the area of obstruction.

If airway appears compromised → call for the most experienced help you can find, get difficult intubation trolley if it exists, and keep calm.

Management

- Determine laryngeal origin of dyspnoea. Clinical clues to this include:
  - inspiratory bradypnoea (prolonged inspiration) is typical of any upper airway obstruction
  - stridor—high-pitched noisy breathing whose timing indicates site of obstruction:
    —inspiratory: obstruction at the larynx or above
    —expiratory: distal obstruction (below trachea)
    —biphasic (on both inspiration and expiration): tracheal obstruction
  - voice change:
    —muffled suggests oro/nasopharyngeal level
    —hoarse suggests glottic, supraglottic level
  - in-drawing: the level of the obstruction is above the level of indrawing area.
- Assess clinical severity of dyspnoea, considering duration, vitals, consciousness level, and clinical cues (in-drawing, inability to complete sentences).
- Take immediate action:
  - Do not force patient to lie down and be careful when using tongue depressor (risk of decompensation if epiglottitis).
  - If the patient is visibly dyspnoeic:
    —Sit patient upright, give oxygen and nebulized epinephrine (adrenaline) and dexamethasone.
    —Consider IV corticosteroid and broad-spectrum antibiotic according to the context.
  - Life-threatening emergency—establish definitive airway (i.e. tube placed in the trachea with cuff inflated below the vocal cords):
    —Endotracheal intubation with rapid sequence intubation: etomidate succinylcholine or ketamine–diazepam..
    —Cricothyrotomy under local or general anaesthesia (see
    ◑ Chapter 50 for definitive guidance).

Paediatric considerations by age group

Newborn

- Bilateral choanal atresia or Pierre Robin syndrome (micrognathia, glossoptosis, cleft palate) are the two main causes of respiratory distress at birth.
- In the presence of significant respiratory distress, inserting an oropharyngeal airway (Guedel cannula) can improve oxygenation.

Infant <6 months

- Congenital laryngomalacia ('floppy larynx') due to laryngeal immaturity is the most common cause of stridor in this age group due to collapse of supraglottic structures on inspiration:
  - Symptoms include intermittent inspiratory stridor exacerbated by feeding and/or crying, and worse during sleep. This condition develops after 6 months of age and usually spontaneously resolves after 2 years of age.
  - Treatment: treat gastroesophageal reflux with a proton pump inhibitor (0.5 mg/kg/day), oxygen if hypoxic, and referral if prolonged apnoeic episodes.
- Subglottic haemangioma (vascular mass):
  - Characterized by a stridor in the first 6 months of life, intermittent to persistent; 50% are associated with cutaneous haemangioma.
  - Diagnosis confirmed by endoscopy if available.
  - Treatment aims to overcome the airway obstruction, typically with steroids and beta blockers. Spontaneous resolution can be seen after several years.

Child >6 months

- Acute laryngitis (laryngotracheobronchitis or subglottitis):
  - Laryngotracheobronchitis (croup) is the most common cause of airway obstruction in children from 6 months to 3 years. It is a viral infection (mainly parainfluenza virus). The most common feature is oedema laryngitis. See ➲ p. 837.
- Epiglottis (obstructive supraglottitis abscess)
  - See ➲ p. 837.
  - (Can be rapidly life-threatening!)

Reference

1. Galletti B, Mannella VK, Santoro R, Rodriguez-Morales AJ, Freni F, Galletti C, et al. ENT involvement in zoonotic diseases. J Infect Dev Ctries 2014;8(1):17–23.

Chronic non-communicable diseases

Philippa Boulle and Tammam Aloudat

Background

The great transition

Non-communicable diseases (NCDs) have become a major cause of morbidity and mortality globally, that has not only been a significant burden to HIC—but also to MIC and LIC. By 2010, almost 80% of global NCD mortality occurred in LIC and MIC, and those same countries saw 29% of their NCD deaths occur among people under the age of 60, a rate that is double that seen in HIC. The rise in NCDs is projected to continue, with the greatest increase expected in sub-Saharan Africa. This epidemiological transition is a combined result of many factors including a global reduction in child mortality and increase in life expectancy, and changes in lifestyle contributed to particularly by urbanization and global trade.

The four key NCDs identified by WHO, which cause 63% of worldwide deaths, are:

- cardiovascular diseases
- cancers
- chronic respiratory diseases
- diabetes.

The major contributory risk factors identified for these and other NCDs include tobacco use, unhealthy diet, and physical inactivity, among others.

Many poorer countries have managed to increase life expectancy, but haven't yet managed to prevent early NCD death nor care for older populations. NCDs cause chronic illness and disability, requiring long-term healthcare, and they disproportionally affect the working-age population in LIC, leading to significant economic and social impacts.

NCDs in the humanitarian context

The profile of humanitarian crises has changed greatly in the past few decades, with many of the conflicts today, with their massive and extended impact on health, happening in MIC where NCDs are an already major burden. Some of the perceived challenges in addressing NCDs in humanitarian settings include competing interests that cover more acute conditions, the high cost of managing some of the NCDs, and the lack of epidemiological understanding of their widespread prevalence and contribution to preventable morbidity and premature mortality.

Nevertheless, engagement in NCDs offers opportunities, including the ability to influence one of the highest global causes of mortality, expand the reach and effect of medical humanitarian assistance, and address medical conditions related to suffering and disability in working-age populations which will contribute to physical and financial recovery post emergency.

General principles

Priorities

NCD care has generally not been a top priority to date, due to the pro-longed nature of most of the illnesses, which commonly have asymptomatic periods. However, as they are an increasing issue confronting humanitarian care providers, it can be useful to consider the different levels of response possible, in order of priority, and to select the appropriate level per situation:

1. Relevant to all situations including first emergency response, is *acute life-saving care* and *management of acute complications*. This includes management of presentations such as diabetic ketoacidosis, hypoglycaemia, and acute myocardial infarction.
2. *Continuation of care* for those who have presented in acute decompensation is a close second priority—enabling patients with diabetes to continue on insulin, for example.
3. Continuity of care should be provided for *patients already diagnosed* and on treatment, to avoid treatment interruptions and prevent consequent decompensation.
4. Screening for new patients is a lesser priority in most humanitarian contexts, and can also involve various levels of comprehensiveness. *Opportunistic case finding* by clinicians with a clinical concern takes priority *over systematic screening* of particular risk groups, e.g. above a certain age.

Local factors

Adapting care to be contextually relevant is a challenge for any humanitarian intervention, and this is particularly the case for chronic diseases, which require patient understanding and self-management. Understanding local concepts of disease, healing, and patient autonomy are very important to be able to have a medically relevant impact with these types of conditions:

- Lifestyle advice should consider what is feasible and realistic—in a refugee camp where patients are given fixed food distributions it may not be useful to advise on high fruit and vegetable intake, and indeed more important to discuss with food distribution programmes about the appropriateness of rations.
- Patient literacy should be considered for education materials, which should include pictures reflective of the local situation.
- The local medical context is also of importance and harmonization with local guidelines and drug lists may be useful, so long as they are evidence based and of sufficient standard.
- Give early consideration to a strategy for local capacity building to facilitate handover of care; include training of local medical staff, advocacy regarding missing elements in local capacity, and potential donation of drugs and equipment.

Challenges in humanitarian settings

Multiple medications

In general, there exist relatively affordable simple drugs for routine NCD care. However, the majority of patients will require multiple medications, due to individual disease requirements or multi-morbidity. Thus, access becomes more complicated due to the need for reliable and affordable availability of many medications.

> The HIV epidemic has provided valuable lessons in terms of the feasibility of providing chronic care in LIC and MIC settings, using simplified protocols, task-shifting, and decentralized care, lessons that can be utilized to enable upscaling of NCD care accessibility.

Model of care

- Task shifting has an important role and routine follow-up care of stable patients can be provided by nurses or trained lower-level staff, particularly if simple protocols or follow-up checklists are provided. Generalist doctors can do most of the routine initiation and adjustment of medications. Patient education can be given by various levels of staff, with trained community health workers able to give general disease information, often in group sessions.
- Having a system for follow-up of patients is very important; appointments for chronic condition patients are useful but it is often helpful to have one clinician dedicated to seeing those with appointments and having another to see acute patients without appointments, if walk-in visits are the norm.
- Investigations can be rationalized, and point-of-care tests used for capillary glucose, haemoglobin (Hb), and creatinine, as well as simple desk-top machines (used by non-laboratory staff), including for glycated haemoglobin (HbA1c), electrolytes, and lipids. As a minimum, stethoscopes, sphygmomanometers, glucometers, and urine dipsticks provide valuable information in the care of NCD patients; measuring tapes, weighing scales, peak flow meters, and ECG machines are also very useful.[1]
- Ideally programme monitoring involves assessment of patient impact, but in some contexts this will not be possible. If you are using simple aggregate data collection, collect patient numbers as well as consultation numbers, and consider adding the variable of new and follow-up patients, to understand whether you are capturing chronic patients returning for review.

Patient support

Patient support, education, and counselling are key components of chronic disease management and aim to improve adherence to treatment, reduce complications, improve quality of life, and provide emotional support. In humanitarian situations, the last is particularly important, as self-management is often compromised by competing priorities—such as addressing basic needs like food and shelter—and by the psychological stress which patients may be suffering.

Cancer

Cancer is a leading cause of disease globally, with increasing proportional mortality in LIC where there are limitations in diagnostics and treatment (see Fig. 46.1). If treatment is unavailable, palliative care may be the only—and very important—option; yet this, too, is often complicated by lack of its prioritization relative to 'life-saving' activities, and by poor availability of opiate drugs due to restrictions on importation and prescription in many countries. However, it should be considered wherever possible, and advocacy for access invoked where necessary. (See ➲ Chapter 47 for more information.)

Cancer prevention is important where feasible, i.e. vaccination for infection-related cancers, such as HPV vaccine for cervical cancer, and hepatitis B vaccination for liver cancer. Screening and treatment of pre-cancerous cervical lesions is another feasible and cost-effective intervention, using visual inspection with acetic acid and lesion management with cryotherapy in one session (with referral for more advanced lesions). This is particularly important in high HIV-burden populations where cervical cancer is more prevalent. Early cancer detection can also play a role, but only where referral for treatment is available. Breast examination, for example, can be included in routine visits in services receiving female patients, especially where mammography is not available.

Treatment options are usually more limited, but when appropriate infrastructure can be ensured, including diagnostic histology and treatment, options may be available for certain cancers, such as Kaposi's sarcoma.

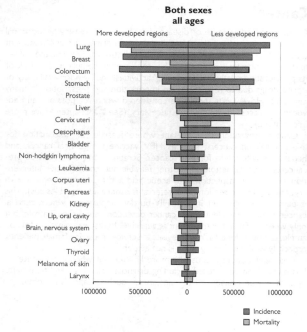

Fig. 46.1 Cancer incidence and mortality in developed and developing countries. Estimated age-standardized incidence and mortality rates: both sexes. Reproduced with permission from Ferlay J., Soerjomataram I., Ervik M., Dikshit R., Eser S., Mathers C., Rebelo M., Parkin D.M., Forman D., Bray, F. GLOBOCAN 2012 v1.0, Cancer Incidence and Mortality Worldwide: IARC CancerBase No. 11 [Internet]. Lyon, France: International Agency for Research on Cancer; 2013. Available from: http://globocan.iarc.fr, accessed on 20/11/2017.

Chronic respiratory disease

Asthma and chronic obstructive pulmonary disease (COPD) are chronic respiratory diseases which can present with cough, difficulty breathing, chest tightness, and/or wheezing. The clinical features and pathophysiology of asthma and COPD overlap, asthma can be a risk factor for COPD, and they can both be present in the same patient.

See ➲ Chapter 37 for specific guidelines for asthma.

Chronic obstructive pulmonary disease

COPD is a common lung condition characterized by airflow limitation interfering with breathing, is not fully reversible, and is usually progressive. Globally, tobacco smoke is the biggest risk factor, but in some low-income settings biomass fuels such as wood smoke play an important contributory role. COPD was responsible for 3 million deaths in 2005, 90% of which occurred in LIC and MIC, where deaths are projected to rise.

Diagnosis
History
Symptoms of breathlessness, chronic cough, or sputum production which are usually:
- in a patient >35 years old with a history of heavy smoking and/or history of heavy and prolonged exposure to burning fossil fuels in an enclosed space, or high exposure to dust in occupational settings
- symptoms which have worsened slowly over a long period
- persistent with little day-to-day variation.

Differential diagnosis
Consider: asthma, TB, heart failure, lung cancer, pulmonary embolus, bronchiectasis asbestosis, and fibrosis

Investigations
- Peak expiratory flow rate: response to bronchodilator <20% makes COPD more likely than asthma.
- Spirometry: demonstrate airflow limitation (forced expiratory volume in 1 second (FEV_1)/forced vital capacity (FVC) <0.7) which is minimally reversible after bronchodilator use.

Chronic management
Objectives
- Symptom management.
- Reduction of risk of severe exacerbations/deteriorations.

Assessment:
- Do lung function testing if possible
  - *Mild* (FEV_1 60–80% predicted): shortness of breath (SOB) on moderate exertion, recurrent chest infections, minimal effect on daily activities.
  - *Moderate* (FEV_1 40–59% predicted): increasing SOB, SOB on level ground, increasing limitation of daily activities, cough and sputum production, exacerbations requiring inhaled corticosteroids/antibiotics.
  - *Severe* (FEV_1 <40% predicted): SOB on minimal exertion, daily activities severely curtailed, experiencing regular sputum, chronic cough.
- Assess for comorbidities which can worsen COPD severity, and should be treated.

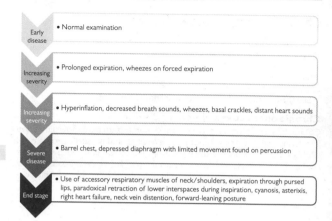

Early disease	• Normal examination
Increasing severity	• Prolonged expiration, wheezes on forced expiration
Increasing severity	• Hyperinflation, decreased breath sounds, wheezes, basal crackles, distant heart sounds
Severe disease	• Barrel chest, depressed diaphragm with limited movement found on percussion
End stage	• Use of accessory respiratory muscles of neck/shoulders, expiration through pursed lips, paradoxical retraction of lower interspaces during inspiration, cyanosis, asterixis, right heart failure, neck vein distention, forward-leaning posture

Fig. 46.2 COPD signs and symptoms.

Interventions
- Reduce irritants:
  - *Smoking cessation*—the most important measure!
  - Cook outside if possible, using wood or carbon; otherwise keep cooking area well ventilated.
  - Avoid occupational exposure to dust or high air pollution.
- Use medications:
  - *Step 1*: bronchodilator (useful even if no spirometric improvement after use):
    —Inhaled short-acting beta agonist (SABA), e.g. salbutamol, 2 puffs PRN, up to four times a day.
    —*Or* inhaled short-acting muscarinic antagonist (SAMA), e.g. ipratropium bromide.
  - *Step 2*: combination of SABA + SAMA.
  - *Step 3*: *if available*: add long-acting beta agonist (LABA) (or long-acting muscarinic antagonist if available).
  - *Step 4*: add inhaled corticosteroid (*note*: beware increased risk of pneumonia in patients treated with inhaled corticosteroid + LABAs—balance against benefits of reduced exacerbations and quality of life).
  - *Step 5*: consider low-dose theophylline if plasma monitoring possible (this may be at an earlier stage depending on other drug availability).
- Further supplement therapies can include physical activity, psychological support, and vaccination.

Palliation of dyspnoea
Opiates may be of benefit in some patients unresponsive to the treatments described—this should be low dose and/or short acting, because of the risk of respiratory depression.

Exacerbations of COPD

The term exacerbation refers to acute episode of worsened respiratory symptoms—cough frequency/severity, sputum volume/character, and/or SOB—beyond day-to-day variations and requiring change in medication:

- 70% of exacerbations are triggered by respiratory infections, especially viral and typical bacterial pathogens.
- 30% are due to environmental pollution, pulmonary embolism, or unknown.

Management

- Assess severity: patients with pulse rate >100, respiratory rate >20, O_2 saturation <92%, use of accessory muscles, and inability to speak complete sentences need immediate treatment and senior clinician review!
- Immediate management:
  - Oxygen if O_2 saturation <92%—*no more than 28%* (2 litres with nasal cannula): higher rates may reduce respiratory drive.
  - Salbutamol via spacer (10 puffs, then 4–6 puffs every 2–4 hours).
- Consider alternative diagnoses: heart failure, pulmonary thromboembolism, pneumonia, and pneumothorax (chest X-ray may be useful if available).
- *Antibiotics*: if clinical signs of airway infection (e.g. increased volume and change of colour of sputum with increased dyspnoea or fever). Options include:
  - 7 days of amoxicillin 500 mg three times daily
  - erythromycin 500 mg four times daily, or
  - doxycycline 200 mg on day 1 then 100 mg daily for 6 days.
- Oral *prednisolone* 30–40 mg daily for 7 days for severe exacerbations.
- *Increase inhaled bronchodilator*: 2 puffs 4-hourly of SABA (± SAMA if available).
- Hospitalize if possible if inadequate response to emergency management, significant increase in dyspnoea over baseline, severe underlying COPD, or clinically unstable.

Diabetes

Type 1 (T1DM), type 2 (T2DM), and gestational diabetes mellitus (GDM) are conditions causing sustained elevation of blood glucose levels.

- *T1DM* is characterized by lack of insulin production by the pancreas. It often presents in childhood with severe hyperglycaemia, but may occur later, especially in sub-Saharan African populations.
- *T2DM* is the most prevalent type of diabetes, due to defective insulin response and progressive insulin resistance. Increasing globally due to obesity and dietary factors, and now occurring in younger age groups.
- *GDM*: a glucose–insulin imbalance in later pregnancy.

Emergency management of hypoglycaemia

Definition : blood sugar <75 mg/dL (4.2 mmol/litre) ± symptoms (autonomic or neurological).

In *conscious patients* (awake; able to eat and drink):
- Give 15 g sugar, e.g. 15 mL (3 teaspoons) sugar dissolved in water, 175 mL (3/4 cup) of juice/soft drink, or 25 mL of 50% glucose.
- Recheck in 15 minutes—retreat if needed; if blood sugar level >4.2 give next meal or snack for slow-release carbohydrate.
- Recheck in 1 hour.
- Try to find a cause: too much insulin (incorrect insulin dose or type), recent weight loss, delayed or missed meal, alcohol, unplanned or extra exercise, or other medications.

In the *unconscious patient* (or unable to drink safely)—glucose is typically <2.8 mmol/litre = 50 mg/dL:
- Ensure IV access and give 25 mL of 50% glucose (children <15 years, give 2–5 mL/kg of 10% glucose IV).
- If no IV access, give 1 mg of glucagon subcutaneously/IM (half dose if <25 kg or <8 years old)
- Recheck in 15 minutes.
- If still <75 mg/dL (4.2 mmol/litre):
  - Unconscious and unable to drink, repeat first step.
  - Lucid and able to drink, give 15 g of sugar by mouth (as above in list) and recheck in 10 minutes.
- If ≥75 mg/dL (4.2 mmol/litre):
  - If conscious and able to eat, give the next meal or snack due or some slow-release carbohydrate. Recheck in 1 hour.
  - If consciousness is still impaired, start an IV infusion of 10% glucose 1 litre over 2 hours (children <15 years: 4–9 kg: 6 mL/kg/h; 10–19 kg: 5 mL/kg/hour; 20–39 kg: 4 mL/kg/hour; 40–59 kg: 3.5 mL/kg/hour; 60–80 kg: 3 mL/kg/hour) and recheck in 1 hour. Stop when conscious and able to drink safely.

> Note: if 10% glucose is not available, make it by adding 10 mL of 50% glucose solution per 100 mL of 5% glucose solution to obtain a 10% glucose solution. Then give 2.5 mL/kg of this 10% glucose solution by IV over 5 minutes.

Emergency management of hyperglycaemia

Suspect if:
- previous diagnosis of diabetes (note: but diabetic ketoacidosis (DKA) may be first presentation)
- vomiting, abdominal pain, flushed cheeks, sweet smell on breath, dehydration and polyuria, rapid evolution over 24 hours → DKA
- polyuria, polydipsia, weight loss, lethargy, focal neurological signs, obtundation, evolution over days → hyperosmolar hyperglycaemic state.

Patients with T1DM can develop a ketoacidosis (DKA) and those with T2DM and extremely high blood sugars are at risk of hyperosmolar hyperglycaemic state. Properly diagnosing and distinguishing these conditions require laboratory facilities that are often not available in humanitarian settings; thus simplified criteria using signs, symptoms, and bedside tests are described. The treatment of DKA and the hyperosmolar hyperglycaemic state are similar, including the administration of insulin and the correction of fluid and electrolyte abnormalities. Management is complex and best undertaken by experienced staff in high-level facilities—refer wherever possible.

Patients requiring urgent hospitalization are those with:
- blood sugar levels >27 mmol/litre (>500 mg/dL) or
- If blood sugar level >11 mmol/litre (>200 mg/dL), plus one or more of:
  - danger signs: dehydration, hypotension, slow, deep breathing (Kussmaul's respiration from ketosis), abdominal pain, nausea and vomiting, fruity breath, focal motor deficits, and/or altered mental status
  - urinary ketones (blood sugar level >22 mmol/litre (>400 mg/dL) + dipstick ketones ≥moderate = DKA).

Before referral, insert IV drip, and give 1 litre of normal (0.9%) saline over 30 minutes–1 hour. Encourage patient to drink water, as much as possible, on the way.

Assessment
- Assess: severity of dehydration (assume 10% if uncertain), level of consciousness, and evidence of infection.
- Check:
  - Blood glucose (glucometer).
  - Ketones (urine dipstick).
  - If laboratory available (according to possibility): blood glucose, blood ketones, electrolytes, HbA1c, urea, creatinine, bicarbonate, Hb, WBC count, venous/arterial pH.

Treatment
- Shock correction:
  - IV/intraosseous fluid 1 litre stat (adults) or 10 mL/kg (children) normal saline 0.9% bolus.
  - If NG tube is used, give same volume over 1 hour of normal saline or ORS.
  - If necessary, repeat with 10 mL/kg boluses, with caution.

- Fluid replacement:
  - Treat decreased peripheral perfusion in children (in absence of shock) with 10 mL/kg 0.9%NaCl in 1 hour.
  - Use normal saline and provide maintenance + replace deficit (*not* urine output) evenly over 48 hours.
  - Add glucose to saline once blood glucose <15 mmol/litre (<270 mg/dL)—use 5% glucose or add 100 mL 50% glucose per litre of saline.
  - Add oral hydration when tolerated.
- Insulin:
  - Start after correction of shock and 1–2 hours after starting fluid replacement to decrease risk of cerebral oedema.
  - IV infusion 0.1 unit/kg/hour via side drip: add 50 units of short-acting (regular) insulin to 500 mL of normal saline (for total of 1 unit per 10 mL).
  - If infusion not possible or not safe, give hourly insulin subcutaneously or IM 0.1 unit/kg rapid insulin (and transfer if possible).
  - Continue until ketones cleared—aim for glucose reduction of about 5 mmol/litre/hour (90 mg/dL/hour).
- Potassium:
  - If unable to measure, do ECG if possible (hypokalaemia—flattened T wave, widened QT, U waves; hyperkalaemia—peaked T waves, shortened QT).
  - Start replacement if necessary, or once patient passing urine.
  - 40 mmol/litre in maintenance fluids or if no IV potassium—ORS, fruit juice, bananas, coconut water.
  - Monitor potassium at least 6-hourly if possible.
- Bicarbonate: do not give; risk of cerebral oedema.
- Infection: if suspected (e.g. fever), give broad-spectrum antibiotics, e.g. ceftriaxone 75 mg/kg/day.
- Cerebral oedema: rare, but often fatal; usually presents 4–24 hours after start of treatment:
  - Risk if too aggressive hydration, use of bicarbonate, initial pH <7.
  - Signs: headache, vomiting, decreased pulse rate plus increased BP; change in neurological status or neurological signs, abnormal respiration, cyanosis.
  - Treat urgently if suspected: reduce fluid administration rate to 75% maintenance and consider mannitol or hypertonic saline only under specialist supervision.
- Transitioning to subcutaneous insulin once hydration corrected, glucose controlled, ketones cleared:
  - First dose 1–2 hours before stopping insulin and glucose infusion(s); give food within 15–30 minutes of the insulin.
  - Patient should have inpatient care until 3 days of stable insulin dose.

Diabetes mellitus testing

Testing for diabetes should be considered in:

- symptomatic patients: polydipsia, polyphagia, polyuria, blurry vision, peripheral neuropathy, unexplained weight loss; also consider if recurrent fungal or urinary tract infections, chronic foot wound
- pregnant women

- those with BMI >25kg/m² and family history in a first-degree relative/ history of large baby or GDM/hypertension/cardiovascular disease/ polycystic ovarian syndrome/on drugs that cause high blood glucose (oral steroids, antiretrovirals, antipsychotics).

Diagnostic criteria (WHO)

In many low-resource settings, capillary glucose may be the only feasible measurement, and point-of-care tests are recommended by WHO if venous glucose testing is not available. *One test is sufficient in symptomatic patients; if asymptomatic, confirm with a second test.* Testing options include:

- random blood glucose (RBG) ≥11.1 mmol/litre (200 mg/dL). Random is defined as the glucose concentration any time of the day without regard to the time since the last meal, *or*
- fasting blood glucose (FBG) ≥7.0 mmol/litre (126 mg/dL). Fasting is defined as nothing to eat or drink except water for at least the past 8 hours, *or*
- HbA1c ≥6.5%, *or*
- in pregnant women: oral glucose tolerance test (OGTT) >11.1 mmol/ litre (200 mg/dL)—2 hours post 75 g glucose (rarely available in humanitarian settings).

Management of T2DM

Most patients will need lifestyle change *and* medication. If the patient is committed, lifestyle change alone can be tried for the first few months. Commonly used oral drugs are as follows:

- Biguanides: metformin—reduces hepatic glucose production and insulin resistance.
- Sulfonylureas: glibenclamide, gliclazide, others—augment insulin secretion (require residual pancreatic beta-cell activity).
- Principles of oral hypoglycaemic drugs:
  - Start with low dose and increase gradually to achieve control. Monitor possible side effects.
  - If blood glucose not controlled, increase up to the maximum tolerated dose.
  - If blood glucose still not controlled, add the next step drug.

Treatment algorithm

- *Step 1*: metformin is used first-line unless renal or hepatic impairment:
  - Start with 500 mg once daily with breakfast, review after 2 weeks.
  - If tolerated, add 500 mg tablet with breakfast, increase by a tablet every 2 weeks, up to a maximum of 3 g daily.
  - To improve adherence, warn patient of likely side effects (i.e. diarrhoea and abdominal discomfort) which can improve with time.
  - Recheck fasting glucose each visit.
  - If blood glucose not controlled add step 2 drug.
- *Step 2*: add a sulfonylurea, once daily before meals (also use as step 1 if metformin contraindicated or not tolerated):
  - Increase as needed by one tablet every 2 weeks (twice daily).
  - Has risk of hypoglycaemia, e.g. in elderly or with kidney disease.
- Sulfonylurea options:
  - Gliclazide: start with 80 mg tablet (or 40 mg in elderly); max. dose 320 mg daily.

- Glibenclamide (longer acting—increased risk of hypoglycaemia): start with 2.5 mg, max. dose 20 mg daily.
- Glimepiride: 1 mg once daily (max. 8 mg), glipizide 2.5–5 mg once daily (max. 40 mg), tolbutamide 0.5 g daily (max. 2 g).
- *Step 3*: if blood glucose not controlled, consider insulin.

Insulin management in T2DM

- Continue oral hypoglycaemic agents, but halve dose of sulfonylurea.
- Start with a single evening injection of NPH (intermediate acting insulin) of 0.2–0.3 units/kg at bedtime: NPH onset of action: 1–2 hours, max. action at 4–12 hours, duration of action: 16–18 hours. (See Fig. 46.3.)
- If self-glucose monitoring is possible, ask patient to record three pre-meal and one bedtime glucose levels per day. Once stable, reduced to testing before each injection and random pre-breakfast.
- Adjust insulin according to fasting blood glucose measurements, 4–10 days after beginning injections

Single dose NPH nocte can be increased up to a maximum of 0.6 units/kg/day if required. If control is not achieved at this level, change to a twice-daily injection regimen, by converting the current insulin dose into two doses: two-thirds in the morning and one-third in the evening 12 hours apart; e.g. if the patient was taking 30 units at bedtime (0.6 units/kg in 50 kg woman), divide this into 20 units in the morning and 10 units in the evening. (See Fig 46.4.)

If the patient still has very poorly controlled blood sugars, despite careful adjustment, counselling, and patient adherence, consider switching to a mixed insulin regimen as for T1DM (see following section).

Management of T1DM

Patients with T1DM require exogenous insulin for survival, with a daily requirement of 0.4–1 U/kg/day.

For insulin initiation, it is suggested to start with a dose of around 0.5 U/kg/day (total daily dose), split between basal insulin and prandial bolus insulin (often 50:50). Two strategies are available: (1) 'intensive' basal/bolus insulin therapy, and (2) 'conventional' (mixed) insulin therapy.

For safe insulin management, patients should be having three meals per day at regular times and two snacks (mid-morning and pre-bed) to help to maintain good blood sugar control and avoid hypos. This may be difficult in some settings; insulin regimens need to be tailored to the individual and may require specialist support. Consider if food support is required.

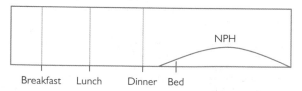

Fig. 46.3 Initial insulin management in type 2 diabetes.

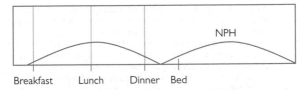

Fig. 46.4 Increased insulin dose in type 2 diabetes.

Insulin product information requires refrigeration for unopened insulin, with room temperature being suitable after opening for up to 28 days. However, various local methods of cooling have proven useful for storage, including clay pots in many African contexts, and in many settings insulin can be managed without refrigeration. Patients must be advised to keep insulin in the coolest part of the house. *Note—freezing destroys insulin, beware of this in the cold chain!*

Follow-up and targets
See Table 46.1.
- Teach patients an injection technique with demonstrations and handouts with pictures; get them to practise with water in front of you.
- If home glucose monitoring is not possible, a urine dipstick can be used for glucose detection—then remember that it reflects what has happened in the body since the patient last urinated. If +++ glucose on urine dipstick, the dose of insulin given 4–6 hours previously should be decreased.
- See patients weekly or more if medication doses were adjusted, or if blood sugar is poorly controlled, then 1–3-monthly when stable.

Insulin in T1DM
Mixed insulin (biphasic)
This is not recommended for T1DM, but is often the most feasible in humanitarian settings, as it requires less self-monitoring and adjustment.
- Fixed combination of NPH (intermediate acting insulin) and short-acting insulin; this comes as pre-mixed formulations, e.g. biphasic 70/30 (70% intermediate and 30% short-acting insulin), or can be mixed by the patient in the syringe immediately prior to injection (drawing 'clear before cloudy'). NPH provides basal insulin action while short-acting insulin provides extra insulin to cover meal times.

Table 46.1 Targets in diabetes

Target	Optimal (especially young patients with longer life expectancy, low risk of hypoglycaemia)	Modified (elderly or significant morbidity)
HbA1c	<7%	<8%
FBG	3.9–7.2 mmol/litre (70–130 mg/dL)	≤10 mmol/litre (180 mg/dL)
RBG	≤11 mmol/litre (200 mg)	≤15 mmol/litre (270 mg/dL)

FBG, fasting blood glucose; HbA1c, glycated haemoglobin; RBG, random blood glucose.
Note: in many settings, patients safety and avoiding hypoglycaemia are the primary objective; higher HbA1cs may be tolerated.

- Start with 0.5 units/kg/day divided in two doses 12 hours apart: two-thirds in the morning 15 minutes before the morning meal and one-third in the evening 15 minutes before the evening meal.
- It is essential that the patient eats after taking the mixed insulin to avoid serious hypoglycaemia. Do not prescribe mixed insulin if the patient does not have access to morning and evening meals.
- Titrate total insulin dose by 20% until blood glucose level is on target. The dose before breakfast is adapted according to the previous dinner blood glucose level and the dose before dinner is adapted according to the pre-breakfast blood glucose level.
- When adjusting, think of the insulin components separately (e.g. 10 units of 70/30 mixed insulin = 7 units of intermediate-acting insulin and 3 units of short-acting insulin).

Intensive/basal–bolus regimen

This is preferred in T1DM as it gives better control, and has been proven to reduce microvascular and macrovascular outcomes:

- Requires self-monitoring of blood glucose (three to four times per day) and adjustment of the dose of the prandial bolus insulin to carbohydrate intake, pre-meal blood glucose, and anticipated physical activity.
- Combines basal insulin (two daily injections of intermediate-acting insulin) with doses of short-acting insulin three or more times daily, at meal times (see Fig. 46.5).
- Basal insulin delivery (50% of daily dose for adults, one-third total daily dose for children): two daily injections of intermediate-acting insulin (NPH): one-half of the dose before breakfast and one-half of the dose before dinner or at bedtime.
- Prandial bolus insulin (50% of the daily dose in adults, two-thirds in children): three daily pre-meal injections of short-acting insulin (regular): one-third of the dose before each meal, adjusted as above.

> 'Dawn phenomenon'—blood glucose level can rise in the early morning; be aware of this when interpreting high morning glucose levels, before increasing the evening NPH, as this can lead to hypoglycaemia in the middle of the night. If suspected, ask patient to check their blood glucose at 2 am.

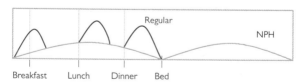

Fig. 46.5 Intensive/basal–bolus regimen.

Insulins

See Table 46.2 for types of insulins and effects.

Table 46.2 Types of insulins

Type of insulin	Onset	Peak	Duration
Rapid-acting[a]	10–30 minute	30–90 minutes	3–5 hours
Short-acting[b]	30 minutes–1 hour	2–4 hours	6–8 hours
Intermediate-acting[c]	1.5–4 hours	4–12 hours	14–18 hours
Long-acting[d]	1–2 hours	No peak	Up to 24 hours

[a,d] Analogue insulins, less often available in humanitarian settings and not on the WHO Essential Medicines List.
[b,c] Human insulins, cheaper than analogue insulins and more commonly in use in humanitarian settings; on the WHO Essential Medicines List.

Thyroid disease

Hypothyroidism

Hypothyroidism is caused by an inability of the thyroid gland to produce enough thyroid hormone to satisfy the metabolic needs of the body. Almost one-third of the world's population lives in areas of iodine deficiency, the most common cause of hypothyroidism globally.

Goitre is endemic when daily intake is <50 mcg, and congenital hypothyroidism is seen at a daily intake of <25 mcg. In iodine sufficient areas, autoimmune disease is most common. Treatment is straightforward, but is life-long and requires monitoring, so consider context prior to initiating therapy.

Assessment

- Assess clinically: symptoms may include fatigue, cold intolerance, weight gain, depression, constipation, dry skin, and muscle pains. Signs include coarse facies, goitre, oedema, bradycardia, hypothermia, and slow relaxation of deep tendon reflexes.
- Measure TSH, if possible:
  - If elevated (>5.5 million IU) → repeat test in 2–4 weeks + measure free T4 if possible:
    —if T4 low → primary hypothyroidism
    —if T4 normal → subclinical hypothyroidism (see ⊃ p. 858)
    —if T4 high → not primary hypothyroidism → endocrinology consult if possible.
  - If normal → euthyroid.
  - If low (<0.35 million IU/litre) → consider hyperthyroidism.

Treatment

- Most patients require lifelong thyroid replacement therapy with synthetic T4, i.e. levothyroxine—average dose is 1.6 mcg/kg body weight per day. (Use a lower dose of 25–50 mcg per day in the elderly/frail/those with symptomatic angina.)
- Take on an empty stomach, usually in the morning 30–60 minutes before eating and do not take within 4 hours of calcium or iron supplements which can interfere with absorption.
- Symptoms usually improve within 2 weeks; increase dose by 25–50 mcg/day until symptoms improve and normal TSH level.
- Initial TSH testing every 6–8 weeks until stable, then check annually.
- If daily administration is difficult, patients can take T4 weekly given its long half-life.

For patients with subclinical hypothyroidism: only treat if TSH >10 million IU/litre, if TSH persistently 5–10 million IU/litre and patient symptomatic, or if patient trying to fall pregnant; continue only if symptomatic benefit, for target TSH of 1–3 million IU/litre.

Hyperthyroidism

Excess synthesis and secretion of thyroid hormones by the thyroid gland leads to the hypermetabolic condition of thyrotoxicosis, and can be caused by autoimmune disease (Graves' disease), toxic multinodular goitre/toxic adenoma, postpartum thyroiditis, and multiple other causes. In humanitarian settings, resources for investigation and management of hyperthyroidism are less likely to be available or be a priority. Symptomatic management with beta blockers may be possible, but diagnosis or specific antithyroid treatments would be less likely to be available in low-resource environments.

Haemoglobinopathies

The genes for Hb disorder traits are present in about 5% of the world's population, with sickle cell disease (SCD) and thalassaemia being most common.

Sickle cell disease

SCD is an inherited autosomal recessive disorder, in which affected children are usually homozygotes for the mutated HBB gene causing Hb S; red blood cells become distorted into a crescent or sickle shape. The sickle cell carrier state confers a survival advantage for falciparum malaria during early childhood, aligning SCD burden with that of malaria. Most patients with SCD are born in low-resource settings, and often die undiagnosed. In sub-Saharan Africa, up to one-third of the population are carriers of the defective gene, with a 1–2% birth prevalence. Only 25% of those born with SCD survive 5 years. Neonatal screening exists, but is not routinely available in much of Africa.

Symptoms

Sickled erythrocytes lead to chronic haemolytic anaemia due to their destruction and painful vaso-occlusive crises due to hindered capillary blood flow. Patients have increased susceptibility to infection with encapsulated organisms (*Pneumococcus, Neisseria meningitidis, Haemophilus influenza, Salmonella*), delayed growth, increased risk of stroke, and organ damage (acute chest syndrome, pulmonary hypertension, avascular necrosis of the femoral head). Vaso-occlusive crises can be precipitated by infections, dehydration, cold, stress, hypoxia, and acidosis.

Investigations

The principal diagnostic means are either not routinely available in low-resource settings (Hb electrophoresis, isoelectric focusing, techniques) or unreliable (microscopy). Unfortunately, a clinical diagnosis is often made when a patient presents with a severe complication. Try to refer for testing where possible.

Management

Regular clinic visits (every 4–8 weeks), education about avoidance of precipitating factors, rapid healthcare seeking for fever or acute pain, need for prophylactic medications, vaccinations, and proper food and hygiene.

Prophylactic medications

- Oral penicillin in children and adolescents (life-long treatment): 50,000–100,000 IU/kg/day in two divided doses (<1 year: 62.5 mg twice daily; 1–5 years: 125 mg twice daily; >5 years: 250 mg twice daily; adolescents: 500 mg twice daily)
- Folate: <1 year old, 2.5 mg daily; >1 year old, 5 mg daily.
- Malaria chemoprophylaxis: in malaria endemic areas, from 6 months to 5 years, e.g. amodiaquine 153 mg + sulfadoxine–pyrimethamine 500 mg/25 mg; <1 year, half a tablet daily; >1 year, one tablet daily.

Immunization
- Pneumococcal: 13-valent if available; 10-valent or 7-valent if not, plus after the age of 2 years, an additional shot with polysaccharide 23-valent vaccine is used.
- Meningococcal: meningococcal conjugate vaccine A from 1 year old; tetravalent conjugant vaccines ACYW-135 from 1–2 years old.
- *Haemophilus influenza* type B: in routine EPI vaccination schedule (pentavalent vaccine).

Management of infection
- Fever >38.5°C should be considered a medical emergency.
- Assess: vital signs, ABCD, pallor, signs of infection, splenic size, neurological examination, malaria test, urine dipstick, chest X-ray.
- Treat: ceftriaxone 100 mg/kg; if child very ill or septic add clindamycin 10 mg/kg/dose every 8 hours for MRSA and anaerobes.

Management of vaso-occlusive crisis
- IV access; ensure adequate hydration.
- Assess for other cause before concluding it is a vaso-occlusive crisis. Chest pain and priapism are always medical emergencies.
- Offer pain management and comfort measures.
- Hydroxycarbamide—increases fetal Hb production which decreases sickling and improves the clinical course of SCD:
  - Use if: more than three vaso-occlusive crisis/painful issues leading to admission yearly; more than two acute painful chest episodes; severe symptomatic anaemia.
  - Starting dose is 15 mg/kg/day PO; increase by 5 mg/kg/day after 6–8 weeks on treatment if insufficient pain control (max. 25 mg/kg/day).
  - Dose is 20 mg/kg/day PO.
  - Stop temporarily if neutrophil count <2000/μL, platelets <80,000/μL, Hb <4.5 g/dL *if* low reticulocytes.

Anaemia
- Emergency blood transfusion in severely symptomatic anaemia, or Hb <7 g/dL with vaso-occlusive crisis, for splenic sequestration, acute chest pain, risk of cerebrovascular accident, or preoperatively.
- Exchange transfusion programmes can be done if there is capacity for chelation to avoid iron overload—otherwise consider hydroxyurea as above.

Thalassaemias

Most common in Asia, the Mediterranean, and the Middle East, thalassaemias are inherited disorders causing a deficit in Hb production, which are managed with regular blood transfusions, iron-chelation therapy, bone marrow transplantation and sometimes splenectomy, and with regular folic acid supplementation, 1–2 mg/day.

In humanitarian settings, clusters of beta thalassaemia patients previously on treatment have been seen by humanitarian actors in MIC such as during the war in Syria. Consider transfusions for diagnosed patients with interrupted treatment. This is life-saving and relatively simple when medical humanitarian infrastructure is in place.

Renal disease

Renal failure

End-stage kidney disease is a leading cause of morbidity and mortality globally, and prevalence is expected to rise due to population ageing and increasing prevalence of hypertension and diabetes. Costs of life-sustaining treatments and renal replacement therapy (dialysis or renal transplantation) remain high, and availability in LIC and MIC is extremely limited. However, where dialysis services exist, supporting them during emergencies to avoid service disruption can be an important life-saving measure. In more stable settings, where renal replacement therapy is not possible, attention should be paid to prevention of end-stage kidney disease, with management of risk factors such as hypertension and diabetes, along with early identification of renal impairment.

Diagnosis

Chronic kidney disease is diagnosed when an estimated or measured glomerular filtration rate (GFR) is <60 mL/min/1.73 m² for ≥3 months with or without evidence of kidney damage

or

there is evidence of kidney damage (albuminuria, non-urological haematuria, structural abnormalities, pathological abnormalities) with or without decreased GFR for ≥3 months.

Staging

See Table 46.3.

- Renal function—and failure severity—can be assessed by calculating GFR or creatinine clearance (CrCl; it exceeds GFR due to creatinine secretion) by comparative measurements of substances in the blood and urine. However, they can be estimated by formulas based on serum creatinine.
- Cockcroft–Gault equation: estimates CrCl using serum creatinine, weight, and age; the Chronic Kidney Disease Epidemiology Collaboration (CKP-EPI) is a newer formula which is more accurate than that of Cockcroft–Gault. It is very complicated without an online calculator or app.

Table 46.3 Staging of kidney disease

Stage		CrCl (mL/min)
1	Normal kidney function	>90
2	Mildly reduced kidney function	60–89
3	Moderately reduced	30–59
4	Severely reduced dysfunction	15–29
5	Very severe/end-stage kidney failure	<15

Management
- Chronic kidney disease is a risk factor for cardiovascular disease: assess patient's overall cardiovascular risk.
- Use an angiotensin-converting enzyme inhibitor to decrease albuminuria and control BP: beware of hyperkalaemia and deteriorating renal function.
- BP should be kept consistently <140/90 mmHg in chronic kidney disease, and <130/80 mmHg if albuminuria (urine ACR >3.5 mg/mmol females, >2.5 mmol males) or diabetes.
- Optimize control of diabetes and lipids.
- Review patient's drugs for those to reduce or avoid (such as antivirals, benzodiazepines, colchicine, digoxin, insulin, lithium, opioids, spironolactone, and sulfonylureas). Use metformin with caution if GFR 30–60 mL/min/1.73 m^2, and not if GFR <30 mL/min/1.73 m^2.
- Stage 4/5: refer to nephrologist or internist if possible.

Reference
1. World Health Organization. Global action plan for the prevention and control of NCDs 2013-2020. Geneva: WHO; 2013. http://www.who.int/nmh/publications/ncd-action-plan/en/

Palliative care

Joseph O'Neill

Introduction

A new vigour has been seen for Hippocrates' admonition to 'Cure some-times, treat often, comfort always' when, on 23 January 2014, the World Health Assembly adopted a resolution that recognized 'palliative care (as) an approach that improves the quality of life of patients (adults and children) and their families facing the problems associated with life-threatening illness, through the prevention and relief of suffering by means of early identification and correct assessment and treatment of pain and other problems, whether physical, psychosocial or spiritual.' The resolution further called upon member states of the WHO to 'develop, strengthen and implement, where appropriate, palliative care policies to support the comprehensive strengthening of health systems to integrate evidence-based, cost-effective and equitable palliative care services in the continuum of care, across all levels.'[1] The WHO has released palliative guidance for first-level health workers.[2]

With no less an authority than the WHO in support, it is clear that humanitarian medicine, if it is to be done well, should encompass palliation in its efforts. How might this be done?

The contemporary discipline of palliative care and the concept of 'total pain' is generally considered to have originated and been defined by Dame Cicely Saunders (a social worker, a nurse, and a physician) at St Christopher's Hospice in the UK in the late 1960s.[3] At the time, and to a great extent now, palliative care's primary focus is cancer and other chronic disease. Increasingly, however, the role of palliative care in acute and emergent situations is being recognized.[4] Even in humanitarian crises engendered by war, displacement, or disaster, palliative care principles can be applied with good effect.

Principles of palliation

Underlying principles of palliative care are universal and should (and often do) underpin humanitarian responses:

- Humans are physical, emotional, and spiritual beings who live in a practical world within a cultural context and have practical needs.
  - All suffering and symptoms have a physical, emotional (psychological), and spiritual dimension.
  - In the palliative care lexicon, this is called a 'total pain' approach.
- Effective care, therefore, is best delivered by an interdisciplinary team that is capable of addressing all aspects of the human experience of suffering in the cultural context relevant to the patient, family, and community.
- The patient *and his/her family* (broadly and non-judgementally defined) are rightly the focus of care.
- Good communication is critically important (and is a skill that can be learned).
- Palliative care begins at the time of diagnosis and continues through the course of the illness up to, and beyond, death (bereavement).
- Spiritual and emotional (psychological) work cannot be effectively done, and the patient's autonomy and dignity are undermined, when physical pain and symptoms are not well controlled.
- Control of symptoms is an art and a science that can be learned.
- Successful palliation gives the patient the information she/he wants, comfort, choice, control, and dignity.

Palliation in low-resource settings

Clearly not all humanitarian relief situations afford the ability to offer a textbook palliative care suite of services to every patient. Creative use of what resources are available can, however, go a long way. There may well be people in the impacted community who have spiritual training or practical skills that can be mobilized to good effect. They should be sought out. Fostering a 'total pain' approach in routine symptom assessment and having the primary provider address this can be very helpful as well.

Through visionary and tenacious efforts of indigenous health providers (supported by health ministries, international donors, and established palliative care and hospice programmes) palliative care has spread well into Africa, Asia, Latin America, and other emerging economic regions. Of course, and as is true for all other health resources, the need for palliative services in developing economies generally far outstrips what is available.

One of the most important means of integrating a palliative component into a humanitarian health response is to seek out and work with what existing palliative resources may be in the region. Local experts will have the best knowledge regarding access to needed medications, local culture and customs, and norms of practice. There are several resources available to assist in identifying local and regional palliative care expertise.[5] The African Palliative Care Association (ℛ http://www.africanpalliativecare.org/), for example, is active across the continent and can assist in identifying palliative care experts in a number of countries and regions.

Practical elements of palliative care

For the medical or nursing professional, there are a number of practical elements of palliative care that are especially important in the humanitarian setting.

• Since ability to cure is often quite limited, it is especially important to institute symptom and pain relief measures early and aggressively. Providers often worry that in doing this they will over-medicate their patients and cause death. It is a generally accepted principle of medical ethics that the intent of an action is the key determinant of its rightness. In the palliative care setting, if the intent of an action is to relieve suffering and due diligence is given to minimize harm, administration of medications in sufficient quantity to relieve suffering, even if it causes death, is ethically sound. This is called the principle of double effect.

• Symptom management as covered in chapters in ➔ Part III, 'Syndromic management', is essential, especially for the dying patient. The provider should be prepared to increase doses, especially of opiates, commensurate with advancing disease.

• Ask about and quantify pain and other symptoms on a scale of 1–10 so that you can follow the impact of therapy.

• Investigate spiritual, practical (economic and other), and psychological sources of all symptoms as you work-up and address physical causes.

• Understand and respect cultural attitudes and practices related to pain, death, grief, and burial.

Guidance for communication

- Communication is critically important in all medical settings especially those touching on matters of life and death. If death is a possibility, it is important to find a way to signal that you are willing to talk about it in an honest and straightforward manner while respecting the cultural context of the patient and their family.
- Try to understand something of the patient's spiritual beliefs, what gives their life meaning, what they value, and what gives them joy.
- If possible, find a quiet, private place to discuss bad news or complicated health issues.
- Whenever possible, sit, rather than stand, when talking with your patient and avoid having a desk or other object between you and the patient during an interview.
- Understand who else (family members, religious counsellor, etc.). needs to be part of the discussion.
- Where appropriate use 'ask, tell, ask' approach in communication of bad, complicated, or difficult news:
  - 'Ask': ask the patient how much information they want to know about what is going on.
  - 'Tell': tell the patient as much as they want to hear honestly, avoiding medical jargon.
  - 'Ask': ask the patient what they understood of what they were told.
- Make sure you give the patient and their family time to speak and for questions. Don't do all the talking. Tolerate silence.
- Understand cultural mores regarding communication of sympathy and empathy and find appropriate ways of demonstrating a compassionate and non-judgemental attitude.
- Avoid using family members to translate unless absolutely necessary.

Special considerations for children

- Children, even neonates, experience pain and must rely on adults to recognize and advocate for pain and symptom relief. There are observational scales that can be helpful in assessing pain in children.[6] In all cases, however, the provider must be alert to the possibility that the child, infant, or newborn they are treating may be experiencing pain or other forms of physical suffering and take appropriate measures to diagnose and relieve it.
- Children should be encouraged to live as normal a life as possible (attend school with friends, play, etc.).
- Children may express their concerns, fears, and understanding of their condition in play, drawings, or other creative ways.
- Answer questions from children simply and honestly in concert with the parent's desires.

Considerations for caregivers

- Recognize that often the best care is provided in the home setting with family members acting as primary caregivers. Some important advice for such caregivers includes the following:
  - Use of extra pillows and more upright positioning in bed, maximizing fresh air, avoiding smoke, and fanning/circulation of air can help relieve dyspnoea.

- Respect that loss of appetite is part of the dying process so let the patient choose what and how much they want to eat. Offer frequent, small meals.
- Small meals, avoidance of cooking near the patient, and warm drinks, especially those containing ginger, can help with nausea and vomiting.
- If the patient has a painful mouth or throat, mouth cleaning with clean, dry cloths to remove bits of food, rinsing the mouth with dilute salt water (should barely taste the salt), or crushed aspirin in water can be helpful. Thickened liquids can often be swallowed more easily than clear liquids
- If constipation is a problem it must be addressed as it can itself be the cause of abdominal pain, delirium, agitation, and other bother-some symptoms. Encourage fluids and fresh fruits, vegetables, and other high-fibre foods. A digital rectal examination can determine if impaction is present. White soft paraffin gently inserted into the rectum can help but digital disimpaction may be necessary.
- Distraction, swaddling, stroking, rocking, and massage are helpful in pain control in children.

Finally, in all cases make sure you don't appear to abandon the dying patient. Be present to them and be aware of your own emotions and support needs. Have a low threshold to seek care and support for yourself.

Pain management

The ability to access strong pain medications is perhaps the thorniest issue complicating provision of palliation in the developing world. Data on global opioid consumption are compelling: Seya et al. made rough estimates of the need for strong pain medications in 188 countries using WHO-derived data and concluded that 'Good access to pain management is rather the exception than the rule: 5.5 billion people (83% of the world's population) live in countries with low to non-existent access, 250 million (4%) have moderate access, and only 460 million people (7%) have adequate access. Insufficient data are available for 430 million (7%).'[7]

If the planning of a humanitarian response to a health crisis is not cognizant of the need for pain management, the necessary financial resources will not be mobilized and targeted to palliation of pain and symptoms. The disparity in access to strong pain medication is, however, not solely the result of a lack of funding.

Often justice, regulatory, and health ministries erect barriers to access out of fear of diversion, addiction, and a lack of understanding of the need for strong pain medication. Practitioners of humanitarian medicine would do well to equip themselves with basic information about access to pain medication in the countries where they are working and be prepared to engage in respectful advocacy when an opportunity presents itself. Bearing in mind that it is understandably difficult to come from a developed country with a high prevalence of opiate misuse to a country where the problem is nearly non-existent and pitch this type of policy change, an approach that is well informed and sympathetic to law enforcement concerns will be most effective. Good resources for these discussions can be found through the earlier-mentioned palliative care resources as well as the World Palliative Care Alliance[8] and the University of Wisconsin's Pain and Policy Study Group.[9]

Management of pain, cough and dyspnoea, and diarrhoea are covered elsewhere in this handbook. Additional resources for clinical palliative practice in resource-constrained regions of the world are available. Among the best of these is the Palliative Care Toolkit published by the Worldwide Palliative Care Alliance and Help the Hospices.[10]

References

1. World Health Assembly. Strengthening of Palliative Care as a Component of Integrated Treatment within the Continuum of Care. 23 January 2014. ℘ http://apps.who.int/gb/ebwha/pdf_files/EB134/B134_R7-en.pdf
2. World Health Organization. Palliative Care: Symptom Management and End-of-life Care. 2004. ℘ http://www.who.int/hiv/pub/imai/genericpalliativecare082004.pdf
3. Saunders C. The evolution of palliative care. J R Soc Med 2001;94:430–2.
4. Institute of Medicine (US) Committee on Guidance for Establishing Standards of Care for Use in Disaster Situations; Altevogt BM, Stroud C, Hanson SL, et al., eds. Guidance for Establishing Crisis Standards of Care for Use in Disaster Situations: A Letter Report. Washington, DC: National Academies Press; 2009. ℘ http://www.ncbi.nlm.nih.gov/books/NBK219954/
5. Clark D, Wright M. The International Observatory on End of Life Care. J Pain Symptom Manage 2007;33(5):542–6.
6. Walker G, Arnold R. Pediatric Pain Assessment Scales. Updated 2015. ℘ https://www.mypcnow.org/blank-kx3g3

7. Seya MJ, Gelders SFAM, Achara OU, Milani B, Scholten WK. A first comparison between the consumption of and the need for opioid analgesics at country, regional and global level. J Pain Palliative Care Pharmacother 2011;25:6–18.
8. Worldwide Hospice Palliative Care Alliance. Resources. ℘ http://www.thewhpca.org/resources
9. Pain & Policy Studies Group. ℘ http://www.painpolicy.wisc.edu/
10. Worldwide Hospice Palliative Care Alliance. Palliative Care Toolkit: Improving Care in Resource Poor Settings. 2015. ℘ http://www.thewhpca.org/resources/palliative-care-toolkit

Part VI

Surgery and procedures

Chapter 48

Major trauma

David Nott

Major trauma in low-resource settings

Especially in low-resource environments, medical providers may be faced with patients with major trauma, which they typically would not see or have to manage in their home practice environment. Even further, the low-resource environment in which they are working may not have access to rapid surgical referral, and so the management decisions made take on even more importance.

This chapter aims to outline the basic management of a trauma patient, from the initial assessment and medical management, to the basic surgical procedures which can be life-saving. Further, this chapter offers guidance as to the limits of management for non-surgeons, when referrals for advanced surgical interventions should occur, and how to optimize management for the best outcome.

Preparations and decision-making in low-resource environments

Major trauma is typically unexpected, and to be prepared for this, emergency rooms should be well stocked with IV fluids and cannulae, both for peripheral and central venous access, chest drains, tourniquets, and field dressings that provide compression as well as cover. Ideally, an operating theatre should be located next to the receiving room, but if this is not possible, a surgical set should be available.

Even with these preparations, the decisions which are made in the initial moments after an injury can be very difficult and have great importance in patient survival and outcome. There are many considerations for determining the best course of action, including, manpower, operating theatre availability, and resources. These decisions are never simple, and the difficult choices need to be made based on the experience of the surgeon and the team. See ➔ Chapter 15 for more information.

Management of major trauma patients

Primary assessment

All cases which present to the emergency department should be assessed with the initial primary survey C, ABCDE:

- Catastrophic haemorrhage control.
- Airway (and cervical spine controlled by appropriate).
- Breathing and ventilation (with oxygen where available).
- Circulation and haemorrhage control.
- Disability or neurological deficit.
- Extremity/environment/exposure.

Catastrophic haemorrhage control

Compressible haemorrhage is controlled by direct pressure or tourniquets applied above the area of bleeding to a pressure greater than systolic arterial pressure, remembering that the initial BP will be low. See ➔ Chapter 50 for further information on controlling active bleeding.

Airway management

The sequence of events is stridor and wheezing, agitation and panic, cyanosis and confusion, followed by unconsciousness.

- Initial airway management includes chin lift and jaw thrust and the passage of an oropharyngeal or nasopharyngeal airway.
- As the patient arrives in the emergency department, if oxygen is available then this must be given by a mask and an oxygen probe inserted onto the finger.

> Think of airway problems if the patient has tachypnoea, grunting, gurgling and snoring sounds from the upper airway, has massive facial trauma or facial burns, or if the patient is unwilling to lie down.

Emergency airways

The indications for emergency intubation or surgical airway are:

- to protect an airway threatened from the loss of protective reflexes in a patient with a GCS score ≤8
- to secure an obstructed or potentially obstructed airway
- to support ventilation in patients who have had a head injury and/or spinal injury causing hypoventilation.

Keep in mind, however, that a ventilator may not be available in this setting and decisions need to be made on the feasibility of endotracheal intubation and hand ventilation with the possibility of transfer or futility of treatment.

If a surgical airway needs to be performed then a cricothyroidotomy is by far and away the best option over a tracheostomy. This is because it is much easier to perform and is safer in less experienced hands. See ➔ Chapter 50 for more information.

Breathing management

Once the airway is secure, the chest is next examined carefully.

The pneumonic TWELVE is useful to use for assessment.

T = trachea, check if central, a deviation away from the midline may indicate a tension pneumothorax—the trachea being pushed away by the overinflated side.

W = wounds, check for all wounds front and back, superficial and deep. Deep may produce a sucking pneumothorax.

E = emphysema, the classical 'rice crispy' feeling, may indicate a pneumothorax.

L = laryngeal injury, think also of the oesophagus.

V = veins, distended veins will indicate a cardiac tamponade.

E = evaluate again, as clinical findings may change rapidly.

Life-threatening conditions can be remembered with the pneumonic *ATOM FC:*

A = airway obstruction.
T = tension pneumothorax.
O = open pneumothorax.
M = massive haemothorax.
F = flail chest.
C = cardiac tamponade.

The specific signs and management of the life-threatening conditions are outlined as follows:

A: airway obstruction
(See ➡ pp. 838–9.)

T: tension pneumothorax
Signs
- Trachea displaced towards the uninjured side.
- A wound probably in the chest.
- Possible subcutaneous emphysema.
- Distended veins.
- May be shocked with cold and clammy skin.
- Hyper-resonant percussion note with decreased and absent breath sounds.

Management
- Urgent treatment is required by placing a large needle into the second intercostal space in the mid-clavicular line as soon as possible followed by immediate chest tube insertion, with the chest tube placed in the fourth intercostal space mid-axillary line.
- This remains until clinically the lung is expanded, which may take days.
- Once the lung can be seen to be fully re-expanded on chest X-ray and there is no further bubbling from the tube when the patient is asked to cough, the chest tube may be removed. See ➡ 'Chest tube insertion' pp. 911–13.

O: open pneumothorax
Signs
There will be an obvious deficit in the chest wall with shortness of breath, tachycardia, and cyanosis.

Management
- All patients, with a pneumothorax need a chest drain placed as soon as possible. See ➜ 'Chest tube insertion' pp. 911–13.
- Those with an open pneumothorax, i.e. a hole in the chest with an entrance into the thoracic cavity, should have an urgent seal placed over the hole. This can be done with either a one-way valve such as an Asherman chest seal or, if not available, then any dressing soaked with lubricant gel should be placed over the defect, with three sides attached so air can escape but not enter the chest. Insert a chest drain immediately.

M: massive haemothorax

Signs/symptoms
- Absent breath sounds.
- Dull to percussion.
- Patient may appear in some stages of shock.
- Remember that respiratory difficulty will be a late symptom.

Management
- As with an open pneumothorax, an urgent chest drain needs urgent placement through the fourth intercostal space, mid-axillary line to allow drainage of the blood.
- The indications for thoracotomy are the initial loss of 1500 mL of blood or 200 mL per hour over the next 4 hours.
- In most low-resource environments, thoracotomy is not feasible, and so autotransfusion is generally recommended, with blood from a chest drain placed in a sterile citrated bag. Autotransfusion can greatly reduce blood loss from the chest, allowing bleeding from intercostals and lung parenchyma to hopefully subside with time.
- Massive uncontrollable bleeding coming from a major pulmonary vessel is probably not containable in this context by any means and therefore thoracotomy should not be attempted unless the surgeon is experienced with this technique and the resources are available, such as postoperative ventilation.

F: flail chest
A flail chest occurs when a segment of the thoracic cage is separated from the rest of the chest wall.

Signs
- Pain.
- Crepitus along the ribs.
- Paradoxical breathing, i.e. indrawing on inspiration and outward movement on expiration.
- Expect associated lung contusion ± haemopneumothorax.

Management
- Analgesia and oxygen breathing on face mask.
- Intercostal nerve block.
- Chest drain for haemopneumothorax.
- Sleep in an upright position in a chair.

C: cardiac tamponade

Signs/symptoms

Patients can present with the classic Beck's triad:
- Hypotension.
- Distended neck veins.
- Muffled heart sounds.

Management

- Cardiac tamponade is almost always the result of penetrating injury to the heart itself. This can be treated with drainage of the pericardial blood and repair of the heart but without an experienced surgeon and intensive care unit (ICU) this should not be undertaken. It is better to accept that some injuries cannot effectively be treated and allocate your resources to those that can be treated effectively. Do not open the chest if you cannot close it.

Circulation management

See ➔ Chapter 18 for complete management guidelines. Quick references to shock in trauma patients are shown on ➔ p. 312 and pp. 313–16. See Table 48.1 for Advanced Trauma Life Support® (ATLS®) classification of haemodynamic shock.

Clinical signs of haemorrhagic shock are:
- tachycardia (be aware that bradycardia is possible with critical hypovolaemia)
- poor peripheral perfusion due to sympathetic overdrive (pale, cold skin with reduced capillary return)
- hypotension
- anxiety and or confusion, or reduced consciousness.
- Tachycardia alone implies the patient is in class 2 shock:
  - The patient has lost up to 1500 mL of blood.
  - ATLS® recommends 3:1 fluid replacement; 4.5 litres of fluid.
  - If possible, try to give blood. If not, then always warm the fluid up to 40°C. Put the IV fluid in a bucket for 30 minutes at a temperature that is just too hot for immersion of hands (that temperature is around 42°C).
- Tachycardic and hypotensive implies class 3 shock:
  - The patient may have lost up to 2000 mL of blood and may require 6 litres of fluid.

The systolic BP can be estimated from the presence of a pulse:
- A carotid pulse implies a BP of >70 mmHg.
- A femoral pulse implies a BP >80 mmHg.
- A radial pulse implies a BP >90 mmHg.

Management notes

- Try to practise hypotensive resuscitation by keeping the systolic BP around 90 mmHg which will maintain adequate perfusion of all organs.
- Normalizing BP is not necessary or even recommended, as increasing the BP too much will disrupt thrombus formation and may cause excessive bleeding. Base your resuscitation on the radial pulse and give 250 mL aliquots of saline as you monitor the changes.
- Measure the haemoglobin as soon as possible to help determine how much blood will be required.

Table 48.1 ATLS® classification of haemodynamic shock

Class	I	II	III	IV
	Up to 750 mL	750–1500 mL	1500–2000 mL	>2000 mL
	(<15% loss)	(15–30% loss)	(30–40% loss)	(>40% loss)
Pulse	<100/min	100–120/min	120–140/min	>140/min
	Full and bounding	Full	Weak	Thready
Systolic blood pressure	120	90–120	<90	<60
	Normal	Radial felt	Radial not felt	Carotid not felt
Pulse pressure	Normal	Narrowed	Greatly decreased	Absent
Capillary refill	Normal	Delayed	Delayed	Absent
Respiratory rate	14–20/min	20–30/min	>30/min	>35/min
	Normal	Mild tachypnoea	Marked tachypnoea	Marked tachypnoea
Urine output	>30 mL/hr	20–30 mL/hour	5–20 mL/hour	Negligible
Mental function	Lucid/thirsty/slightly anxious	Anxious/frightened/irritable	Hostile/irritable/confused	Confused/lethargic/unresponsive
Physiological status	Fully compensated	Peripheral vasoconstriction	Compensation fails, classical clinical picture	Immediately life-threatening

Reproduced from War Surgery: working with limited resources in armed conflict and other situations of violence, Volume 1, Christos Giannou, Marco Baldan. Geneva: ICRC; 2009. Table 8.2, page 179, with permission.

Disability

An important part of the primary survey is to obtain an accurate assessment of conscious level using either the Glasgow Coma Scale (GCS) or AVPU.

Glasgow Coma Scale

The GCS is based on 13 responses of eye opening, verbal response, and motor response and is very useful for monitoring the progress of a patient.
- A GCS score of 14–15 is classified as having mild head injury; they have a 2% chance of having a brain lesion. The brain lesion can be a contusion, subarachnoid, subdural, or extradural haematoma.
- A GCS score of 9–13 indicates a moderate head injury, and patients have a 20% chance of a lesion in the brain.
- A GCS score of 3–8 indicates a severe head injury with a 50% chance of a lesion in the brain.

Without computed tomography, one has to observe sequential neurological observations, unless signs of raised intracranial pressure such as a fracture over the temporal bone with a third cranial nerve palsy (pupil wide and unresponsive and eyeball rotated down and out) mandate an urgent burr hole to evacuate an extradural haematoma.

AVPU

This is an easier assessment based on four responses, mainly used by first responders (see Table 48.2).

Exposure and environment control

In the primary survey, always make sure the patient is completely undressed but prevent hypothermia. Remember: exposure means logrolling the patient, look at the back, feel all the spineless processes for alignment ending with the coccyx, and examine the anus with emphasis on anal tone.

Hospital transfer

Handover

It is very important that a handover is given from the pre-hospital staff to those in hospital and the best method of transfer of knowledge is by using the *ATMIST* handover. With this information, it is possible to standardize the handover from pre-hospital to hospital, or interhospital between medical and nursing staff:
- A= age of patient.
- T = time from injury or time of injury.
- M = mechanism of injury, e.g. gunshot wound, fragment from a bomb, mine injury.

Table 48.2 AVPU

Level of consciousness	Mortality (%)	Approximates to GCS score of
A = alert	11.5	15
V = responsive to voice	33.3	12
P = respond to pain	79.1	8
U = unconscious/coma	100	3

- I = injury. Where on the body is the injury?
- S= signs and symptoms:
  - respiratory rate, normal, rapid or depressed
  - SpO_2
  - pulse rate
  - BP, if measured, if not is there a radial or femoral pulse?
  - GCS or AVPU.
- T = treatment given. Has a tourniquet been applied? How much saline or blood has been given? Has a chest drain been placed?

Once the patient is safely transferred to an appropriate facility, and after the ATMIST handover, the emergency physician will assume care of the patient and if necessary hand over to the surgeon if theatre is necessary.

Medical management of the surgical abdomen

Massey Beveridge and Marco Baldan

Introduction to medical management of the surgical abdomen

> *Vita brevis, ars longa, occasio praeceps, experimentum periculosum, iudicium difficile.*
>
> Life is short, the Art long, opportunity fleeting, experience perilous and decision difficult.
>
> Hippocrates

Physicians working in humanitarian emergencies may find themselves having to deal with abdominal problems of a surgical nature when surgical referral is desirable but difficult or impossible. This chapter is designed as advice for the non-surgeon working in an environment where there is no surgeon, transport to a surgical facility is hazardous or impossible, there is little if any diagnostic radiology or blood bank, no operating theatre, and no ICU. It does not describe optimal treatment for the surgical abdomen but aims to offer some practical advice about what may be done to temporize when definitive surgical care is not available.

There is no circumstance in which an untrained operator should open the abdomen. Bad surgery performed by the inexperienced in unsterile, poorly equipped facilities inflicts more suffering than good first aid and nursing care. It also consumes time, human, and material resources that may better be used elsewhere. Even, perhaps especially, in the dying patient, 'bush' laparotomy by an untrained operator is *not* advised. To do so is to inflict more suffering on an already gravely ill patient and create potentially serious concerns in the host community about the reputation of the medical team. It is much better to provide basic resuscitation with IV fluids, antibiotics, analgesia, and comfort measures.

Keep it simple. There are only six fundamental reasons for emergent laparotomy:
• Bleeding
• Obstruction
• Perforation
• Inflammation
• Infection
• Ischaemia.

Even if definitive surgery cannot be performed, for each of these situations there is much that can be done with sound medical management. IV fluids, antibiotics, blood, and drugs can all help abate the fundamental processes of dehydration leading to renal failure, organ infarction, and infection that underlie many abdominal surgical illnesses. *The absence of a clear diagnosis should not delay prompt fluid resuscitation and treatment of suspected infection.* This chapter aims to provide advice about what *can* be done for such surgical patients to normalize their physiology, keep them comfortable, and give them the best chance of surviving.

Diagnosis of acute abdominal problems

Accurate diagnosis of acute abdominal problems in situations where diagnostic resources are scarce can be difficult. Where there are few diagnostic tools available, pay close attention to the patient's story. The history will usually suggest the nature of the problem and the physical examination its location and severity. A pain history should include location, severity, quality, onset, duration, changes, associated symptoms such as nausea, vomiting, and change in bowel function, and exacerbating and relieving features. Pay special attention to function: energy level, appetite, weight change, bowel, bladder, and reproductive function. In women, it is important to know about possible pregnancy and to get an accurate idea of menstrual bleeding. Be aware of local endemic diseases. Trauma may bring on a bout of acute falciparum malaria in those with a chronic parasitaemia, causing a fever that muddies the diagnostic picture. Chronic anaemia, parasites, and poor nutritional status compromise baseline health and should be taken into consideration. Diabetes, hypertension, and coronary artery disease are all becoming increasingly common worldwide and may be undiagnosed or under-treated.

Diagnostic clues

- *Sudden onset* of or change in pain suggests a mechanical issue such as obstruction or perforation, whereas the *gradual onset* of pain over time suggests something inflammatory or neoplastic.
- *Visceral pain* in tubular organs of the gut is typically crampy and intermittent and localizes to the midline. The exception is biliary tract pain which is usually severe, constant, and often is felt right of the midline.
- *Foregut* pain originating between the oesophagus and the duodenum localizes to the epigastrium, *midgut* pain from the distal duodenum to the transverse colon localizes to the umbilical region, and *hindgut* pain from the transverse colon to the rectum localizes to the suprapubic region.
- Those with a problem affecting the small bowel will almost always have *diminished appetite, nausea,* and *vomiting.* The presence of hunger is a good sign.
- As the process driving the visceral pain progresses and local inflammation begins to affect the surrounding peritoneal surfaces, parietal or somatic pain emerges. It is typically constant, localized, and the abdominal musculature tenses to protect the inflamed parts from the examining hand. This is the abdominal 'guarding' that signifies serious underlying inflammation.
- Those with *peritonitis* lie very still and move very carefully if at all, whereas those with *renal colic* have waves of severe pain and writhe around in pain unable to find a comfortable position.

Clinical examination

- Do an old-fashioned physical examination. Observe first their *general condition, level of consciousness, temperature, colour, state of hydration, nutritional status, and vital signs.* Search for signs of chronic systemic illness. Marks and bruises from traditional treatments such as hot poultices, cupping, and coining (rubbing the edge of a coin along the edges of the ribs) can yield clues to chronicity.

- Check for *lymphadenopathy*, listen to the *chest*, and percuss the *lung bases* if you suspect pleural effusion.
- *Observe* the belly for signs of trauma, previous operations, splinting, distension, hernias, and visible loops of bowel. Ask them to 'blow-out your abdomen and suck in really fast, in and out'. If this can be done without pain there is not much peritoneal irritation. Jiggle the bed to see if motion causes pain. If they can jump up and down they probably do not have peritonitis.
- *Listen* for bowel sounds. High-pitched rushes of tinkling bowel sounds suggest obstruction, especially if the belly is distended and the patient has vomited. Rock the patient back and forth while listening over the stomach for a succussion splash if you suspect gastric outlet obstruction. A silent abdomen, especially in a sick patient with abdominal tenderness, suggests inflammation sufficient to produce an ileus of the small bowel and can be an ominous sign.
- *Palpate* each quadrant carefully looking for tenderness, masses, and involuntary guarding. Try to feel the liver edge looking for masses. It may help to roll the patient on their left side, particularly while examining the right lower quadrant in suspected appendicitis. Be aware of and don't be fooled by tropical splenomegaly where the spleen may extend to the right lower quadrant. Faecal masses can usually be indented. A right lower quadrant mass in a child could be a bolus of worms. Umbilical hernias are very common so check carefully for tenderness and reducibility.
- *Percuss* (gently) looking for subtle tenderness, and listening for the hollow sound of air (or distended gut) or the solid notes of fluid or solid organs. Thump each flank to check for renal tenderness.
- *Move the hips* in extension and internal/external rotation to look for irritation of the psoas and obturator muscles in the retroperitoneum suggesting by deep inflammation or abscess.
- *Check the groin* for hernias and hydroceles. Large incarcerated hernias are obvious, but smaller hernias are best checked with the patient standing. Invaginating the scrotum with your finger, gently slide it up the inguinal canal and ask the patient to cough. A small hernia will produce a distinctive impulse.
- *Do a rectal exam:* inspect for fissure, fistulas, and haemorrhoids then gently insert a gloved and lubricated finger. Check the prostate or cervix, feel for tumour, masses, tenderness, and check for blood. Melena stool suggests a more proximal source of bleeding, but bright red blood can come from either a fast upper GI bleed or something lower down.
- Consider performing a *vaginal exam* in women.

Investigations of acute abdominal problems

If available, laboratory and imaging tests are very useful.

Lab testing

- Complete blood count, chemistry including liver and renal function and urine analysis are universally helpful.
- If blood cultures are available, it is wise to draw the blood before starting antibiotics.
- Women of childbearing age with abdominal presentations should always have a pregnancy test.
- Testing for malaria, sickle cells, schistosomiasis, or HIV will be appropriate in some populations.
- Stool may be examined for parasites, bacteria, and viruses depending on the available facilities.

Imaging

- An upright *chest X-ray* is helpful to look for air under the diaphragm (suggesting perforated viscus) and for seeing pleural fluid and pulmonary consolidation that may be a reaction to a neighbouring abdominal process. Pulmonary metastases indicate an advanced malignancy of which knowledge is useful in both diagnosis and prognosis.
- A supine view of the abdomen may show foreign bodies or distended loops of bowel, but either an *upright or a lateral decubitus view* are needed to see the air–fluid levels characteristic of bowel obstruction. Some kidney stones can be spotted on plain film as can bladder stones.
- *Ultrasound* is very helpful in experienced hands but is highly operator dependent (see ➋ Chapter 55.) The increasing availability of ultrasound for guidance opens the possibility of percutaneous drainage of deep abscesses which can be very useful. (See ➋ Chapter 55 for more information.)

Communication systems in humanitarian emergencies are improving steadily and it is often possible to get advice from an experienced surgeon by telephone or email. Any organization sending non-surgeons into situations where surgical referral is known to be difficult should make arrangements for reliable tele-consultation.

Managing the surgical abdomen

There are only six reasons for urgent or emergent abdominal operation:
- bleeding (which is by far the most urgent)
- obstruction
- perforation
- inflammation
- infection
- ischaemia.

Each of these situations is at least partially treatable without actual surgery. Good first aid and medical resuscitation will alleviate suffering, buy time, and save lives. When definitive care is not possible, it is well worthwhile providing IV fluids, analgesia (morphine), appropriate antibiotics, simple wound care (cleaning with saline or potable water and a bulky gauze dressing), warmth, and if possible, nutrition.

Bleeding

Bleeding is the most urgently life-threatening problem. The first sign of haemorrhagic shock is anxiety in the young and confusion in the elderly. A pale, shocked, anxious patient with a thready pulse and hypotension has lost 30%–40% of the circulating blood volume and is at high risk of imminent death. See ➲ Chapter 38 and Chapter 48 for more information.

Internal bleeding

Internal bleeding may be into the lumen of the gut, reproductive or urinary tracts, or it may be contained in a body cavity. The thorax, peritoneum, retroperitoneum, and thigh can each hide several litres of blood. Blunt trauma causes solid organ disruption (liver, spleen, kidney) and retroperitoneal haematomas from pelvic fractures and penetrating trauma of the abdomen often combine bleeding and perforation of the gut. The best treatment is to stop the bleeding directly, but if that is not possible, there is still much that can be done.

Fluid resuscitation

- If serious bleeding is suspected establish two large-bore IV lines, draw blood for type and cross match, CBC, and electrolytes.
- Blood is the best resuscitation fluid, but typically is scarce in the environments we are considering. When it is available, but in short supply, ensure the bleeding has stopped before giving the blood. There should be a transfusion policy that is understood and agreed upon by all medical staff. See ➲ Chapter 54 for more information.
- Give an initial fluid challenge of 1–2 litres of Ringer's lactate over 30 minutes. Then assess the patient's response. If the patient does not respond to this initial fluid challenge, transfuse blood if available.
- Titrate fluid resuscitation fluids to maintain a palpable radial pulse, keep the systolic BP >90 mmHg, the pulse <120 bpm, and maintain the urine flow around 0.5 mL/kg/hour.
- >2 litres of IV fluid given in a short period will thin the blood leading to dilution of clotting factors and may elevate the BP just enough to blow a nascent clot off the vessel. Avoid 'cyclic hyper-resuscitation' with crystalloids.

Diagnostics
- Ultrasound, if available, can help diagnose free blood in the peritoneal cavity in blunt trauma. Look behind the liver, around the spleen, and in the pelvis. Ultrasound can also detect fluid in the chest and pericardium. Reliability is operator dependent.
- Diagnostic peritoneal lavage is unlikely to change management and carries risks of inadvertent injury, false positives, misinterpretation, and spreading any spilled enteric contents all over the peritoneal cavity.

Management guidance
- *Penetrating wounds below the nipple* are associated with abdominal injury as well as chest injury, both of which can cause internal bleeding. Intra-abdominal bleeding should be suspected in both penetrating and blunt trauma and, given optimal supportive care, may stop on its own.
- Many *hepatic and splenic injuries* will clot with time, the one thing that is always available. If you suspect such an injury, prescribe bed rest and maintenance fluid sufficient to maintain urine output. Transfuse blood judiciously.
- Open-book pelvic fractures, usually resulting from blunt trauma, may cause massive *retroperitoneal haematoma*. Check by grasping the patient's anterior superior iliac spines and testing gently for bony instability of the pelvis. Do not repeat this test unnecessarily and cause more bleeding. Bleeding from such a fracture may be reduced by wrapping the pelvis in a bed sheet and tying it tightly around the patient. This will also splint the fracture and reduce pain when the patient is moved. If the urethra is intact, place a bladder catheter. Treat with bedrest, physiotherapy, a good diet, and iron supplements. Avoid bedsores with padding and frequent turning until patient can mobilize.
- *Urethral disruption* may accompany such fractures and is suggested by *blood at the meatus,* a high lying, mobile prostate, and a scrotal haematoma/urinoma. Without imaging (ultrasound), it is hard to know if the suprapubic swelling is caused by the haematoma or by a distended bladder. Passing a spinal needle into the bladder just above the symphysis may help make this distinction.
- *Ectopic pregnancy* is a life-threatening source of intraperitoneal bleeding. Not all bleeding ectopics are ruptured, sometimes blood leaks out through the fallopian tube and causes a gradual haemorrhage. (See ➲ Chapter 41 for more information.)

Gastrointestinal bleeding
GI bleeding is common and difficult to sort out without endoscopy, but fortunately often settles by itself. Search carefully for risk factors in the history that may guide you.
- *Vomiting a large amount of blood* suggests peptic ulcer, varices, or stomach cancer. Treat for the peptic ulcer with proton pump inhibitors (double dose by IV if possible) and *Helicobacter pylori* eradication with antibiotics.
- The diagnosis of *variceal haemorrhage* may be suggested by signs of hepatic failure and portal hypertension and is a leading cause of death in hepatic schistosomiasis and alcoholic cirrhosis, not least because of the associated coagulopathy. If blood is scarce, do not pour it into someone with end-stage liver disease and ongoing bleeding.

- *Bleeding per rectum* is harder to sort out. Examine the stool volume, colour, and consistency. Acute bloody diarrhoea may be acute amoebic colitis. Digital rectal exam may help diagnose bleeding fissure-in-ano, haemorrhoids, and suggest malignancy in the pelvis if there is a rectal mass, adnexal mass, or metastases in the pouch of Douglas. Blood mixed in with the stool suggests colitis or cancer. Melena or clots suggest a more proximal source. Pass a NG tube and aspirate the stomach. If there is blood, treat with antacids and antibiotics for *H. pylori*. If neither blood nor bile is present, the duodenum could still be the source and the test is suggestive but non-diagnostic. If there is visible bile without blood in the return then it is fairly certain that the bleeding source is distal to the duodenum and so most likely in the colon as serious bleeding from the small bowel is uncommon. Lower GI bleeding will often settle with bowel rest and time.

See ◗ Chapter 38 for more information.

Obstruction

GI obstruction, unresolved, is ultimately *but not immediately* fatal. In general, death is usually from dehydration and renal failure, sometimes combined with sepsis from gangrenous bowel. Fluid resuscitation and medical measures effectively prevent the fatal dehydration and can buy time, either for the problem to resolve itself, or for referral to a surgical facility.

Upper gastrointestinal obstruction

- *Oesophageal food bolus obstruction* is diagnosed by history and the inability to swallow water or saliva. It usually results from a bolus of incompletely chewed meat lodging at the gastro-oesophageal junction. It will often resolve spontaneously if the patient can urge or vomit and dislodge the bolus. Keep them hydrated with IV fluids and try to wait it out. It may be tempting to attempt passage of a NG tube but this risks oesophageal perforation and the risk increases with the time the obstruction has been present. More often than not there is no underlying pathology, but if the patient gives a history of reflux, antacid medication given once the obstruction has passed (H_2 blockers or proton pump inhibitors) may help reduce inflammation and lower the chance of recurrence.
- *Malignant oesophageal obstruction* is also usually clear on history, with *progressive dysphagia first for solids, then liquids*, and is not susceptible to treatment in these environments. A barium swallow will usually confirm the diagnosis. Prescribe morphine elixir if they can still swallow liquids and palliation.
- *Gastric outlet obstruction*, sometimes from malignancy but more commonly due to a peptic ulcer lying in the pyloric channel can cause tremendously painful dilatation of the stomach, presenting as upper abdomen and/or chest, and shoulder pain mimicking cardiac pain. The distension should be evident on examination, percussion will yield a drum-like tone, and a succussion splash (fluid sloshing about in the stomach) should be audible with the stethoscope. Decompression with a NG tube and treatment with proton pump inhibitors and *H. pylori* eradication is indicated and may yield dramatic resolution. Check their electrolytes. Beware of hypokalaemia and consider carefully giving potassium in the IV fluid.

Biliary obstruction

- Severe epigastric pain and tenderness in the right upper quadrant suggest *biliary colic* progressing to *acute cholecystitis*. Analgesics combined with either hyoscine butylbromide or atropine may help and it would be prudent to add antibiotics if the patient is febrile. Hold food until the pain and tenderness resolve. Most episodes will settle with IV fluids and antibiotics for 24–48 hours followed by gentle progression to a low-fat diet.
- Jaundice associated with acute pain and tenderness in the right upper quadrant suggests *choledocholithiasis*, gall stones stuck in the common bile duct (or *Ascaris* in the bile duct), and may resolve if the patient is kept nil by mouth and given IV fluids. Once accompanied by fever, it constitutes Charcot's triad and the clinical diagnosis is of *ascending cholangitis*. IV antibiotics are mandatory and may help control or resolve the sepsis.
- Painless jaundice accompanied by a palpable gallbladder and weight loss is highly suggestive of *carcinoma of the head of the pancreas*. Steady deterioration over a few weeks helps confirm the diagnosis. Palliation is about all there is to do.
- Jaundice with malaise is more likely *viral hepatitis* and should resolve with time. If viral hepatitis is suspected, make sure staff use appropriate precautions so they are not infected.

Small bowel obstruction

Small bowel obstruction has many causes but one final common path if not relieved—death from dehydration and renal failure or sepsis. Some hernias can be reduced and many *small bowel obstructions due to adhesions* will resolve on their own with NG suction, fluid resuscitation, and time

Diagnostics

- The diagnosis is based on the presence of crampy periumbilical pain, vomiting, distension, borborygmi (rushes of high-pitched tinkling bowel sounds), and dehydration. Profound dehydration and distended loops of small bowel visible through the abdominal wall with a fine white dusting of urea on the skin are late and ominous signs. The higher the obstruction lies, the less the distension. Think of causes in the lumen (foreign body, helminths), in the wall (Crohn's disease, typhoid, intussusception) and outside the wall of the bowel (hernia, adhesions, volvulus). Look for the scar of a previous abdominal operation.
- Look for distended loops of bowel with air/fluid levels on the upright or decubitus *abdominal films*. Sometimes you can see a bolus of worms in the terminal ileum, or foreign bodies causing the obstruction.
- Search carefully for *hernias* and know how to distinguish hernia from hydrocele. A *hydrocele* will have been there for a while, is uncomfortable but is not acutely tender, the examining fingers can get around its 'neck' below the inguinal ring, and it will transilluminate nicely with a torch. Hydroceles never cause bowel obstruction, hernias do. An *incarcerated hernia* will be bigger than it was before, very tender, and the thickening extends right up into the inguinal canal. It does not transilluminate.

Management guidance

- The amount of IV fluid required to rehydrate a person with a small bowel obstruction is commonly underestimated. An adult with a complete small bowel obstruction for several days will need a large volume of crystalloid to reverse dehydration and preserve renal function. Calculate 2.5 litres deficit for each day they have been obstructed plus the amount they have vomited. As in burns, give half the deficit in the first 8 hours and the remainder over the next 16 hours in addition to ongoing maintenance 2.5 litres/day). Titrate the fluid to thirst and urine output. Replace volume lost in NG drainage. Monitor electrolytes. Sometimes simply replenishing the patient's fluid deficit helps relieve the obstruction.

- NG tube placement: a NG tube must be in the stomach to do any good and once it is inserted, it should be aspirated to ensure that it is draining stomach contents. Tape it firmly in position and check regularly to make sure it does not come out. Be aware that hypokalaemia can result from both vomiting and NG suction. Monitor electrolytes and adjust the IV solutions accordingly.

- *Hernia reduction*. With a head-down position, gentle sedation, and accurate technique many groin hernias can be reduced. Apply pressure to the bowel in the hernia with one hand while guiding its reduction up the inguinal canal with the other. Use firm, continuous pressure over a few minutes. First there is a gurgling as the gas or liquid in the bowel reduce, then the oedema goes down, and finally the bowel itself slithers back inside.

- With luck and patience, a patient with small bowel obstruction will report their crampy pains abating, the NG drainage will diminish, and they will start to pass first gas then stool per rectum. When they pass gas, the *NG tube* may be removed and they can start drinking clear fluids.

Special considerations

- A *functional ileus* (where the bowel stops working without actual physical obstruction) commonly accompanies any process that irritates the peritoneum or retroperitoneum: bleeding, inflammation or infection, as well as spinal cord injury. Patients do not eat, and vomit, but do not have the severe crampy pain and distension that characterize a mechanical bowel obstruction. There are no bowel sounds on auscultation. X-rays will show modest distension of the bowel but few or no air/fluid levels. This will usually resolve when the underlying process is treated and can be managed with adequate fluids. Try to get them up and walking.

- *Helminth obstruction* of the terminal ileum, typically seen in children, is suspected on the basis of a vermicular mass in the right lower quadrant (it feels like a bag of worms) and sometimes the vomiting of worms. Give mineral oil by mouth or NG tube to lubricate the mass of worms and wait for the obstruction to resolve before giving anthelminthic medication: live worms pass more easily than dead ones.

- *Intussusception* refers to the intestine invaginating into itself, usually in the vicinity of the terminal ileum, and is the most common cause of bowel obstruction in infants and small children. Typical presentations include sudden-onset lower abdominal pain, red jelly stool, and bilious vomiting associated with tenderness and perhaps a mass in the right iliac fossa. Hydrostatic reduction with saline or pneumatic reduction with air under ultrasound control is easier and less risky if done early in the course of the illness. Few other than paediatric radiologists will have personal experience with this procedure, but where there is no alternative, it may prove worth the risk to try. Keep in mind the complications of electrolyte imbalance, failed or partial reduction, and frank perforation, all of which grow more common the longer the process has gone on.

Large bowel obstruction

Large bowel obstruction may be hard to differentiate from small bowel obstruction except that the pain tends to be more suprapubic than periumbilical and there may be relatively more distension. When advanced, it carries the risk of colon rupture which is fatal if not treated.

- *Constipation* can be very painful and mimics bowel obstruction. Manually disimpact any rock-hard faeces in the rectum and start enemas and dietary modification.
- *Sigmoid volvulus* is a common cause in Africa and Central Asia and may affect young healthy individuals. Massive abdominal distension of fairly rapid onset in the absence of hernia is suggestive. The rectum is usually empty. Try to pass a large blunt tube (a chest tube, for instance) per rectum with the aid of a rigid sigmoidoscope. If it gets through the twisted part of the bowel it may deflate the volvulus, allowing it to de-tort. Success in this procedure can be explosive. Fluid resuscitation, NG decompression, antibiotics, and analgesia may buy time and prevent infarction of the bowel, but if it does not resolve the prognosis is grim.
- *Colon and rectal cancer* is becoming more common in developing countries and is usually accompanied by at least some blood in the stool. Look for a history of obstructive symptoms, change in the size, shape or frequency of bowel motions, blood in the stool, loss of energy, anaemia, and fatigue. Examine the rectum and palpate the belly carefully for masses. Significant weight loss suggests liver metastases and ultrasound may show them. A chest X-ray may show metastases or a pleural effusion and will help establish prognosis. A low-residue diet may reduce symptoms and appropriate analgesia helps with palliation.

Urinary obstruction

Bladder outlet obstruction

- Bladder outlet obstruction causes urinary retention particularly in men. Typically the bladder is huge and tensely distended. Check their prostate. Causes include prostatic hypertrophy or tumour, urethral stricture (usually related to recurrent STDs), and stones. Try to pass a catheter with the benefit of lubricant containing local anaesthetic. Be prepared to try several different shapes and sizes of catheter.
- If it is not possible to catheterize the urethra and appropriate equipment is available, place a suprapubic catheter. It may be wise to look with ultrasound to confirm the presence of a distended bladder before poking it. Alternately, pass a spinal needle just above the symphysis pubis and make sure that urine returns.

- A bladder that has been very distended and then drains can bleed, so once 600 mL has drained from the catheter, clamp it for a few minutes before releasing the next 600 mL, and so on.
- Beware of the possibility of acute kidney injury if the patient has been obstructed for long and order appropriate lab work.
- They may get a post-obstructive diuresis that requires careful management of fluids and electrolytes until it resolves.

Ureteric stones
- Renal colic from an obstructing ureteric stone is suspected in a patient with severe flank pain and a trace of blood in the urine. They often give a history of previous similar attacks. Many renal and ureteric stones will pass on their own so analgesia, spasmolytics, and patience are advised.
- The real problem emerges when infection develops in the blocked kidney, mandating drainage. This can be averted or delayed by the use of appropriate antibiotics.

See ➲ Chapter 40 for more information.

Perforation

Perforation of the intestine may be due to non-traumatic visceral causes (i.e. obstruction or neoplasm) or trauma. The body's natural response to perforation is to wall off and isolate the leak in an abscess or collection. Such an abscess may eventually drain to the skin surface and if there is a persistent communication with the lumen of the gut this is known as an enterocutaneous fistula. If you cannot fix the perforation directly, you can still successfully help the body *contain the leak, fight the infection, and control the fistula*. The immediate aim should be to get the patient well enough that they can eat because nutrition will become the life-limiting factor.

Non-traumatic visceral perforations
Non-traumatic visceral perforation is usually associated with either an obstructive, inflammatory, or malignant process. Causes include perforated duodenal ulcer, perforated gallbladder, typhoid perforation of the terminal ileum, perforated appendicitis, or diverticular perforation of colon. If there is sufficient inflammation before the viscus actually ruptures, the leak may be contained by omentum, bowel, or mesentery. In these cases, the prognosis is a little more hopeful. The history usually begins with pain, becoming localized and more intense, fever or chills, dehydration, and a functional bowel obstruction (ileus). If the guarding seems localized to one quadrant, the spill is probably localized and walled-off, but if the peritonitis is general, so too probably is the contamination.

Management guidance
- Start IV fluids, correct electrolyte imbalances, insert a urinary catheter to monitor urine output, and give fluid until the patient is making >0.5 mL/kg/hour of urine.
- If you suspect perforation distal to the duodenum, it is reasonable to place a NG tube to reduce ongoing leakage. If the NG tube is not draining, check its position and irrigate it to remove any blockage. If it is patent and in a good position but still not draining, it is serving no purpose and should be removed.

- Antibiotics should be administered by the IV route. Ampicillin, gentamicin, and metronidazole or a combination of a third-generation cephalosporin and metronidazole are both reasonable choices and provide broad-spectrum coverage of Gram-positive, Gram-negative, and anaerobic organisms. It is prudent not to start gentamicin until urine is running clear because of its potential nephrotoxicity.
- Control the fistula. Many GI fistulas will close spontaneously if infection is drained, there is no foreign body trapped in the wound, no distal bowel obstruction, no cancer, and the track is not so old that it has become lined with epithelium. Enteric contents, especially from the small bowel, irritate the skin so much that patients learn not to eat. Use either a colostomy appliance or a catheter (or both) to keep the enteric flow off the surrounding skin.
- *Analgesia* is appropriate in all such cases and the generous use of morphine may be the single kindest thing to do for the patient.

Special consideration
- *Typhoid* is a disease characterized by a flu-like prodrome going on to a protracted febrile illness with abdominal pain, malaise, and sometimes a fine rose-coloured rash and clouding of consciousness. Knowledge of local antibiotic resistance patterns is helpful as there is marked resistance to the usual fluoroquinolones in many areas. In the second or third week of the illness, increasing abdominal tenderness may be caused by perforation of the terminal ileum and plain films may show free air. The perforations may seal off with omentum and if laparotomy is not possible, IV fluid and antibiotics may help. Use both broad-spectrum drugs to cover the perforation and specific treatment for the typhoid, depending on local susceptibility patterns.
- *Acute appendicitis* can settle with IV fluid, antibiotics, and rest. If it goes on to form a palpable mass in the right iliac fossa, especially if a fluid collection can be seen on ultrasound, *appendiceal abscess* is suspected. Percutaneous drainage of the associated abscess with local anaesthesia and ultrasound guidance may be considered.

Penetrating injuries
Penetrating abdominal wounds often combine bleeding and perforation of the gut.

Management guidance
- Start resuscitation with IV fluids and broad-spectrum antibiotics.
- Do not forget *tetanus* prophylaxis.
- Examine the wounds to see what structures are involved. Use local anaesthetic if necessary and put your sterile gloved finger in the wound. Some may not actually transgress the peritoneum, others will drain gut contents or blood. The presence of food suggests a perforated stomach, dark green bile comes from the bile ducts, yellow green fluid is usually from the small bowel, and stool from the colon. Blood and pus can be from anywhere but a faecal smell strongly suggests a colon injury.

Small holes

Small holes caused by stab wounds or low-velocity projectiles may be plugged with a Foley catheter with its balloon inflated beneath the fascia.

Bowel perforation from penetrating wounds

These injuries are likely to cause widespread contamination but the wound tract itself provides an avenue that can be exploited for drainage if it is kept open with a soft rubber drain or Foley catheter. The wound may slowly organize around the drain and form a discrete drainage tract or 'controlled' fistula. If there is much drainage of any sort, place a soft Foley catheter or other drain in the wound and secure it to the skin. Cover the wound with a dressing or with a stoma appliance if it drains around the catheter. Once the infection settles you must start feeding the patient.

Eviscerated omentum can be left to plug the hole and covered with a dressing. Eviscerated bowel should be reduced as otherwise it will desiccate or strangulate. If protruding bowel is not perforated, and not yet gangrenous, wash it with saline and push it back inside. Plug the hole with a single strip of paraffin gauze and apply a sturdy dressing. Change the dressing every day or two and be very careful not to tear the surface of the bowel. Do not use multiple pieces of gauze in your dressing because of the risk of losing them into the belly.

Gangrenous eviscerations

If eviscerated gut is already gangrenous, do not try to put it back in the belly. If there is no prospect of early referral and the bowel seems stuck to the abdominal wall so it will not retract inside, it may be incised with a scalpel or scissors to create a stoma thus relieving the associated obstruction. Fit an ostomy bag over the protruding bowel.

Large defect eviscerations

Eviscerations of abdominal contents through large defects should be washed with saline and covered with a large plastic sheet to prevent desiccation of the bowel. A plastic IV bag can be cut open to make a sheet and sutured to the skin edges to contain and protect the bowel (Bogota bag).

Special considerations

• When the perforating instrument (knife, arrow, spear) is still in the wound, most surgeons would elect to remove it under controlled conditions in the operating theatre; however, if this is not possible it may be judiciously extracted, understanding that significant bleeding may ensue. Consider replacing the blade with packing in soft tissue or a soft drain if the wound extends into the peritoneum.

• Wounds containing barbed arrows can be treated with antibiotics and allowed to suppurate for a few days until there is sufficient pus to lubricate the weapon and permit its removal with a gentle twisting action.

• In case of established enterocutaneous fistula, correct the electrolyte imbalance, treat infection, put a colostomy bag over the external opening, and protect the skin from enteric spillage. Feed them with a high-protein, low-residue diet (soup, eggs, low fibre). Many will eventually close, or at least become easier to manage.

- In the case of rupture of the bladder or penetrating trauma through the bladder, a urinary catheter inserted per urethra will collapse the bladder, sometimes allowing the hole to seal itself.

Inflammation

Inflammatory conditions of the abdomen including esophagitis, gastritis, duodenitis, cholecystitis, pancreatitis, Crohn's disease, and infectious colitis may mimic more serious problems and may be difficult to distinguish from them without modern diagnostic aids. That said, inflammation will often resolve with non-operative management.

Management guidance

- Inflammation of the *oesophagus, stomach*, and *duodenum* will often settle with antacids or proton pump inhibitors.
- *Pancreatitis* may be suspected in a patient presenting with severe pain in the epigastrium or left upper quadrant radiating to the back, dehydration, and a tender abdomen. Such patients may be more comfortable sitting up than lying down. Generous fluid resuscitation, analgesia, and bowel rest are the mainstays of treatment. Where the diagnosis can be confirmed with biochemistry and imaging, antibiotics are often withheld unless there is radiological evidence of abscess formation in the pancreatic bed, but where that is not possible it seems reasonable to give antibiotics if fever develops.
- *Crohn's and ulcerative colitis* usually respond to medical treatment with steroids, anti-inflammatories, and antibiotics which may be given if there is reasonable clinical certainty regarding the diagnosis.

See ➔ Chapter 38 for more information.

Infection

Bacterial peritonitis

This is the final result of any number of pathological processes, most often bacterial contamination from perforations of the GI tract or penetrating trauma. The story will include evolving pain, fever, nausea, anorexia, and obstipation with tenderness, guarding, and distension. It may be localized to one region of the abdomen, or general, involving the entire abdominal cavity.

- Septic shock from generalized peritonitis is typically characterized by hypotension and peripheral vasodilation (as opposed to peripheral vasoconstriction in hypovolaemic shock). The patient may respond to fluids and antibiotics but the prognosis without immediate treatment of the underlying cause is grave. Palliation may be the kindest course.
- A localized peritonitis suggests the contamination has not spread all over and has been walled off by adjacent peritoneal surfaces and omentum as the body tries to isolate the infection. Based in well-vascularized surrounding tissue, the immune system fights the infection, the debris collects as liquid pus, and an inflammatory rind develops. Abscesses have a natural tendency to find their way to the surface and eventually drain. While treatment with antibiotics will not get rid of the abscess itself, it can certainly tip the balance against the bacteria, and perhaps even convert the abscess to a sterile collection.

A *psoas abscess* may result from retroperitoneal perforation of an abdominal organ and, if neglected long enough, may point in the anterior thigh below the inguinal ligament lateral to the femoral ring. If the diagnosis is clear (swelling, flexed thigh, painful abdomen, often fever) and can be differentiated from a hernia, it is reasonable to incise the skin to facilitate drainage while avoiding the femoral vessels and nerve. If in doubt, consider needle aspiration first.

If an intra-abdominal abscess points at the skin, incise and drain it as best you can.

Perianal abscesses

These should be incised and drained. With a cooperative patient this may be done with benefit of local anaesthesia. (See ➔ Chapter 50 for advice on incision and drainage.)

> Abdominal infections are usually bacterial but *TB peritonitis* (see ➔ Chapter 38) and parasitic infections such as *amoebic liver abscess* and *echinococcal cysts* of the liver should be remembered. The latter two could be drained under ultrasound guidance.

Ischaemia

Bowel ischaemia and infarction result from strangulated internal or external hernia, tight adhesions, volvulus of the gut, or vascular embolism. Severe pain out of proportion to the physical findings is suggestive of embolism and a sharp increase in the severity of pain being experienced by someone with a small bowel obstruction suggests infarcted bowel. If indeed the bowel is infarcted, there is little you can do save treat the pain.

Sometimes severe dehydration can cause a highly reversible *mucosal ischaemia* of the watershed region of the transverse colon between the territories of the middle and left colic artery. It manifests as crampy pain and bloody stool very similar to an acute ulcerative colitis with significant left-sided tenderness. Treatment with IV fluids and antibiotics is often very successful.

Testicular torsion is found in pre-pubertal and adolescent males and un-treated goes on to cause testicular necrosis. They present with an extremely tender, red, swollen, hemi-scrotum and elevation of the testicle. Ultrasound showing diminished or absent testicular blood flow on Doppler confirms the diagnosis. Manual detorsion may be successful. External rotation of the testicle should be tried first. Conscious sedation is strongly advised. See ➔ Chapter 40 for more information.

Abdominal admissions

Case admission orders ('DAVIIDDDD')

The initial non-surgical management of abdominal cases is fairly uniform and it is worth re-iterating that institution of treatment does not need to wait on a definitive diagnosis. What follows is a general method for admission of cases with abdominal problems of a presumed surgical nature. Think about each of these points as you admit the patient and you will cover all the basics. Get the patient resuscitated and follow-up on the investigations. Serial clinical examination will help narrow the diagnosis.

D: diet

- Most abdominal cases should be kept nil by mouth at least until the diagnosis is apparent. It is prudent to give clear fluids before solid food.
- Remember that ongoing physiological stress from infection increases metabolic requirements. For those who can eat, a high-protein diet with vitamin supplementation should help.
- Consider using a NG tube for both fluid maintenance and nutrition, especially in children with difficult IV access.

A: activity

Order an appropriate level of activity and any special positioning needs, e.g. elevate head of bed.

V: vitals

Order pulse, temperature, BP, and urine output to be recorded at appropriate intervals

II: IVs and investigations

IV fluids

- Estimate the patient's fluid deficiency and aim to replace it in the first 12–24 hours with Ringer's lactate. Small children should receive some glucose with their initial fluid resuscitation.
- When the fluid deficit has been replaced, provide a maintenance IV including glucose. A simple way to do this in an adult is to specify 2 litres of 5% glucose and 1 litre of either Ringer's lactate or normal saline per 24 hours. Thirst is nature's guide to hydration so let it guide you. Urine output of 0.5 mL/kg/hour is a reasonable target to guide fluid resuscitation.

Investigations

- Complete blood count and electrolytes and any other appropriate lab work.
- Cross-match blood if required.
- Urinalysis.
- Appropriate X-rays (usually upright chest X-ray, supine and upright or decubitus views of the abdomen). Look for free air, bowel distension, air-fluid levels in the bowel, and foreign bodies.
- Ultrasound (depending on availability and capability).

DDDD: drugs, drains, dressings, and DVTs
Drugs
- Empiric broad-spectrum antibiotic coverage is appropriate if you suspect bacterial contamination or infection in the chest or abdomen. Cefazolin, metronidazole, and gentamicin is a traditional cocktail, but choice will depend on availability. Hold on the gentamicin until you know the kidneys are functioning normally.
- Consider analgesics/antinauseants.
- Add any specific treatments—i.e. proton pump inhibitor, iron supplements ± anthelminthics

Drains
Consider requirements for NG tube, urinary catheter, chest tube, wound drains, etc.

Dressings
Specify the type and frequency of dressings.

DVTs
Consider thromboprophylaxis.

Planning for definitive care
When planning a humanitarian intervention, consideration should be given to mechanisms for transfer of patients whose needs exceed those of the index facility. It is important to establish the current local referral options and the condition of local referral centres as soon as possible upon arrival at a site.
- The decision of which patients to transfer out for surgical care is a triage decision and should be based on who has the best chance of making a good recovery given the time necessary for transport and the level of care available at the referral hospital, not on who is sickest.
- A clear transfer note in an appropriate language describing the clinical history and treatments initiated should accompany the patient.
- Provision should be made for a relative or friend to accompany the patient.
- Medication for the journey should also be provided, particularly analgesics and antiemetics, and an attendant capable of administering that medication should accompany the patient.

Chapter 50

Wound care and minor surgical procedures

Massey Beveridge

Introduction to wound care and minor surgical procedures

In humanitarian settings, medical providers will inevitably be faced with conditions such as abscesses, wounds, or bleeding, which in well-resourced settings might be dealt with by a quick page to the surgical resident on call. In the field setting, there may be no surgical team, and the reality is that many of these conditions can adequately be dealt with by a primary care provider. Most of the time, these providers will actually have had experience in such management during their own education or training. This chapter is intended as a brief refresher in the management of minor surgical conditions with special attention to humanitarian settings. All providers will need to make the individual judgement as to their own experience level and proficiency with such procedures. All recommendations provided imply adequate training by the provider in question, the necessity of such procedures for patient management, and the understanding and consent of the patient.

Active external bleeding

Fools rush in where angels fear to tread

And the angels are all in Heaven, but few of the fools are dead.
                                                        James Thurber

Primary survey

Make your primary trauma survey as you control the bleeding. Major external bleeding may distract the examiner from other less obvious sources of blood loss and associated injuries. Remember the most obvious injury may not be the only one. Always suspect the possibility of internal bleeding, especially in blunt trauma, and beware not to underestimate the potential blood loss from extremity wounds

Control the bleeding

- Use direct digital pressure from a gauze pad held in a gloved hand and maintained for 5–10 minutes by the clock. Get your hand right into the wound, clean out clot and debris, try and see or feel where it is bleeding, and press with a gauze pad.
- Consider which structure is bleeding. Can you see it? Is it arterial or venous bleeding? Keep the pressure constant for 5 minutes, then check, carefully. Roll the gauze off the wound bed to see where the bleeding is coming from. Dab with gauze rather than wiping, so as not to dislodge a nascent clot. Analgesia and suction can help. Reapply pressure as required.
- Point compression of the proximal artery will help to reduce inflow and allow a clot to form where the vessels are ruptured.
- There are an increasing number of *advanced haemostatic wound dressings* available and it is logical to use them if they are available. Follow product-specific directions.
- *Deep wound tracts* may be packed tightly with a single, long piece of gauze. Use forceps if there are bone or shrapnel fragments in the wound, otherwise a gloved finger is perfectly good.

Tourniquets

- A field tourniquet may be useful for arterial bleeding if evacuation to definitive surgical care is available within a couple of hours.
- Use a wide belt, not a rope.
- Apply it over the muscle belly and avoid bony prominences and superficial nerves such as the common peroneal at the fibular head.
- They are better placed on the proximal extremity (arm, thigh) than distally where it is more difficult to compress the vessels between the double bones.
- Use the opportunity to get better control of the bleeding, then deflate the tourniquet as soon as possible.
- A tourniquet left in place for 3 hours will already be causing ischaemic injury to all distal tissues.
- Never leave a tourniquet on any longer than absolutely necessary and assess the limb's perfusion after it is removed.

Risks of using a tourniquet
- Too loose and it occludes venous return, not arterial inflow, thus increasing the bleeding.
- Too tight and it causes direct injury to underlying muscle and nerve.
- Too long leads to ischaemia of the distal limb, compartment syndrome, local tissue damage, and higher levels of amputation. Release of a tourniquet that has been on too long causes reperfusion injury.

Dress the wound
- When the bleeding subsides, assess the wound(s) and decide the plan of action.
- *Cover the wound* completely with a clean dressing. Many would use gauze dipped in povidone-iodine, but don't use alcohol-based solutions as they will sting, a lot.
- Then wrap the dressing in a compressive bandage.
- Splint and elevate it.
- Pre-fabricated splints and plaster back slabs may be used.
- Examine the distal limb for pulse, function, and compartment syndrome.

Fluid resuscitation
- Establish IV access, draw blood for complete blood count, and cross-match.
- Blood is by far the best resuscitation fluid but is seldom available.
- Alternatively, give up to 2 litres of Ringer's lactate, then maintenance fluid until the patient is drinking well.
- *Clinical guides to fluid resuscitation in haemorrhagic shock are the return of normal mentation, a palpable radial pulse, a systolic BP of 80–90 mmHg, and urine output of 0.5 mL/kg/hour.*

Be aware that a haemoglobin level taken during the bleeding episode does not reflect the extent of the haemorrhage.

In acute haemorrhage, the *haemoglobin level* will not change until interstitial fluid (or IV fluid) reaches the intravascular space, causing dilution. After the bleeding stops, it then takes some time for the haemoglobin level in the circulation to stabilize.

A drop in systolic BP implies loss of at least 45% of the circulating volume.

Chronic anaemia is often prevalent in populations affected by humanitarian emergencies, especially children <5 years old and women of childbearing age. Keep this in mind when evaluating laboratory haemoglobin results so as not to overestimate the extent of bleeding. Healthy young people, already acclimatized to chronic anaemia, survive with surprisingly low haemoglobin levels. Give a good diet, oral iron, and multivitamin supplementation ± anthelminthics.

Wound care

Providers in humanitarian settings will invariably be faced with wounds of varying shapes and sizes and medical providers should be proficient in the principles and procedures for their care. The extent of wound exploration will involve individual discretion, depending upon the provider's skills and the context in which they are working.

Principles of wound management

- In humanitarian settings, most wounds are not clean, the patients may be malnourished, the environment is full of tetanus spores, and tetanus vaccination coverage is spotty. In these circumstances, any practitioner reaching for a suture set should feel on the back of their neck, the stern cold gaze of a ghostly surgeon demanding to know *why* they are suturing a dirty wound.
- It is *much* more important to clean wounds than to close them. Even small wounds are prone to infection so in most situations it is better to clean the wound and close it later.
- Basic hygiene is essential to human comfort but is often forgotten. Wounded patients in humanitarian emergencies will truly appreciate a thorough wash with lots of soap and water as soon as practical after admission—and it will reduce wound infections.
- Every significantly wounded patient should receive antibiotics. The ICRC antibiotic protocols are shown in ◗ Table 50.1 p. 918.
- Those with incomplete or uncertain tetanus vaccination history and anything more than clean minor wounds require human tetanus immune globulin (TIG) *and* tetanus toxoid (Td) with wound cleaning and antibiotics. (See Box 50.1).

Overview of wound management principles

Establish and maintain the environment in which the body has the best chance of healing the wound. Much can be accomplished by cleaning and immobilizing a wound and allowing infection to drain. These simple measures combined with good hygiene, pain control, antibiotics, warmth, and nourishment will buy considerable time.

- Stop the bleeding.
- Cover the wound.
- Clean the patient.
- Give tetanus prophylaxis.
- Give appropriate antibiotics.
- (Re-) Examine the patient and the wound.
- Debride foreign material and non-viable tissue.
- Immobilize fractures.
- Leave the skin open (except clean, minor lacerations <6 hours old).
- Pack with a bulky gauze dressing.
- Splint and elevate the limb.
- Delated primary closure in 3–5 days if no sign of infection.
- Analgesia.
- Nutrition.

Box 50.1 Tetanus prophylaxis

Tetanus prophylaxis for war wounds

All patients whatever their immunization status:

1. Tetanus toxoid vaccine 0.5 mL IM (5 LF units)—this is a booster dose in a previously vaccinated patient.
2. Penicillin.
3. Thorough excision of the wound.

Non-immunized patients or those in whom immunization status is in doubt, addition of:

4. Human tetanus immunoglobulin 500 IU IM (adults) or 250 IU (children under 15 years of age)—also known as human anti-tetanus serum.
5. Tetanus toxoid 0.5 mL IM to be repeated at 4 weeks and again at 6 months.

Please note: vaccine and immunoglobulin should be administered through separate syringes and at separate sites.

Reproduced with permission from War Surgery: working with limited resources in armed conflict and other situations of violence, Volume 1. Christos Giannou, Marco Baldan. Geneva: ICRC; 2009. p261.

Decision-making

Once the patient is clean and has had fluid, analgesics, tetanus prophylaxis, and antibiotics it is time to make some decisions:

- Assess *general condition* with attention to *function*.
- Test distal *pulses, motor function, and sensation*.
- Check for bony stability: if there is a *fracture*, is it open or closed?
- Remove the dressing, gently clean around the edges, and inspect the wound. Sniff.
- Note the size and number of *skin defects*, areas of necrosis, de-gloving, blistering, embedded grit, burns, and inflammation.
- Does the wound penetrate deep fascia so you can see muscle? High-velocity gunshot wounds may cause massive *cavitation wounds* to muscle, especially in the thigh.
- Are nerves, vessels, tendons, or other vital structures involved?
- Is the wound fresh or old and contaminated? Are there signs of *established infection*?
- If you suspect *gas gangrene*, put a stethoscope on the skin and palpate the vicinity—listen for the 'velcro' sound of crackling gas bubbles in the tissue.
- Look out for *compartment syndrome*.
- Cover with povidone iodine gauze pending definitive dressing.

Wound exploration

Wounds that you are confident exploring with the benefit of local anaesthetic or ketamine

The objective is to clean the wound, remove debris, and excise dead tissue which acts as a culture medium for infection. Most such wounds should be left open and dressed for 3–5 days before delayed primary closure. Consider the magnitude of the wound, your own experience, the anaesthetic resources available, and the facilities at your disposal before proceeding.

Serial debridement with local anaesthetic may be considered with large wounds where surgical and anaesthetic resources are insufficient for a definitive procedure. At a minimum, try to ensure that pus can drain, even if you cannot get at the source of the infection.

Procedure

- Get good light.
- Protect yourself and your staff with waterproof apron, boots, gown, gloves, mask, and eye protection.
- Get an assistant for larger cases.
- Consider using a pneumatic tourniquet for the extremities. They work best placed on the proximal extremity as vessels travel between two bones in the distal extremity, making compression less effective. Elevate the extremity for a couple of minutes to drain it of blood, wrap the muscle belly where you will put the tourniquet with soft gauze to protect the skin, then apply the tourniquet and inflate it to 50 mmHg above the patient's systolic BP, or (in adults) 250 mmHg at the thigh and 150 mmHg at the arm.
- For hands—a surgical glove can be wrapped around the wrist in a wide band and held with a small artery forceps or clamp.
- When finished, remove the tourniquet and watch for a few minutes *before* dressing the wound to make sure there are no bleeding points that have been missed. Never leave a tourniquet inflated more than an hour. If you need more time, release it for 5 minutes before continuing.
- Prep the skin and drape the wound.
- Inject local anaesthetic, remembering the nerve endings are in the skin, not the fat. Use a scalpel to trim ragged skin edges, lift the skin and look underneath for further damage.
- Extend the skin defect proximally and distally to see the base of the wound.
- Visualize the local anatomy identify and try not to cut important structures.
- Disrupted fascia may be opened in line with its fibres to inspect the underlying muscle. Go layer by layer through the tissue. Sturdy curved scissor are good for excising dead and macerated tissue.
- The gloved finger is the best instrument for exploring wounds but avoid this if you suspect bone fragments, which can be razor sharp.
- Upstream pressure controls most bleeding and enables you to see exactly what is bleeding. With satisfactory visualization you can put a small artery clamp on small bleeding points. Twist it once and leave it for a few minutes. Figure-of-eight suture ligation with absorbable material is usually the best choice if it continues to bleed. Pick up the tissue with the first bite and see exactly where to put the second bite. *If you cannot see, do not suture.* Use pressure, suction, swabs, and an assistant with retractors and try to get a better look.
- Excise damaged, contaminated, or necrotic material, loose bone fragments, and debris in the wound.
- Bullets and metal fragments do not need removal unless they cause problems, but cloth, vegetation, and dirt must be removed.

- *Wash the wound* with a large volume of saline or drinkable water. A large syringe (60 mL) connected to a large (e.g. 16 G) cannula is an efficient way to irrigate small wounds. A large jug is good for larger wounds. Wear boots. Surgical scrub brushes are good for removing superficial debris and gravel embedded in the skin.
- *Apply a dressing.* Cover the base of the wound with a sheet of gauze, pack the cavity with a generous amount of fluffed gauze (to absorb exudate), and secure it in place with bandage rolls and tape.

Wound closure

- After 3 days, the dressing may be removed and the wound inspected. If it is clean and closed with a dry scab and no sign of infection, no suturing may be required at all.
- If it is clean and open, you may perform delayed primary closure, suturing the skin edges with interrupted stitches of non-absorbable suture material. Use a cutting needle.
- If the wound edges do not come easily together, do not close them under tension: sometimes partial wound closure is all that can be done. Continue dressings—many such wounds will fill in with time if there is no infection whereas some may require eventual skin grafting.
- *Minor lacerations* that are truly clean, with no underlying tissue damage and are <6 hours old may be sutured, preferably with non-absorbable material on a cutting needle. All others should be cleaned, dressed, and re-examined in 3 days. If then it is found to have closed with a dry scab, no suturing may be required at all.

Larger wounds you are not confidant exploring

Treatment of larger wounds really depends on surgical expertise and the availability of safe anaesthesia. Given those constraints, do the best you can to clean out the wound, excise damaged skin edges and subcutaneous fat, remove foreign material, debride non-viable muscle and loose bone fragments, then irrigate it with lots of saline (or drinking water).

If the wound tract is deep and there is infection or tissue damage you cannot reach, place a soft rubber drain (Penrose or Foley catheter) in the wound track to allow free drainage of pus and debris from its depths. Incorporate the outside end in a bulky absorbent dressing.

Chest tube insertion

Chest tube insertion for acute symptomatic tension pneumothorax is life-saving and should be performed immediately on the basis of clinical findings, without waiting for a chest X-ray.

In the acute emergency, a long, large-bore IV cannula may be inserted in the second intercostal space in the mid-clavicular line while you prepare to insert the chest tube. Expect to observe a rush of air from the needle and easing of respiratory distress if there was a tension pneumothorax. Hang on to it and keep it pressed in or it will fall out. Once you have poked the pleural cavity (and possibly the lung) with this needle, a chest tube is considered mandatory.

In less acute situations it often wise to get a chest X-ray first.

Indications
- Pneumothorax.
- Haemothorax.
- Empyema.

Equipment required
- Sterile gloves, gown, and mask.
- Skin prep and sterile towels.
- Local anaesthetic and syringe.
- Scalpel (#10 blade).
- Large Kelly clamps (× 2).
- Heavy suture on cutting needle.
- Needle driver.
- Scissors.
- Large-bore chest tube. (e.g. 32 Fr, do not use a trocar even if one comes with the tube).
- Drainage bottle with underwater seal or flutter valve cut from a glove finger.
- Dressing and lots of tape.

Technique

Preparations
- Normally chest tubes are easy to put in, but beware patients with a history of pulmonary TB, previous empyema, or other longstanding pulmonary problems that may have caused pleural adhesions. Lung tissue stuck to the parietal pleura may tear.
- Explain what you are going to do and obtain the patient's consent.
- Sedation (fentanyl, midazolam, etc.), can be used if oxygen saturation monitoring is available.
- Before applying the drapes, position patient on their side with the affected side up.
- Mark the insertion site by making an indentation in the skin with a metal instrument (ink washes off).

Procedure
- Prepare for an incision on the top of the rib below to avoid the intercostal vessels and nerve. (See Fig. 50.1.)
- Inject local anaesthetic in the skin, into the intercostal muscle and a little into the pleural space. Withdraw on the syringe when in the pleural space to confirm the presence of air, blood, or pus.
- Make a transverse skin incision about 4 cm long completely through the skin and subcutaneous tissue. Clamp the outboard end of the tube with the first Kelly clamp.
- With a guiding finger atop the second Kelly clamp, palpate the muscle above the fifth rib. Warn the patient this will hurt and push the point of the clamp through the intercostal muscle into the pleural space. Pushing requires more force than most appreciate and a guiding finger atop the Kelley clamp will prevent going too deep. A rush of air/blood indicates pleural space decompression.
- Using both hands to open the jaws of the clamp parallel to the ribs to spread the intercostal muscle fibres.
- Put a gloved index finger through the hole and confirm position in the pleural cavity, not chest wall, liver, ventricle, or lung.
- Feel for adhesions and if they are dense, consider trying another site.

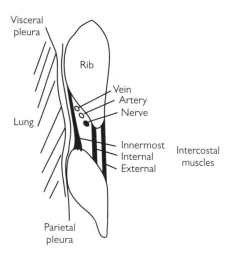

Fig. 50.1 Chest tube insertion anatomy. Reproduced from McLatchie, Greg, Borley, Neil, Chikwe, Jo, Oxford Handbook of Clinical Surgery 4th ed. (2013), with permission from Oxford University Press.

- Grasping the inside end of the chest tube in the jaws of the second Kelly clamp and using a finger to find the defect you have created in the intercostal muscles, use the Kelly to guide the chest tube into the pleural space.
  - In general, it should lie behind the lung pointing towards the apex. Once it is in, it should not hurt much.
  - If the patient complains of undue pain it may be tenting up the apex of the pleura. Pull it back a few centimetres.
  - Remove the first Kelly from the chest tube and connect an underwater drainage system. If none is available, a flutter valve can be constructed from a Penrose drain or the finger of a glove.
- Place a heavy suture through each side of the skin incision and tie it securely, leaving the ends long to be tied around the tube itself.
  - A second heavy suture can be used to close the skin around the tube.
- Apply some gauze around the insertion site and make an airtight secure dressing over the tube using waterproof tape.
- Tape the joins in the tubing so they don't come apart.

Chest tube monitoring

- Confirm position via chest X-ray if available. Otherwise, confirm function by the presence of bloody drainage and air bubbles in the bottle. Bubbling should subside as the lung re-expands. If the lung has been collapsed for a long time it may take a while to re-expand and bubbling may persist with coughing. If the bubbling still persists there is a leak in the lung (bronchopleural fistula), which may close with time.
- Monitor carefully, milk the tubing of clots, and observe the normal respiratory fluctuation of the fluid level in the tube. Ask the patient to cough and watch for bubbles. Bubbling subsides with lung re-expansion and closure of the bronchopleural fistula.
- Chest tubes should be left in as long as they either bubble or drain and be removed if blocked (no respiratory fluctuation, visible clot stuck in tube) or when drainage is <100 mL per 12 hours.
- The drainage bottle should be kept lower than the patient so fluid does not flow back into the chest.
- Chest tubes should never be clamped except on direct medical order.

To remove a chest tube

- Explain to the patient what you are about to do. It will not hurt nearly as much as it did going in.
- Position the patient on their side, remove dressings, and snip the suture
- Ask the patient to take a big breath and hold it.
  - While they are holding their breath, gently slide the tube out and cover the hole with a plug of petroleum jelly/paraffin gauze. Then allow the patient to breathe.
- Apply an airtight dressing.
- Take a chest X-ray an hour after removing the chest tube and look at it to ensure there is no residual or recurrent pneumothorax.

Abscess drainage

Never let the sun set on un-drained pus

Abscesses are common, painful, and do not respond to antibiotics alone. Pus, once present, must be drained. The immuno-compromised require drainage of pus more urgently than the immunocompetent. The most common errors are incomplete drainage or an incision made too small that closes over the cavity before it has had time to heal from its base.

Diagnosis

- The diagnosis is easy: pain, redness, swelling, and local heat all point to infection.
- Check for fluctuance which indicates liquid pus in the wound:
  - If this is not detectable, either the infection has yet to suppurate and you should wait, or the abscess is deep.
  - Insertion of an 18 G needle will usually help sort this out.
  - Ultrasound may help.

Equipment
- Sterile gloves.
- Skin prep.
- A sterile towel.
- Local anaesthetic and syringe.
- Syringe with finder needle (18 G).
- Scalpel (#11 blades are pointed and good for this).
- Haemostat for breaking down loculations.
- Large syringe with saline for irrigation.
- Forceps for packing.
- Gauze.
- A bowel to collect the pus.
- Take precautions to prevent spread of infection to the environment. Do not drain abscesses in the obstetrical delivery room.

Technique

- Before embarking, remind yourself of the local anatomy and the structures to avoid.
- Local anaesthetic does not work so well in inflamed tissue and is painful to inject so explain this to the patient.
  - In some cases, the least painful route may be a swift incision without local anaesthetic.
  - If you use local anaesthetic, infiltrate it in the skin around the abscess, not directly into the swelling then go away and do something else for 20 minutes while it takes effect.
- Position the patient appropriately and prep the skin.
- Steady the tissue with your non-dominant hand, then firmly insert the blade at the edge of the abscess and cut up through its roof. If a larger incision is required, excise an ellipse of skin or make the incision in the shape of an 'X'.

- Probe the wound with haemostats to break down any loculations and use digital pressure to express all the pus from the wound. Irrigate the wound.
- Direct digital pressure will stop most bleeding, but if necessary, pack the cavity with a single, long piece of gauze. Never put more than one piece of gauze into a deep wound or you risk infection from retained pieces of gauze that got lost in the wound.
- Cover with a dry dressing.
- Unless there is significant surrounding cellulitis, systemic antibiotics are not generally required.
- Change wound packing daily for about 1 week.
- Infiltration of the packing with local anaesthetic 20 minutes before will mitigate the discomfort of dressing changes.

Special considerations

- Pus in an old surgical incision: remove the sutures to drain the pus.
- Breast abscess: if daily observation is possible, consider aspiration of the pus with a large syringe and antibiotics instead of formal open drainage.
- Perianal abscess: always try to examine per rectum to feel location of abscess. May be easier for the patient after you have injected local anaesthetic in the anal sphincter. The natural history may sometimes lead to fistula-in-ano. Aftercare involves rinsing the wound three times a day. This can be accomplished with either a 'sitz bath' where the patient sits in a large plastic bowl and rinses their bottom, or with a hose or telephone shower apparatus.
- Neck lesions: consider tumour.
- Midline facial swelling in children: make sure not to incise an encephalocoele on the bridge of the nose.
- Groin abscess: think psoas abscess, but make sure not to incise a hernia or worse, a femoral aneurysm.
- Hand abscesses: may be drained through small incisions in the palm after which the arm should be splinted and elevated for a few days while the patient receives antibiotics.
- Foot abscesses: should be drained through lateral or medial incisions where possible, not through the sole of the foot. It is very difficult to anesthetize the sole of the foot with local agents and scars on the sole of the foot can be very painful.
- To drain a pilonidal abscess: place your incision away from the midline.

Emergency cricothyroidotomy

> *Caution*: the decision to place a definitive airway in the type of austere medical environments this book is designed for is a very complicated decision, and one that depends mostly on what can be done with the patient after the airway is in. Unless there are provisions for immediate removal of the patient to an operating room, ICU, or transport where there is proper supervision of the airway, it is probably better not to attempt intubation, let alone a surgical airway. The conditions in which intubation may be performed should be worked out in advance and all members of the medical team should understand when it may be appropriate and when it is not.

Indications

- The indications for a surgical airway are the same as for intubation, except it is done when you cannot intubate via the orotracheal or nasotracheal routes:
    - It is almost always worth trying the orotracheal route for intubation first, and only if that fails should a surgical airway be attempted.
- In an emergency, the cricothyroid route into the trachea is the only route to be considered.
- *Tracheostomy is not suitable for emergency airways and certainly should not be undertaken by the inexperienced.*

The following guidance is provided for those with sufficient skills when a surgical airway is necessary.

Equipment

(Gather this as soon as you know a surgical airway may be necessary.)
- Suction.
- #10 scalpel.
- Sharp, pointy towel clips.
- Haemostats or artery forceps.
- Toothed forceps.
- Heavy sutures (non-absorbable).
- Endotracheal tubes with cuffs (sizes 5, 6, 7), or tracheostomy tubes:
    - Beware that tracheostomy tube sizing is sometimes different from endotracheal tube sizing.
- Bag valve mask or ventilator.

Procedure

By the time you have decided to do a surgical airway, there are usually only a couple of minutes before the patient dies so you must work fast. In these circumstances, don't fuss over prepping and draping or anaesthetic.
- With the patient supine, place a pillow behind their shoulders, extend their neck, and get an assistant to hold the head.
    - Palpate the cricothyroid membrane which lies just below the thyroid cartilage and above the cricoid. (See Fig. 50.2.)

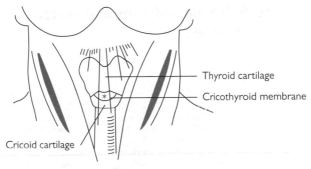

Fig. 50.2 Anatomy of the cricothyroid membrane. Reproduced from Wyatt, J.P. et al. (1999). Oxford Handbook of Accident and Emergency Medicine, 1st edn, Chapter 8, p. 345, with permission from Oxford University Press.

- Make a generous (6–8 cm) vertical midline incision centred over the cricothyroid membrane.
  - This will bleed, but less than a transverse incision. Once the airway is in, the bleeding will subside.
  - Suction blood away so you can see.
- Keep the trachea fixed between the fingers of your non-cutting hand.
- Keep cutting in the midline until you see cartilage.
- Palpate the rings of the trachea and grasp one with the sharp towel clip, drawing it up into the wound.
- Identify the cricothyroid membrane, poke the scalpel blade through it then turn the blade 90° to enlarge the hole
- Still holding the trachea with the towel clip, pass the largest endotracheal tube you can through the hole and down the trachea. A tracheostomy tube works too if one is available.
  - Make sure you see the tube enter the trachea.
  - Inflate the balloon.
- Auscultate for bilateral breath sounds and if possible confirm position and ventilation with CO_2 monitoring.
- Start bagging the patient, and administer 100% oxygen.
- Suction the airways as needed.
- Inspect for haemostasis in the wound and suture or ligate any bleeding points, suture the tube in place, and close the skin with interrupted sutures.
  - Do not use cautery as oxygen leaking around the tube can cause a fire in the wound.
- Prepare for transport to a critical care facility.

Protocols for wound care and minor surgical procedures

See Table 50.1.

Table 50.1 ICRC antibiotic protocol

Injury	Antibiotic	Remarks
Minor soft-tissue wounds, uncomplicated Grade 1	Phenoxymethylpenicillin tablets 500 mg QID for five days	Anti-tetanus measures for all weapon-injured patients
Compound fractures Traumatic amputations Major soft-tissue wounds (Grades 2 and 3)	Benzylpenicillin 5 MIU i.v. QID for 48 hours Follow with phenoxymethylpenicillin tablets 500 mg QID until DPC	Continue phenoxymethylpenicillin for 5 days if closure is performed with a split skin graft
Compound fractures or major soft-tissue wounds with delay of more than 72 hours Anti-personnel landmine injuries to limbs whatever the delay	Benzylpenicillin 5 MIU i.v. QID and metronidazole 500 mg i.v. TID for 48 hours Follow with phenoxymethylpenicillin tablets 500 mg QID and metronidazole tablets 500 mg TID until DPC	If redebridement is performed instead of DPC: stop antibiotic unless there are signs of systemic infection or active local inflammation – in latter case, add metronidazole 500 mg i.v. TID and gentamicin 80 mg i.v. TID
Haemothorax	Ampicillin 1 g i.v. QID for 48 hours, followed by amoxicillin orally 500 mg QID	Continue until two days after removal of the chest tube
Penetrating cranio-cerebral wounds	Benzylpenicillin 5 MIU i.v. QID and chloramphenicol 1 g IV TID for at least 72 hours	Continue i.v. or orally according to patient's condition for a total of 10 days
Brain abscess	Same regime as for penetrating cranio-cerebral wounds plus metronidazole 500 mg i.v. TID	Continue i.v. or orally according to patient's condition for a total of 10 days
Penetrating eye injuries	Benzylpenicillin 5 MIU IV QID and chloramphenicol 1 g i.v. TID for 48 hours	Continue i.v. or orally according to patient's condition for a total of 10 days Local instillation of antibiotic eye-drops
Maxillo-facial wounds	Ampicillin 1 g i.v. QID and metronidazole 500 mg i.v. TID for 48 hours	Continue i.v. or orally according to patient's condition for a total of 5 days

(Continued)

Table 50.1 (*Contd.*)

Injury	Antibiotic	Remarks
Abdominal wounds: 1. solid organs only; liver, spleen, kidney; or isolated bladder injury	Benzylpenicillin 5 MIU i.v. QID	Continue for 3 days depending on drainage
2. stomach, small intestines	Ampicillin 1 g i.v QID and metronidazole 500 mg i.v. TID	
3. colon, rectum, anus	Ampicillin 1 g i.v. QID and metronidazole 500 mg i.v. TID and gentamicin 80 mg i.v. TID	

MIU = million international units; QID = quater in die (4 x day); TID = ter in die (3 x day).
Please note: This protocol was established by the ICRC Master Surgeons Workshop held in Geneva in 2002.
Reproduced with permission from War Surgery, working with limited resources in armed conflict and other situations of violence, Volume 1. Christos Giannou, Marco Baldan. Geneva: ICRC; 2009. Annex 13A, page 266.

Burns

Massey Beveridge

Introduction to burns

Burns, especially in children, are common and although major 'metabolic' burns have a poor prognosis outside a burn unit, the vast majority of burns are not lethal and much subsequent disability can be averted with simple dressings, supplementary nutrition, proper splinting, scar stretching, and early mobilization. Surgery to remove necrotic skin and close the wounds with skin grafts reduces mortality in larger burns and disability in smaller burns, but much can still be achieved without it. Significant burns should be referred to an experienced surgeon or burn unit, but where that is not possible, much can still be accomplished. A clean, granulating wound, splinted against contracture, in an active, well-nourished patient, is not such a bad outcome, and such a patient will be able to tolerate the wait for eventual surgery. Some will actually go on to heal though that may take up to a year.

Mortality from burn injury comes in three phases:

• In the first few days, inhalation injury, renal failure, and the systemic immune response to massive burns are the main causes of death.

• After the first week, infection becomes the main source of mortality and this phase lasts until the wounds are closed.

• The third phase of mortality, often occurring months or years later, comes from the chronic debilitation, malnutrition and immunosuppression caused by large, chronic, open wounds.

Burn care is a team endeavour and if you are going to undertake it, it is well to engage the support of senior nurses, a dietician, and a physiotherapist. Caring for a burn patient is a long-term commitment and involves tremendous dedication on the part of nursing staff. The assiduous physician will set an example and encourage the nurses, who all too often have seen bad results from burns.

Burn mechanisms

Flame burns

These are the most common burns, usually deep in the middle with feathered edges of partial thickness and superficial burn surrounding. They are often sooty or charred. (See Fig. 51.1.)

Scald burns

These are the next most common burn, typically seen with well-demarcated edges. These often will prove to be deeper when examined on the third day than they had previously seemed. (See Fig. 51.2.)

Contact burns

These bear the imprint of a hot object coming in contact with the skin. These burns are often very deep in the centre and may destroy the underlying muscle. (See Fig. 51.3.)

Electrical flash burns

These are caused by the intense flash of radiant energy from a high-voltage electrical arc. Typically affecting the face and hands, the flash may also set clothing alight, adding an additional component of flame burn. (See Fig. 51.4.)

Electrical conduction burns

Involve conduction of high voltage (>1000 V) electricity through the body. (See Fig. 51.5 and Fig. 51.6.) Small entry and exit wounds may conceal massive underlying muscle necrosis, compartment syndrome, myoglobinuria, and acute kidney injury.

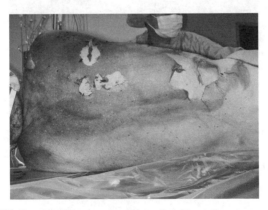

Fig. 51.1 Flame burn. Photo courtesy of Massey Beveridge.

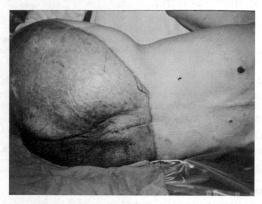

Fig. 51.2 Full-thickness scald burn. Photo courtesy of Massey Beveridge.

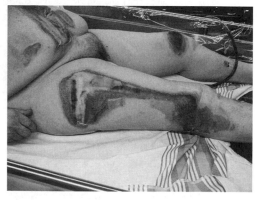

Fig. 51.3 Contact burn. Photo courtesy of Massey Beveridge.

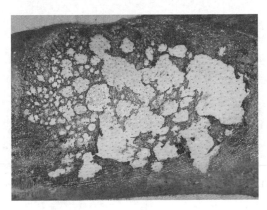

Fig. 51.4 Full-thickness electrical flash burn. Note spackling. Typically involves hands and face. Photo courtesy of Massey Beveridge.

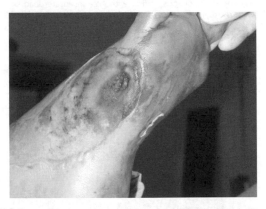

Fig. 51.5 Electrical conduction burns. Small exit wounds mask huge underlying tissue injury. Photo courtesy of Massey Beveridge.

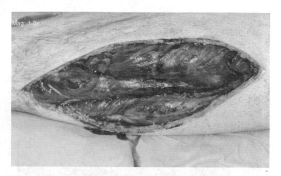

Fig. 51.6 Massive underlying muscle injury in a conduction burn. Photo courtesy of Massey Beveridge.

Chemical burns

Result in the destruction of tissue due to exposure to a chemical. If you suspect chemical burns, protect yourself and your staff (gowns/gloves/masks/goggles) before approaching the patient. Brush off any dry or powdered chemical and as quickly as possible get the patient to a shower where they need to wash off the burning chemical for at least 45 minutes. Irrigate the eyes thoroughly if they are affected. Acid coagulates the tissue and acid burns may appear innocuous at first with grey insensate dead skin. They will, however, usually go on to full-thickness skin loss. (See Fig. 51.7 and Fig. 51.8.)

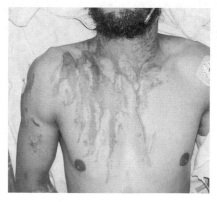

Fig. 51.7 Fresh sulphuric acid burn. Photo courtesy of Massey Beveridge.

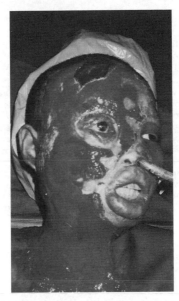

Fig. 51.8 Facial acid burn presenting 2 months post injury. Photo courtesy of Massey Beveridge.

Assessment of burns

Immediate first aid

- Cool the burn and stop the burning process:
  - Apply cool, clean water copiously to the burned part as fast as possible in the field.
  - Wrap the wound in clean, wet towels and keep it elevated.
- Remove smouldering, contaminated, or constricting clothing and any rings, necklaces, or bracelets.
- In cold climates do not let your enthusiasm to cool the burn freeze the patient. 20 minutes in a cold, wet towel is enough to stop the burning process. Thereafter pay attention to maintaining the patient's core temperature in transport.
- If there is a suggestion of smoke inhalation or carbon monoxide poisoning, give as much oxygen as possible.
- *Chemical burns* should be immersed in water or washed in running water for 45 minutes as soon as they are identified in the field.

Assessment

- Establish *the time elapsed* since the burn.
- In acute burns, look to the *ABCs* and remember that burns can easily distract the examiner from other associated injuries.
- Examine the *nose and mouth* looking for singed hairs and soot indicative of inhalation injury.
- Examine the eyes looking for lid and corneal injury. Use fluorescein dye if possible.
- Wash the patient with surgical scrub solution or soap and water while you examine the burns. This will enable a much more accurate assessment of their depth and extent and reduces the probability of infection. Note areas of *circumferential burn*. Do they require *escharotomy*?

All burns require tetanus prophylaxis.

Inhalation injury

- Smoke inhalation injury should be suspected in any case with a history of a *fire in an enclosed space*.
- Loss of consciousness is highly suggestive.
- Look for signs of singed nasal hairs and soot in the nose and mouth.

Components of inhalation injury

Laryngeal swelling

This is found in those who have inhaled a lot of smoke, but also large burns, >30% of total body surface area (TBSA), and in smaller burns of the anterior chest, neck, and face and can lead to airway compromise, stridor, and death. Endotracheal intubation with the largest possible sized tube, left long and not cut off at the mouth, is indicated if you suspect laryngeal swelling, but is not always practical. In an emergency, cricothyroidotomy may be necessary if the skills and resources are available.

Carbon monoxide poisoning

Should be suspected in anyone with a diminished level of consciousness and a history of a burn in an enclosed space. A good arterial oxygen saturation reading on the pulse oximeter does not rule out carbon monoxide poisoning and the classic cherry-red appearance is a very late sign. Carbon monoxide is eliminated by providing 100% oxygen preferably via an endotracheal tube.

Chemical pneumonitis

This generally becomes apparent on chest X-ray by the third day with bilateral infiltrates and sometimes pleural effusions. It can be difficult to distinguish from acute lung injury and management requires intensive care.

Estimating burns

Burn extent

- It is common to overestimate the size and underestimate the depth. Use the *rule of nines* in adults (Fig. 51.9) or a Lund–Browder diagram in children (Fig. 51.10) to estimate TBSA affected.
- The palmar surface of hand/fingers is ~1% body surface area.
- Count only second- and third-degree burns, not first-degree burns.
- Make a burn diagram and add up the percentage of second- and third-degree burns to calculate the TBSA involved.

Burn depth

Think of a burn as a three-dimensional pancake of injured tissue.

Superficial (first-degree) burns

- Are painful, erythematous, and not blistered—like sunburn.
- Will heal by themselves and have minimal metabolic effect.
- Water-based skin moisturizing cream is usually sufficient.
- If a patient has fresh scald burns, have them return to clinic in 3 days for a check—the burns may have grown much deeper.

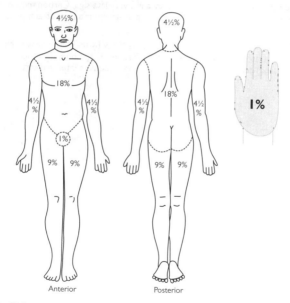

Anterior   Posterior

Fig. 51.9 The rule of nines. Reproduced with permission from Philip Downing, *Emergencies in Adult Nursing*, Oxford University Press, 2009. Figure 10.1.

Partial-thickness (second-degree) burns
- Will often go on to heal but the deeper the injury, the worse will be the resulting scar. The healing process is a combination of re-epithelialization and contracture, and the balance between processes determines the severity of scarring and contracture formation.
- Skin is blistered and the base of the blisters is exquisitely sensitive, moist, and usually blanches to digital pressure. If the base is dry and stained dull red, it is deeper.
- Most experienced practitioners withhold judgement on depth of partial-thickness burns for 3 days, as some areas may convert to deeper injury and others may show early signs of healing.
- Small, clear, durable burn *blisters* may be left intact—just cover for protection. When a blister bursts, trim away the blister membrane and cover its base with a dressing. Blisters containing cloudy fluid, frank pus, or blood should be unroofed and trimmed as should those affecting joint function along with big floppy blisters of doubtful durability.

Full-thickness (third-degree) burns
- Involve the entire thickness of the skin.
- May show charring and are generally painless to fine touch and pinprick as the nerve endings have been destroyed.
- The outer layer of skin will be dull and waxy; hairs will pull out easily. This layer may peel off, leaving grey dead dermis beneath.
- Thrombosed subcutaneous veins may be visible.

Burn hyperaemia
Fresh burns typically are surrounded by a ribbon of inflamed, hyperaemic, red, blanching skin known as burn hyperaemia. This is normal, does not initially imply infection, and usually fades in a few days. If, however, the surrounding inflammation increases, it may herald burn wound infection. Check daily and mark the border of inflammation with a pen.

(a)

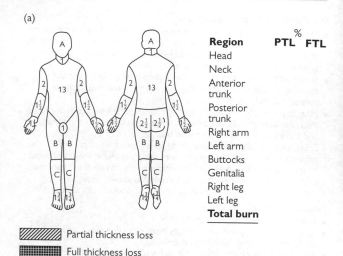

Region	PTL	% FTL
Head		
Neck		
Anterior trunk		
Posterior trunk		
Right arm		
Left arm		
Buttocks		
Genitalia		
Right leg		
Left leg		
Total burn		

▨ Partial thickness loss

▦ Full thickness loss

(b) Relative percentage of body surface area affected by growth

AREA	AGE 0	AGE 1	AGE 5	AGE 10	AGE 15	ADULT
A = ½ of head	9½	8½	6½	5½	4½	3½
B = ½ of the thigh	2¾	3¼	4	4½	4½	4¾
C = ½ of one leg	2½	2½	2¾	3	3¼	3½

Fig. 51.10 Calculation of burn surface area in children. (The infant's head is relatively larger than the adult's and the legs relatively smaller.) Reproduced with permission from Philip Downing, Emergencies in Adult Nursing, Oxford University Press, 2009. Figure 10.2a,b.

Initial management of burns

Fluid resuscitation

Burns cause local tissue swelling, drawing fluid from the intravascular compartment. In small- and medium-sized burns this is localized to the burned area, but when the burn involves >25–30% of the body surface area, the inflammatory reaction to the burn becomes generalized and capillary permeability increases throughout the body. This can result in third-space fluid loss and, untreated, the blood eventually sludges, causing renal failure, respiratory failure, intestinal ischaemia, coma, and death. This is avoided by giving fluid resuscitation to maintain the patient's circulating volume and tissue oxygenation. Over-resuscitation has its own perils including massive swelling, and truncal compartment syndrome.

> ### Parkland formula
>
> Ringer's lactate 2–4 mL/kg/%TBSA.
>
> - The *Parkland formula* gives a suggested range of fluid volume required *in addition to maintenance fluid* in the first 24 hours after a moderate or severe burn.
> - This indicates the fluid amount the patient should receive in the first 24 hours, beginning at the time of injury, not of presentation.
> - For partial-thickness burns, start with the lower number and for full-thickness burns use the higher number.
> - When burns present later than 24 hours it is really a clinical judgement of their state of hydration that governs how much fluid they need.
> - The Parkland formula is only a guide and individual fluid requirements will vary; infusion rate should be titrated clinically for good peripheral perfusion and adequate, but not excessive urine output.
> - *Children under five should always receive some dextrose in their resuscitation fluid to prevent hypoglycaemia.*

Additional points

- Small burns (less than about 15% TBSA) do not necessarily require IV fluid, and where IV access is logistically difficult it is quite reasonable to give ORS, either orally or via a NG tube to those with even moderate-sized burns. The latter is often helpful with infants.
- The presence of inhalation injury may increase fluid requirements by as much as 50%.
- Those burned while intoxicated with alcohol may have a deceptively high initial urine output (alcohol diuresis) but will end up dry if this is not compensated for with supplemental fluids.
- Most surgeons would start giving fluid as soon as they recognized a major burn. Start with a 1-litre bolus of Ringer's lactate while assessing the burn.
- In each case, titrate the infusions downward while keeping the patient well filled and hydrated. If available, colloid solutions may have some value after the first 24–48 hours in larger burns.

Examples
Consider the following examples:

A 20 kg child presents with a 5% partial-thickness scald burn to her hand and forearm
Parkland: 2–4 mL × 20 kg × 5% = 200–400 mL.
   She does not need an IV line and her fluid requirements can easily be met by encouraging her to drink. ORS is a good choice.

A 12 kg, 3-year-old toddler presents with partial-thickness burns involving 20% TBSA
Parkland: 2–4 mL × 12 kg × 20 = 480–960 mL in 24 hours.
- Start at 30 mL/hour × 8 hours (240 mL) then reduce to 15 mL/hour × 16 hours.
- Maintenance fluid in a 12 kg child (4:2:1 rule)* is 44 mL/hour. Remember to add glucose to fluid to prevent hypoglycaemia.
- Total 74 mL/hour × 8 hours then 59 mL/hour for the next 16 hours. This is probably more than the child can drink so either the IV or NG tube routes would be suitable. 5% glucose in Ringer's lactate or 0.45% saline would be an appropriate choice of IV fluid. ORS would be appropriate for the NG route.

A 70 kg adult presents with 30% full-thickness burns to both legs
Parkland: 2–4 mL × 70 kg × 30% = 4200–8400 mL.
- Because the burns appear full thickness, use the larger number.
- Give Ringer's lactate 525 mL/hour × 8 hours, then 263 mL/hour for the next 16 hours plus maintenance fluid of 100 mL/hour. This is only a guide and fluid should be adjusted to maintain good peripheral perfusion and urine output between 0.5 and 1.0 mL/kg/hour.

Analgesia

Burns are exquisitely painful and even in the most basic circumstances it is usually possible to alleviate the pain. *Where you can do nothing else, you can treat pain.* Exposed partial-thickness wounds are the most painful and should be covered as soon as possible if only with a cool damp towel.

> In a serious acute burn, give IV morphine as soon as possible and titrate the dose *to effect*. In other words, if the patient is awake with a reasonable BP and complaining of pain, *give more morphine*.

Background pain
Is best treated with a combination of different classes of analgesic given on a regular schedule, i.e. opioid + paracetamol + NSAID. Long-acting narcotics are an excellent choice when available; use generously as with pain control patients will eat better and mobilize sooner.

Breakthrough pain
Order additional aliquots of PRN (by patient request) opioids for sporadic episodes of pain. Count up the additional doses required and modify the level of regular opioid as necessary.

* 4 mg/kg/hour for each of the first 10 kg; 2 mg/kg/hour for each of the next 10 kg, and 1 mg/kg/hour for each kg over 20.

Procedural pain

Dressing changes, wound debridement, and vital stretching exercises should all be done with pre-medication.

Neurogenic pain

Can be significant and may increases with time. Anticonvulsants (gabapentin, carbamazepine) and antidepressants may help.

Itching

Burns can be terribly itchy as they heal, especially under dressings in hot climates. Antihistamines are good and the sleepiness they bring on is not altogether a bad thing.

To admit or not?

- Admission criteria will be different in humanitarian emergencies than in civilian practice and depend not only on the size, depth, and location of the burn, the patient's age, and associated medical issues, but on the resources and environment in the hospital.
- Try not to admit a clean burn to a ward full of infected wounds; also, do not put a badly infected burn in the clean surgical ward.
- Infection is a major issue in burns and if the home environment seems cleaner than the hospital, arrange outpatient care as soon as feasible.

Outpatient care

Outpatient care for smaller burns is often a good solution if the home situation is reasonable and caregivers can bring the patient for regular dressing changes and wound checks. Analgesia, nutrition, splints, and scar care all still require attention.

Inpatient care

Burns are complicated injuries, and many require the intensive environment of hospitalization to get proper care. If the patient is to be admitted, Box 51.1 outlines the considerations when admitting a burn patient. Obviously those with smaller burns require fewer interventions

Box 51.1 Burn case admission orders ('DAVIIDDDD')

D: diet

- Encourage patients to drink and eat as soon as possible.
- Estimate calorie and protein requirements and consider NG feeding in those who do not take enough by mouth.
- Patients with older burns and chronic wounds may be frankly malnourished; consult a nutritionist.

A: activity

- Includes splinting, positioning, and physiotherapy.
- Elevate burned extremities on pillows to alleviate swelling.
- Avoid pillows for anterior neck burns.

V: vitals

- Record pulse, temperature, BP, and urine output regularly.

II: IVs and investigations

IV fluid

- Parkland formula plus maintenance fluid if >15% TBSA.
- Monitor urine output until the patient is euvolaemic and drinking well.

Investigations

- Complete blood count and electrolytes and any other appropriate lab work.
- Urinalysis.
- Baseline chest X-ray if inhalation suspected.

DDDD: drugs, drains, dressings, and DVTs

Drugs

- Prophylactic antibiotics in burns probably do more harm than good, as burns are notorious for chronic multimicrobial infection and evolving resistance to antibiotics.
- Evidence of serious local or systemic infection should prompt treatment that is as specific as possible.
- Analgesics—see above in box for recommendations; for a major burn order medication for:
  - Background pain.
  - Breakthrough pain.
  - Procedural pain.
  - Neuropathic pain. Not usually necessary at time of admission:
    —Nausea, i.e. dimenhydrinate or metoclopramide.
  - Eye drops or ointment for corneal injuries.
  - Antacid or H_2 blocker or proton pump inhibitor to prevent ulcers.
  - Iron, calcium, folic acid, and multivitamins.
  - ± anthelmintics for anaemia and malnutrition.
  - Tetanus prophylaxis; DVT or thromboprophylaxis.

Drains

- Consider the need for a NG tube or bladder catheter.

Dressings

- Specify the type and frequency of dressings.

Dressings for burns

- Dressings maintain a moist, clean, and comfortable wound healing environment and isolate the wound from environmental contamination while also reducing cross contamination *from* the wound.
- The choice of dressing material and schedule of dressing changes must be practical, considering material and nursing resources available.
- Adding antibiotics to the dressings suppresses bacterial growth but is no substitute for physical removal of dead tissue.
- Burn dressings should be changed daily or when soiled. The burns may be gently debrided with forceps and scissors at dressing change.
- There is no substitute for close sequential observation of burn wounds to help you decide what is working and what is not.

Dressing components

All dressings have three layers: the contact layer, the absorbing layer, and the holding layer.

Contact layer

The *contact layer* should be non-adherent so it does not stick to the wound and dressing changes are less painful:

- *Silver sulfadiazine* (SSD) cream is excellent for full-thickness burns, but is expensive and when scarce, should be reserved for infected burns.
- Aqueous silver nitrate solution (0.5%) is cheap and effective but stains everything black.
- If petroleum jelly or paraffin gauze is available, it is an excellent choice for clean, partial-thickness burns, particularly if a *topical antibiotic ointment* (bacitracin/polymyxin) is added.
- Plain gauze can be saturated with white petroleum jelly or mineral oil and applied to uninfected burns.

Honey and ghee dressings have been used successfully for thousands of years with success and, where the ingredients are more readily available than medication, is a good choice for burns. Honey possesses some anti-bacterial properties and may contain epithelial growth factors. The ghee provides the greasiness so the dressing does not stick. Take equal parts of butter and honey. Melt the butter and cook gently until it turns golden brown then add the honey and stir well. Open large sheets of gauze on a shallow pan and pour the mixture over the gauze, spreading it around evenly. Cover tightly and use as the contact layer for the dressing. If there is no butter, cooking oil or mineral oil could probably be substituted.

The absorbing layer

- Usually made of gauze and absorbent pads.
- Fluffed gauze works better than gauze sheets.
- This layer should be thick enough to contain the exudate that accumulates between dressing changes.

The holding layer

- Usually made from rolled gauze bandage followed by elastic bandage.
- A splint may be incorporated under the elastic bandage.
- Tape at the edges will stop the bandages from rolling up at their edges.

Applying a dressing

Dressing changes are painful, so pre-medicate. Have everything open and ready with the gauze pre-treated before removing the old dressing and minimize the time the wounds are open. Maintain sterility and be particularly vigilant not to cause cross-contamination between patients.

Equipment

- Dressing tray.
- Sterile towels/disposable plastic sheets.
- Basin containing sterile saline.
- Material for all three layers—unwrapped and ready to apply.
- Scissors.
- Tape.
- Gloves, gowns, and masks for caregiver(s).

Procedure

- To save time, apply your medication to the gauze before starting. Use large pieces of gauze (i.e. laparotomy pads), moisten them with saline, lay them flat, and apply SSD with a sterile tongue depressor.
- Lay out towels, drapes, or clean plastic sheet beneath the burned part and carefully remove the old dressing, moistening adherent bits with saline and noting signs and smells of infection.
- Dispose of the old dressing carefully, clean and inspect the burn, gently debriding loose, necrotic tissue with scissors.
- Apply the prepared sheets of medicated gauze, and cover with a substantial absorbing layer of gauze.
- Finally wrap the dressing with rolled bandage and/or tape.
- Leave tips of fingers and toes exposed so you can check circulation.

It is advisable to wash the burns periodically with running water but avoid immersion in unsterile tubs. Disinfect the shower thoroughly both before and after the burn patient is in it. An alternative, where climate permits, is to cover a stretcher with disposable plastic sheets, wheel it outside, and wash the patient there.

The exposure method

Sadly, there remain situations where no dressings are available. If you find yourself in such a place it is just as well to know what to do:

- 'Dressing the wound with air' only works in warm environments.
- Isolate the patient from infection at all times. Use gloves and gowns. Place a sterile, waterproof sheet on the bed covered with a sterile drape. Put the clean, dry patient on the sheet and cover them with another sterile sheet draped over a burn frame and, where appropriate, a mosquito net. Change the sheets if they appear soiled.
- Any clothing should be strictly clean if not absolutely sterile.
- Keep the room warm and moist.
- Prevent the patient from lying on their burns. Turn them every 2 hours.
- Splint and elevate the burned part appropriately.
- Leave the crusts intact. In 2 or 3 weeks the crust will lift off partial-thickness burns revealing pink, healing skin beneath. Areas of full-thickness eschar will slowly separate as a result of bacterial activity beneath the eschar. This may be accelerated by soaking areas of eschar in saline and gentle sharp debridement.

Escharotomy

With full-thickness burns, the dermal layer can become stiff, forming an eschar which can cause the skin to shrink and become hard and leathery. This dreaded complication in circumferential full-thickness burns can lead to ischaemia, compartment syndrome, gangrene, and limb loss. Incision of the eschar, escharotomy, can be limb-saving.

To recognize the pending need for escharotomy:

- Be particularly vigilant in fresh acute burn of an extremity with circumferential regions of deep partial or full thickness in a patient who is about to receive a significant volume of fluid resuscitation.
- Diminution of distal pulses should prompt immediate action.

If required, it should be done promptly.

Equipment

- Gloves/gowns/masks.
- Dressing tray.
- Skin prep.
- Scalpel or diathermy machine.
- Small artery forceps.
- Needle driver.
- Absorbable suture material.
- Scissors.
- Dressing materials.

Technique

Though cutting through full-thickness dead burn eschar is theoretically pain-less, there may be shoals of partial-thickness injury where nerve endings are preserved so experience dictates that anaesthesia is helpful, be it ketamine or conscious sedation with fentanyl, midazolam, or propofol.

- Prep and drape the affected part.
- Draw out your incisions in the mid-medial and mid-lateral axes of the limb. (See Fig. 51.11.) Never cut viable skin!
- Draw 'T's at the end of each incision, 1–2 cm long, where burn meets unburned skin that allow the apex of the incision to open and so prevent constriction. (See Fig. 51.12.)
- Using a scalpel or diathermy, incise along the marked lines down into subcutaneous fat, deep enough so the skin spreads, releasing the tension in the limb, but not into deep fascia or muscle.
- The cut burn edge will not bleed (if it is a full-thickness burn) but subcutaneous veins will. They may be grasped and either cauterized or ligated.
- Once the release is satisfactory, check the muscle compartments which should be soft and viable.
- Finally apply a suitable dressing (SSD) and keep the limb splinted and elevated. Monitor distal circulation and sensation.

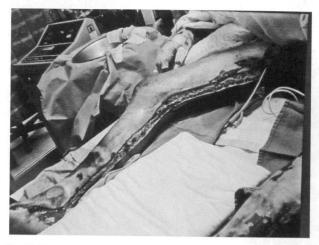

Fig. 51.11 Escharotomy of the leg. Note how the burn spreads open, releasing the pressure in the limb. Photo courtesy of Massey Beveridge.

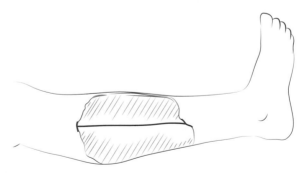

Fig. 51.12 Make small 'T's' at the ends of limb escharotomy incisions which spread as the wound gapes and reduce constriction at the apex of the incision. Image courtesy of Massey Beveridge.

Nutrition for burns

- Apart from appropriate surgery, aggressive nutritional supplementation likely has the most impact on outcome in moderate-sized burns.
- Acute major burns more than double the patient's normal calorie requirements and increase their daily protein requirement three- to fourfold.
- Persistent open burn wounds ooze protein and people with old burns will already be nutritionally depleted when they present.
- Early supplement nutrition reduces complications such as Curling's ulcers (acute duodenal ulceration or haemorrhagic gastritis in burns), as does the addition of antacid medication to the feeding solution.
- Many children will be carrying significant loads of intestinal parasites so early de-worming is a good idea.
- Burn patients (especially children) do not feel well enough to eat as much as they need so a NG tube is very helpful for feedings. Divide the 24-hour volume into six or eight feedings throughout the day and give with a clean syringe and clamp the tube for a while after each feed. If residual volumes are high, consider adding a prokinetic such as metoclopramide.

Calculating nutritional requirements

Calorie requirements = basal energy expenditure × stress factor × activity factor

(See Table 51.1 and Table 51.2.)

Basal energy expenditure

= 66 + (14 × weight in kg) + (5 × height in cm) − (6.8 × age in years)

Stress factors
- Minor procedures: 1.3.
- Orthopaedic trauma: 1.35.
- Systemic sepsis: 1.6.
- Major burns: 2.1.

Activity factors
- Bed rest: 1.2.
- Mobilizing: 1.3.

Table 51.1 Protein and carbohydrate requirements (g/kg/day)

	Adults	Children
Protein	2	3
Glucose	6	6

Table 51.2 Caloric content

	Kcal/g
Protein	4
Fat	9
Glucose	4

Example

A 20-year-old male, 50 kg, 160 cm tall, with a major burn, now mobilizing.

> Calorie requirements = basal energy expenditure × stress factor × activity factor
> = $(66 + (14 × 50) + (5 × 160) − (6.8 × 20)) × 2.1 × 1.3$
> = $(66 + 700 + 800 − 136) × 2.1 × 1.3$
> = 3904 kcal

The patient needs:
- protein 100 g/day and as that also supplies calories (4 kcal/g), it will contribute 400 kcal
- glucose 300 g/day. Glucose provides 4 kcal/g so that will contribute another 1200 kcal
- the remaining 2300 kcal to be of fat which supplies 9 kcal/g. 2300/9 kcal = 256 g of fat.

For volume, each litre of the feeding solution in Table 51.3 contains roughly 40 g protein, 80 g fat, and 120 g of glucose and 1415 kcal.
- Volume = requirements (3900 kcal)/nutritional value per litre (1415 kcal/litre). So in this example, 2.75 litres of feeding solution will provide 3900 kcal, 110 g protein, 220 g fat, and 330 g glucose.
- 3 litres per day is manageable for most adults.

Table 51.3 Making a high-energy feeding solution for burn patients

Ingredients	Glucose (g)	Protein (g)	Fat (g)	kcal
Skimmed milk powder 110 g (244 mL)	44	40		385
Edible oil 80 g (80 mL)			80	720
Sugar 50 g (50 mL)	50			200
1 Banana (15 mEQ potassium)	25			110
Add:				
Salt 3 g.				
Calcium-containing antacid: 3 tablets.				
Multivitamin tablet: 1 daily.				
Ferrous sulfate + folic acid tablets.				
Codeine 30–60 mg per litre provides analgesia and reduces diarrhoea.				
Eggs contain 15 g of protein each: beware of salmonellosis from raw eggs.				
Supplement tube feeds with cooked eggs fed by mouth when possible.				
Boiled and filtered water to make 1000 mL of solution				Total: 1415 kcal per litre

Splinting, physiotherapy, and mobilization for burns

- Correct elevation, splinting, stretching, and mobilization of burns can diminish the resulting burn contracture and consequent disability.
- Elevate the burn after the splint is applied to relieve swelling and pain.
- Splinting and mobilization are complementary treatments. Splint all burns affecting joints until joints can be mobilized, at which point, mobilize with exercises during the day and maintain in splints at night.
- Stretching the burns daily to keep joints moving and expand the overlying scar is very important to prevent subsequent disability from contracture. Gentle massage can reduce swelling.
- Stretch the involved joint passively, release and repeat for 30 minutes. Add active stretching as soon as the patient is able.
- It hurts, and both patients and staff will rebel if they regard the pain as intolerable, so pre-medication with narcotics is advisable.
- When the wound is solid enough, try to apply pressure to reduce hypertrophic scar formation. A simple elastic bandage can be useful, as is Coban™, a self-adherent elastic tape used for wrapping fingers and hands to reduce swelling and scar thickening.

Making a simple plaster splint

Thermo-plastic splinting material is ideal, but perfectly adequate splints can be fashioned from plaster of Paris. (See Fig. 51.13.)

- Measure the length of the splint to provide adequate support
- Select an appropriate width of plaster, either rolls or sheets will do. Make a pile as long as you need and about 1 cm thick. Big splints should be thicker.
- Cut a piece of stockinette about 15 cm longer than the plaster so you can fold over the ends.
- Prepare a bucket of warm water lined with a plastic bag.
- Grasping the plaster pile in a gloved hand, submerge it and then slide it between the fingers of your other hand to squeeze out the wetness, but not too much plaster. Then pull the stockinette over the hand holding the plaster until it is covered.
- Fold the ends in and make it tidy. Apply it to the outside of the dressing and secure it with elastic bandage.

Splinting positions

Neck burns

Neck burns should be kept in extension. (See Fig. 51.14.) Do not allow use of a pillow. A thermoplastic moulded neck splint is ideal, but a similar splint can be made of plaster and a hard cervical collar can if absolutely necessary.

Axillary burns

Axillary burns may fuse the arm to the torso. (See Fig. 51.15.) Position with the axilla extended. (See Fig. 51.16.) Keep the shoulder in abduction with an 'airplane splint' moulded to the chest wall and medial arm and supported with a strut. The splint is secured with bandages around the chest and arm.

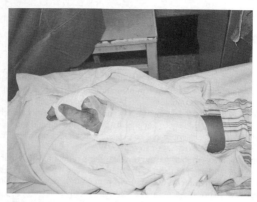

Fig. 51.13 Simple plaster of Paris splint for the hand. Photo courtesy of Massey Beveridge.

Elbows and knees and hips
Should be splinted in extension (see Fig. 51.17) except in the most extreme cases where splinting in flexion for function could be considered.

Hand burns
Should be supported with a plaster splint with wrist slightly dorsiflexed, metacarpophalangeal joints at 90° and interphalangeal joints straight. (See Fig. 51.18.)

Ankles
Ankle burns should be splinted at 90°, or use a foot board on the bed and get the patient to keep their foot pressed against it. (See Fig. 51.19.)

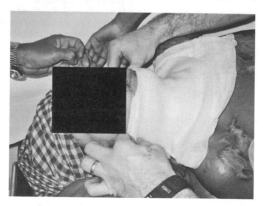

Fig. 51.14 Anterior neck splint. Photo courtesy of Massey Beveridge

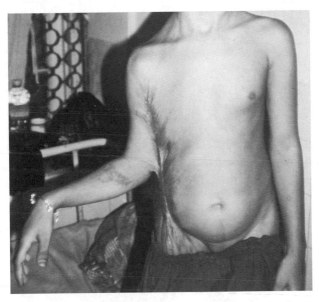

Fig. 51.15 Much of this contracture could have been avoided with proper splinting. Photo courtesy of Massey Beveridge.

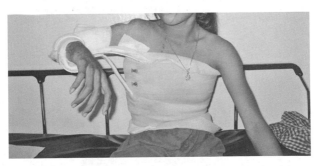

Fig. 51.16 Airplane splint for axillary burn. Photo courtesy of Massey Beveridge.

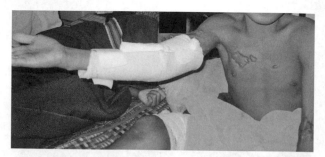

Fig. 51.17 Splint extremities in extension. Photo courtesy of Massey Beveridge.

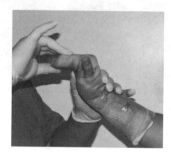

Fig. 51.18 The correct position for splinting a hand. Wrist slightly dorsiflexed, metacarpophalangeal joints at 90 degrees, interphalangeal joints as straight as possible, fingers spread and thumb abducted. Photo courtesy of Massey Beveridge.

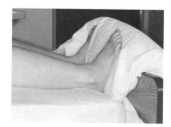

Fig. 51.19 Keep ankles at 90°. Photo courtesy of Massey Beveridge.

Special situations for burns

Old burns

- Healing burns can cause a relative immune suppression that precipitates other infections complicated by malnutrition and disability.
- When faced with a patient with an old wound, clean the wound gently and trim away bits of necrotic tissue.
- Look for a fine grey, slightly shiny film of epidermal cells which appear in partial-thickness burns as tiny 'epithelial pearls' of grey tissue. As they grow thicker they acquire the patient's natural pigmentation. These are a good sign and indicate healing in that part of the burn.
- Red raspberries of granulation tissue growing between interstices of basal dermis, or in a carpet across the wound indicate a deep burn that will *not* heal by re-epithelialization but rather through contraction of the wound. Good nutrition and wound care can maintain the patient's overall condition until such time as the wounds can be closed by surgery.
- Chronic granulating wounds may persist for decades and occasionally develop aggressive form of squamous cell cancer (Marjolin's ulcer).

Dressing

- The principles to follow on chronic granulating wounds are to try to dry up the wet wounds and to moisten the dry wounds. While there remain patches of un-separated eschar, SSD is a good choice.
- Once the wounds are clean, a simple petroleum jelly (paraffin) gauze dressing that completely covers the wound and prevents desiccation is adequate. It should be light enough not to hinder physiotherapy.
- Healed areas benefit from frequent application of water-based hand cream.

Scarring

- Burn healing through the process of wound contraction and scar maturation can take a year or more and contraction is relentlessly progressive.
- In children, this may be compounded by normal bone growth that pushes on a joint while the contracting skin is pulling on it.
- Some patients will present with older burns that are healing but with severe hypertrophic scarring and disabling contractures. Physiotherapy with stretching, splinting, and scar massage may still help and analgesics will aid compliance. Elective referral for surgical reconstruction is usually needed.

Facial burns

- The skin of the face (except the eyelids) is thick, especially in bearded adults, and has an excellent blood supply, both factors which mitigate for healing.
- Clean the wounds and cover with topical antibiotic ointment.
- Three times a day, or when the wounds get crusty, apply warm, moist saline gauze compresses and clean the exudate and crust, then re-apply a thin coat of antibiotic ointment.

In men with burns to the hair-bearing part of the face
- Start shaving them on the second or third day. In places where beards are subject to cultural sensitivities, always get permission.
- It is very difficult to control the crusting of the burn through beards and shaving should be regarded as medically necessary.
- Soak the face very well in warm wet towels and use the best quality razor and shaving cream available.
- When done, re-apply a thin coat of antibiotic ointment.

The eyes are vulnerable and burns to the thin skin of the eyelids usually cause contractures of the lids and ectropion
- Use antibiotic ointment on the lids.
- Benign lubricating ophthalmic drops or ointment should be applied often to prevent desiccation of the cornea and allow abrasions to heal.
- Keeping a moist cloth over the eyes helps, but avoid contact with cornea.

Scalp burns
- Use clippers to trim the hair around the burn.
- The skin of the scalp is thick and epithelial cells penetrate deep in the hair follicles so they will almost always heal.
- Either occlusive gauze and SSD dressings or face care can be used.

Hand dressings
- Proper hand dressings with each finger individually wrapped are difficult and time-consuming. A *plastic bag method* is a useful alternative.
- Wash the hands, apply SSD, and cover the hand with either a plastic bag or a large surgical glove secured at the wrist.
- Make a volar plaster splint to keep the hand in the safety position (wrist slightly dorsiflexed, metacarpophalangeal joints at 90° and interphalangeal joints straight) and use elastic bandage to attach the splint.
- Keep the hand elevated and start the patient moving their metacarpophalangeal joints in the dressing as soon as they can.

Further reading
Cotton M. Primary Surgery (Vol. I: Non-Trauma). Rev ed. 2016. ℬ http://global-help.org/products/primary-surgery/
Giannou C, Baldan M. War Surgery: Working with Limited Resources in Armed Conflict and other Situations of Violence. ICRC; 2009. ℬ http://www.icrc.org/eng/resources/documents/publication/p0973.htm
King M. Primary Surgery (Vol. II: Trauma). 1st ed. 1990. ℬ https://www.ghdonline.org/uploads/Primary_Surgery_Vol_2_-_Trauma_ch_50-83.pdf

Orthopaedics and limb injuries

David Rowley

Introduction to orthopaedics and limb injuries

Pluralitas non est ponenda sine necessitate
(Plurality should not be posited without necessity)

William of Ockham (1285–1347/49) – or Occam's razor.

In this chapter, an attempt has been made to cover the generality of bone and joint trauma and infection on the assumption that something can be done where facilities allow. The level of expertise is always a vexed issue. It takes 6 years to become a doctor, a further 4 years or so to train in the generality of surgery, followed by another 6 years to become an orthopaedic and trauma specialist! Many of the injuries and conditions described here would challenge the best trained orthopaedic surgeons with access to state-of-the-art facilities. What we hope the chapter will do is delineate the possible and demonstrate that many simple techniques can be applied by any doctor and many by nurses and clinical practitioners with limited training. Common sense and a bit of humility all round is a thread you will find running through the text.

Most musculoskeletal problems encountered in humanitarian settings are traumatic in origin and however much deformity, especially in children, or severe degenerative disorders will be encountered in the elderly, there are, sadly, real risks in making things worse if you are over-ambitious! Therefore, only perform procedures in which you have been trained.

A few general principles:

- No one dies from most orthopaedic conditions. Controlling any consequent bleeding and preventing infections are priorities.
- Open wounds associated with fractures imply a high risk of infection but also indicate high-energy injuries with challenging soft tissue problems.
- Blunt trauma to long bones involves a lot of soft tissue damage and do not underrate occult blood loss early on. Assume that these patients will become anaemic and pay attention to their diet, giving iron supplements if available.
- Gunshot wounds behave differently to blunt trauma open fractures and often the bone heals easily because the tissue damage is usually highly localized. Obey the rules of wound toilet and avoiding infection as even high-velocity missile wounds do respond to the core principles described here.
- Dislocations present a terrible problem unless you have access to good-quality anaesthesia. Analgesia alone is seldom enough to relocate a joint without the risk of doing more damage.
- In massive limb injury, amputation may be the only recourse but always think twice because of the consequences of leaving an amputee in an environment which, even when equipped with a prosthetic limb, poses formidable challenges to a person and their dependants.
- Finally always look for the simplest solution—never forget Occam's razor!

Wound management for orthopaedics and limb injuries

The general principles of wound management are covered in ➜ Chapter 50, but there are specific considerations for open wounds associated with fractures—confusingly called 'compound' fractures or more logically termed 'open fractures'.

- These remain a challenge even in a sophisticated medical environment.
- Aim to stabilize the wound early and deal with the fracture when time best allows. If there is no vascular compromise, the rule that all open fractures need immediate attention is not borne out by evidence. It is better to find time when the patient is a bit better and you are rested.
- Always give an antibiotic where there are open wounds and penicillin in large doses is fine. Also give appropriate anti-tetanus prophylaxis providing either passive or active immunity.
- To reduce the likelihood of infection, prevent unnecessarily opening and closing of cleaned and dressed wounds by taking and referencing a digital picture to complement the X-ray.
- Once life-threatening situations have been addressed, the patient can be taken to the operating theatre and under proper anaesthesia, surgeons can take time to explore the wound.
- After surgical exploration, keep the limb splinted as this relieves pain and muscle spasm and also helps in (for want of a better word) 'resting' the tissues and begins a process of recovery.

Dislocations

Some things never change. For dislocations (as well as fractures), the old maxim which remains true is:

- put the parts back where they belong (reduction)
- keep them there until they are stable enough to carry load without deforming again (holding)
- rehabilitate to achieve as much normal function as is possible.

The key is to do so safely and without adding any new complications.

A dislocated joint is one of the most painful injuries imaginable, and if left untreated the short-term peripheral blood supply may be prejudiced either by arterial compression or impaired venous return. In the longer term, an unreduced dislocation leads to high levels of disability and can take a patient off their feet permanently.

It is imperative to relocate dislocated joints early as muscle spasm and swelling will rapidly reduce the chances of successful treatment. Even dislocated minor joints in the foot and hand can leave individuals with significant impairment and so these injuries take priority over fractures.

Clinical presentation

- Pain, typically severe, plus the inability to move the affected joint should be the mainstay of clinical suspicion.
- Deformity may be obvious, but, for example, in a shoulder or hip which is deeply covered in muscle, the signs may be more subtle.

Assessment

- Examine patients first to ensure viable blood and nerve supply.
- Motor nerves often run adjacent to bones and so loss of functions beyond the dislocation should be checked. For example, the sciatic nerve is just behind the hip joint and loss of lower limb movement and indeed changed sensation should ring alarm bells.
- The complete loss of a pulse or intermittent loss means that arteries are at risk and increases the level of the emergency. The first thing to do is to relocate the joint.

Management principles

> You may read that adequate analgesia might result in spontaneous reduction especially if gravity is recruited to help by 'dangling' the limb. *Do not try this.* In >30 years of practice this author can think of no instances where this actually worked! Rendering a dislocated limb dependent (i.e. suspended), will only contribute to swelling which is a major impediment to subsequent success.

- Sedation with a reasonably profound level of analgesia is necessary to relax muscle spasm. This correctly implies that a full anaesthetic is the best way forward; this could be general anaesthesia or regional, depending on available expertise.
- In general, a joint can be relocated by pulling it in the opposite direction to the deformity observed either directly or on X-rays. For example, hip dislocation is almost always posteriorly in a flexed position—so you need to pull the flexed hip forward and *then* extend the limb.

- Once relocated it needs treating like a closed fracture as the surrounding ligaments and soft tissues need to heal. As with fractures, rest them in splints that provide stability and maintain the limb in a functional position.
- Test that the joint is stable by *gently* trying to dislocate it again while you still have anaesthesia. If you have a fairly stable and reduced joint then early and controlled active movement will help joint rehabilitation.
- Look to mobilize the joint once it does stabilize and first use active movements under supervision.

What could go wrong?

Immediate consequences and complications

Nerve palsies

If there are palsies beforehand, ensure splintage and rehabilitation maintains any peripheral nerve supply issues until the nerve recovers.

Nerves injured simply by being stretched and crushed but not cut (injuries in continuity) are very likely to recover eventually. If they appear after your treatment then you may need to reconsider the holding position you achieved and alter it.

Compromised blood supply

Loss of blood supply in a dislocation is usually caused by arterial stretching and spasm; rarely it may be due to end-arterial damage. Reduce the dislocation and wait at least a little time but with the absent of arterial imaging or surgical expertise this could leave an impossible situation to resolve.

Fracture

It is possible you could cause a fracture or displace an undetected fracture. Always get a postoperative radiograph to confirm that all is well.

Later complications

There is a small risk of bone death—avascular necrosis—which occurs in the proximal head of a joint. This is rare but does occur especially in the femur. If it does occur, the head will revascularize in time but may result in non-union and pain. There is little to be done other than to control pain and encourage active movement if this occurs.

Fractures

The aims of fracture management are to stabilize the limb in a functional position and allow the broken bone to heal. There is no magic wand that makes fractures heal any quicker than nature intends—the bone must be allowed to 'knit'.

A few tips:

- Remember Occam's razor—the simplest solutions are typically the best.
- Open reduction and internal fixation is fraught with hazard and best avoided in circumstances where resources and/or expertise are limited.
- Get the limb in a functional position through closed manipulation as early as possible before soft tissue swelling. Delaying this may be complicated by scar formation, which prevents easy manipulation. Getting the bone position correct and managing any wound should go on in parallel.
- What is a functional position?
  - The nearer the fracture is to a joint, then the more likely it is that any residual deformity will affect long-term function and risk arthritis.
  - The nearer to the centre of a long bone, then the more tolerable is some deformity, although reasonable attempts to restore alignment, get rid of shortening, and correct angulation still apply.
- In the upper limb, plaster of Paris (POP) casts provide adequate splintage.
- In the lower limb, choices include casts for injuries below the knee and traction for injuries above the knee including the femur and hip.

Clinical presentation

- The cardinal features are pain, deformity, swelling, and loss of function. Although obvious in the periphery of the limbs, this is more challenging to detect in deeper bones and joints in and around the pelvis and shoulder girdle where the surrounding soft tissues may mask features.
- In moderate-resources circumstances, rely on radiographs to confirm the fracture and to plan management.

Assessment

- With or without X-rays you must examine patients carefully.
- Look for the cardinal features and specifically check for any disturbance in arterial supply via the peripheral pulses and the presence of pallor or impeded venous return which can cause the limb to be discoloured—deep red or blue and very swollen.
- Check whether the nerve supply to the skin and muscles distal to the suspected injury are working properly.

Any change in sensation may be temporary but it is useful to note it, not least to be sure you have not caused it by your treatment! Similarly, loss of power or function may simply be affected by pain and so specific examination of the territory of the peripheral nerves is helpful.

Management of fractures

Reducing and holding fractures

- The general rule (as with dislocation) is to reverse the direction of the deforming force as you assess it on the radiograph. This can be deceptive because the fragments will be subject to new and unbalanced muscle forces. Essentially refer to the rules laid out for dislocations with the caveat that you may need to distract the fragments by pulling distally on the lower fragment and the rest of the limb. If you have muscle relaxation, this is a movement of finesse and not of brute force! For example, a high fracture of the femur will result in the proximal fragment being in flexion from psoas and abduction under the influence of the gluteal muscles, and the distal fragment will externally rotate through gravity.
- If you do not have X-rays you might simply have to manipulate the fracture until looks 'right'. Signs of success are improvement in colour, reduction of swelling over a day or so, and some improvement in discomfort for your patient.

Reducing fractures

- As with dislocations, the process should be gentle and purposeful. The need for fracture surgeons to have the build (and brains) of a gorilla is (I am pleased to say) a myth.
- It is always best to have full anaesthesia; heavy sedation does not overcome muscle spasm.
- Once the muscles are relaxed, you need to apply sufficient force on the distal fragment to disengage the fragment ends and then place the distal fragment back on the proximal fragment, allowing for the known unbalanced muscle forces. Doing this under sedation and/or inadequate analgesia is unnecessarily cruel and risks further damage—such short cuts are never justified.
  - Once this position is achieved, there may be sufficient fragment engagement to hold the fracture in a proper functional position.
  - Sometimes, however the distorting forces might re-deform the fracture and so any holding position might involve a short period of the distal fragment being in a non-functional position.
  - A balance between holding a reduction and achieving a functional position requires judgement.

Skeletal traction is a holding method is to make use of resting muscle tone to hold and mould the broken fragments. The reality is that while skeletal traction can be very effective, it is extremely complicated to manage in humanitarian and low-resource settings. In those settings in which skeletal traction is feasible, there will likely be sufficient resources to have the necessary expertise and resources for the procedure.

Using plaster casts

- The principle is simple—the wet cast is applied to the limb as a holding device after reduction of the fracture:
  - POP is anhydrous calcium sulphate which, with water, forms crystals which stiffen the material and produce heat.

- The cast is held in position until the chemical reaction of the POP on its cotton mesh substrate forms a stiff and custom-fitting support.
  - To maintain position, the cast should include joints above and below the broken bone, with position accounting for future function.
  - For example, an elbow is best flexed so that the mouth and the perineum can be reached for cleaning and the lower limb with some flexion at the knee and the foot at right angles to the leg at the ankle.
- POP can be a challenge to store in warm and humid climates and supplies should be provided in waterproof wrapping and kept dry.
- Because the POP construct becomes very stiff and indeed quite brittle, then if it completely envelops the limb there is a risk that subsequent swelling may constrict venous return or even arterial supply or encourage a compartment syndrome.
  - For this reason, an initial treatment with incomplete POP slabs held by non-elastic bandages which can easily be split is advocated.
  - The dressing may need to be cut if there is any suspicion of any swelling restricting the limb in any way.
- Definitive use of casts for most closed upper limb and below-the-knee injuries should be reserved until swelling has settled and in any case a change of cast is helpful at this stage both for maintaining the reduction and ensuring a good fit and so preventing friction sores.

What could go wrong?

Immediate consequences
- Even in well-applied casts, soft tissue swelling can cause a compartment syndrome. Look for:
  - pain that is disproportionate or requires increasing analgesia
  - pain on passive movement of the fingers or toes.
- Be aware that the following are often, but not *necessarily* present in compartment syndrome:
  - Distal numbness—common, but absence does not exclude diagnosis
  - Sluggish venous return—again, common, but not always required.
  - Lack of pulse—*a pulse may remain present.*
- Treat any suspicions and split any wool or dressings down to the skin. Have a very low threshold for performing a fasciotomy if you have the facilities and expertise.

Early and later complications
- Any complaint of cast soreness or burning requires temporary removal of the cast. Pressure or movement can cause friction and sores. New nerve palsies can indicate excessive pressure from the splint and at least temporary removal of the cast might be required.
- If there is a known wound under the cast and it has a bad smell, the wound needs to be explored in the operating room at the first opportunity.
- Prolonged casting will leave muscles wasted and joints stiff. Encourage the patient to take every opportunity to exercise, even in the cast.

Applying plaster of Paris casts

Casting with POP is a versatile method and is indicated in all upper limb injuries and lower injuries below the knee. The technique for initial splintage is described using back slabs as this permits easy access to wounds, and accommodates swelling and splitting of bandages without affecting the effectiveness of the back slab.

- Select material and cut it to the length required by measuring off the normal limb.
- Make two slabs using either rolls or special slab material with at least six layers of the material.
- Use an under-splint padding over any wound dressings. Mark it on the splint at the end of the process.
- Wet the slabs but do not squeeze them out excessively so as not to wash off the plaster material from the bandage.
- Apply them crosswise with the intersection at the back of the knee or elbow joint. This is the area of most weakness. Finish off with one starting distal on the outside and the other distally on the inside of the limb so that the opposite is true proximally. (See Fig. 52.1.)
- Take care to hold your new cast still until dry. Remember the POP reaction is exothermic and can get warm. *Do not use* hot water to form the cast or skin burns can occur
- Place the final cast on a pillow covered by a plastic bag until it has dried out.
- Give clear instructions to check the distal sensation and circulation.

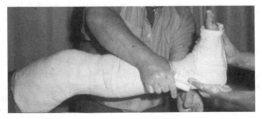

Fig. 52.1 Here the cast is crossing behind the knee and the foot is held at 90° to the leg at the ankle. Apply the finishing bandages smoothly to avoid ridges.

Outcomes for orthopaedics and limb injuries

Rehabilitation

- Encouraging early mobilization of both the specific limb and whole person is the responsibility of the whole team. The aim is to keep immobilization as short as possible in order to achieve bone and joint healing in positions of function. Compensations for deformity (or the disaster of amputation) for individuals who have to continue to live and work in deprived environments is difficult to overemphasize.
- Fracture management is considerably enhanced if there is a physiotherapist in the team who can supervise traction, check casts, and follow up on fracture care. The value of a physiotherapist should not be underestimated.
- Mobility is also important to reduce the risks associated with post-injury hyperthrombotic state.
- Injuries, such as high-velocity gunshots, can have heal remarkably quickly and immobilization should only be maintained for a maximum of 3–6 weeks, after which patients should move on to mobilizing in braces and simple splints.
- Closed nerve injuries are more likely to recover than not. The part supplied by the injured nerve should be exercised passively and splinted in positions where joints cannot go stiff and develop contractures.

Amputations

In the face of massive injury such as by landmines then sadly the decision would be already made at the time of injury and amputation is a lifesaving operation. If the limb is badly mangled and contaminated, trying to save it as distally as possible is likely to fail through poor blood supply and high risks of infection. In major below-knee injuries which are frequently caused by ricocheting bullets, major road traffic events, or crushing under falling buildings, the decision may not be as obvious. In simpler open injuries involving bone, particularly in the periphery of limbs, very careful choices are required.

The decision to amputate is always a grave one. However, if the limb is clearly severely mangled or has no peripheral pulses beyond the severe wound with grey and non-bleeding tissues then there is little choice. If the injury is old and patient is clearly unwell with a rapid pulse and a high temperature, then infection is a high possibility. In these situations, however grave the consequences, amputation becomes life-saving. *Always* seek another person on your team with some experience and try and reach a mutually agreed decision. Occam's razor and common sense will take you a long way in such a fraught situation

Bone and joint infection

Musculoskeletal infection is a challenge, even in the best resourced settings. Some general principles to remember:

- Prevention is most definitely superior to cure.
- In children, always consider musculoskeletal infections as quite a few fevers may be accounted for by septic arthritis or acute osteomyelitis.
- In open fractures, a clean wound with a good blood supply heals much better and reduces the infection risk.
- Left with an unstable and infected fracture wound, then the potential for fracture healing is severely limited. If the infection is untreated, bone union is unlikely, and amputation may be the only solution.
- If there is a proven collection of pus, dead material, or foreign material then surgery is essential.

> It should be noted that in a modern medical context most such infections are caused by surgical intervention, followed distantly by war injury. This again stresses the need to limit surgery (especially in otherwise closed injuries), and to do so only in circumstances where appropriate levels of expertise, sterilization, and infection control are possible. Acute infections in the absence of wounds occur mainly in children, and across age groups, chronic infections with, for example, TB remain prevalent and this is also a surrogate for the overall health of an affected population. Antibiotics are an essential adjuvant to any management plan

Acute osteomyelitis and septic arthritis

In the absence of surgical site infection this is mainly a disease of children, which needs to be actively excluded:

- Diagnosis starts with suspicion of local signs of inflammation or unwillingness to move the affected limb.
- X-rays are often normal and if there are signs of periosteal reaction, then the risk of an accumulation of pus is increased commensurately.
- The first line of treatment is high doses of antibiotics primarily covering *Staphylococcus* and *Streptococcus* such as penicillin or flucloxacillin given preferably IV (or much less kindly IM).
- Monitor if tenderness and fever abate, but still continue antibiotics. There is no rush to repeat X-rays, clinical progress counts most.
- If you have the capabilities, and a joint infection is suspected, then consider aspiration of the joint under operating room conditions:
  - Any turbid synovial fluid is abnormal and would confirm diagnosis.
  - Repeated aspiration prevents the build-up of pus which could form an abscess and destroy the articular surface. With antibiotics, it can help cure the condition.
- If the child continues to be ill, further intervention is indicated if:
  - repeat X-rays show ongoing periosteal or joint swelling
  - a normal X-ray should not put you off as radiographic changes will occasionally lag behind the clinical picture
  - if a bone remains hot and tender, in which case, a limited surgical intervention is justified.

Chronic bone and joint sepsis, excluding TB

The most common scenario in chronic bone or joint sepsis is a failed healing of a trauma wound. It is possible to see discharging sinuses, often erroneously referred to as fistulas (a fistula connects two epithelial surfaces).

- The presence of dead bone or other foreign material in a wound, can act as a focus for bacteria to accumulate and form a glutinous biofilm.
- Biofilms often contain different types of bacteria including anaerobes and allow the bacteria then to live with low rates of reproduction, thus making antibiotics less effective in many.
- Unless the biofilm and any associated dead or foreign material is removed, no antibiotic on earth will help. Chronic sepsis almost *always* requires surgery.

The principles of treatment for bone and joint infection apply to all medicine, and still sometimes defeat well-resourced and expert teams:

- Isolating the pathogens (often more than one!) improves success.
- Lacking access to microbiological labs, use a cocktail of antibiotics tailored on local prevalence and knowledge.
- Finding the dead or foreign stuff can be tricky but a good-quality X-ray is certainly better than nothing. Dead bone looks dense and white, and metal is even denser and has an irregular or manufactured shape.
- With a little cooperation from a radiographer, a little urography contrast medium used for pyelograms can massively improve your ability to trace the origins of a sinus. See Box 52.1 for guidance.
- Infections associated with an unstable fracture are formidable problems:
  - Consider how to achieve a stable fracture environment, such as plasters with windows in them, which give you access to the wound site.
  - Failure in this situation will be common and life will always rule over limb, but the consequences for individuals are far reaching.

Box 52.1 Sinus visualization: a sinogram for beginners!

Many settings which have X-ray capabilities do have injectable radiocontrast medium available. Using a sterile technique, prepare a 50% diluted solution with sterile saline of your contrast medium and draw it into a bladder syringe.

- Make sure the radiographer prepares with two radiographic cassettes ready to take quick anteroposterior and lateral films.
- Use an 8 or 10 mm Foley type catheter with a 5 mL balloon.
- Under sterile conditions, gently insert the catheter through the wound sinus far enough to safely inflate the catheter bulb.
- Gently inject a few millilitres of the contrast medium ensuring it does not leak out onto the skin or dressings which would confuse the picture.
- After looking at the resultant X-rays you may need to insert the catheter further (first deflating the balloon!) and repeat the process.

Further reading

Cotton M. Primary Surgery (Vol. I: Non-Trauma). Rev ed. 2016. http://global-help.org/products/primary-surgery/
Giannou C, Baldan M. War Surgery: Working with Limited Resources in Armed Conflict and other Situations of Violence. ICRC; 2009. http://www.icrc.org/eng/resources/documents/publication/p0973.htm
King M. Primary Surgery (Vol. II: Trauma). 1st ed. 1990. https://www.ghdonline.org/uploads/Primary_Surgery_Vol_2_-_Trauma_ch_50-83.pdf

Part VII

Investigations and studies

Laboratory

Cara Kosack

Introduction to the laboratory

Laboratory services have a fundamental role in the diagnosis, management, surveillance, and control of diseases. However, a laboratory is not a substitute for clinical skills. Medical staff should rely first on their clinical acumen. Taking a patient's history and performing a physical examination are the first steps in reaching a diagnosis. The role of the laboratory should be to increase or decrease the pre-test probability for a certain disease or monitoring.

The diagnostic tests available will depend on the context. Rapid diagnostic-tests (RDTs) are available for the diagnosis of infectious diseases such as malaria, to confirm a pregnancy or as urine-dipsticks. These type of tests are easy to perform and can be carried out without much infrastructure required. However, when it comes to the provision of more complex diagnostic techniques such as those requiring a microscope or blood transfusion services, a laboratory infrastructure is required.

Regardless of where diagnostic tests are carried out, providers should be trained in how to perform testing and know about the limitations of a certain procedure. Clinical management decisions for medical staff in humanitarian emergency situations can be greatly enhanced by a well-functioning laboratory and good-quality diagnostic services. All staff conducting diagnostic testing should have standard operating procedures available and be able to perform quality control.

Quality assurance in the laboratory

A laboratory cannot deliver accurate and dependable results without a well-functioning approach to quality assurance. A basic understanding of quality control is essential, and providers should work with the laboratory to ensure that standardized procedures for the pre-analytic, analytic, and post-analytic phases as well as human resource management are in place.

Standard operating procedures

Standard operating procedures provide laboratory staff with written instructions on how to perform laboratory tests consistently to an acceptable standard. They also promote safe laboratory practice.

- Standard operating procedures must be applicable and achievable in the laboratory by adaptation to the available equipment and consumables.
- They should be clearly written, easy to understand, and easily accessible.
- They must be available for every test performed in the laboratory and must be updated regularly.

Human resource management

Assessment of workload and human resource needs in the laboratory must be assessed and monitored by the supervisor. The WHO has developed a workload indicator for staffing needs (ℜ http://whqlibdoc.who.int/publications/2010/9789241500197_users_eng.pdf).

Internal quality control

Reagents

Commercial quality control reagents are available for most handheld and bench top analysers. Quality control reagents can be purchased from the same manufacturer of the analyser or as universal control reagents. Most often these are available in liquid form or as freeze-dried reagents. Be aware: often they must be stored in a refrigerator.

Blinded second readings

Blinded second reading of a percentage of randomly selected slides for microscopy is an easy quality control system that can be arranged in house or between laboratories. The percentage of slides for quality control readings should be approximately 5–10%; however, the absolute number of slides should not exceed 20 per month per disease to prevent over-burdening the system. The agreement between the two readers should be >90%, if below this, the causes for the discrepancy should be investigated.

External quality control

A laboratory may receive specimens to analyse in their laboratory from an external laboratory. After the analysis, the laboratory reports the results back to the external or reference laboratory where results will be compared and reported back. Alternatively, a laboratory can send specimens with their measured results to a reference or external laboratory where the analysis will be repeated to compare the results.

Malaria testing

Malaria testing is performed by either RDTs or microscopy, two techniques which have advantages in various settings. RDTs have the advantage that they do not require an equipped laboratory or highly trained staff, and are therefore suitable for remote settings. Furthermore, a result is available within minutes and is highly accurate. In contrast, microscopy requires a laboratory, well trained technicians, and more time; it can, however, distinguish between all *Plasmodium* species and is suitable for monitoring treatment response.

Malaria RDTs

These days, malaria RDTs are preferred over microscopy in emergency settings as they are highly accurate, easy to perform, and do not require a trained microscopist.

Generally speaking, a drop of capillary blood is placed with a transfer device on the rapid test. Then a few drops of buffer are added to allow for migration of the blood on the test device. After the incubation period (outlined in the package insert), a control line should appear on the test strip. Do not interpret the test if the control line cannot be observed. If a test is positive for malaria infection, a second line appears on the test device.

Please be aware that some RDTs can have two testing lines. These tests allow for differentiation of some malaria species.

Information on good practices for selecting and procuring RDTs for malaria is available from WHO (% http://whqlibdoc.who.int/publications/2011/9789241501125_eng.pdf).

Malaria smear microscopy with Giemsa stain

Equipment and materials required
- Microscope.
- Giemsa solution.
- Methanol for fixing the thin smear.
- Buffer tablets pH 7.2 and/or pH paper.
- Staining rack.
- Transfer pipettes.
- Microscopy slides.
- Microscopy/immersion oil.
- Tally counter.

Procedure for slide preparation
Place one to two drops of blood in two places on the slide to prepare a thick and a thin smear. (See Fig. 53.1.)

Procedure for thin blood film preparation
- Place one to two drops of blood on one side of the slide.
- Use a second slide to spread the blood at a 45° angle over the slide.
- Allow the thin film to fully dry before staining. The slide can be warmed gently to accelerate drying, but do not place against a hot surface or use a spirit lamp.
- Fix the blood with methanol by holding the slide up and let a few drops run over the dried blood film. Allow to dry.

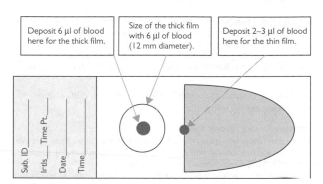

Fig. 53.1 A template for thick and thins smear on microscopy slides.

Reproduced with permission from Research Malaria Microscopy Standards Working Group (2015). Microscopy for the detection, identification and quantification of malaria parasites on stained thick and thin films. Geneva: World Health Organization.http://apps.who.int/iris/bitstream/10665/163782/1/9789241549219_eng.pdf

Procedure for thick blood film preparation
- Place one to two drops of blood on the slide.
- Use the corner of the spreader to mix the three drops. Using a circular motion, prepare a thick film. It should be just possible to read newsprint through the thick film while it is still wet.
- Allow the thick film to fully dry before staining. The slide can be warmed gently to accelerate drying but do not place against a hot surface or use a spirit lamp.

Procedure for slide staining
- Place the slides horizontally on the staining rack, cover with the freshly prepared stain (1:10 (v/v) dilution Giemsa with a 7.2 pH buffer solution, e.g. 1 mL Giemsa in 9 mL buffer) and leave undisturbed for 5–15 minutes.
- Wash the slides with filtered water in a horizontal position on the staining rack by using a Pasteur pipette with filtered water and adding it to one end of the slide so that the stain is removed from the slide.
- Note: try to wash with buffer solution of pH 7.2 instead of filtered water to improve colouration.
- Allow slides to dry in a vertical position.

Procedure for slide reading: thick film
- Examine the thick film using the ×10 objective to check the quality of the film and to scan the film for trophozoites.
- Then examine the thick film using the ×100 oil immersion objective. Each field has usually about 8–20 white blood cells (WBC).
- Use two tally counters and count the number of parasites seen on one tally counter and the number of WBCs on the other.
- Count up to 200 WBC, if 100 or more parasites are found, the results should be recorded on the form in terms of number of parasites per 200 WBCs. If, after 200 WBCs have been counted, the number of parasites is 99 or fewer, counting should be continued up to 500 WBCs.

- Note: some parasitaemias are so heavy that hundreds of parasites are counted per oil immersion field. In this situation, counting up to 100 WBCs or the total number in about five oil-immersion fields (assuming about 15 WBCs per thick film field) would be appropriate.
- Calculate the number of 'parasites per microlitre of blood' using the following formula:

    (Number of parasites counted × 8000)/number of WBC counted = parasites per microlitre

Procedure for slide reading: thin film
- The thin film is only examined if the thick film is positive. In all positive cases, examine the thin film using the ×100 oil immersion for species identification, if not obvious in the thick film.
- Refer to bench aids or a parasitology atlas for assistance in identification of malarial parasites. Colour charts for malaria parasite identification should always be available close to microscopes and are available at ᴪ http://www.who.int/malaria/publications/atoz/9241545240/en/index.html.

Procedure for reporting
- Report the number of parasites per microlitre.
- Report the species identified.
- Count and report the presence of schizonts separately.
- Report the presence of gametocytes.

Urine examinations

Usually the bladder and urinary tract are sterile. The urethra may contain a few organisms that can contaminate the urine when collecting it. Thus cleaning of the collection area is necessary. The ideal urine to examine is morning mid-stream urine. If the urine cannot be examined immediately, it can be stored for up to 2 hours in a refrigerator (2–8°C). Colour and turbidity should be included on the report of any urine examination.

Urine dipsticks

Urine dipsticks are used for a wide range of indications, most commonly for screening for bacterial infections in the urinary tract, gestational diabetes, and gestosis.

Urine dipsticks are a cheap and easy-to-use method to examine urine for a wide range of biochemical and physiological components. Usually a dipstick with nine parameters covers the following parameters: leucocytes, nitrite, pH, protein, glucose, ketone bodies, urobilinogen, bilirubin, and blood/erythrocytes.

Procedure
- Mix the urine sample thoroughly and completely immerse the reagent area of the strip in urine for 1 second and remove.
  - Gently tap the edge of the strip against the inside of the urine container to remove excess urine.
- Read each test colouration at the exact time specified by the manufacturer:
  - Compare the test areas with the colour on the colour scale provided with the dipsticks.
  - Do not report colours that develop after the specified time.

Urine microscopically

Microscopy cannot measure chemical components but can provide direct visualization of an infectious agent or cells. Centrifuged urine is examined as a wet preparation to detect an excess of, e.g. WBCs, red blood cells (RBCs), bacteria, yeast cells, casts, *T. vaginalis*, and *S. haematobium* eggs.

Equipment and materials required
- Microscope.
- Tubes with conical bottom.
- Microscopy slides and cover slips.

Procedure
- Transfer 10 mL of urine into a conical tube and centrifuge at 1000 g (i.e. approx. 3000 rpm (rounds per minute) depending on centrifuge being used) for 5 minutes.
- Discharge the supernatant fluid.
- Remix the sediment and transfer one drop on a slide and cover with a cover glass.
- Then examine the preparation using the ×10 and ×40 objectives with the condenser down and sufficiently closed to provide contrast.
- Report on presence of (i.e. few, moderate, many) bacteria, WBCs, RBCs, casts, epithelial cells, yeast, *T. vaginalis*, and *S. haematobium* eggs, etc.

Stool examinations

Most often diarrhoea is self-limiting. However, in cases with persisting diarrhoea, stool examinations are carried out to determine causes of infectious diarrhoeal diseases. For individual diagnosis, wet preparations of stool samples are made to diagnose symptomatic amoebic dysentery, giardiasis, or other parasitic infections. (See Fig. 53.2.)

> To investigate suspicion of outbreaks (e.g. cholera, shigellosis), microbiological examinations (i.e. culture) may be necessary. For this, samples should be transferred in appropriate medium to a specialized laboratory.

Equipment and materials required
- Microscope.
- Wooden applicator and/or Pasteur pipettes or transfer pipettes (plastic).
- Saline/NaCl 0.9% solution.
- Lugol's iodine solution and/or eosin solution (0.5 g eosin powder in 100 mL distilled water stored in a dark bottle).
- Microscope slides and cover slips.

Procedure for Lugol wet mount
- Place a drop of saline at one end of a slide and a drop of Lugol's iodine at the other.
- Add from the most abnormal part of the stool an equivalent amount to each drop (use a Pasteur pipette if stool is liquid) and mix using an applicator stick.
- Place a cover slip on each of the two preparations and examine using the ×10 and ×40 objectives.
- The iodine wet mount is to examine stool for amoebic and flagella cysts and ova. It assists in defining the morphology of the parasites.

Procedure for eosin stain
- Place a drop of saline at one end of a slide and a drop of eosin solution at the other.
- Add from the most abnormal part of the stool an equivalent amount to each drop (use a Pasteur pipette if stool is liquid) and mix using an applicator stick.
- Place a cover slip on each of the two preparations and examine using the ×10 and ×40 objectives.
- The eosin examination is to examine identify motile trophozoites, e.g. *Entamoeba histolytica* amoeba or *Giardia lamblia* flagellates.

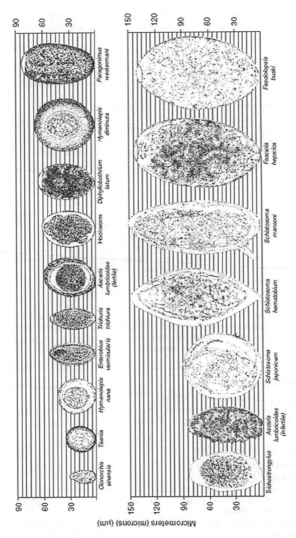

Fig. 53.2 Protozoan trophozoites, cysts, oocysts, and helminth eggs by size. Reproduced with permission from Manual of Clinical Microbiology, Eleventh Edition, James H. Jorgensen, American Society for Microbiology, 2015, chapter 143, p2449. http://www.asmscience.org/content/book/10.1128/9781555817381.mcm11.ch143

Cerebrospinal fluid examinations

Cerebrospinal fluid (CSF) is most often examined when meningitis is suspected. Symptoms include fever, headache, stiff neck, and intolerance of light. In addition, vomiting, convulsions, and lethargy can be observed.

Meningitis can be caused by viruses, bacteria, parasites, or fungi. The most common pathogens found differ by age group:

- Neonates: group B *Streptococcus, Escherichia coli, Listeria monocytogenes.*
- Infants and children: *Streptococcus pneumoniae, Neisseria meningitidis, Haemophilus influenzae* type b.
- Adolescents and young adults: *Neisseria meningitidis, Streptococcus pneumoniae.*
- Older adults: *Streptococcus pneumoniae, Neisseria meningitidis, Listeria monocytogenes.*
- HIV patients: cryptococcal *neoformans, Mycobacterium tuberculosis.*

Diagnosis of meningitis is made from investigations of CSF, starting with the reporting of appearance and followed by procedures including Gram stain, cell count, and biochemical investigations (Table 53.1).

When examining CSF in patients suspected of meningitis, start with describing the appearance, performing a cell count, and a Pandy test (Table 53.2). In addition, perform a RDT or an Indian ink examination for *Cryptococcus neoformans* in HIV-infected patients.

If any abnormal parameters are found (i.e. CSF is cloudy, cell count is ≥6 cells/μL, or the Pandy test is positive), proceed with the following examinations based on the findings in the cell count:

- If neutrophils > lymphocytes: perform a Gram stain.
- If lymphocytes > neutrophils: perform a Ziehl–Neelsen or auramine stain.

> If a meningitis outbreak is suspected, CSF samples must be sent to a reference laboratory for culture in order to prepare and adjust the response programme (i.e. treatment and vaccination). See ➋ 'Transport of specimens' p. 979.

Appearance of CSF

- A normal CSF is clear and colourless.
- A CSF from a patient with a bacterial infection is purulent and/or cloudy.
- In viral, tuberculous, or cryptococcal infections, the CSF can appear clear or slightly turbid.

White cell count in CSF

Equipment and materials required

- Microscope.
- Fuchs–Rosenthal chamber with special cover slips (standard cover slips as used for e.g. urine examinations see page 1100 are NOT suitable to be used on chamber).
- Pipette yellow: 10–100 μL with tips, Pasteur pipette or capillary tube.
- Toluidine blue solution (0.1 g toluidine blue powder in 100 mL sodium/chloride/saline/NaCl 0.85 g).
- Tally counter.

Table 53.1 Findings in cerebrospinal fluid investigations

CSF	Appearance	Cells	Microscopy	Protein	Glucose
Normal	Clear, colourless	<5 × 10⁶ cells/litre, lymphocytes	–	Normal: 0.15–0.4 g/litre Pandy test: negative	2.5–4.0 mmol/litre or 45–72 mg/dL
Bacterial	Purulent or cloudy	Many neutrophils	Gram-stained bacteria visible	Protein: high Pandy test: positive	Very low
Viral	Clear or slightly turbid	Raised lymphocytes	–	Protein: normal or increased Pandy: negative or positive	Usually normal
Tuberculous	Clear or slightly turbid	Raised lymphocytes	Ziehl–Neelsen; AFB but may be difficult to find	Protein: high Pandy test: positive	Reduced
Cryptococcal	Clear or slightly turbid	Raised lymphocytes	Indian ink encapsulated yeast. May be also seen in Gram stain	Protein: usually increased Pandy: positive	Normal or reduced

Table 53.2 Examination of cerebrospinal fluid

	Normal CSF	Abnormal CSF
Appearance	Clear	Cloudy
Cell count	0–5 cells/μL	≥6 cells/μL
Pandy test	Negative	Positive
Cryptococcus test	Negative	ositive

Procedure for cell count
- Cover a clean Fuchs–Rosenthal counting chamber with a clean special cover glass for counting chambers.
- Mix the CSF with toluidine blue with a 1:2 ratio (i.e. one drop of CSF with two drops of toluidine blue).
- Fill the Fuchs–Rosenthal chamber with a small quantity of the prepared fluid, using an automatic pipette, a fine-bore Pasteur pipette, or a capillary tube.
- Leave the counting chamber on the bench in a moist chamber for 2 minutes, to allow the cells to settle.
- Place the Fuchs–Rosenthal chamber on the microscope stage and count the cells of five large squares, using the ×10 objective.
- Close the condenser iris to give good contrast.

- If necessary, use the ×40 objective to ensure that the cells counted are leucocytes.
  - Estimate the percentage of lymphocytes and neutrophils.
- Calculate the number of cells in CSF as follows:
  - (No. of counted cells in 5 squares) × 2 (dilution factor) × 10^6 cells/litre.
  - Example: cell count in 5 large squares = 240.
  - Calculation: 240 × 2 × 10^6 cells/litre.
  - Report: 480 × 10^6 cells/litre.
  - When no white cells are seen, report the count as: <5 × 10^6 cells/litre.
  - A normal CSF can contain up to 5 × 10^6 cells/litre. If white cells are present, estimate which cell type (neutrophils vs lymphocytes) is dominant in order to differentiate the cause of the meningitis.

Note: if it is too difficult for the microscopist to differentiate between the cell types, a drop of the sediment can be put on a slide and stained with a Giemsa stain (see ➲ 'White blood cell differentiation' p. 982).

Note: if the CSF is contaminated with blood, it may be easier to use Türk's solution to be sure that leucocytes are being counted and not red cells. When the CSF contains too much blood and a result is not possible to obtain, a new CSF sample can be collected.

Protein measurement/Pandy reaction in CSF

Protein levels can be measured with a spectrophotometer (see ➲ 'spectrophotometer' p. 981) or by Pandy reaction, which can detect increased amounts of protein.

Equipment and materials required
- Phenol crystals.
- Distilled water.
- Reagent tube 15 mL.
- Plastic transfer pipette or automated pipette 100–1000 µL with tips.

Procedure for Pandy reaction
- Dissolve 2 g phenol crystals in 30 mL distilled water (i.e. saturated phenol solution).
- Pipette 1 mL of the saturated phenol solution in a reagent tube.
- Hold the tube at eye level against a dark background and add one drop of CSF.
- Do not mix.
- If high levels of globulin are present in the CSF, cloudiness appears immediately after adding the CSF to the phenol.

Cryptococcus neoformans testing in CSF

C. neoformans can be detected via a RDT detecting cryptococcal antigen or by the Indian ink method.

Equipment and materials required for Indian ink on CSF
- Centrifuge.
- Microscope slides and cover slips.
- Pasteur pipette.
- Indian ink.
- KOH 10%.

Procedure Indian ink
- Centrifuge the CSF at 1500 g (~4000 rpm) for 20 minutes.
- Carefully transfer the supernatant to a second sterile tube as appropriate. Take extreme care not to disturb the sediment during this step.
- Re-suspend the sediment by gentle agitation or with a Pasteur pipette.
- Transfer one drop of the sediment to a clean slide.
- Add an equal sized drop of black Indian ink.
- Place a cover slip over the suspension and press gently.
- Examine the preparation using the ×40 objective at reduced light. *C. neoformans* appears as an encapsulated cell surrounded by a clear zone, 2–10 μL in diameter. Budding can often be seen in some cells.
- For positive findings: to distinguish between fat droplets (false-positive) and *C. neoformans*, add a second drop of the CSF sediment to a slide, add one drop of 10 % KOH, mix, allow to stand for 30 seconds, then add one drop of Indian ink. *C. neoformans* will remain detectable whereas the KOH will dissolve fat droplets.
- Report the presence or absence of *C. neoformans*. If positive report the number of cryptococci seen (i.e. # per field, # per 10 fields, etc.)

Gram stain in CSF

Equipment and materials required
- Microscope.
- Potentially centrifuge.
- Pasteur pipette.
- Gram stain kit.
- Heat fixing, e.g. via a Bunsen burner or a spirit lamp.
- Microscope slides.
- Immersion/microscope oil.

Preparation of CSF for Gram stain
A Gram-stained smear should be done when the CSF appears purulent or cloudy. This can also provide useful information when a CSF sample is unsuitable for cell counting or biochemical testing, e.g. when heavily blood stained.
- If CSF is purulent, prepare a Gram smear from an uncentrifuged sample.
- If CSF is clear, centrifuge the CSF at ~1000 g (~3000 rpm; manual of centrifuge must be checked) for 5–10 minutes. (Leave a small amount of CSF uncentrifuged for a cell count.)
  - After centrifugation, transfer the supernatant into another tube to be used for glucose and protein measurements.
  - Re-suspend the sediment and transfer several drops of the sediment to a microscopy slide with a Pasteur pipette.
  - Do not make the smear too thick, as it will not decolourize properly.
  - Allow the smear to air dry.

Procedure for Gram stain
- Transfer one drop of the sample on a slide and spread it out. Allow to air dry.
- Fix the smear through heat.

- Cover the smear with crystal violet stain for 30–60 seconds and wash the slide with clean water after.
- Tip of all water and cover smear in Lugol's iodine for 30–60 seconds. Wash the iodine off with water.
- Decolorize for a few seconds with acetone-alcohol and wash immediately with clean water.
- Cover smear with safranine or neutral red for 30–60 seconds and rinse with water.
- Put slide vertically and let air dry.
- Examine the smear with the ×40 objective first in order to get an overview of the smear and then with oil and the ×100 objective.
- Report on presence of bacteria (i.e. scanty, few, moderate, many), Gram reaction (i.e. positive, negative), and morphology (e.g. cocci, diplococcic, streptococci, rods, coccobacilli).

Suspected tuberculous meningitis

The WHO recommends that the *Xpert® MTB/RIF* (see Box 53.1) test should be used as the initial diagnostic test in testing CSF from patients presumed to have tuberculous meningitis. The Xpert® system is an automated real-time nucleic acid amplification technology for rapid and simultaneous detection of tuberculosis and rifampicin resistance.

A Ziehl–Neelsen stain should be performed if TB meningitis is suspected and Xpert® MTB/RIF test is not available. To do so, a drop of the sediment should be placed on a slide and then stained. See ⯈ 'Sputum examinations' pp. 977–8 for details of staining technique.

Box 53.1 Xpert® MTB/RIF

The Xpert® system (Cepheid, CA, USA) is an automated real-time nucleic acid amplification technology for rapid and simultaneous detection of TB and rifampicin resistance. However, implementation of Xpert® requires a high level of infrastructure and may not be routinely available in emergency settings. Further information can be found at ℛ http://www.who.int/tb/publications/Xpert_factsheet.pdf.

Sputum examinations

- Ziehl–Neelsen stain is the most common stain performed for TB.
- A Gram stain of sputum is usually not useful because many organisms that will be seen belong to the normal flora and a Gram stain cannot determine whether these are pathogenic or not.
- The WHO recommends the use of Xpert® MTB/RIF as the initial diagnostic test to detect pulmonary TB and rifampicin resistance, instead of conventional microscopy, phenotypic culture and drug susceptibility testing (DST), for all patients with signs and symptoms of TB (see ➔ Box 53.1 p. 976). However, implementation may be hindered by logistical constraints such as need for stable uninterruptable electrical supply, ambient operating temperature of the instrument should not exceed 30°C, cartridges must be stored below 28°C etc.

Ziehl–Neelsen stain

Each slide needs to be examined for ~15 minutes (300 fields) before a negative result can be given. Thus, one technician can only read 20–25 slides a day otherwise the quality will be reduced.

Equipment and materials required

- Microscope.
- Microscope slides.
- Wooden applicator.
- Carbol–Fuchsin solution.
- Acid-alcohol solution (hydrochloric acid 37% and 95% ethanol).
- Methylene blue solution (methylene blue powder and distilled water).
- Spirit lamp or Bunsen burner.
- Distilled water.
- Reagent tube 15 mL.
- Plastic transfer pipette or automated pipette 100–1000 µL with tips.

Procedure for Ziehl–Neelsen stain

- Prepare a smear of the most mucopurulent part of the sputum sample with a wooden applicator and let it air dry.
- Then heat-fix the smear by passing the slide over a flame three to five times.
- Place the heat-fixed smear horizontally on a staining rack.
- Filter Carbol–Fuchsin working solution (mix of 10 mL solution A with 90 mL solution B; must stand for a few days before use) directly onto the slide using a funnel and filter paper:
  - The slide should be completely covered with stain.
  - Heat the slide until it steams without boiling.
- Allow it to stand for 5 minutes.
- Gently wash with filtered tap water.
- Flood the slide with acid-alcohol (prepared by adding 30 mL of concentrated hydrochloric acid very slowly to 970 mL of 95 % ethanol).
- Incubate for 3 minutes.
- Then wash with tap water.
  - If the slide is red, or partially red, reapply acid-alcohol for 1–3 minutes and rinse gently with tap water.

- Counter stain with methylene blue (3 g methylene blue in 1 litre distilled water) for 1 minute.
- Gently wash with filtered tap water.
- Allow slide to dry vertically.
- Examine the slide systematically for acid-fast bacilli (AFB) using the ×100 objective.
  - Report the macroscopic appearance of the sample and the number of AFB seen.

The main scale for AFB in use is the WHO-IUATLD (International Union Against Tuberculosis and Lung Disease) scale (Table 53.3).

Sputum collection

The most important factor in the pre-analytical phase contributing to TB diagnosis is the quality of the sputum production and its collection. During sputum collection, medical staff present should wear a mask/respirator to prevent bacilli inhalation. These respirators are not typical surgical masks but specially designed high-filtration masks (e.g. N95 certified).

Two sputum samples are to be collected from each patient, in an isolated and designated area for sputum expectoration (preferably in open air away from other people).

- The first sample is taken on the spot, right after the consultation.
  - If the patient has recently eaten, the mouth must be rinsed with water to avoid the presence of food in the sample.
- The second sample is collected the next day in the morning at home, right after waking up before eating.
  - The patient then has to bring the second sputum back to the healthcare facility for examination.
  - Alternatively, the second sample can be collected an hour after the first samples has been taken. This is called front-loaded microscopy.

Collection technique

- The patient has to take a deep breath and hold the air in his/her lungs for a few seconds and then exhale. This needs to be repeated two to three times and the patient needs to cough.
- It can help to clap the patient on the chest for a few minutes to make the sputum production easier.
- The sputum brought up (minimum of 3 mL) from the lungs after a productive cough must be collected in the labelled sputum containers. The container must be hermetically sealed.

Table 53.3 WHO-IUATLD scale for acid-fast bacilli

Number of AFB	×100 magnification	Report
0	In 100 fields	AFB [−] not seen
1–9	In 100 fields	Exact number/100 fields
10–99	In 100 filds	1 +
1–10	per field	2 +
>10	per field	3 +

Transport of specimens

Transport of samples to a higher-level laboratory can be useful in outbreak situations to guide a programmatic response and for surveillance reasons. Also in cases of unusual presentations and diseases with unknown origin, examination at larger laboratory can be useful. When samples are transported to a reference or external laboratory, ensure that the package can be tracked during shipment and notification is given on arrival, especially when shipping across borders.

The triple layers in summary (see Fig. 53.3):
- The first layer is the specimen container (such as the blood tube or the stool plastic cup).
- The specimen container is placed in a second plastic container with shock and liquid adsorbent (such as cotton wool).
- The second layer is placed in an outer box properly identified with infectious material symbols and codes UN 3373 (biological sample) or UN 2814 (infectious sample) depending on the infectious risk of the substances being transported).

UN 3373

Most samples fall under UN 3373 regulations for biological samples e.g. stool sample, sputum sample, blood samples. UN 3373 shipments are usually easily accepted by international carriers such as DHL. The outer layer must be labelled 'UN 3373 – biological sample'.

UN 2814

Samples of higher infectious potential include those samples from patients with suspected haemorrhagic fever and pre-cultured second-line sputum samples on an agar with grown bacteria (e.g. Loewenstein–Jensen agar). The outer layer must be labelled with 'UN 2814 – infectious sample'. It is often difficult to get a UN 2814 sample accepted for shipment so work with the logistician to get agreement.

See WHO's 'Guidance on Regulations for the Transport of Infectious Substances' (ℰ http://www.who.int/ihr/publications/who_hse_ihr_2015.2/en/).

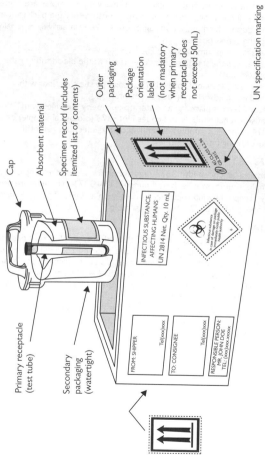

Fig. 53.3 Triple transport box for transporting specimens. Reproduced with permission from International Air Transport Association (IATA).

Blood examinations: clinical chemistry

Handheld analysers and point-of-care analysers

Handheld and point-of-care analysers are available for a various number of analyses starting with a simple glucometer to more complex clinical chemistry analysers including blood gases and electrolyte analysis.

- Most important when using any of these analysers is proper supply chain management and regular quality control.
- The costs of the analysers are usually relatively cheap; however, each cartridge/strip is relatively costly. So, weighing the needs of the programme, the supply in country, and the availability of laboratory staff, should influence the choice of analysers.
- Regular maintenance, besides daily quality control, is for most small handheld and point-of-care analysers not necessary. Repair, once defective, is often costly and time-consuming, thus it is more cost-effective to replace these small handheld analysers with a new one.

Spectrophotometer

- A spectrophotometer is an instrument to measure clinical chemistry parameters, such as enzyme activity, or levels of biochemical substances in the human body.
- The measurement of enzymes requires careful attention as they are usually present in very small amounts and sensitive to temperature, pH changes etc. Small errors of technique can lead to grossly unreliable and misleading results.
- In places with a high workload for clinical chemistry analysis or at secondary healthcare level (i.e. hospital), a spectrophotometer is recommended.
- The choice of analyser should be made based on availability and technical support in country, access to trained staff, and need for type of analysis.
- Most commonly measured parameters are haemoglobin, glucose, glutamate pyruvate transaminase, creatinine, bilirubin, and C reactive protein.

Quality control for clinical chemistry tests performed with a spectrophotometer

- Of utmost important is daily performance of internal quality control, the establishment of Levy–Jenning charts, and the use of Westgard rules for their interpretation.
- Quality control procedures are required to detect and minimize errors in the performance of tests and to keep imprecision and inaccuracy errors to a minimum. When performing quality control in clinical chemistry, the accuracy and precision of a method is checked for.
- Before a test method is used routinely, the laboratory must first ensure that the method is working reliably and that it can be performed within acceptable limits of variability. After the test is introduced, it must be adequately controlled.
- A trained laboratory technician in clinical chemistry or a clinical chemist should establish the use of Levy–Jenning charts and Westgard rules in a laboratory for clinical chemistry and haematology analysers.

Blood examinations: haematology

White blood cell differentiation

White blood cell differentiation (WBCD) is performed to investigate infections, unexplained fevers, inflammation, and allergies, among others. A WBCD includes the percentages of neutrophils, lymphocytes, monocytes, eosinophils, and basophils. The WBCD determines if the cells are present in a normal proportion to one another, if one cell type is increased or decreased, or if immature cells are present.

Equipment and materials required
- Microscope.
- Slides.
- Methanol.
- Filtered water.
- Giemsa stain.
- Buffer tables pH 7.2.
- Immersion/microscopy oil.
- WBCD counter, alternatively hand written on a piece of paper.

Procedure
- Prepare a thin blood smear on a slide and once dried, fix it with 100% methanol.
- Then prepare a 1:10 dilution of the Giemsa stain using the buffer solution (i.e. 1 mL Giemsa in 9 mL pH 7.2 buffer).
- Place the slides horizontally on the staining rack, cover with the freshly prepared stain for 10–15 minutes.
- Wash the stain off with washing solution (i.e. water pH 7.2 adjusted) to one end of the slide so that the stain overflows the slide.
- Keep adding washing solution until all the Giemsa has been removed and the fluid leaving the slide is colourless.
- Let the slide dry vertically.
- Place a drop of immersion oil on the slide and count the different blood cells in an area of the smear where the cells lie nicely next to each other and do not overlap using the ×100 objective. Count until 100 WBCs are reached using the battlement technique.

Erythrocytes (red blood cells)

When carrying out a WBCD, RBC appearance is reported together with the WBCD. Report at least on the following:
- Colour (i.e. normo-, or hypochromic or polychromatic)
- Size (normo-, micro-, macrocytic or anisocytosis).
- Shape: abnormal cell shapes are: acanthocytes, target cells, elliptocytes, tear drop cells, spherocytes etc.
- Red cell inclusions are Howell–Jolly bodies, Pappenheimer bodies, or basophilic stippling etc. If they are seen, then report them.

White blood cell count

A WBC count is performed to investigate infections and unexplained fevers, and to monitor treatments which can cause leucopenia.

Equipment and materials required
- Microscope.
- Improved Neubauer chamber with special cover slips.
- Pipette 'blue': 100–1,000 µL with tips.
- Pipette 'yellow': 10–100 µL with tips.
- Small tubes.
- Türk solution.
- Tally counter.

Procedure
- Put the special cover glass for chamber counting with slight pressure in the centre of the Neubauer chamber covering the two counting chambers. When the cover glass is properly in place, Newton rings (i.e. a rainbow effect) will appear.
- Put 380 µL of Türk's solution into a small tube.
- Add 20 µL of the well mixed venous blood sample or capillary blood to the tube. Mix the tube well.
- Then fill one of the Neubauer chambers with the diluted blood sample using a Pasteur or automatic pipette. No bubbles or overflow into the ditches are allowed. Do not under-fill either. Allow the cells to settle for a few minutes.
- Place the improved Neubauer counting chamber on the microscope stage. Select the ×10 objective and focus on the ruled area.
- Count the cells in the four big corner squares. Count all the cells inside the ruled areas plus any cells touching the top and left outside border. Do not count the cells touching the bottom and right outside border. (See Fig. 53.4 and Fig. 53.5.)

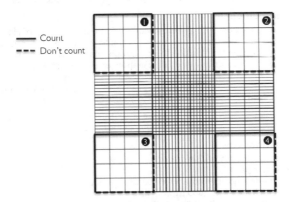

Fig. 53.4 Improved Neubauer chamber. Cells in the four big corner squares are counted for a white blood cell count. Reproduced with permission from http://www.hemocytometer.org/tag/neubauer-chamber/.

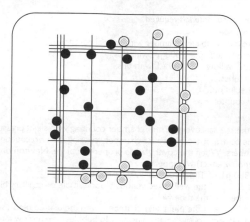

Fig. 53.5 Corner square of improved Neubauer chamber: only count the cells inside the square and touching the left and top border. Reproduced with permission from Dr. Oscar Bastidas, Celeromics Technologies, S.L. Available from www. celeromics.com/en/resources/Technical%20Notes/cells-chamber-counting.php.

Calculation
- For the new improved Neubauer chamber, the quick calculation for WBC/mm³ is: total cells counted in 4 squares × 50.
- Reported as WBC × 10^9/litre or WBC/mm³.
- Wash the chamber and the cover glass immediately after each use.

Haemoglobin

Hb can be measured using various methods. As the measurement of Hb is an essential laboratory parameter, it is important to have a handheld analyser, a haematology bench-top analyser, a spectrophotometer, or similar available. The choice depends on workload, availability of trained staff, and cost.
- The oxyhaemoglobin or methaemoglobin method requires a spectrophotometer. A haematology analyser can be used as alternative.
- Handheld Hb measuring devices for tropical climates are available.

Note: methods such as WHO colour scale, Sahli method, or the Lovibond comparator are *not* recommended due to their inaccuracy.

Thrombocytes

Equipment and materials required:
- Microscope.
- Fuchs–Rosenthal chamber with special cover slips.
- Pipette 'blue': 100-1,000 µL with tips.
- Pipette 'yellow': 10 - 100 µL with tips.
- Small tubes.
- Ammonium oxalate solution (1 g ammonium oxalate in 100 mL distilled water).
- Tally counter.

Procedure

- Put the special cover glass with slight pressure in the centre of the Neubauer chamber covering the two counting chambers. When the cover glass is properly in place, Newton rings (i.e. a rainbow effect) will appear.
- Transfer 380 µL of ammonium oxalate solution to a small tube and add 20 µL of well-mixed venous whole blood sample to the tube and mix well.
- Then fill one of the Neubauer chambers with the diluted blood sample using a Pasteur or automatic pipette. No bubbles or overflow into the ditches are allowed. Do not under-fill either. Allow the cells to settle for a few minutes.
- Place the improved Neubauer counting chamber on the microscope stage. Using the ×10 objective, focus on the ruled area, then select the ×40 objective and fine-focus on the central set of squares.
- The platelets appear as small refractile cells without a nucleus, particularly when the condenser is lowered to reduce the light passing through the counting chamber.
- There are 25 group squares in the central set of squares. Count the cells in five of these group squares including the ones touching the top and left outside border (see Fig. 53.6). Do not count the cells touching the bottom and right outside border.
- Reference range: 150,000–400,000/mm³.
- Wash the chamber and the cover glass immediately after use.

Formula for platelet count/mm³ = total cells counted in 5 group squares × 1000.

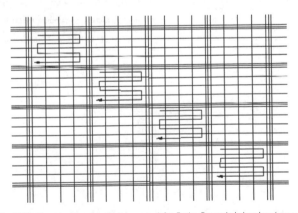

Fig. 53.6 Counting directions (follow arrow) for Fuchs–Rosenthal chamber (upper diagram). As for the Neubauer chamber, count the cells in the square and those which touch the top and left border (·). Do not count the ones touching the right and lower border. Reproduced with permission from Lavens and Sorgeloos, Manual on the production and use of live food for aquaculture, Food and Agriculture Organization of the United Nations (FAO), 1996. Available from http://www.fao.org/docrep/003/w3732e/w3732e0b.htm.

Further reading

The US Centers for Disease Control and Prevention has excellent online material including bench aids with images on the diagnosis of parasitic diseases. ℘ http://www.cdc.gov/dpdx/diagnosticProcedures/stool/index.html

The WHO has published a guideline, 'Good Clinical Laboratory Practice' (2009), which also addresses quality assurance systems for laboratories. ℘ http://www.who.int/tdr/publications/documents/gclp-web.pdf

The WHO has published bench aids, 'Bench aids for the diagnosis of malaria infections'. ℘ http://apps.who.int/iris/bitstream/handle/10665/42195/9241545240.pdf;jsessionid=BFE92D5CBE8453540077617382A817BA?sequence=1

Monica Cheesbrough has published two textbooks: 'District Laboratory Practice in Tropical Countries'. Part 1 and 2.

The WHO has published a guideline, 'Guidelines for the collection of clinical specimens during field investigation of outbreaks'. ℘ http://apps.who.int/iris/bitstream/handle/10665/66348/WHO_CDS_CSR_EDC_2000.4.pdf?sequence=1

The WHO has published a guideline, 'Laboratory quality management system: handbook'. ℘ http://www.who.int/ihr/publications/lqms_en.pdf

The WHO has published a guideline, 'Good Clinical Laboratory Practice'. ℘ http://www.who.int/tdr/publications/documents/gclp-web.pdf?ua=1

The WHO has published a guideline, 'Good Clinical Laboratory Practice' (2009), which also addresses quality assurance systems for laboratories. ℘ http://www.who.int/tdr/publications/documents/gclp-web.pdf

The WHO published a policy update, 'Xpert MTB/RIF assay for the diagnosis of pulmonary and extrapulmonary TB in adults and children'. ℘ http://apps.who.int/iris/bitstream/handle/10665/112472/9789241506335_eng.pdf?sequence=1

The WHO published an implementation guide 'Xpert MTB/RIF implementation manual. Technical and operational 'how-to': practical considerations'. ℘ http://apps.who.int/iris/bitstream/handle/10665/112469/9789241506700_eng.pdf?sequence=1

The WHO published a checklist: 'Prerequisites to country implementation of Xpert MTB/RIF and key action points at country level'. ℘ http://www.who.int/tb/publications/WHO_HTM_TB_2011_12/en/

The WHO published a book, 'Basic laboratory procedures in clinical bacteriology'. ℘ http://apps.who.int/iris/handle/10665/42696

The International Federation of Clinical Chemistry (IFCC) published, 'Fundamentals for External Quality Assessment (EQA). Guidelines for Improving Analytical Quality by Establishing and Managing EQA schemes. Examples from basic chemistry using limited resources.' ℘ http://www.ifcc.org/ifccfiles/docs/fundamentals-for-eqa.pdf

Blood transfusion

Cara Kosack and Monique Guegen

Overview of blood transfusion

Blood transfusion can be a lifesaving activity but should only be performed when absolutely indicated due to the risks of an adverse reaction and infection.

Direct transfusion versus blood bank

In resource-constrained settings, the choice of direct transfusions versus the set-up of a blood bank depends on the need for transfusions in the area of the healthcare facility and its capacity. A hospital which receives a lot of trauma patients requires blood units more regularly than a small hospital with a few in-patient beds. Most often, however, a direct transfusion service is easier to manage than an entire blood bank, especially because an uninterrupted electricity supply is essential to ensure proper storage of the blood units but is often difficult to guarantee in resource-constrained settings.

Direct transfusion needs the active mobilization of family members, the constant availability of staff to select and test the potential donors, and is only possible when the need for blood is not urgent. It is common to have to wait between 1 and 2 hours between making a transfusion decision and when the blood is ready.

Transfusion indications

- Anaemia results in reduced oxygen-carrying capacity which is often well tolerated. Blood transfusion is indicated only if anaemia is no longer compensated, often with signs that include tachycardia, respiratory distress, altered mental status, heart failure, or shock. (See Table 54.1.)
- The most common events that cause an indication for blood transfusion are uncompensated anaemia, e.g. caused by malaria, or through major haemorrhage, e.g. caused by trauma or obstetric complications.

Table 54.1 Transfusion thresholds (except for hereditary anaemia such as sickle cell disease)

Patient group	Transfusion is indicated if	Remarks
Children	Hb <4 g/dL	Transfusion is not indicated if Hb is 4–6 g/dL unless there are signs of decompensation
Pregnant women <36 weeks	Hb <5 g/dL	Transfusion is indicated if Hb <7 g/dL *and* malaria, pneumonia, other serious bacterial infection, or a pre-existing heart disease is present
Pregnant women >36 weeks	Hb <6 g/dL	Transfusion is indicated if Hb <8 g/dL *and* malaria, pneumonia, other serious bacterial infection, or a pre-existing heart disease is present
Adults	Hb <7 g/dL	Consider patients with severe malaria

Notes: During delivery the blood loss is usually 500 mL for a vaginal delivery and 1000 mL for a caesarean section. If the Hb is 10 g/dL before delivery, transfusion is rarely indicated.

Clinical signs of decompensation include: respiratory distress, tachycardia, altered consciousness, heart failure or coronary insufficiency or signs of shock.

Data sourced from Clinical Use of Blood, WHO; Geneva, 2005. http://www.who.int/bloodsafety/clinical_use/en/Handbook_EN.pdf

Donor selection for blood transfusion

- All blood donations must be voluntary and non-remunerated.
- 'Professional' donors should not be recruited as they have a higher risk of being affected by transfusion-transmissible infections (TTIs).
- The risk of TTIs is also higher in donations from friends or relatives as family pressure may force potential donors to give false information during the selection process. Sometimes, however, if no other donor can be found, this may be the only available option.
- The minimal interval between two donations is 2 months. Men can donate blood four times/year if their haemoglobin (Hb) level is >13.5 g/dL and women three times/year if Hb >12.5 g/dL.
- Every potential donor should fulfil pre-selection criteria including a confidential pre-donation questionnaire about their medical history, TTI risk exposure, and current health.
- A nurse or physician should carry out a physical examination including body temperature, heart rate, and BP with examination of conjunctive, lymph nodes (i.e. cervical, axillary, inguinal), skin for rash, and mouth (e.g. oral thrush).

Contraindications

Age <15 and >65 years, weight <45 kg, last donation <2 months before, Hb level <11 g/dL, current pregnancy and <6 months after delivery or miscarriage, and exclusive breastfeeding are absolute contraindications for blood donation. Chronic diseases including HIV, hepatitis, severe asthma, haemopathy/haemoglobinopathy, epilepsy, insulin-dependent diabetes, and cancer are permanent contraindications. History of blood transfusion and unexplained jaundice are also permanent contraindications.

Temporary reasons that contraindicate blood donation include surgery or endoscopy <6 months before; history of acute adverse reaction, TB, Q fever, osteomyelitis until 2 years after cure; history of syphilis cured <1 year before, other STI cured <4 months before; unprotected casual sex, rape, IV drug use, scarifications, tattoo, piercing in the past 6 months; root treatment or extraction in the past week; current cutaneous infection; and axillary temperature above 37.5°C.

Systolic BP <100 or >180 mmHg, or pulse <50 or >100/minute or irregular contraindicate blood donation.

Refer to the physician for advice in case of mixed breastfeeding, current treatment, fever within the last 3 weeks, recent vaccination, swollen lymph nodes, or skin rash.

Donor screening and blood grouping

Screening every donor's Hb and testing for TTIs is essential before collecting blood. If a particular donor blood group is needed, blood grouping also needs to be carried out before donation.

HIV

Even if antibody screening is negative, blood may still contain HIV due to the window period. In order to reduce the risk of transfusing HIV positive blood, the interview and examination of donors is crucial.

Hepatitis B and C

The average window period for HBsAg is 30 days (range 7–63 days). The average window period for HCV antibody detection is 82 days (range 54–192 days) after infection. Donor interview and examination is important to judge residual risk.

Treponema pallidum (syphilis)

Treponema pallidum-positive blood may be transfused at the physician's discretion combined with treatment if no other blood donor is available.

Malaria

In low endemic areas (or areas with seasonal malaria)

Donors with a positive malaria test should receive an effective antimalarial therapy. Blood should not be collected, unless transfusion is needed urgently and no other donor is available. All recipients of malaria-positive blood should be treated with a full, effective antimalarial treatment.

In high endemic areas

- Option 1: malaria screening is omitted and effective antimalarial treatment is routinely administered to all recipients.
- Option 2: systematic screening is performed but positive blood is not necessarily excluded. It can be labelled and stored separately and when transfused, the recipient receives antimalarial treatment.

In all cases, transfusion of malaria-positive blood to pregnant women and children <5 years old is not recommended and should be avoided unless there is no alternative.

Chagas disease

Screening may be required if you are in an endemic area.

Human T-cell lymphotropic virus

Screening may be required if you are in an endemic area.

ABO blood grouping

The ABO blood grouping system is the most important blood system. Natural antibodies (i.e. anti-A and anti-B antibodies) develop in the first year of life. The blood group determines which type of blood the patient can receive. Only transfuse ABO-compatible blood—see Table 54.2.
   Persons with:
- blood group A have anti-B antibodies
- blood group B have anti-A antibodies
- blood group AB have neither anti-A nor anti-B antibodies
- blood group O have anti-A and anti-B antibodies.

Table 54.2 Blood group to use

ABO group of patient	Choice of blood			
	1st choice	2nd choice	3rd choice	4th choice
O	O			
A	A	O		
B	B	O		
AB	AB	A	B	O

Transfuse only ABO-compatible blood
and
Prefer ABO identical blood.

If non-ABO identical blood is used, preferably transfuse packed red blood cells, or the least amount of plasma possible.

Reproduced with permission from Monica Cheesbrough, District Laboratory Practice in Tropical Countries, Second Edition, (2006), Cambridge University Press.

Rhesus grouping

In contrast to the ABO blood grouping system, there are no naturally occurring rhesus (Rh) antibodies. Rh antibodies are always acquired through transfusion or during pregnancy and are developed by individuals who do not express the corresponding antigen. Incompatibility occurs when a Rh-D negative recipient acquires anti-D antibodies which destroy the Rh-D positive transfused red cells. Rh antibodies often cause mild and/or delayed haemolysis, and rarely immediate severe haemolysis.

Situations may occur when Rh-D identical transfusion is not possible due to a shortage of blood. The following two occasions may occur:

Rh-D negative blood to Rh-D positive recipient
Rh-D negative blood may be transfused to Rh-D positive recipient without immunological risk, but only as a second choice. Rh-D negative blood is rare and should be reserved for Rh-D negative recipients.

Rh-D positive blood to Rh-D negative recipient
Rh-D positive blood may be transfused to Rh-D negative recipient, but only in the event of absolute emergency. No immediate transfusion reaction is expected in Rh-D negative men and nulliparous women who have never been transfused before. Incompatibility accidents may occur if the recipient has developed acquired anti-D antibodies through previous transfusion or pregnancy. Since a simple cross-match procedure cannot detect a recipient's anti-D antibodies, the risk of an immediate transfusion reaction and ineffective transfusion is unpredictable. Therefore, the decision to transfuse Rh-D positive blood to Rh-D negative patients must be a well-considered medical decision, taking into account not only the immediate risks but also the potential consequences:

- The recipient has a high likelihood of developing anti-D antibodies and their future transfusions may be put at risk.
- Rh-D negative women are likely to experience obstetrical complications if they subsequently conceive Rh-D positive children.

Important: do not administer anti-D immunoglobulin to a Rh-D negative patient who received Rh-positive blood as high doses of anti-D immuno-globulin would be required to prevent anti-D alloimmunization and the anti-D immunoglobulin could even destroy the transfused red cells.

Testing and procedures: ABO and Rh blood grouping—tile method
The blood donor and recipient must undergo ABO and Rh blood grouping. Blood grouping should be carried out in a designated area in the healthcare facility, ideally a laboratory, by a laboratory technician, or a trained medical doctor or clinician.

Materials required
- Blood collection materials.
- Donor and recipient's blood sample.
- Commercial monoclonal antibody reagents: anti-A (blue solution), anti-B (yellow solution), anti-AB antibodies (colourless), anti Rh D (colourless), and a Rh negative control.
- Physiological saline.
- Blood grouping tile.
- Transfer pipette, plastic, non-sterile.
- Applicators.

Procedure steps
- Label a blood grouping tile with the patient/donor's name or identification number and mark a sequence of squares or wells for anti-A, anti-B, anti-AB, anti-D and Rh-D negative control.
- Add to each of the corresponding square/well 1 drop of anti-A, 1 drop of anti-B, 1 drop of anti-AB, 1 drop of anti-D, and 1 drop of Rh-D negative control.
- Using a transfer pipette add 1 drop of whole blood or 30–40% blood suspension with saline to each of the five reaction areas next to the blood grouping reagents.
- Mix each of the five reagents with the blood using an applicator. Use a clean applicator, or a new part of the applicator, before proceeding to the next test area.
- Gently rock the grouping tile to further mix the red cells suspended in the reagents, for 1–2 minutes. Reactions may develop at different rates and to different extents.
- Interpretation: look for agglutination. Agglutinates form progressively and leave the background free of red cells. When the mixture remains homogeneous, no agglutination is present. The interpretation is possible only if the reaction with the Rh-D negative control is clearly negative.
- Record the results.

Other blood group systems, e.g. Kelly, Duffy, and Kidd, may cause severe transfusion reactions but they generally cannot be tested for in resource-constrained settings.

Blood collection, storage and cross-matching

After the donor has been selected and all TTI tests were negative and the Hb level meets the donor requirements, blood can be drawn.

If a direct transfusion is planned, choose the appropriate blood collection bag in order to only collect the amount that is needed.

The total amount of collected blood should be limited to 500 mL in an adult >50 kg.

Work under aseptic conditions as the collection procedure carries the risk of bacterial contamination and this puts the recipient at risk of receiving contaminated blood.

Procedure

- Place the donor in a semi-sitting or lying position.
- Prepare the blood bag. Close the clamp on the giving line.
- Prepare the puncture site. Disinfect twice and let it air dry. Do not touch the puncture site again!
- Perform the puncture and open the clamp.
- When the bag starts filling, gently tilt the bag so that the blood can be mixed with the anticoagulant.
- Stop the collection once the correct volume according to the blood bag size is reached, ideally measured with a scale.
- Close the clamp before removing the needle as otherwise air can enter the blood bag and cause contamination.
- Ask the donor to press the puncture site with a compress.
- Tighten a knot close to the needle after the needle has been protected.
- Cut the blood bag giving line close to the knot at the distal end of the knot. In case donation testing is performed after blood has been collected, collect the blood from the cut-off piece into a labelled EDTA tube
- Place approximately four tight knots in the giving line at intervals of 10–15 cm distance to allow further testing, such as a second HIV test and second blood grouping and cross-matching on the segments.

Storage of blood

- If the blood is not transfused immediately, it must be stored in electric refrigerators that are strictly temperature monitored between 2–8°C.
- A special refrigerator for storing blood units must be used.
- Allow the blood to cool down for 2–4 hours after the donation at room temperature <25°C before storing it in the blood refrigerator.
- Within the refrigerator the blood should be stored by blood group and expiry date. The shelf-life of the blood depends on the preservative solution used in the blood bags (the most commonly used solution is CPDA-1 which allows whole blood and packed RBCs to be stored for up to 35 days).
- The blood units should be stored in an upright position with giving line and transfusion outlets facing down.
  - This technique is very useful as the RBCs sediment to the bottom of the blood bag. It allows transfusing only the sedimented red cells, which is the preferred blood component for patients with normovolaemia. The preparation of packed RBCs by centrifugation is not feasible in resource-constrained settings.

Cross-matching: tile method

- When blood is cross-matched, the donor's RBCs are brought in contact with the recipient's plasma to predict a potential transfusion reaction.
- Only negatively cross-matched blood units may be transfused!
- Although generally the only method accessible to verify compatibility between donor and recipient, cross-matching on a tile at room temperature does not detect all clinically significant immune blood group antibodies (e.g. to Rh, Kell, Duffy, Kidd, Ss systems).
- Transfusion reactions are low risk for patients who receive blood for the first time. If patients are poly-transfused, the risk for a transfusion reaction increases.

Testing and procedures: cross-matching—tile method

Materials required

- Blood collection materials.
- Donor blood unit and recipient's blood sample.
- Centrifuge.
- Tube, plastic.
- Test tube rack.
- Automatic pipette 10–100 μL plus pipette tips or transfer pipette.
- Blood grouping tile.
- Applicator.

Procedure steps

- Label the tile with the blood unit number and the recipient's identification number.
- Cut the distal segment of the blood bag giving line and empty the contents of the segment into the plastic tube. The segment may contain clots from which red cells can be extracted.
- Place a tip on the pipette and extract 50 μL of free red cells and deposit on the tile.
- Drop 100 μL of recipient's plasma next to the red cells on the tile.
- Mix in a circle of 3 cm diameter with an applicator.
- Rock the tile gently, for 2 minutes, while observing the reaction. If there is no agglutination: the cross-match is negative. If there is agglutination: the cross-match is positive.

A positive cross-match indicates that the donated blood is incompatible with the recipient, i.e. the recipient has antibodies directed against the blood unit red cells which could provoke a haemolytic reaction. The blood must not be transfused to the patient.

The blood transfusion process

Once the blood unit is delivered to the ward or operating theatre, the ABO blood group of donor and recipient must be verified with a bed-side test card, i.e. ABO compatibility card, in order to verify compatible blood groups immediately before the transfusion. This procedure is carried out on a card which is pre-coated with dried anti-A and anti-B sera. Once the testing is finalized and the card is dried, it has to be kept in the patient's file.

- Once the bed-side test shows compatibility, the blood transfusion can be connected to the patient's IV line and be slowly started.
- Allow the blood unit to reach room temperature, approximately 10 minutes, if it comes directly from the refrigerator as quick transfusion of cold blood can cause cardiac arrest.
- Blood should always be transfused through a blood-giving set with a filter mesh of 200 μm.
- Connect the blood-giving set to the blood unit outlet and let the giving set tubing fill. Then connect the tubing to the catheter.
- Set the transfusion rate. Typically, 1 mL of blood equals 15 drops.

Monitoring transfusion

A transfusion monitoring form should be filled out with every transfusion. The following information should be collected on the form:
- Date and name of nurse/physician monitoring patient.
- Patient information: ID, name, weight, sex, blood group (ABO, Rh).
- Blood unit information: blood unit number and blood group (ABO, Rh).
- Bed-side test result.
- Transfusion information: start time, rate of transfusion (drops per minute), and end time of transfusion.

Temperature, pulse, BP, and respiratory rate should be recorded before transfusion, at 5, 15, 30, 45, and 60 minutes. Thereafter the same should be recorded every 30 minutes until the transfusion is finalized and then again at 4–6 hours after transfusion. In addition, urine output should be recorded at 1, 2, 3 and 4 hours after the start of transfusion.

Transfusion volumes and rates in children and infants

The recommended volume of packed RBCs is 15 mL/kg and whole blood is 20 mL/kg at an hourly rate of 5 mL/kg in the absence of hypovolaemia or shock.

Intraosseous transfusion

Intraosseous transfusion is indicated in young children when IV placement is unsuccessful, i.e. after three attempts. The puncture must be carried out under sterile conditions, and is best at the flat anteromedial part of the tibia.

Procedure

- Flex the knee and put the leg in a stable position.
- Identify the puncture site: palpate tibial tuberosity and move 1–3 cm down to the anteromedial part of the tibia.
- Disinfect your own hands and put on sterile gloves.
- Disinfect the skin and allow for drying. Repeat.
- Inject a local anaesthetic in the skin and move to the periosteum in a conscious child. No local anaesthesia is necessary if the child is unconscious.
- Insert the intraosseous needle (14–18 G) at 90° to the skin and slightly caudal to avoid the epiphyseal growth plate.
- Advance the needle with a drilling motion until the needle penetrates the bone. Remove the inner trocar and aspirate some bone marrow with a 5 mL syringe to confirm correct positioning.
- If the needle does not aspirate, it can be blocked. Slowly inject 0.9% NaCl with a 10 mL syringe to check correct positioning and unblock. Ensure the limb does not swell. If the procedure is unsuccessful, remove the needle and move to the other tibia.
- Secure needle and connect blood-giving set to the intraosseous needle.
- Transfusion can be given under slight pressure, e.g. with a BP cuff around the blood bag.
- Remove the intraosseous needle immediately once the transfusion is finished.

Contraindications are osteomyelitis and fractions of the bone at the access site and femur fracture on the ipsilateral side. Complications are fracture of bone (especially in neonates), osteomyelitis, skin necrosis, and cellulitis (<1% if aseptic technique is used).

Transfusion reactions

Most severe transfusion reactions are caused by clerical error. Therefore the identification of the patient/recipient and donors, the correct recording of the test results, and the identification of the blood units must be checked at every stage of the procedure. The use of a bed-side test, i.e. ABO compatibility card, is compulsory and leaves evidence in the patient's medical file that ABO compatibility has been checked at bedside before transfusion.

Causes

The most serious, often fatal transfusion reactions are caused by the following:

- Transfusion of ABO-incompatible blood due to patient misidentification, incorrect labelling of specimens, or other clerical errors.
- Transfusing bacterial infected blood, commonly caused by inadequate cleaning of the vein puncture site when collecting donor blood.
- Transfusing blood which has expired, has been haemolysed by being stored next to the freezing compartment of a refrigerator, or has been stored at temperatures >8°C.
- Other reasons:
  - A severely anaemic person may react adversely to a blood transfusion when blood is transfused too quickly or when too much whole blood is transfused causing circulatory overload. Most reactions to transfused blood are minor non-haemolytic febrile reactions causing shivering and a slight rise of temperature.
  - Occasionally allergic anaphylactic reactions occur with urticaria and bronchial spasm due to hypersensitivity to plasma protein antigens.
  - Malaria parasites will often cause a temperature rise and also antibodies to leucocytes or platelets.

Patient management in transfusion reactions

- Stop transfusion but keep IV line open with saline.
- Check vital parameters.
- See Table 54.3 for recognition and management of transfusion reactions.

Laboratory management in transfusion reactions

- Identification of clerical errors.
- Repeat laboratory ABO compatibility tests with patient and donor blood and repeat cross-matching.
- Examination of the blood for bacterial contamination by checking its colour change, and via a Gram-stained smear.
- Check for haemolysis by centrifuging a new blood sample and staining blood film and check for spherocytes and red cell fragmentation. Also, check the urine for haemoglobin with a urine dipstick.
- Check for disseminated intravascular coagulation with a D-dimer test.

Further reading

Cheesbrough, M. District Laboratory Practice in Tropical Countries. Part 2. 2nd ed. Cambridge: Cambridge University Press; 2005.

Transfusion reactions: ℘ https://www.pathology.med.umich.edu/blood-bank/blood-transfusion-policies

World Health Organization. The Clinical Use of Blood. 2002. ℘ http://www.who.int/bloodsafety/clinical_use/en/Handbook_EN.pdf

Table 54.3 Transfusion reactions

Type reaction	Symptoms	Occurrence	Treatment: adult	Follow-up
Allergic: urticaria	Laryngeal oedema, bronchospasm	1% of recipients	Antihistamines, corticosteroids and oxygen as required	
Allergic: anaphylaxis	Dyspnoea or stridor. Cardiovascular instability, e.g. hypotension, tachycardia, loss of consciousness, cardiac arrhythmia, shock, and cardiac arrest	Rare Occurs within seconds to minutes after starting the transfusion. However, also later anaphylactic reactions may occur	Epinephrine (adrenaline) in addition to antihistamines, corticosteroids, oxygen, crystalloids as required	Treat shock if appears
Acute haemolytic	Patient shows anxiety, fever, chills, lumbar pain, tachycardia, hypotension, haemoglobinuria. Oliguria can occur, followed by renal failure	Occur within minutes of starting transfusion but may occur later during transfusion Rare	Maintain BP and renal flow (e.g. furosemide if necessary)	
Non-haemolytic febrile transfusion reaction	Fever	Within 4 hours of transfusion 1 in 8 transfusions	Paracetamol	
Septic transfusion reaction	Patient has fever or hypothermia, tachycardia, drop or rise in systolic BP ≥30 mmHg, nausea, vomiting, oliguria or anuria in sepsis	Within 4 hours of transfusion	Administer immediately broad-spectrum antibiotic (e.g. ciprofloxacin+ gentamicin or amoxicillin + gentamicin)	
TRALI (transfusion-related acute lung injury)	Rapid onset with hypoxaemia and dyspnoea, cough	During or within 6 hours of transfusion Rare	Oxygen and mechanical ventilation	Most cases of TRALI resolve within 72 hours although fatalities may occur in ~10% of cases
TACO (transfusion-associated circulatory overload)	Respiratory distress with cough, tachycardia, raised JVP (jugular venous pressure), peripheral oedema	During or within 6 hours of transfusion	Furosemide	

Ultrasound

Matthew Lyon and W. Ted Kuhn

Context for ultrasound

Humanitarian medicine is a rapidly changing specialty and advancing technology such as ultrasound can play a crucial role in the right hands. In most humanitarian emergencies, advanced capabilities are likely not available and plain X-ray, CT, and MRI may not be at a provider's disposal. Point-of-care ultrasound can be of enormous benefit in these situations. High-quality, portable ultrasound units are now increasingly available at a more affordable cost. They are the size and weight of a laptop computer and are easily available and transported in a backpack. These small portable machines can operate in remote locations and can be moved from one village to another while being operated on battery power. Point-of-care ultrasound is an important adjunct for diagnosis of many of the illnesses and injuries common in humanitarian emergencies in the immediate, continuation, and recovery phases.

Skilled sonographers can be of enormous benefit while an unskilled sonographer can lead to diagnostic and therapeutic misadventures. Ultrasound in any clinical environment, emergent or not, resource poor or not, is best performed following prior formal training and apprenticeship. The eye does not see what the mind does not know. Some scans are more easily mastered (e.g. focused assessment with sonography in trauma (FAST)) but all must be correctly performed for correct results.

Mastery of ultrasound is not feasible with this chapter alone. Ideally, you should obtain training prior to a mission while practising, improving, and maintaining your skill during your daily practice. Use of ultrasound in a humanitarian emergency will have additional challenges beyond that in your normal controlled practice environment. This chapter will provide guidance on how to incorporate the ultrasound skills into a humanitarian mission and includes a description of the three essential components of clinical ultrasound:

- Image acquisition—obtaining appropriate images using ultrasound.
- Image interpretation—determining normal from abnormal structures on the ultrasound image.
- Clinical integration—incorporating ultrasound results into your clinical practice.

Understanding ultrasound

Basic principles

- Ultrasound uses sound waves of a very high frequency, those beyond human hearing, to create pictures of internal body structures. The pictures are created as the sound wave, transmitted into the body by the ultrasound transducer, strikes an interface.
- When the sound wave strikes the interface, part of the sound wave is sent deeper into the body to image deeper body structures and part of the wave is sent back towards the transducer. It is these reflected waves which are used to image interfaces of the body structures.
- Interfaces are, in a general sense, any structure that has a different density to the adjacent structure. This can be the blood vessel wall, the blood in the vessel, or the surrounding fat or muscle, which all have different densities and can be imaged using ultrasound.
- An easy way to interpret an ultrasound image is to compare the darkness of the image to the amount of fluid or blood the structure contains:
  - The more water-like (or blood-like) a structure, the darker the image.
  - *Anechoic* refers to a structure with no echoes at all and is consistent with fluids such as blood, urine, pus, ascites, etc.
  - As the percentage of blood or fluid decreases, the brighter the structure is represented on the screen. For example, the liver is hypoechoic, or darker, than the gallbladder wall which is hyperechoic or bright.
- The only structures which do not follow this pattern are bone and air. Bone and air are very hyperechoic and produce a shadowing effect. The shadowing effect prevents imaging of deeper body structures.
  - Bones and foreign bodies produce a deep dark shadow; whereas air or gas produces a grey ('dirty') shadow. Bone and air are enemies of ultrasound as they prevent imaging of the structures behind them.

Key terms

- *Anechoic*: producing no echoes at all. The resulting image is therefore completely black.
- *Echogenic*: a material that produces echoes. The more echogenic a substance is, the whiter the image appears.
- *Echolucent*: a material that does not produce echoes. The more echolucent a substance is, the blacker the image it produces.
- *Hyperechoic*: more echogenic (therefore whiter/brighter) than surrounding tissue.
- *Hypoechoic*: less echogenic (therefore darker) than surrounding tissue.
- *Longitudinal or long axis*: these terms refer to the longest dimension of the structure being imaged. The term may refer to an up and down orientation to the body (sagittal and coronal planes).
- *Transverse axis or cross-section*: these terms refer to the shortest dimension of the structure being imaged. This image is typically 90° offset from the longitudinal axis. The term may also refer to a cross-section of the body, similar to a CT image.
- *Acoustic window*: area where the ultrasound image can be transmitted, allowing for visualization of body structures. Ultrasound imaging is prevented by bone, air, and distance.

Common ultrasound transducers and uses

- *Curvilinear transducer*: low-frequency transducer (2–5 MHz) with a curved face. It produces low-resolution images but can image deeply into the body (up to 30 cm or more). This transducer produces a spectrum of shades of grey and is typically used for abdominal imaging.
- *Linear transducer*: high-frequency transducer (5–12 MHz) with a flat face. It produces a high-resolution image but will not image deeply into the body (maximum depth is around 10 cm). This is typically used for evaluation of superficial structures such as skin abscesses, vessels, and nerves as well as for ultrasound guidance of procedures.
- *Phased array transducer*: low-frequency transducer (1–5 MHz) with a very small face (footprint). The image produced is pie shaped as the field of view widens as the depth increases. This has less shades of grey than the curvilinear transducer, but because it produces a pie-shaped image, it can image structures through a narrow window such as between the ribs. This is typically used for cardiac imaging, but because it is capable of imaging deeply into the body, this transducer may also be used in the abdomen.
- *Endocavitary transducer*: specialized transducer used typically for imaging in small confines such as the vagina. It has a medium frequency (4–8 MHz) and as such produces an image that has both good resolution and moderate depth. The field of view is extremely wide, more than 180°, making it unsuitable for general abdominal imaging.

Key machine controls

- *On/off switch*: improper shutdown can cause loss of stored data.
- *Depth*: depth control is generally well marked on the ultrasound system. Place the structure of interest in the centre of the ultrasound screen by increasing or decreasing the depth.
- *Gain*: gain is the overall brightness of the ultrasound image. As the gain increases, shades of grey are lost, leading to a less detailed image. Typically the best image is one where fluid-filled structures, such as blood vessels, are completely anechoic.

Logistics of ultrasound in resource-limited settings

Electricity

- All portable ultrasound machines will run on batteries but usually for only 20–60 minutes per charge. Extra batteries are available but are relatively expensive and heavy so a better solution is to use a generator.
- If a generator is not available, then a lithium battery can be charged by solar power. One or two folding 40–70 watt solar panels can be carried in a backpack and weigh <9 kg (20 pounds). The lithium battery can be charged when not in use and if required, an inverter can convert 12 V battery power to 110 V power to run the ultrasound. A charged lithium battery should run most portable ultrasounds for a minimum of 1–4 hours per charge depending on the watts required for the individual machine.

Ultrasound gel

If ultrasound gel is not available, simple surgical lubricant can be substituted. While perhaps not acoustically as good, it is quite adequate for most uses. Water can also be used to fill an air-space gap.

Abdomen: FAST examination

Initial response: trauma

Once patients are identified as suffering from acute trauma, life-threatening conditions need immediate diagnosis and attention if possible. Ultrasound can provide a reliable assessment of many bodily structures that can each be performed within a few minutes during the initial assessment. Ultrasound has been shown in trauma situations to be a useful, reliable tool in both the diagnosis of injury as well as in the triage of patients. Therefore, the use of ultrasound in these settings should be considered for all patients, regardless of the apparent injuries in order to expedite diagnosis and management.

Focused assessment with sonography in trauma (FAST) exam goal

The goal is the rapid evaluation of free intra-abdominal fluid which is presumed to be blood in a trauma patient.

Transducer selection

Curvilinear abdominal transducer or phased array cardiac transducer.

Image interpretation

- All fluid appears hypoechoic or anechoic using ultrasound.
- Fluid can be of any variety, but is assumed to be blood in the scenario of trauma.
- The identity of the fluid can be confirmed as blood by performing a paracentesis or diagnostic peritoneal lavage.

Areas of focus of FAST exam

A FAST exam consists of four areas of evaluation:

Hepatorenal recess (Morrison's pouch)

(See Fig. 55.1.)

Image acquisition

- The transducer is placed longitudinally with respect to the body on the right flank at the level of the eighth to eleventh ribs.
- Image obtained of the liver is in long axis adjacent to the kidney.

Image interpretation

- The liver and kidney should not appear separated; the liver and the kidney should be directly opposed to one another with only a bright, echogenic, line demarcating the liver from the kidney.
- Fluid appears as a black or hypoechoic line or stripe between the liver and kidney, superior to the liver edge, or at the inferior pole of the kidney (Fig. 55.2). The two surfaces, the liver capsule and the capsule around the kidney, which formed the bright echogenic line, will be separated by the black anechoic fluid.
- The thickness of the stripe is relatively proportional to the amount of free fluid (blood) in the peritoneum. A 1 cm stripe is equivalent to 1 litre of fluid (blood) and a 0.5 cm stripe is equivalent to 0.5 litres of blood.

Splenorenal recess

(See Fig. 55.3.)

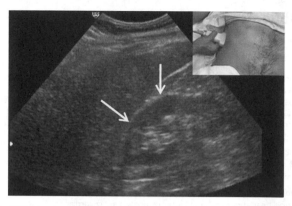

Fig. 55.1 Negative right upper quadrant (RUQ) FAST exam. White arrows mark Morrison's pouch.

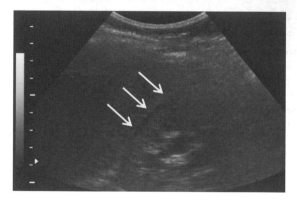

Fig. 55.2 Positive RUQ FAST exam with fluid in Morrison's pouch. White arrows delineate the fluid in Morrison's pouch.

Image acquisition
- The transducer is placed longitudinally on the left flank at the level of the ribs similar to Morrison's pouch.
- As the spleen is smaller than the liver, in order to visualize the spleen–kidney interface, the transducer will need to be placed more posterior and angled up towards the abdominal surface.
- Image obtained of the spleen is in long axis adjacent to the kidney.

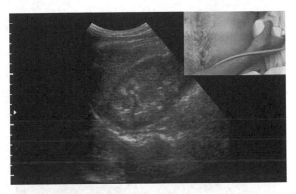

Fig. 55.3 Negative LUQ FAST scan.

Image interpretation

- Fluid (anechoic stripe) in the left upper quadrant (LUQ) most often collects above the spleen (between the spleen and the hyperechoic diaphragm).
- Care should be taken to distinguish this from a pleural effusion or haemothorax, which is above the diaphragm.
- Rarely, fluid will collect between the spleen and kidney (Fig. 55.4).

Pelvis

(See Fig. 55.5.)

Image acquisition

- The transducer is placed horizontally (cross-section to body) just above the symphysis pubis.
- If the bladder is empty, the transducer may need to be tilted inferiorly to visualize the bladder.
- The transducer is rotated in long axis to the body to visualize the bladder in long axis.
- Image obtained of the bladder is in cross-section (bladder appears as a circle or trapezoid depending on how much the bladder is filled).

Image interpretation

- Posterior to the bladder will be the vagina (hypoechoic oval structure) in females and the prostate (hypoechoic oval structure) in males with the transducer in a transverse axis to the body orientation.
- In an orientation of long axis to the body, the bladder will appear as a triangle and the vagina and uterus in a female will appear as a hypoechoic structure posterior to the bladder and usually in close contact with the superior (intra-abdominal) surface of the bladder.
- Fluid (anechoic stripe) will collect between the bladder and the uterus or posterior to the cervix (cul-de-sac) in females and posterior to the bladder superior to the prostate in males (Fig. 55.6).

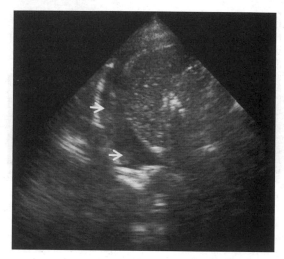

Fig. 55.4 Positive LUQ FAST scan—blood.

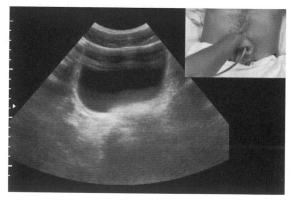

Fig. 55.5 Negative (no fluid) on pelvic FAST exam.

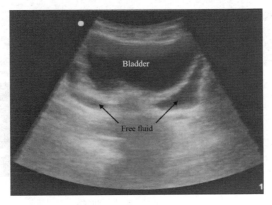

Fig. 55.6 Positive pelvic fluid on FAST exam.

Cardiac view
(See Figure 55.7.)

Image acquisition
- The transducer is placed horizontally in the subxiphoid region (cross-section to body).
- The heart is visualized by placing the transducer as flat as possible under the ribs angling superiorly. The liver is used as an acoustic window with the heart appearing on the lower part of the image. Increase the depth of the image to visualize the pericardium.

Image interpretation
- Evaluate for the presence of a pericardial effusion which will appear as a hypoechoic or anechoic collection of fluid between the heart and the pericardium (diaphragm/liver) (Fig. 55.8).
- Evaluation for cardiac tamponade will be covered in the next section.

Pearls and pitfalls
- Be aware that a small stripe of fluid correlates to a large amount of fluid in the abdomen.
- The location of the fluid (blood) does not indicate the location of the injury. In the supine patient, fluid most often collects in Morrison's pouch (independent of the source of blood). In the ambulatory or erect patient, fluid most often collects in the pelvis as this is the dependent portion of the abdomen.
- Not all fluid is blood. The assumption is that fluid in the abdomen is blood when a trauma has occurred. However, all fluid is visualized as hypoechoic on ultrasound and cannot be differentiated based on appearance (e.g. blood, ascites, urine, and pus).
- Ultrasound cannot detect solid organ injuries that are not associated with free intra-abdominal blood. For example, you cannot detect liver haematomas, which are subcapsular.
- Ultrasound cannot detect bowel injuries.

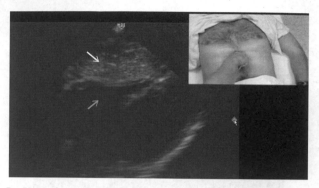

Fig. 55.7 No pericardial effusion on FAST exam—subcostal view. White arrow points to the liver. Green arrow points to the right ventricle.

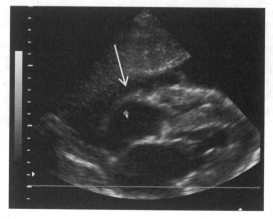

Fig. 55.8 Positive for pericardial effusion on FAST exam. White arrow points to the pericardial space with an effusion.

Thorax: eFAST examination

Extended FAST (eFAST) exam goals

The goals are twofold:

- To evaluate for free intrathoracic fluid which is presumed to be blood in a trauma patient.
- To evaluate for the presence of a pneumothorax.

Transducer selection

Curvilinear abdominal transducer or phased array cardiac transducer for evaluation of a haemothorax and the curvilinear or the linear transducer for evaluation for a pneumothorax.

Evaluation for haemothorax

Patient position

The patient is generally in the supine (trauma patient) position; however, if the patient can be in a semi-recumbent or placed in a head-up incline position, the sensitivity of the exam increases.

Transducer position

The transducer is placed in same position in the right and left flank as in the FAST exam in a longitudinal (to the body) axis.

Image acquisition

- Identify the liver/kidney or spleen/kidney interface.
- Angle the transducer towardS the head or move it vertically up the ribs towards the head until the superior portion of the liver or spleen is visible.

Image interpretation

- Just superior to the liver or spleen is a bright (hyperechoic) line that is the diaphragm (see ➔ Fig. 55.3 p. 1007). Above the diaphragm is the hemithorax.
- Typically, the normal lung tissue cannot be imaged and a mirror reflection (artefact) of the liver (or spleen) is visualized above the diaphragm which appears as if there is a liver above the diaphragm in the chest. If this reflection is seen, the lungs are normal and there is no haemothorax (or pleural effusion).
- If a hypoechoic stripe is seen, this is consistent with fluid, presumed to be blood in the trauma setting (Fig. 55.9).

Evaluation for pneumothorax

Patient position

The patient must be absolutely supine with no head elevation.

Transducer position

- The transducer is placed on the anterior chest wall adjacent to the sternum, in an axis longitudinal to the body.
- Start the evaluation in fourth to fifth intercostal space; however, always evaluate from the second to the sixth intercostal space to ensure that a small pneumothorax is not missed.
- Repeat the examination for the other lung on the opposite side of the chest.

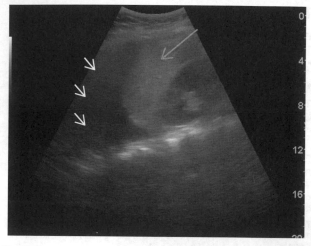

Fig. 55.9 Haemothorax. The green arrow is on the spleen. White arrows define the haemothorax.

Image acquisition
- Normal lung tissue is not visible by ultrasound. However, the pleural surfaces (as with the diaphragm) are visible.
- A potential space can be present between the visceral and parietal pleura. When air (i.e. pneumothorax) is between these surfaces, the deeper visceral pleura cannot be imaged as ultrasound does not image through an air interface.

Image interpretation
- Normal pleura (i.e. no pneumothorax) appears as a bright, hyperechoic line just deep to the ribs in cross-section. When visualized with the gain decreased on the ultrasound machine, this line appears to have fine, black (hypoechoic) structures sliding along the line.
  - These structures are actually small defects in the two pleural surfaces which can be seen to slide relative to one another due to the two pleural surfaces' relative movement. This indicates there is not air between the pleural surfaces at this location and called the 'sliding lung sign'.
- If the heart is visualized, there is no pneumothorax at this location, as ultrasound cannot image structures deep to an air interface.
- With a pneumothorax, or air between the pleural surfaces, the deeper pleural surface (visceral pleura) is not imaged. Hence the hypoechoic defects of the parietal pleura are the only ones visualized and they do not move relative to the single pleural surface (Fig. 55.10).

- M-mode ultrasound imaging aids in the identification of the presence or absence of the 'sliding lung sign':
  - Using the same transducer position, the M-mode line is placed between the ribs in cross-section. M-mode imaging is activated, demonstrating movement of the pleura over time:
    —When a pneumothorax is not present, the M-mode image will show a 'seashore sign' with horizontal lines representing the waves and the static, snowstorm image representing a sandy beach.
    —With a pneumothorax, only horizontal bright lines will be seen, the waves and the sandy beach will not be seen.

Pearls and pitfalls

- As with the FAST exam, the fluid seen in the chest may not be blood. The clinical scenario must be taken into account in order to make the correct diagnosis (e.g. haemothorax, pleural effusion, or empyema).
- Compressed lung may be seen 'floating' in the hypoechoic fluid. This may be compressive atelectasis. Pus will appear as linear strands or a mass of hyperechoic strands in the dependent portion of the lung field. TB may produce a thick-walled pleural effusion similar to Swiss cheese that is known as a caseous pleural effusion.
- When visualizing the left chest for pneumothorax, if the heart is visualized, there is no pneumothorax (i.e. the visceral pleura will not be seen but the heart will, but in either case there is no air present between the heart and chest wall or between the two pleura).
- Occasionally, lung sliding may not be seen over a lung bleb. Use clinical judgement to distinguish between these clinical entities.
- A tension pneumothorax should be identified clinically.
- In ballistic penetrating injuries of the chest or in 'sucking' chest wounds, a pneumothorax may not be demonstrated by ultrasound. This is because the open chest allows the plural surfaces to become adjacent and the air to escape from the open wound.

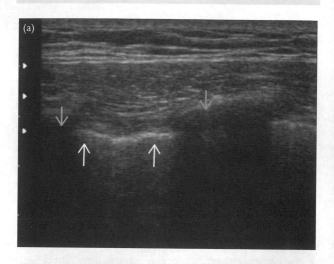

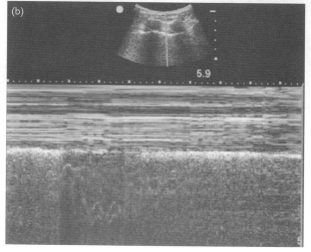

Fig. 55.10 A) No pneumothorax (sliding lung sign present). White arrow shows sliding lung and green arrows are on the rib shadows. B) No pneumothorax, M- mode showing seashore sign.

Soft tissue injuries and fractures

Goal

The goal is to evaluate superficial structures for foreign bodies, soft tissue infections, and bone fractures.

Transducer selection

Linear transducer.

Image acquisition

- Image the area of interest in at least two planes, 90° apart.
- Scan slowly, using light pressure to prevent pain.
- A bucket or a basin filled with water can be used to image distal superficial structures. This 'water bath' can aid in imaging by increasing the distance from the transducer to the skin surface. The structure is placed underwater and the transducer is placed near the object.

Image interpretation

- Normal soft tissues have differing appearances:
  - Fat: hypoechoic with hyperechoic surrounding septae.
  - Muscle: hypoechoic with linear hyperechoic striations.
  - Tendons: hyperechoic with linear striations.
  - Bone: hyperechoic with shadowing posterior to the anterior surface of the bone (Fig. 55.11).
- Oedema or cellulitis can be seen by visualization of fluid in tissues which will appear as hypoechoic striations between the fat lobules (in the area of the septae).
  - As the fluid amount increases, the fat becomes more hyperechoic and the septa are replaced by the hypoechoic fluid (i.e. cobble stone appearance) (Fig. 55.12).
- Abscesses appear as a localized fluid collection (i.e. hypoechoic sphere or ovoid shape) (Fig. 55.13).
  - They are usually encapsulated by a relatively hyperechoic capsule. Pus in the abscess may be hyperechoic and will move with transducer pressure (i.e. squish sign). Septations may be seen.
- Foreign bodies such as wood, metal, and glass are generally hyperechoic:
  - All demonstrate some degree of posterior shadowing.
  - Wood after a few days will become hypoechoic in the soft tissue because it absorbs water, making identification more difficult.
- Fractures appear as discontinuity of the hyperechoic cortex of the bone (Fig. 55.14).
  - If the fracture is displaced, the linear cortex will also be displaced on the ultrasound.
  - Growth plates appear as hypoechoic lines perpendicular to the cortex of the bone.
  - Growth plate injuries which are not displaced (obvious fracture) may demonstrate hypoechoic fluid (blood) at the growth plate.

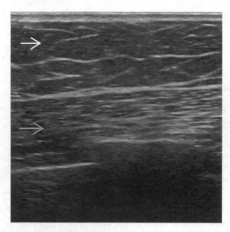

Fig. 55.11 Normal soft tissue scan. White arrow points to fat, and green arrow points to muscle.

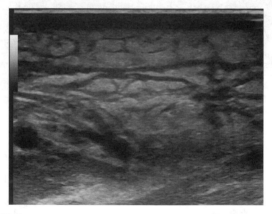

Fig. 55.12 Cellulitis.

Pearls and pitfalls

- Superficial structures (e.g. cellulitis, abscesses, foreign bodies, etc.) may not be visible unless a *standoff* is used:
  - A standoff is a sonographically neutral (i.e. does not affect the ultra-sound beam) object which allows for an increased distance between the transducer and the skin surface.
  - A standoff can be made from a water-filled glove. However, the standoff effect can also be accomplished by using a large amount of gel and 'floating' the transducer in the gel (i.e. not touching the skin surface) or by placing the object of interest (e.g. hand) into a bucket of water with the transducer suspended above the skin surface.
- Foreign bodies can be difficult to remove using ultrasound as a guide, however it is possible to use ultrasound to place a hypodermic needle adjacent to the foreign body and dissect down the needle to the foreign body.
- For fractures, growth plates, and cellulitis, compare to the opposite side of the body or an unaffected area if unsure if pathology exists.

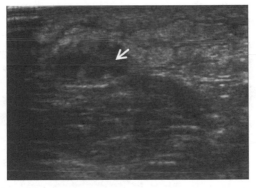

Fig. 55.13 Abscess. Arrow points to the abscess. There is also some surrounding cellulitis.

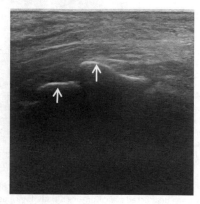

Fig. 55.14 Fracture. This is a fracture of the distal fibula. The white arrows mark the proximal and distal fragments of the bone.

Medical emergencies in ultrasound

Evaluation of the hypotensive or unresponsive patient is a common scenario in a humanitarian emergency. Underlying conditions such as severe malnutrition, TB, and HIV complicate the evaluation of patients based solely on history and physical examination. Differentiation of the type of shock present and guiding resuscitation is possible using ultrasound techniques. Patient evaluation usually begins with determining the central venous pressure (CVP) through evaluation of the inferior vena cava (IVC) size and collapsibility with ultrasound. Adding other ultrasound examinations such as a cardiac evaluation further refines the diagnosis.

Assessment of inferior vena cava

Goal
The IVC is a corollary to the CVP as well as the circulating blood volume. By evaluating the IVC collapse with respiration, the CVP can be estimated and combined with other clinical information, the IVC can be used to classify the type of shock present and guide resuscitation (see Table 55.1).

Transducer
Curvilinear abdominal transducer or phased array cardiac transducer.

Patient position
The preferred position is with the patient supine with no head elevation if possible.

Image acquisition
• IVC is visualized with the transducer longitudinal to the body placed in the subxiphoid location.
• The liver should be identified along with the hepatic veins as they enter the IVC just before the IVC enters the diaphragm and right atrium.
• If the hepatic veins are not visualized, ensure that the aorta is not being visualized (the aorta does not travel through the liver).

Image interpretation
• Evaluate collapse of the IVC at the IVC–hepatic vein junction (Fig. 55.15).

Clinical integration
• The IVC is a great tool in differentiating the cause of shock in a hypotensive patient (see Table 55.2).
• The IVC can be used to guide fluid resuscitation as well as other shock management.

Evaluation for altered mental status or coma

Goal
Elevations in intracranial pressure (ICP) can be determined via ultrasound of the optic nerve sheath (ONS) or by determining the presence of papilloedema by ultrasound visualization of the optic nerve head. See ➜ 'Headache' pp. 675–6 for causes of elevated ICP.

Transducer
Linear transducer.

Patient position
The patient may be in any position for this exam, but is easier to perform with the patient in the supine or semi-recumbent position.

Image acquisition
- Using a small amount of ultrasound gel, place the transducer horizontally across the patient's closed eye.
- ONS: visualize the globe as a hypoechoic spherical structure. Posterior to the globe will be a hypoechoic linear structure exiting the globe (ONS) (Fig. 55.16).
  - Adjust the transducer orientation until the border of the ONS is well-defined.

Image interpretation
- Measure 3 mm back from the posterior globe (retina) and the width of the ONS. A value exceeding the maximum ONS width is associated with increased ICP. (See Table 55.3.)
- Note that the ONS should be dilated bilaterally in the setting of elevated ICP. If only one ONS is dilated, then other causes such as optic neuritis should be considered.

Papilloedema
- The optic nerve head is located at the junction of the ONS and the retina (posterior globe) (Fig. 55.17).
- The retina and optic nerve head should be flat (i.e. no elevation).
- With subacute elevations in the ICP, the optic nerve head will swell into the globe (i.e. papilloedema). This will appear on the ultrasound image as a doming of the optic nerve head into the globe using ultrasound.
- Since the lateral sides of a sphere are difficult to visualize, a swollen optic nerve head may appear as a linear hyperechoic structure parallel to the retina.

Pearls and pitfalls
- Dilation of the ONS will occur immediately with the elevation in ICP.
- Dilation of the ONS is not proportional to the amount of elevation in ICP.
- Papilloedema takes time to develop and may not be present with acute elevations in ICP.
- Dilated ONS should always be present with papilloedema.

Table 55.1 IVC diameter in expiration and inspiration to CVP comparison

IVC diameter expiration	IVC diameter inspiration	CVP (approximate pressure in cmH$_2$O)
Small, slit like	Complete collapse	Very low (0–4)
Small to normal size	Complete collapse	Low (4–8)
Normal size	Collapses 25–75%	Normal (8–12)
Large (approaching 20–25 mm)	Collapses <25%	High (12–18)
Large (maximal size)	No collapse	Very high (>20)

Table 55.2 Use of the IVC diameter in shock

IVC	CVP	Other findings	Potential cause
Small Complete collapse	Low	Hx. Vomiting/diarrhoea Hyperdynamic LV	Dehydration
Small Complete collapse	Low	Hx. Trauma Blood in peritoneum	Haemorrhage
Small Complete collapse	Low	Hx. Fever Hyperdynamic LV	Septic shock
Small Complete collapse	Low	Hx. Weakness Pale conjunctiva/palms	Severe anaemia
Dilated Little collapse	High	Hx. Uraemia or TB Pericardial effusion	Pericardial tamponade
Dilated Little collapse	High	Hx. Chest pain Hypodynamic LV	Cardiogenic shock
Dilated Little collapse	High	Hx. Acute dyspnoea Dilated RV/RA	Massive PE
Dilated Little collapse	High	Hx. Renal failure	Volume overload

Hx, history; LV, left ventricle; PE, pulmonary embolism; RA, right atrium; RV, right ventricle.

Table 55.3 Optic nerve sheath width — upper limit of the ONS diameter (measured 3 mm posterior to the retina)

Age	Maximum ONS width (mm)
Adult	5.0–5.7
Child	4.5
Infant	4.0

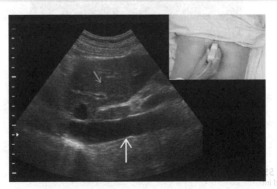

Fig. 55.15 IVC. White arrow points to the vena cava. Green arrow points to the liver.

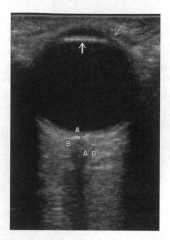

Fig. 55.16 Optic nerve sheath (ONS) measurement. A to A equals 3 mm and B to B is the width of the ONS, in this case 4.3 mm. Green arrow points to the cornea and white arrow points to the iris.

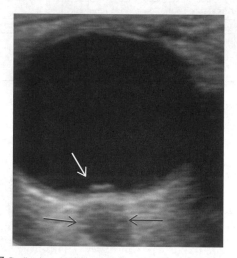

Fig. 55.17 Papilloedema. White arrow demonstrates doming of the optic nerve head into the vitreous. Green arrows show a widened optic nerve sheath.

Evaluation of pregnancy: ultrasound

There is frequently a large population of pregnant women before, during, and after the acute emergency (as well as during chronic emergencies) and their need for obstetric care continues regardless of the external circumstances. Recognizing life-threatening emergencies for the fetus or mother ahead of time can be critical for saving the life of mother and/or child.

There are several life-threatening conditions in the first and third trimester that can be evaluated by ultrasound. Accurate and rapid assessment of intrauterine verses extrauterine pregnancy, identifying the number of fetuses, fetal health, and fetal position, as well as placental location are all critical for successful delivery and maternal and fetal well-being.

Goal

The goal of ultrasound of the pregnant patient is to recognize the most common life-threatening conditions for both mother and fetus.

Transducer

Curvilinear abdominal transducer and/or transvaginal transducer. Also referred to as an endocavity transducer.

Patient position

Supine

Image acquisition

- As in the FAST exam, identify the bladder and the vagina/uterus posterior and superior (intra-abdominal).
- If present, the fetus should be within the uterus (Fig. 55.18).

Determining location of the pregnancy

A positive pregnancy test without evidence for an intrauterine pregnancy should raise suspicion for an ectopic pregnancy:

- The first sign of intrauterine pregnancy is the double decidual sign which can be present as early as 4.5 weeks after the last menstrual period. This appears as a double ring involving the two layers of the decidua with the gestational sac in the centre.
  - The double decidual sign should not be used as the only evidence for location of the pregnancy.
- The identification of a yolk sac is the earliest indicator of pregnancy and used to determine location (Fig. 55.19).
- If a yolk sac or a fetal pole cannot be identified in the uterus, then the location of the pregnancy cannot be determined.
  - If a yolk sac, fetal pole, or fetal pole with heart motion is identified outside the uterus, then an ectopic pregnancy can be confirmed.

Pearls

- A double decidual sign with a yolk sac or embryo inside the gestational sac confirms an intrauterine pregnancy.
- A gestational sac or double decidual sign should be visible on transabdominal ultrasound by the sixth week after a missed menses and by 5.5 weeks on transvaginal ultrasound

- If the mean gestational sac diameter (calculated by measuring the three dimensions of the gestational sac in centimetres and dividing by 3) is >20 mm without a yolk sac, the outcome of the pregnancy is abnormal 100% of the time
- If the mean gestational sac diameter is >25 mm without an embryo, the outcome is abnormal 100% of the time.

Pitfalls

- A pregnancy less than 5.5 weeks will give you a positive pregnancy test but no gestational sac or double decidual sign. If the patient is stable without vaginal bleeding or pain, repeat the scan in 1 week.

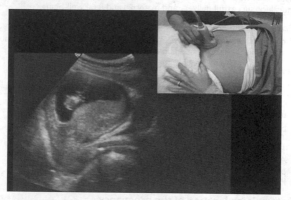

Fig. 55.18 Trans-abdominal view of a normal pregnancy.

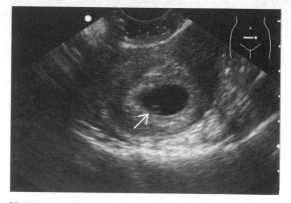

Fig. 55.19 Arrow pointing to the yolk sac in patient with early pregnancy and a double decidual sign (yolk sac, white arrow, inside the gestational sac).

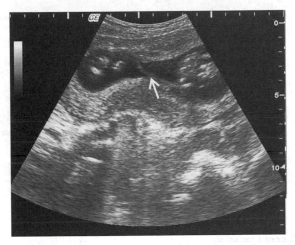

Fig. 55.20 First-trimester twin pregnancy. Arrow points to the amniotic membrane separating the twins.

- A miscarriage will also give the sonographer a positive pregnancy test without a gestational sac.
- A molar pregnancy will give a positive pregnancy test without a viable pregnancy.

Number of fetuses

While a singleton pregnancy often can be delivered by an inexperienced birth attendant, multiple pregnancies present a need for more supervised care at the time of delivery. The most accurate time to evaluate for the number of fetuses is in the first trimester (Fig. 55.20).

Gestational age of the fetus

In cases where there is a need to emergently deliver the baby due to fetal emergency or maternal complications, ultrasound can be useful in determining the gestation age and gives an indication if the fetus will survive if delivered. A fetus delivered prematurely is not likely to survive the rigors of a humanitarian emergency without access to sophisticated neonatal care. Accurate calculations of fetal age are critical to determine the necessity for referral and sophisticated neonatal care and resuscitation.

- Gestational age best correlates to true gestational age when measured using biparietal diameter (BPD) in the first trimester and femur length in the second and third trimesters (Figs 55.21–55.23).
  - Crown–rump length (CRL) is the most accurate estimation of the gestational age in early pregnancy. The CRL is the length of the embryo from the top of its head to the bottom of the torso (Fig. 55.21).
    —The CRL is the largest dimension of the embryo. Do not include the yolk sac.
    —Cardiac activity should be present in an embryo with a CRL >7 mm.

- BPD is measured outer edge to inside edge of the calvarium at the level of the thalami perpendicular to the falx (Fig. 55.22).
  —The BPD is best found by finding an image of the fetal head where the falx runs directly through the centre of the fetal head and both thalami are symmetrically situated on each side of the falx.
  —The BPD is measured in the centre of the skull, through both thalami and perpendicular to the falx from the outside of the skull on one side to the inside of the skull on the other side. The ultrasound machine will provide the gestational age for you.
- Femur length must be measured perpendicular to the transducer and not oblique, excluding the distal epiphysis. An oblique measurement will be inaccurate secondary to foreshortening (Fig. 55.23).
- CRL can be used to determine age in the first trimester. It is most accurate when the CRL is between 10 and 84 mm. Between 12 and 14 weeks, the CRL and the BPD are similar in accuracy. If the CRL is >84 mm, the BPD should be used for gestational age determination. In the second or third trimester, a combination of biometric parameters (BPD and femur length) should be used to determine gestational age.

Placenta location

A placenta previa or placenta partially covering the cervical os is a recipe for disaster in a resource-limited setting without access to caesarean section or blood transfusion services. Every attempt should be made to refer to a medical facility with these resources prior to delivery.

Image acquisition
- The placenta will appear as a lobulated, hyperechoic but also often mixed echogenic structure attached to the uterus.
- In the late third trimester, the placenta becomes more lobulated and the venous lakes (hypoechoic) become more prominent.

Image interpretation
- If the placenta overlies the os in the late third trimester, this is considered a placenta previa and is an obstetric emergency.
- A partial placenta previa or a low-lying placenta in late second or early third trimester will 'migrate' up and away from the os as the uterus enlarges.
- If the placenta partially overlies the os in the second trimester, it still has time to pull away from the os as the uterus enlarges with the increasing gestational age of the pregnancy, thus it is best to wait until the third trimester before deciding that there is a complete placenta previa (Fig. 55.24).

Fetal position

Fetal position is usually ascertained by physical examination. If there is doubt, ultrasound can easily diagnose breech or transverse lie, which requires a supervised delivery.

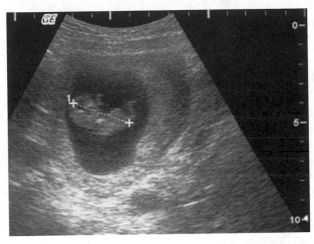

Fig. 55.21 Measurement of crown–rump length (CRL) in first-trimester pregnancy.

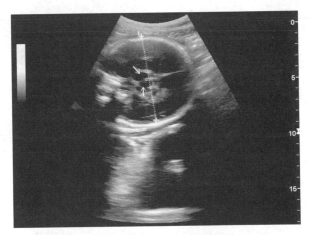

Fig. 55.22 BPD gestational age—can be done by BPD or femur length depending on the trimester of the pregnancy. BPD is more accurate in first trimester and femur length in the second and third trimesters. Measure outer table of the skull to inner table of the skull at 90° to falx through the pared thalami. Each white arrow points to one of the paired thalami.

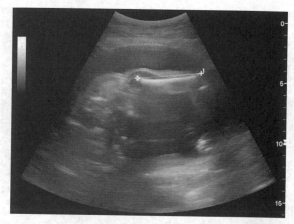

Fig. 55.23 Femur length. Ultrasound beam must be perpendicular to the femur shaft to prevent foreshortening and an inaccurate measurement.

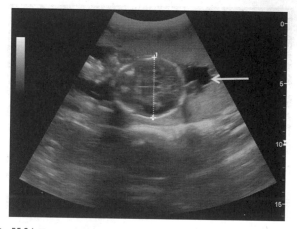

Fig. 55.24 Measuring gestational age in a fetus with the placenta covering the entirety of the cervical os. This is a complete placenta previa. White arrow points in the direction of the cervical os with the placenta overlying the os.

Part VIII

Water, sanitation, and waste

Chapter 56

Water, sanitation, and hygiene

Peter Maes, Rafael Van Den Bergh and Joos Van Den Noortgate

Introduction to water, sanitation, and hygiene (WASH)

Safe water and sanitation, which enable proper hygiene, are essential determinants of health, quality of life, as well as human dignity. As the most essential element of life, water is protected by international law. The UN General Assembly explicitly recognized the right to water and sanitation, and acknowledged that clean drinking water and sanitation are essential to the realization of all human rights. Additionally, in situations of conflict, the Geneva Conventions stipulate that water supplies essential for the survival of the civilian population must be protected from attack.

However, a large part of the world's population does not have access to these essential services. More than 780 million people today lack safe drinking water, and some 2.5 billion—>35% of the world's population—lack improved sanitation. As a consequence, more than a million people, most of them children, die every year from diseases associated with the lack of access to safe drinking water, inadequate sanitation, and poor hygiene. In many contexts where humanitarian crises commonly occur, where water, sanitation, and hygiene (WASH) infrastructure vital for public health might have been under fire, where people are under constant threat and have experienced years of conflict and/or have had to flee their home, the risk of diseases or epidemics is even greater. Consequently, the need for WASH interventions to prevent and control such diseases is also greater.

This chapter aims to provide the health worker with the necessary information to appropriately prioritize WASH, understand the process of primary prevention of WASH-related diseases, identify best practices for different contexts, and recognize when specialized assistance might be required.

As the full complexity of WASH, particularly in low-resource settings, may be beyond the scope of this work, readers interested in further information are referred to the comprehensive field-oriented handbook 'Public Health Engineering in Precarious Situations'.[1] This freely accessible manual provides detailed information on the subject, including narratives per technical domain and detailed guidance for implementation of basic WASH activities in the field.

WASH as public health intervention

Non-improved hygiene, inadequate sanitation, and insufficient and unsafe drinking water account for 7% of the total disease burden and 19% of child mortality worldwide.[2] WASH interventions are highly cost-effective, and are capable of preventing a large part of this devastating disease burden and are a cornerstone of primary prevention.

While perennially in the shadow of the 'big three' of the international public health community—HIV/AIDS, TB, and malaria—one disease alone kills more young children each year than all three combined—diarrhoea[3]—and the key to its control is WASH. Evidence suggests that adequate WASH interventions such as improved excreta disposal and/or a surge in handwashing with soap by the affected population and/or rehabilitation of improper water infrastructures may be capable of reducing the prevalence of diarrhoeal disease by 30% under operational conditions. A more pronounced impact (up to 63% reduction) may be associated with water piped to one or more taps on a property.

Universal access to safe drinking water, adequate sanitation, and improved hygiene is steadily increasing; and the level and quality of services continues to grow, but progress is painfully slow in many LIC. Despite having identified the cause, and having the technology and means to eliminate this cause, countless children in the world continue to die each year from easily preventable diseases. In industrialized countries, much of the early drive to provide WASH came from the medical community rather than falling under a variety of governmental departments. In LIC, the health sector could play a similar crucial and much more prominent role in providing universal access.

Although involvement in WASH may seem like an added burden for an overtaxed, under-resourced health system, it actually represents a highly cost-effective strategy. It may represent an added upfront investment burden, but it reduces downstream costs, due to the decreased morbidity and mortality burden, as well as time saved.

Breaking the cycle of infectious disease transmission

Transmission of infectious diseases is not random, but results from a complex interaction between the environment, pathogen, and host. The reservoir of an infectious agent is the habitat or host in which the agent commonly lives and the most appropriate primary prevention strategy is reducing the environmental reservoir, and/or blocking the transmission routes to a new host. This blocking of transmission can be achieved by applying general WASH principles in a context-specific manner.

The F-diagram in Fig. 56.1 illustrates how appropriate primary prevention interventions can halt faecal–oral disease transmission, primarily by promoting the safe disposal of faeces, improving the quantity and quality of the water supply, and improving hygiene. The scope of WASH, however, goes far beyond prevention of faecal–oral transmission. Primary prevention interventions to break other transmission pathways have been developed for other diseases in a multitude of contexts. (See Table 56.1 for environmental classification of water- and excreta-related infections.[3,4])

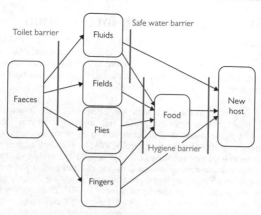

Fig. 56.1 F-diagram.

Hardware and software components

WASH activities enable the promotion of hygiene practices that prevent and control infectious diseases. In all WASH activities, a distinction can be made between complementary 'hardware' and 'software' components:

- 'Hardware' generally refers to technical activities such as the supply, construction, or installation of specific equipment (with tangible outputs such as the construction of culturally appropriate latrines).
- 'Software' includes activities such as health promotion, education, and community involvement, which generally concern context-specific social and cultural factors aiming to achieve behavioural change (with tangible outputs such as the appropriate use of the aforementioned latrines).

Effective WASH-driven public health interventions in the field require complementary hardware and software components (e.g. an impregnated bed net only protects against malaria if used correctly). Considering that motivators to adopt primary prevention measures are not necessarily health related, the importance of providing appropriate/context-adapted 'software' (health promotion, training) must be emphasized.

Table 56.1. Environmental classification of water- and excreta-related infections

Category	Examples	Control strategies
A. Faecal–oral diseases Potentially: *water-borne* (= enteric infections spread through faecal contamination of drinking water) or *water-washed* (= infections that spread in communities that have insufficient water for personal hygiene)	*Viral* Hepatitis A, E, and F Poliomyelitis Viral diarrhoeas *Bacterial* Campylobacteriosis Cholera Salmonellosis Typhoid, paratyphoid *Protozoal* Amoebiasis Cryptosporidiosis Giardiasis	Improve water quality (to prevent water-borne transmission), improve water availability, hygiene promotion (to prevent water washed transmission)
B. Purely water-washed diseases	*Skin and eye infections* Scabies Conjunctivitis Trachoma *Louse-born infections* Relapsing fever Typhus	Improve water availability, hygiene promotion
C. Soil-helminth diseases	Ascariasis Trichuriasis Hookworm infection	Sanitation, hygiene promotion, treatment of excreta before re-use for agricultural purposes
D. Tapeworm diseases	*Taenia solium* infection *Taenia saginata* infection	As for C above, plus meat inspection and cooking
E. Water-based diseases (= diseases where the causative organism requires part of its lifecycle to be spent in an intermediate aquatic host)	*Helminthic* Schistosomiasis Clonorchiasis Dracunculiasis	Reduce contact with/ consumption of infected water, sanitation, treatment of excreta before re-use for agricultural purposes
F. Insect-vector diseases	*Water related* Dengue Yellow fever Malaria West African trypanosomiasis *Excreta related* Bancroftian filariasis Trachoma Fly- and cockroach-borne excreted infections[a]	Reduce the number of potential breeding sites and contact opportunities, improve surface water drainage, use repellent/ insecticide where appropriate

(Continued)

Table 56.1 (*Contd.*)

Category	Examples	Control strategies
G. Rodent-borne diseases	*Rodent-borne excreted infections*[a] Leptospirosis Lassa fever Tularaemia	Rodent control, hygiene promotion, reduce contact with infected water

All diseases in categories A, C, and D, most helminthic diseases in E, and diseases labelled with [a] together comprise 'excreted infections'.

WASH activities

The collection, treatment, and distribution of potable water

Water source

Identification of the best water resources should include all stakeholders, in collaboration with local, national, and international partners. Typically, the preferred choice is a protected ground water source, extracted via a pump-equipped borehole. However, other options can be considered as well (see Table 56.2). To ensure access to potable water, various parameters need to be considered:

- The source needs to be self-contained, independent of the variations of climate or outside factors.
- A physical, chemical, and microbiological analysis of the water should systematically be performed prior to the initial supply to the population.
- Optimal sources are free of microbiological contamination and have a low turbidity (the amount of suspended particles in the water will have an impact on the chlorination efficacy).
- Water sources should have a low concentration of toxic chemical products, which can be naturally occurring (e.g. arsenic, documented in Bangladesh, or fluoride causing dental or skeletal fluorosis in Niger), or the consequence of human activities (e.g. by mercury, a toxic heavy metal from gold mining; or nitrates/nitrites, from agriculture).
- Although with a limited effect on health, factors such as salinity, colour, odour, and taste have a role in the acceptability by the consumers.
- Accessibility of water, including distance, altitude differences, and queuing at the supply point, largely determine water utilization.

Water intake

To be usable, water is collected from a source through *an intake* which transports the water from the source either to treatment and/or storage, or in some cases directly to the user. The water intake has to be:
- well chosen (e.g. avoid rivers with a fluctuating water level and ensure the intake is set below the minimum water level of the river)
- well designed, to avoid loss and further contamination of the water. Water moves through the intake either by gravity or by lifting (e.g. wells with a hand pump, or a deep well with a solar submersible pump)
- well maintained, an unexpected challenge as demonstrated by the plethora of broken hand pumps around the world.

Atypical intakes have been developed in response to specific extenuating circumstances, such as in Libya, when the water supply was cut off and acute insecurity made movement outside the health structures impossible. In this case, condensation water was harvested from the multiple air conditioners working at full capacity with all the windows open. Another example was in Sudan, during an emergency situation, when a gigantic plastic sheet was spread out on the ground, leading rainwater to a ditch equipped with a pump that transferred the water to a storage reservoir.

Water treatment

- Water treatment at *household level* reduces the risk of recontamination during transport and storage, but raises difficulties in the mass distribution of the products/material and teaching the population how to use them correctly.
- *Community-level* water treatment, in rural settings, is easier for distribution and training as less people are involved, but might not be possible for small isolated pockets of people or for populations on the move.
- *Centralized* water treatment is especially suited for big populations in cities (e.g. slums) and larger refugee camps.

See Table 56.3 for the various treatment methods for the elimination of microbiological pathogens.[1]

When there is suspicion of salt intrusion (a major concern in coastal aquifers) or chemical pollution (e.g. quality decreases drastically in gold mining areas), it is in general advisable to change the water source. To ensure elimination of salt and chemical intoxicants, more elaborate methods are required to obtain potable water such as reversed osmosis or filtration on resins. These methods are expensive, high tech, and more difficult to operate and maintain in resource-poor settings.

Table 56.2 Advantages and disadvantages of different water sources

Source	Advantages	Disadvantages	Practical
Surface water (e.g. river water, lake)	Relatively big quantities, Easier extractions, Easy to discover	Usually contaminated and considered unsafe, Always need for treatment (see ➜ p. xxx)	Often used in (acute) emergencies, Avoid swamp and pond water if possible as they are often difficult to disinfect effectively
Groundwater[a] (e.g. borehole, hand-dug well (Fig. 56.2), spring)	Of good microbiological quality if correctly protected	May be subject to chemical contamination, Needs to be extracted, except for springs	Often preferred option in the longer term if acceptable chemical water quality, Construction know-how often locally available
Precipitation (e.g. rainwater collected from roofs and stored in ferro-cement tanks)	Drinking quality (rural) if correctly collected, Easy to collect	Significant variability in quantity, Needs big storage capacity to cover dry period	An important source in emergencies during the rainy season, Considered a welcome additional long-term source

[a] An aquifer <3 m deep has the characteristics of surface water.

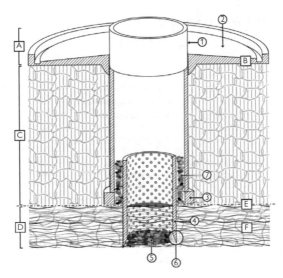

Fig. 56.2 Description of a hand-dug well. Reproduced with permission from Médecins Sans Frontières (MSF)—Public Health Engineering In Precarious Situations (2010, 2nd edition).

Key

Hand-dug well with telescoping principle

A. Wellhead (with lid/lifting mechanism)

B. Apron with protective kerb and anchorage

C. Shaft

D. Intake with graded aggregate filter

E. Water table (static water level)

F. Aquifer

1. Impermeable concrete rings or sealed masonry lining

2. Reinforced concrete slab with anchorage

3. Foundation anchorage

4. Perforated/permeable concrete rings (or open-jointed masonry lining)

5. Graded aggregate filter (cleaned gravel)

6. Cutting ring

7. Backfilling (cleaned gravel)

Water distribution, transport, and storage

Transport, storage, and distribution of water can result in recontamination of the water prior to its consumption, so special attention should go to the following:

- The internal cleanliness of pumps, pipes, water trucks, reservoirs, and tap stands. Consider that pressure in the distribution network can be intermittent and as a consequence, contaminated surface water can be sucked into the pipe in case of leaks in the network.

Table 56.3 Water treatment methods

Method	Advantages	Disadvantages	Context
Boiling	Easy to do Effective (also for turbid water)	High amount of combustibles needed Loss of water Bad taste of the water Risk of post-contamination	Household treatment only
UV radiation[a]	Easy to do Effective	Only for low water turbidity Risk of post-contamination	Household level (UV of sun) Community/centralized level
Filtration	Relatively simple (Rather) effective	(Rather) expensive Risk of post-contamination	Household/community/centralized level
Chemical disinfection (chlorine)[a]	Lower risk of post-contamination (remnant effect)	No protection against cysts and helminth (eggs) Taste/odour Only for low water turbidity	Household/community/centralized level

[a] Methods requiring low water turbidity—UV radiation and chlorine disinfection—require an initial step removing the suspended particles in the water, by assisted sedimentation and/or sand or membrane filtration.

- The cleanliness and appropriate use of household recipients of the collected water. In emergency contexts, quickly-deployed distribution of jerry cans or buckets can be important, in particular during outbreaks of infectious diseases (e.g. cholera in rural areas).
  - Jerry cans with a small opening reduce the risk of people putting their hands inside, but render their cleaning difficult.
  - Buckets with special lids having a small opening are ideal, as they allow safe taking of water for everyday use, and allow occasional internal cleaning.

Excreta disposal facilities

Management of excreta disposal is of paramount importance in keeping the environment, and thus the water sources, safe. This is particularly true in contexts with large population concentrations (e.g. refugee camps, urban slums), or where the usual sanitation infrastructures are destroyed (e.g. natural disasters). Though often overlooked as a priority during emergencies, it is essential to immediately provide and maintain simple temporary toilet facilities (e.g. trench latrines—Fig. 56.3). Over time, the temporary solution should be upgraded (e.g. improved trench latrines) and replaced progressively by more suitable structures as the situation develops into a chronic emergency (e.g. simple pit latrines—Fig. 56.4) and a stabilized situation (e.g. ventilated improved pit latrines).

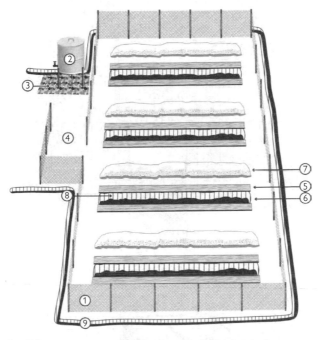

Fig. 56.3 Description of a trench latrine. Reproduced with permission from Médecins Sans Frontières (MSF)—Public Health Engineering In Precarious Situations (2010, 2nd edition).

Key

1. Fence (e.g. plastic sheeting)

2. Closed water container with tap/ soap or ash

3. Infiltration system for wastewater (e.g. gravel pit)

4. Zigzag entrance

5. Planks

6. Trenches (0.3 m wide)

7. Soil for burying excreta

8. Band of plastic sheeting (optional)

9. Runoff drainage

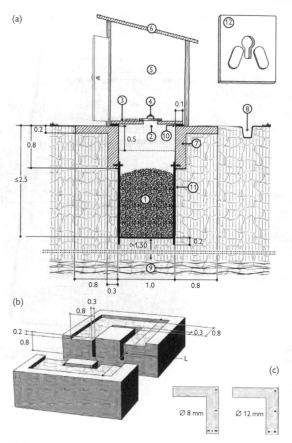

Fig. 56.4 Simple pit latrine. Reproduced with permission from Medecins sans frontiers (MSF)—Public Health Engineering In Precarious Situations (2010, 2nd edition).

Key

A. Vertical cut of the simple pit latrine
B. Excavation for the concrete base
C. Detail of the base reinforcements
1. Pit (partly filled with excreta)
2. Defecation hole
3. Slab with footrests
4. Cover
5. Superstructure

6. Roof
7. Concrete base
8. Drainage channel (at the sides and back of the latrine)
9. Aquifer (water table)
10. Mortar layer (at least 10 mm thick)
11. Perforated corrugated iron sheets (pit reinforcement)
12. Example of a slab: concrete, plastic, (wood)

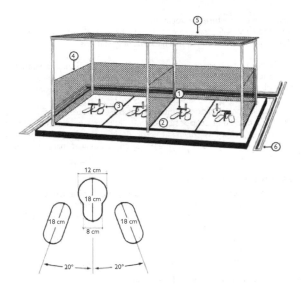

Fig. 56.5 Children's pit latrines. Reproduced with permission from Médecins Sans Frontières (MSF)—Public Health Engineering In Precarious Situations (2010, 2nd edition).

Key

1. Handle bar (for a child to hold on to when squatting)
2. Slab with adapted footrests
3. Defecation holes (adapted size for children) with lid
4. Open superstructure
5. Roof
6. Drainage channel

In these later phases, users should be consulted in order to better meet their needs. Small children might have problems using normal pit latrines because of the big size of the drop hole, the position of the foot rests, or fear of the closed structure of a normal pit latrine, and so a modified children's pit latrine should be used (Fig. 56.5).

Toilet facilities should meet basic criteria, including the following:

• Not posing a public health threat, such as attracting disease vectors.
• Offering users a certain level of comfort, taking into account local beliefs and incorporating cultural requirements
• Offering the frequently overlooked requirements for appropriate menstrual hygiene management in humanitarian emergencies.
• Offering a minimum of privacy, with separated facilities for men and women.

- Being safe in structure and location.
- Adapted to specific users (e.g. disabled, children, elderly, women).
- Have some form of functional handwashing stations.

In addition to the hygiene aspects, provision of safe sanitation can have significant social and security benefits. Some areas with high levels of poverty and a lack of law enforcement can make venturing out at night in search of a place to go to the toilet risky for all, particularly women who face the additional and documented threat of sexual violence. Further, for girls, the provision of school sanitation facilities means that they are less likely to miss school by staying at home during menstruation. The proximity to the dwelling results in time not spent queuing at shared sanitation facilities or walking.

Waste management

Management of domestic waste, on a household as well as a collective level, aims to reduce the risk of pollution, poisoning, fire, and/or the proliferation of insects and rodents. The process includes temporary storage, collection, transport, potential treatment (e.g. incineration, composting), and final disposal. Staff involved in the collective disposal of waste require appropriate protective clothing. See ◎ Chapter 57 for more information on waste management in medical facilities.

Wastewater drainage and disposal

Stagnant water, originating from rainwater or wastewater, requires effective wastewater disposal systems to contain smells, proliferation of insect larval breeding sites, contamination of water sources, and spread of pathogens. Wastewater disposal can include:

- rudimentary soak away pits (see Fig. 56.6) for infiltration of limited amounts of wastewater into permeable soil during an emergency intervention
- more elaborate infiltration trenches (see Fig. 56.7), which serve as dispersal systems with infiltration pipes, typically installed in a later phase
- evapo-transpiration areas, suitable in hot, windy, arid, or semi-arid climates.

Once collected and before wastewater infiltrates into the ground, the solid faecal matter coming from toilets should be removed by a septic tank. The solid materials, grease and fat coming from kitchens/showers/sinks, should be separated from the wastewater by a grease trap in order to avoid very quick clogging of an infiltration system.

Dead body management

It is a common misconception that dead bodies that are not cared for immediately will lead to outbreaks of infectious diseases. In general, the management of human remains is more a matter of respect and of providing a culturally appropriate response.

However, for some highly contagious infectious diseases, the correct management of human remains is an important component of the outbreak response. In contexts of haemorrhagic fevers (e.g. Ebola, Marburg, Lassa fever) or of faecal–oral epidemics (e.g. cholera), culturally appropriate adaptations need to be made during the management of the human remains to avoid contact with infectious bodily fluids. In the context of

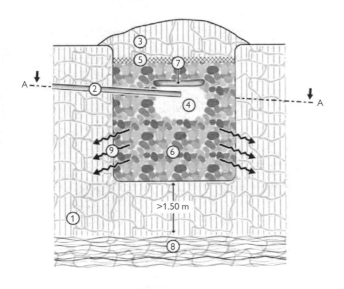

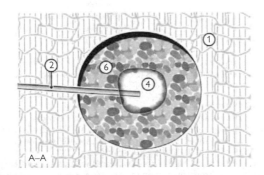

Fig. 56.6 Soak away pits. Reproduced with permission from Médecins Sans Frontières (MSF)—Public Health Engineering In Precarious Situations (2010, 2nd edition).

Key

1. Permeable soil
2. Incoming pipe (min. diameter 100 mm)
3. Compacted earth
4. Cleared space at the end of the pipe

5. Geo-textile or perforated plastic sheeting
6. Clean stones (boulders)
7. Flat stone or concrete slab
8. Water table
9. Wastewater infiltrating in the soil

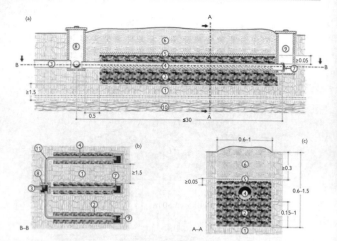

Fig. 56.7 Infiltration trenches. Reproduced with permission from Médecins Sans Frontières (MSF) - Public Health Engineering In Precarious Situations (2010, 2nd edition).

Key

A. Longitudinal section

B. Bird's view of the multiple trench system

C. Cross section

1. Permeable soil

2. Clean gravel

3. Incoming pipe

4. Drain pipe

5. Geo-textile or perforated plastic sheeting

6. Compacted earth

7. Plug at the end of the drain pipe

8. Distribution box

9. Manhole (optional)

10. Water table

11. Union pipes with elbow

Measurements are indicated in metres.

louse-borne (e.g. relapsing fever, typhus) or flea borne (e.g. plague) infections, the transfer of infected insects to non-infected individuals needs to be avoided with timely and context-specific effective vector control measures.

Vector control

Vector control aims at reducing the morbidity and mortality due to vector-transmitted diseases, and strategies are generally tailored to the vectors' context-specific behaviour. The vector control response is an integral part of the WASH responsibility and measures include:

- preventive actions (drainage of stagnant water, waste collection, etc.)
- distribution of personal protection methods (e.g. repellents, insecticide-treated mosquito nets, etc.)
- chemical control (e.g. insecticide residual and space spraying, insecticidal dusting, use of larvicides in water bodies, rodenticide application, etc.)
- other innovative vector control methods (e.g. sterile insect technology).

Hygiene/health promotion

People's motivation to change their hygiene behavior not always relates to health but can depend as well on other drivers of human behavior like convenience and self-respect. To have any impact, it's important to have a better understanding of the target population as well as their preferred communication ways in a given context. Simple education/information sharing might be sufficient during acute emergencies as people might be receptive to the hygiene/health messages because they might be afraid to get ill of a specific outbreak, whereas for chronic emergencies and stabilized situations other reasons might have to be highlighted (e.g. promote ownership of a latrine as a status symbol). Some people will prefer face-to-face communication (e.g. participatory exercises) which is normally limited to rather small groups but has the advantage that potential questions can be addressed immediately. Mini-media (e.g. theatre, puppet show, video) offers the advantage to reach already a bigger audience, whilst their immediate feedback is still possible. Mass-media (e.g. newspapers, radio, television) is more suited for spreading relevant information to big numbers of people, but goes mainly in one direction, thus additional monitoring for correct comprehension is required.

Context-related WASH

In health structures

Nosocomial or healthcare-associated infections are a global burden and represent a safety concern for patients, visitors, healthcare professionals, and nearby communities alike. Healthcare-associated infections are very diverse and include diarrhoeal diseases, hepatitis B and C, HIV/AIDS, wound infections, urinary tract infections, and chest infections. The prevalence varies considerably from hospital to hospital, with an incidence range in HIC reported between 5% and 15%, with a broader range of 5.7–45.8% reported in sub-Saharan Africa where little is known about the overall epidemiology.[5]

The reality in many LIC is one of insufficient personal washing or hand hygiene implementation, improper cleaning and/or sterilization of medical and surgical apparatus and equipment, insufficient drinking water and washing water safety, poor provision of sanitation, poor medical practices (such as unsafe injections), lack of vector control measures, as well as risky medical waste and wastewater disposal. Many of these issues are integrated within the standard precautions, and the provision of WASH elements to any healthcare system is an essential requirement. In particular, in the context of highly contagious diseases, context-specific WASH interventions play a crucial role.

In populations

An elder in South Sudan, when asked about the health needs of his community said: 'Why are you giving me medicine to cure my diarrhoea—that I must swallow with the same water that made me ill?'

WASH activities are essential at all phases of health provision, from acute emergencies to more stable environments. In acute or chronic emergencies and post-conflict situations, or in the aftermath of a natural disaster, WASH services in LIC are often dysfunctional or non-existent. To prevent excess morbidity and mortality in the affected population, services need to be (re-) established as soon as possible.

Rather than a 'one-size-fits-all' approach which tracks universal coverage indicators, giving priority to 'transmission' hotspots amenable by adequate WASH interventions is often preferable as a strategy in, e.g. large-scale cholera or malaria outbreaks. The type, size, extension, and focus of WASH activities should be adapted to the contexts, and medical goals set in the multidisciplinary evolution of the public health problem. The response should be geared towards tools for fast deployment in the acute phase, and foreseeing transition to more sustainable, less resource-heavy technology in the post-emergency phase.

Example of a WASH response in populations after acute emergencies
A relevant WASH intervention in natural catastrophes such as floods is the massive cleaning and disinfection of all flooded water points such as wells and boreholes, which needs to be conducted once the waters retreat.

Future and innovation in the WASH sector

Interestingly, while WASH interventions are among the most crucial in public health, the evidence base on the impact of WASH interventions on health outcomes in humanitarian crises is sparse, and numerous methodological limitations undermine the ability to determine associative, let alone causal, relationships. The challenging contexts where the WASH sector operates, often characterized by life-or-death situations, overwhelming constraints, and competing priorities, tend to be a fertile environment for the development of innovative strategies and tools that greatly benefit the populations in need and strengthen the WASH sector's expertise. However, despite this continuous innovation, rigorous documentation and publication of both innovative and long-standing empirical WASH interventions remain sparse, and generation of evidence through, e.g. operational research, continues to lag behind.

The further translation of WASH innovations into policy adaptation and wider implementation in the field thus remains an important area for improvement. The interface and communication between the WASH sector and global policymakers needs to be strengthened, in order to assure that it is accorded at least the same importance as other activities in humanitarian interventions and in the research sphere—the absence of an industrial lobby behind WASH should not mean that it is absent from the operational decision-making table.

References

1. Van Den Noortgate J, Maes P. Public Health Engineering in Precarious Situations. Paris: Médecins Sans Frontières; 2010 http://refbooks.msf.org/msf_docs/en/public_health/public_health_en.pdf.
2. Prüs-Üstün A, Bos R, Gore F, Bartram J. Safer Water, Better Health: Cost, Benefits and Sustainability of Interventions to Protect and Promote Health. Geneva: World Health Organization; 2008.
3. Bartram J, Cairncross S. Hygiene, sanitation, and water: forgotten foundations of health. PLoS Med 2010;7:e1000367.
4. Mara DD. Unitary environmental classification of water and excreta-related diseases. J Environ Engineering 1999;125(4):335.
5. Bagheri Nejad S, Allegranzi B, Syed SB, Ellis B, Pittet D. Health-care-associated infection in Africa: a systematic review. Bull World Health Organ 2011;89:757–65.

Further reading

Cairncross S, Feachem R. Environmental Health Engineering in the Tropics. Chichester: Wiley; 1993.
Cook GC. Thomas Southwood Smith FRCP (1788–1861): leading exponent of diseases of poverty, and pioneer of sanitary reform in the mid-nineteenth century. J Med Biog 2002;10:194–205.
Davis J, Lambert R. Engineering in Emergencies: A Practical Guide for Relief Workers Intermediate Technology. 2nd rev ed. London: ITDG Publishing; 2002
Ferron S, Morgan J, O'Reilly M. Hygiene Promotion. A Practical Manual for Relief and Development. 2nd ed. Rugby: Practical Action Publishing; 2007.
PAHO/WHO/IFRC/ICRC. Management of Dead Bodies after Disasters: A Field Manual for First Responders. Washington, DC: PAHO; 2006.
Porter D. Health, Civilization, and the State: A History of Public Health from Ancient to Modern Times. London: Routledge; 1999.
Rozendaal J. Vector Control: Methods for Use by Individuals and Communities. Geneva: World Health Organization; 1997.
The Lancet. Keeping sanitation in the international spotlight. Lancet 2008;371:1045.
Thomson M. Disease Prevention through Vector Control: Guidelines for Relief Organisations. Oxford: Oxfam Publication; 1995.
Wagner EG, Lanoix JN. Excreta Disposal in Rural Areas and Small Communities. Geneva: World Health Organization; 1958.

Medical waste management

Joos Van Den Noortgate, Rafael Van den Bergh and Peter Maes

Introduction to medical waste management

Healthcare waste refers to all 'waste' generated in the different types of healthcare structures, including excreta, wastewater, and *medical (-related) waste*. The manner in which these types of waste are dealt with should be according to the national legislation (if existing for waste), local context, and constraints. Improper disposal of medical waste can cause environmental pollution, and lead to health risks in various ways:

- Direct contact: contact with the waste can result in pathogens entering the body through a puncture or abrasion of the skin, mucous membranes (e.g. ocular contact), ingestion, or inhalation.
- Air pollution: hazardous smoke emissions with thermoresistant pathogens and toxic by-products can occur when medical waste is incinerated improperly (i.e. burned at low temperatures or not properly conducted).
- Pollution of the soil and water resources: untreated medical waste can contaminate the soil and ground/surface water with pathogens or chemical substances.
- Increased presence of vectors: proliferation of vectors (e.g. flies, mosquitoes, rodents) in poorly discarded medical waste.

The multiple routes of transmission provide risk to (para-) medical staff, cleaners and healthcare waste personnel, patients (in particular if immuno-compromised) and visitors, and the community, especially children and waste scavengers (in the vicinity where waste is improperly dumped or left adjacent to incinerators).

Typical guidelines are very extensive and impossible to reproduce in a concise handbook. In addition, in the field of medical waste management, many guidelines/publications describe systems that are pertinent for HIC and MIC, but the reality shows that they are often less suited for LIC (e.g. too complex, too expensive). As such, they are often inadequately executed in these contexts.

The medical waste management principles described in this chapter are developed to be as pragmatic as possible, based on years of experience in low-resource settings. They don't always fully adhere to the procedures as described in other established guidelines. However, over the years, organizations such as the WHO and ICRC have, next to other established standards, integrated some of the facilities/principles in their guidelines on healthcare waste management.

Waste management approach

Objectives of healthcare waste management

Health structures should be responsible for ensuring that all their healthcare waste is harmless to all people potentially at risk. Good healthcare waste management (HCWM) results in waste being non-infectious and/or inaccessible for the population/vectors.

Correct hygiene and HCWM should be implemented and promoted in all health structures, from the smallest health post to the biggest hospital. Furthermore, this should be done in all situations, from acute to chronic emergencies throughout stabilized situations (with the management system adapted to the actual stage of the intervention). HCWM should also be considered as part of emergency preparedness.

Approach

Disposal methods in HIC are typically complicated and very expensive, so it is preferable to use more pragmatic, comprehensible, affordable, and efficient methods in low-resource contexts. The treatment and final disposal should preferably be done at the health centre itself, in a well-defined area: the waste zone.[1] This allows the treatment to be under the control of the staff of the medical facility and to be performed by clearly defined, well-trained, trustworthy, and supervised persons, equipped with the right protective gear.

Medical-related wastes are classified based on their 'common disposal properties'.[1] The three main categories of medical waste that will be found in nearly every medical facility are sharps, 'soft' waste, and organic waste. Hazardous wastes are less frequent, but demand extra attention because of the technical requirements for disposal. Waste generated by the patients and visitors can be considered as domestic waste as it is non-infectious, and as such can be discarded potentially outside the healthcare structure within available facilities (e.g. landfill).

- *Sharps*: objects that can be responsible for perforations or cuts of the skin, including needles, auto-disable (AD) syringes, scalpels, blades, empty ampoules and vials, and (broken) glass.
- *Soft waste*: comprises all 'solid' medical waste that can be easily burnt, including dressings, latex or nitrile gloves, respirators, and syringes without needles. Separation between contaminated and non-contaminated soft waste, often difficult to distinguish in reality, is normally not required in low-resource settings as they can be incinerated together.
- *Organic waste*: containing a lot of fluid, able to decompose by itself. Includes placentas, aborted fetuses, amputated limbs, organs, body fluids, and potentially food residues. Although technically speaking, human dead bodies could be considered as organic waste, this may be very controversial from an ethical, legal, and/or cultural point of view. Therefore, they fall out of the scope of this chapter, but more information can be found in ⊃ Chapter 56 of this handbook.

- *Hazardous waste*: consists mainly of dangerous chemicals and biohazardous waste. A distinction is made between recurrently generated hazardous waste (which should be dealt with immediately if quantities and hazardousness permit) and expired/inappropriate hazardous products (which should be taken care of in special elimination campaigns possibly outside of the health structure (e.g. once every 6 months). Hazardous waste includes the following subcategories:
  - Laboratory waste: diagnostic test kits/products, chemical reagents.
  - Biological hazardous waste: this includes most body fluids (samples) from potentially infected patients, laboratory cultures.
  - Pharmaceutical waste[2]: opened but unused drugs, cold chain damaged vaccines, expired and/or unwanted drugs.
  - Expired disinfectant solutions: all prepared solutions have an expiry period (e.g. 0.05% chlorine solution expires after 1 day, 1% chlorine solution expires after about a week).
  - X-ray-related waste.
  - Insecticides: left overs, expired and unwanted products.
  - Specific hazardous waste—some examples include:
    —material used to prepare and administer cytotoxic drugs
    —waste with heavy metal content (e.g. batteries, thermometers, and blood pressure gauges containing mercury)
    —pressurized containers (although these are mainly reused).

Medical waste management process

To achieve correct medical waste management, several technical steps must be taken into account: segregation, collection and possible temporary storage, treatment, and/or final disposal (see Table 57.1). The steps to be included in the entire technical process are fixed and depend on the waste category. Hazardous waste has a case-by-case management and can therefore not be represented in this simple schedule.

Segregation

Medical waste should be segregated according to the different categories at the time when and at the place where it is generated by the person generating it, thus most often the (para-) medical staff.

- Sharps waste:
  - Needles should not be re-sheathed, and must be discarded in the sharps container without the syringe as the latter will help the combustion of other soft waste. The exceptions are AD syringes used in immunization, which should be put in safety boxes.
  - The sharps containers should be available in each room where sharps are generated, must be puncture resistant, and must have a lid with a hole small enough to prevent this waste from spilling out.
  - Glass can be segregated from the other sharps if it is bulky and don't fit in the regular sharps container, and/or when it is generated in large amounts.
- Soft waste: although plastic disposable bags are often considered convenient for soft waste collection, concerns include expense and poor combustion (due to insufficient air/combustible gas circulation between the primary and secondary combustion chambers of some incinerators). A good alternative is large plastic quality buckets (i.e. 20–60 litres) with lids, which can be reused after cleaning and disinfection (with chlorine solution).
- Medical organic waste: this can be put in plastic bags, although plastic buckets with a well-fitting lid can again be a very good alternative (with a different colour than those for soft waste, for clear recognition).

> Empty, sturdy plastic drug containers, often readily available in LIC, can be recycled into regular sharps containers. A small triangular opening can be made in the lid that should be tightly screwed or glued to the container in order that the sharps contents cannot be tampered with.

Table 57.1 Medical waste management

Segregation	Sharps	Soft waste	Organic waste
Temporary storage	Yes	Yes	No
Treatment (burning/incineration)	No (except AD-syringes, potential glass crushing)	Yes	No (only very exceptionally)
Final disposal	Sharps pit	Residues pit	Organic pit

Collection and temporary storage

The medical waste collection should be done by one or two waste managers who are responsible for and specialized in HCWM, or their delegated cleaners.

The frequency of medical waste collection depends on the type of waste category, with the waste container being replaced by an empty one:

- Sharps container: when three-quarters full, it should be collected by the waste managers and transported to the waste zone.
- Soft waste bucket: at least once a day, it must be brought to the roofed part of the waste zone for storage prior to being burnt/incinerated. Storage should be <24 hours in hot regions and <48 hours elsewhere (<72 hours in winter).[1,3,4]
- Organic waste: collected as soon as possible after the medical intervention.[1]

Treatment

Burning or preferably incineration currently remains often the most suitable waste treatment method in LIC, at least for soft waste. Possible exceptions include urban situations where space to build an incinerator is limited and/or the smoke generated would not be acceptable, or small rural health structures with limited production of medical waste and sufficient space for on-site land filling.

Options for treatment include:

- permanent (auto-combustion) incinerators in heat-resistant materials which have high performance and durability (see Fig. 57.1)
- temporary volume reducers, often modified fuel drums, which are more easily available (see Fig. 57.2).

Organic waste contains a lot of liquids, making it very difficult/expensive to incinerate. This should be disposed of in a ventilated organic waste pit (see ➔ p. 1056).

Metal sharps will only melt at temperatures well above what can be reached with standard field equipment and stay therefore sharp and dangerous after the treatment. Glass sharps might explode and cause injuries, or result in damage to the incinerator.[4] Hence, treatment of sharps by combustion is strongly discouraged for LIC, where a sharps pit should be used (see ➔ p. 1056).

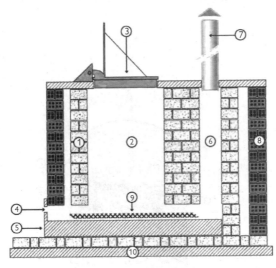

Fig. 57.1 Incinerator (De Montfort). Note: never modify existing plans/models on your own initiative! Reproduced with permission from Médecins Sans Frontières (MSF) - Public Health Engineering In Precarious Situations (2010, 2nd edition).

Key

1. Refractory bricks
2. Primary combustion chamber
3. Loading door with handle
4. Air inlet
5. Ashtray/door

6. Secondary combustion chamber
7. Chimney with head cap
8. External wall (e.g. bricks, metal hull)
9. Grate
10. Concrete slab

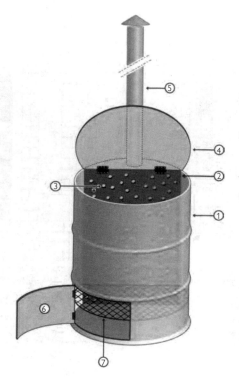

Fig. 57.2 Volume reducer. Reproduced with permission from Médecins Sans Frontières (MSF) - Public Health Engineering In Precarious Situations (2010, 2nd edition).

Key

1. Metal drum, 200 litres
2. Perforated metal plate
3. Perforations in the metal plate for draught

4. Loading door
5. Chimney with head cap
6. Ash door
7. Metal grating (or heavy mesh)

Final disposal

If possible, every health structure should have a waste zone where the waste can be treated and/or disposed of (see Fig. 57.3). This zone should comprise several facilities:

- A temporary storage area for the soft waste.
- An incinerator or (temporary) volume reducer.
- Different waste pits: sharps pit[1,3–5] equipped or not with a safety box reducer[1] (see Fig. 57.4) and a glass crusher that reduces the volume of glass ampoules and vials; residues (ash) pits[1] (see Fig. 57.5) and organic waste pits[1,3,4] (see Fig. 57.6).
- Wash area for empty waste containers, with wastewater facilities.
- A small storage space for the cleaned waste containers, wood to pre-heat the incinerator/volume reducer, the personal protective equipment, cleaning material, and consumables.

The size of the waste zone depends on the amount of waste that is generated, thus on the size of the health structure itself and on the number of patients that are treated each day. The quantity of medical waste generated daily in LIC varies normally between 0.3 and 1.5 kg/bed (or 2–3 litres/bed) although the quantity per category can vary between health structures.

Recommendations for final disposal by category of waste

- Sharps:
  - The intact, unopened sharps containers should be disposed of directly into the sharps pit without prior treatment.
  - Safety boxes containing AD syringes: to reduce the volume of the syringes and safety boxes, it is recommended that these are burnt in a safety box reducer standing on top of a (second) sharps pit. This allows the residue to fall directly into the pit without contact.
  - Glass waste: if collected separately, the volume can be reduced by a specifically designed glass-crusher mounted over a sharps pit.

A sharps pit is an encapsulation technique made out of a concrete lined (sealed) pit for long-term interventions (e.g. a concrete closed foundation, concrete rings for the vertical lining, and a concrete slab on top with a vertical pipe in its centre). In emergency situations, or in cases with insufficient burial space (e.g. a health centre in a slum), a sharps pit can be made from a 200-litre drum or plastic container.

- Soft waste: after burning or incineration, the residues should be disposed of in a residues (ash) pit, and covered with soil (in acute emergencies) or preferably a lid.
- Organic waste:
  - Should be disposed of immediately in the ventilated organic waste pit. Some wood ashes can be added to the pit before its lid is closed, in order to reduce the decomposition odour.
  - Food residues: can be disposed of in the organic waste pit if produced in small quantities (<10 litres/day), otherwise the pit will fill up too fast.

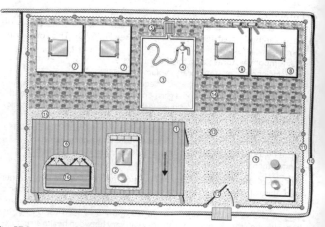

Fig. 57.3 Waste zone. Reproduced with permission from Médecins Sans Frontières (MSF) - Public Health Engineering In Precarious Situations (2010, 2nd edition).

Key

1. Waste bins' temporary storage place
2. Incinerator/volume reducer
3. Washing area
4. Water supply
5. Grid leading to a wastewater system
6. Roof
7. Residues (ash) pits
8. Organic waste pits
9. Sharps pit
10. Runoff water drains
11. Fence
12. Door (with padlock)
13. Concrete floor
14. Gravel (or concrete)
15. Parking place for a possible pushcart
16. Closed storage space

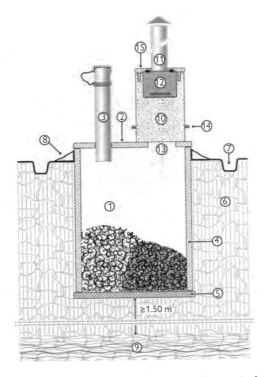

Fig. 57.4 Sharps pit with safety box reducer. Reproduced with permission from Médecins Sans Frontières (MSF) - Public Health Engineering In Precarious Situations (2010, 2nd edition).

Key

1. Pit
2. Concrete slab
3. Drop pipe with cover
4. Sealed lining (e.g. concrete)
5. Sealed (closed) concrete foundation
6. Soil
7. Drainage ditch
8. Impermeable layer (mortar)
9. Water table
10. Safety box reducer (in heat resistant bricks)
11. Chimney with head cap
12. Vertical loading door
13. Disposal hole for residues to fall in the pit
14. Grid
15. Metallic cover

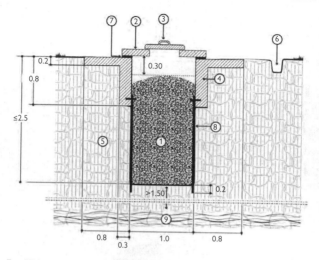

Fig. 57.5 Residues (ash) pit. Reproduced with permission from Médecins Sans Frontières (MSF) - Public Health Engineering In Precarious Situations (2010, 2nd edition).

Key

1. Pit
2. Slab (concrete)
3. Lid
4. Base (concrete)/lining
5. Soil

6. Drainage channel
7. Mortar layer (at least 10 mm thick)
8. Corrugated iron sheets
9. Water table

Dimensions are indicated in metres

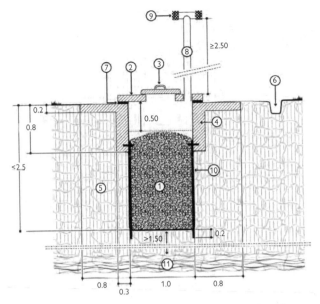

Fig. 57.6 Organic waste pit. Reproduced with permission from Médecins Sans Frontières (MSF) - Public Health Engineering In Precarious Situations (2010, 2nd edition).

Key

1. Pit
2. Slab (concrete)
3. Lid
4. Base (concrete)/lining
5. Permeable soil
6. Drainage channel

7. Mortar layer (at least 10 mm thick)
8. Ventilation pipe (e.g. PVC)
9. Tee with mosquito netting
10. Corrugated iron sheets (perforated)
11. Water table

Dimensions are indicated in metres

Hazardous waste

Incorrect elimination of hazardous waste can be extremely harmful to the environment, and represents a serious public health hazard. Recurrently generated hazardous waste has to be managed on a case-by-case basis based on the following principles:

- Small amounts of used X-ray developing and fixing products can be mixed and the neutralized solution stored for at least 1 day before being diluted with clean water and discarded into a closed sewer system.[4]
- Biohazardous waste such as TB sputum, bacteria cultures, and blood samples should be incinerated by adding sufficient combustibles, preferably with pre-autoclaving while still in the laboratory.
- Glass bottles containing (bio-) hazardous samples or opened vials still containing vaccines should be disposed of in a completely lined sharps pit or be encapsulated.[2]
- Urine and stools can be disposed of in pit latrines, after having been chemically disinfected (e.g. lime milk, not chlorine) or after having been sterilized in an autoclave specifically reserved for waste management.[4]
- Disinfectant solutions can be 'reused' for cleaning the floors of non-critical areas (e.g. *not* for an operating theatre).
- Prepared but leftover insecticides that have been used for spraying health structures indoors can be utilized to treat the latrines.

Inappropriate/expired hazardous products have to be eliminated according to the national legislation (if existing) or during specially organized (6-monthly) campaigns. As this is quite complicated, it is best to ask for advice from a specialist. In general, the following steps will always have to be respected:

- Hazardous waste needs to be isolated from the other still valid products in a separate room that can be closed with a key. Incompatible products must be placed in different rooms (e.g. inflammable and toxic products).
- A record should be kept of all the hazardous products that need elimination, which can be used to negotiate with the authorities or elimination companies, or to ask for advice from specialists.
- The most appropriate elimination procedure per product has to be looked for, depending on its composition, amount, and context. In case there are specialized institutions/companies that have been accredited, they should be contacted to check if they can deal with the hazardous waste. There are additional specialized disposal options possible, depending on the product, but this will require expert input.
- The elimination procedures have to be prepared, with potential transport of the hazardous waste, and implemented.

Organization and planning

The main objective of a HCWM system is to improve safety. However, technical solutions alone are not sufficient and organizational planning should follow the different steps of the 'project cycle':

- For acute emergencies, the *essential medical waste requirements* can often be implemented immediately after an initial assessment (see Box 57.1).
- For chronic emergencies and stabilized situations, an additional in-depth assessment should be performed for context-specific implementation.
- It is recommended that a site-specific medical waste management strategy (ideally formalized in a memorandum of understanding) is prepared by formation of a hygiene committee (see Box 57.2).
- A waste management system must be adapted to the needs, habits, culture and other constraints of the users.
- Technical solutions must be complemented by technical trainings for medical and non-medical staff, and health promotion for patients and visitors.
- A budget will be required.
- The general recommendations provided in this text are normally sufficient for hospitals up to 100 beds although scaling up of the recommendations may be required as bed numbers increase. For 300 beds and more, other solutions are probably required (e.g. semi-industrial incinerators).
- It is recommended to vaccinate the medical and non-medical staff who are potentially exposed to medical waste, at least against hepatitis A/B and tetanus.[1, 4]
- Once the waste management system is in place, continuous monitoring should be performed to see if everything is on track, followed by a regular evaluation (every 3–6 months, at least once a year) to check if the objectives are reached.

Box.57.1 Essential requirements for medical waste management

Goal:

to provide a safe and secure segregation, collection and temporary storage, potential treatment, and final disposal of all waste.[1]

General measures

- Install waste containers for patients/visitors at a maximum of 5–20 metres' walking distance from where the waste is generated.
- Ensure three (single-use) sharp containers, three soft waste containers, and three organic waste containers per ward (with maximum of 20 beds)/treatment room.

All waste containers should be available in quantities of three to allow one for use, one for rotation (kept in the waste zone after cleaning and disinfection), and one for spare (kept in the ward/treatment room).

Operating theatre

Near the operating table, install:

- two sharps containers: one for the surgeon, one for the anaesthetist
- two soft waste containers of 20 litres, one for the surgeon, one for the anaesthetist

- one big soft waste container of 60 litres
- one big organic waste container.

Ensure availability of waste containers in quantities of three.

Sharps
- Provide appropriate sharps containers in convenient locations and ensure regular collection and disposal.
- If many empty ampoules and vials are generated, separate glass collection can be done, with safe glass crushing afterwards.
- Provide an appropriate sharps pit.

Soft waste
- Provide appropriate soft waste containers in convenient locations.
- Ensure at least daily collection of the soft waste, with safe temporary storage before treatment.
- Ensure cleaning and disinfection of the emptied soft waste containers.
- Provide appropriate treatment and/or disposal facilities:
  - In an acute emergency, this would include a drum volume reducer and ash/residues pit.
  - In chronic emergencies and stabilized situations, a double combustion incinerator with two ash/residue pits.
  - A covered pit (without treatment) should only be used if a (very) small quantity of waste is generated and/or a lot of space is available.

Organic waste
- Provide appropriate organic waste containers in convenient locations, including delivery room and operating theatre.
- Ensure immediate collection and disposal of the organic waste.
- Ensure cleaning and disinfection of the emptied waste containers.
- Provide appropriate final disposal facilities:
  - In an acute emergency: an organic waste pit (closed pit, or open pit with contents covered with soil) can be used.
  - In chronic emergencies and stabilized situations: two organic waste pits, each with a fixed cover and a ventilation pipe.

Hazardous waste
- Ensure that all hazardous waste is disposed of legally, and disposal practices and methods comply with or exceed the country legislation.
- Ensure that all hazardous waste is disposed of safely (according to the WHO recommendations).[2,3,4]

Waste zone
- Provide a defined waste zone with soft waste storage and all appropriate treatment and disposal facilities.
- Install a fence around the waste zone.
- Install a washing area with water point within the waste zone.
- Install facilities for wastewater evacuation via a grease trap to an appropriate disposal system.
- Ensure management and supervision by trained person(s).
- The waste zone should be at a distance >50 metres from water sources.
- The complete waste zone must be maintained daily.

Box.57.2 Suggested composition of a hygiene committee

- The hospital director.
- The head nurse.
- The administrator (ad hoc)
- The head of the technical services.
- The head cleaner.
- A health authority representative.
- A (local) government representative.
- A community representative.
- A NGO/aid-agency representative.

References

1. Van Den Noortgate J, Maes P. Public Health Engineering in Precarious Situations. Paris: Médecins Sans Frontières; 2010
2. World Health Organization. Guidelines for Safe Disposal of Unwanted Pharmaceuticals in and after Emergencies. 1999. ℘ http://apps.who.int/medicinedocs/en/d/Jwhozip51e/
3. World Health Organization. Management of Solid Health-Care Waste of Primary Health-Care Centres. Geneva: WHO; 2005.
4. Chartier Y, Emmanuel J, Pieper U, Prüss A, Rushbrook P, Stringer R, et al. Safe Management of Wastes from Health-Care Activities. 2nd ed. Geneva: World Health Organization; 2014
5. International Committee of the Red Cross. Medical Waste Management. Geneva: ICRC; 2011.

Index

Note: Tables, figures, and boxes are indicated by an italic *t* , *f* , and *b* following the page number.